HAEMATOLOGICAL ASPECTS OF SYSTEMIC DISEASE

Edited by

I.W. DELAMORE
Consultant Physician, The Royal Infirmary, Manchester, UK

and

J.A. LIU YIN
Consultant Haematologist, The Royal Infirmary, Manchester, UK

Baillière Tindall
London   Philadelphia   Sydney   Tokyo   Toronto

This book is printed on acid free paper. ∞

Baillière Tindall 24–28 Oval Road
W. B. Saunders London NW1 7DX

The Curtis Center, Independence Square West
Philadelphia, PA 19106-3399, USA

55 Horner Avenue
Toronto, Ontario M8Z 4X6, Canada

Harcourt Brace Jovanovich Group (Australia) Pty Ltd
30–52 Smidmore St, Marrickville, NSW 2204, Australia

Harcourt Brace Jovanovich Japan, Inc.
Ichibancho Central Building, 22–1 Ichibancho
Chiyoda-ku, Tokyo 102, Japan

First published 1990

British Library Cataloguing in Publication Data is available

ISBN 0–7020–1408–7

Typeset by Columns of Reading
Printed in Great Britain by the University Press, Cambridge

Contents

Contributors

R.P. BRETTLE MB ChB, FRCP(Ed)
Consultant Physician, Infectious Diseases Unit, City Hospital, Greenbank
Drive, Edinburgh EH10 5SB, UK

H. COHEN MB ChB, MRCP, MRCPath
Clinical Lecturer in Haematology, Department of Haematology, University
College and Middlesex School of Medicine, Mortimer Street, London W1N
8AA, UK

I.W. DELAMORE PhD(Ed), MB ChB, FRCP(Ed), FRCPath
Consultant Physician, Department of Haematology, Manchester Royal
Infirmary, Oxford Road, Manchester M13 9WL, UK

J. FLETCHER MD, FRCP
Consultant Physician, Nottingham City Hospital and Clinical Teacher,
Nottingham Medical School, Nottingham, UK

C.D. FORBES MD, DSc, FRCP
Professor and Hon. Consultant Physician, Department of Haematology,
Ninewells Hospital and Medical School, Dundee, UK

E.C. GORDON-SMITH MA, BM BCh, FRCP, FRCPath
Professor of Haematology, St George's Hospital, Blackshaw Road, London
SW17, UK

D.I. GOZZARD MB ChB, MRCP, MRCPath
Consultant Haematologist, Ysbyty Glan Clwyd, Bodelwyddan, UK

T.J. HAMBLIN DM, FRCP, FRCPath
Professor of Immunohaematology, Southampton University, Consultant
Haematologist, Royal Victoria Hospital, Shelley Road, Bournemouth BH1
4JG, UK

J.L. HANSLIP MB ChB, MRCP
Lecturer in Ageing and Health, Department of Medicine, Ninewells Hospital
and Medical School, Dundee, UK

A.V. HOFFBRAND DSc, MD, FRCP, FRCPath
Professor of Haematology, Department of Haematology, Royal Free
Hospital, London, UK

J.M. HOWS MSc, MD, MRCP, MRCPath
Senior Lecturer in Haematology, Department of Haematology, Royal
Postgraduate Medical School, Hammersmith Hospital, London W12 0HS,
UK

P.R. KELSEY MBBS, MRCP, MRCPath
Consultant Haematologist, Victoria Hospital, Blackpool, UK

A. KRUGER MRCP, MRCPath
Senior Registrar in Haematology, Southampton General Hospital,
Southampton, UK

ROBERT A. KYLE MD
Chairman, Division of Haematology and Internal Medicine, Mayo Clinic and
Mayo Foundation, William H. Donner Professor of Medicine and Laboratory
Medicine, Mayo Medical School, Rochester, Minnesota 55905, USA

S.J. MACHIN MBChB, MRCPath
Consultant Haematologist, University College and Middlesex School of
Medicine, Mortimer Street, London W1N 8AA, UK

N.T.J. O'CONNOR MD, MRCP, MRCPath
Consultant Haematologist, Royal Shrewsbury Hospital, Shrewsbury,
Shropshire, UK

T.C. PEARSON MD, FRCPath
Reader, Division of Haematology, United Medical and Dental Schools of
Guy's and St Thomas's Hospitals, London SE1 7EH, UK

J.D.M. RICHARDS MA, MD, FRCP, FRCP(Ed), MRCS, FRCPath
Consultant Haematologist and Physician, Department of Haematology,
University College Hospital, London, UK

STEPHEN J. RUSSELL MBChB, MRCP
Clinical Research Fellow, Department of Cell and Molecular Biology,
Chester Beatty Research Institute, London, UK

J. STUART MD, FRCP, FRCPath
Professor of Haematology, Department of Haematology, Medical School,
University of Birmingham, Birmingham B15 2TJ, UK

D.F. TREACHER MA, BS, MRCP
Consultant Physician, Intensive Therapy Unit, St Thomas's Hospital,
Lambeth Palace Road, London SE1 7EH, UK

HELEN WALKER BSc
Senior Cytogeneticist, Department of Haematology, University College
Hospital, London, UK

JOHN T. WHICHER MA, MSc, MB, MRCPath
Professor of Chemical Pathology, Department of Chemical Pathology, Old
Medical School, University of Leeds, Leeds LS2 9JT, UK

J.A. LIU YIN MRCP, MRCPath
Consultant Haematologist, Manchester Royal Infirmary, Oxford Road,
Manchester M13 9WL, UK

Preface

The modern haematologist should have a working knowledge not only of the primary haematological disorders but also of those changes which occur in the blood secondary to other systemic diseases, and should be able to differentiate between the two. Many haematological changes such as thrombocytopenia or polycythaemia should not be regarded as primary disorders until all underlying causes have been eliminated. A careful study of the blood film down the microscope may be the first clue to a wide variety of diagnoses such as lead poisoning, malaria, mycoplasma pneumonia and the hyperviscosity syndrome. Some of the changes that one sees down the microscope may reflect the end-product of a number of disease processes and it is the duty of the haematologist to advise on the appropriate investigations to elucidate the precise cause.

The object of this book is to describe those changes both clinical and laboratory which may first present themselves to the haematologist but yet which reflect systemic disease. We have attempted to give a clear account of the changes themselves, of how they may be recognized and what investigations should be set in hand. We have not dealt in detail with the management of such disorders since this is a book which is much more concerned with pathogenesis and diagnosis than actual management. Mention has been made of management procedures where this flows naturally from the previous text and where such procedures have a diagnostic element to them. It will be apparent that the contents should be of interest not only to haematologists but also to general physicians, and a wide variety of specialists such as endocrinologists, gastroenterologists, immunologists, microbiologists and nephrologists.

We have been fortunate to obtain the services of many distinguished authors and we believe that they have provided an accurate and up-to-date account of an area of haematology which is often neglected. We trust that the reader will find the text both interesting and helpful and that it will prove to be an invaluable aid in the detective work which is an indispensable part of modern day medical practice.

We are particularly indebted to all the authors who have participated to produce this book. Special thanks must go to Mrs Margaret Power for the hours of endeavour that she has contributed to the preparation of the manuscript and to Dr Peter Johnson for a careful reading of the manuscript and for his constructive comments.

I.W. DELAMORE
J.A. LIU YIN

Blood film and marrow

P.R. Kelsey
Consultant Haematologist, Victoria Hospital, Blackpool, UK

INTRODUCTION

Changes in the formed elements of the blood and bone marrow are seen very frequently in patients with various underlying systemic diseases. These changes may vary from such non-specific features as a neutrophil leucocytosis to much more specific appearances such as the leuco-erythroblastic anaemia of malignancy.

It is important to be aware that changes in the blood may sometimes be the first sign of an underlying disease – a good example of this is the thrombocytopenia which sometimes precedes other features of systemic lupus erythematosus. For both the physician and the haematologist an awareness of the association between haematological changes and systemic disease is important.

In this chapter some of the more frequent of these associations are outlined. Many of the changes described will be covered in more detail in other chapters of this book and are simply collected together here to give an overview.

In addition to examining the haematological associations of various types of disease it is useful to look at the major causes of common changes seen in the blood and some of these are tabulated in Tables 1.1 and 1.2.

MALIGNANT DISEASE

Anaemia

Changes in the formed elements of the blood are seen frequently in association with malignant disease (Table 1.3) and the commonest finding is the anaemia of chronic disorders (see below). This may occur with virtually all kinds of tumour both localized and disseminated, although there is a slight correlation between the extent of spread and the level of haemo-globin.[1] Anaemia of this type is not responsive to haematinics, but may be corrected by surgical removal of the underlying tumour.

Acute or chronic blood loss is another important cause of anaemia in patients with malignant disease, particularly of the gastrointestinal tract. Tumours of the genito-urinary tract and respiratory tract are less common causes of haemorrhage. In cases of chronic blood loss the blood film

Table 1.1 Some Underlying Causes of Anaemia

Normochromic/normocytic	Microcytic/hypochromic	Macrocytic
Anaemia of chronic disorders	Iron deficiency	Vitamin B$_{12}$ deficiency
Malignancy	Blood loss	Pernicious anaemia
Collagen disease	Increased demands	Post-gastrectomy
Chronic infection	Dietary inadequacy	Ileal disease
Uraemia	Malabsorption	Blind loop syndromes
Endocrine disease	Thalassaemia	Vegan diet
Haemolysis	Sideroblastic anaemia[a]	Folate deficiency
Aplasia		Malabsorption
Acute blood loss		Dietary inadequacy
		Alcoholism
		Hypothyroidism
		Anti-convulsant therapy
		Haemolysis
		Myelodysplasia
		Sideroblastic anaemia[a]

[a] In sideroblastic anaemia there is a population of hypochromic microcytic red cells but the anaemia is dimorphic and the mean corpuscular volume is frequently raised.

appearances of iron deficiency may be associated with a mild thrombocytosis.

The most characteristic blood picture associated with disseminated malignancy is *leucoerythroblastic anaemia*, and this appearance is highly suggestive of bone marrow infiltration. The blood film shows the presence of immature myeloid cells and nucleated red cells, sometimes in large numbers (Fig. 1.1). Other features vary from case to case, but anisocytosis, poikilocytosis and polychromasia are usually present. A moderate reticulocytosis of up to 10% is often seen. The white cell count is usually moderately raised or normal and a 'left shift' with the appearance of metamyelocytes, myelocytes and occasional blast cells in the peripheral blood is typical. The main causes of leucoerythroblastic anaemia are listed in Table 1.4. It is important to realize that nucleated red cells and immature white cells can appear in the peripheral blood in situations other than marrow infiltration (e.g. severe haemolytic anaemia, severe acute blood loss, severe megaloblastic anaemia). The most important differential diagnosis is primary myelofibrosis although this can usually be differentiated by the presence of splenomegaly, which is uncommon in patients with disseminated carcinoma.

A less common cause of anaemia sometimes seen in disseminated malignancy is *microangiopathic haemolysis*. The hallmark of this condition is the presence of schistocytes in the peripheral blood. These represent cellular fragments which have resealed their membranes following damage and partial loss. Spherocytes are also characteristically present, in addition to the usual features of increased erythropoiesis (Fig. 1.2). The anaemia is usually quite severe, of abrupt onset and associated with a very poor prognosis.[2] Thrombocytopenia is usually present and evidence of disseminated

Table 1.2 Systemic Diseases Associated With Changes in the Leucocyte Count

Neutrophilia
  Inflammation
  Infection
  Haemolysis
  Haemorrhage
  Trauma
  Burns
  Malignancy
  Myeloproliferative disease
  Corticosteroids

Neutropenia
  Infections
  Drugs
  Megaloblastic anaemia
  Marrow infiltration
  Hypersplenism
  Radiation and cytoxic drugs
  Autoimmune (e.g. in SLE)

Eosinophilia
  Allergic reactions
  Parasitic infections
  Drugs
  Skin Diseases
  Carcinoma, Hodgkin's disease
  Irradiation
  Polyarteritis nodosa
  Hypereosinophilic syndrome
  Sarcoidosis

Eosinopenia
  Corticosteroids
  Cushing's syndrome
  Acute infections ('stress')

Basophilia
  Infections (viral)
  Myxoedema
  Ulcerative colitis
  Myeloproliferative disease

Reduced basophils may accompany eosinopenia in disorders above

Lymphocytosis
  Acute infections
    Infectious mononucleosis
    Infectious lymphocytosis
    Mumps
    Rubella
    Pertussis
  Chronic infections
    Tuberculosis
    Syphilis
    Brucella
    Infectious hepatitis
  Thyrotoxicosis
  Lymphoproliferative disorder

Lymphopenia
  Corticosteroids
  HIV infection
  Hodgkin's disease
  Thoracic duct fistula
  Intestinal lymphangiectasia

Monocytosis
  Chronic bacterial infections
    Tuberculosis
    Infective endocarditis
    Brucella
  Other infections
    Malaria
    Kala-azar
    Typhus
  Malignancy
    Hodgkin's disease
    Carcinoma
    Leukaemia

Monocytopenia
  Cytotoxic drugs

Table 1.3   Major Haematological Associations of Malignant Disease

Red cell changes	Commonly associated neoplasms
Anaemia of chronic disorders	All types
Iron deficiency anaemia	Gastrointestinal, uterus (others)
Leucoerythroblastic anaemia	All types: most commonly bronchus, prostate, breast, kidney, stomach, thyroid
Microangiopathic haemolytic anaemia	Stomach, breast, ovary, bronchus
Megaloblastic anaemia	Stomach, rarely others
Pure red cell aplasia	Thymoma, lymphoma, bronchus
Autoimmune haemolytic anaemia	Lymphoma, ovary, rarely others
Sideroblastic anaemia	Myeloproliferative disorders, other carcinomas
Hypersplenism	Haematological malignancies, rarely others
Polycythaemia	Renal, lung, uterus, liver, cerebellum

intravascular coagulation is common. Whilst microangiopathic haemolytic anaemia (MAHA) has been described in association with many types of tumour, in particular mucin-secreting adenocarcinomas, gastric carcinoma is most frequently involved.[2] It is important to be aware that a similar syndrome may be precipitated by chemotherapeutic agents (in particular mitomycin) in some patients with cancer.[3]

Autoimmune haemolytic anaemia (AIHA) of the warm antibody type is often associated with neoplastic disorders, particularly lymphoproliferative disease. The blood film is characterized by spherocytosis, anisocytosis and polychromasia (Fig. 1.3). In severe cases nucleated red cells and immature myeloid cells may be present. Autoagglutination of red cells *in vitro* is seen occasionally if the haemolytic process is very severe. As mentioned above, lymphoid neoplasms are frequently associated with AIHA, and in chronic lymphocytic leukaemia (CLL) this complication develops most frequently. It has been estimated that up to 25% of patients with CLL will develop AIHA at some time during the course of their disease.[4] In Hodgkin's and non-Hodgkin's lymphoma a lower incidence of around 2–3% has been reported.[5,6]

In addition to haematological malignancy, AIHA occasionally develops in association with solid tumours. Anaemia may be the first symptom of occult cancer, and it has been suggested that all patients over 60 years of age who present with AIHA should be investigated for an underlying malignancy.[7] There is an interesting association between ovarian tumours and AIHA.[8] In most cases the tumour is a benign dermoid and the haemolysis ceases when the tumour is excised.

AIHA of cold antibody type is also encountered in association with malignancy, again particularly with lymphoid neoplasms. The characteristic

Table 1.4 Causes of Leucoerythroblastic Blood Picture

Marrow infiltration
  Metastatic carcinoma involving the bone marrow (by far the commonest cause)
  Haematological malignancies (e.g. myelofibrosis, myeloma, lymphoma, leukaemias)
  Lipid storage disorders (e.g. Gaucher's disease, Niemann–Pick disease)
  Histiocytosis X
  Osteopetrosis

Without marrow infiltration
  Severe haemolysis
  Severe acute haemorrhage
  Severe megaloblastic anaemia

---

feature in the blood film is the agglutination of red cells (Fig. 1.4). The association of non-haematological malignancy and cold antibody AIHA is not common, but is probably more than a chance association.[9,10]

Pure red cell aplasia (PRCA) is characterized by anaemia, reticulocytopenia and selective bone marrow erythroid hypoplasia. The blood film usually shows a normochromic normocytic anaemia. An association between thymic tumours and PRCA has long been recognized, [11,12] and is sufficiently strong that it is advisable to search for a thymoma in any patient in whom PRCA is diagnosed. Clinically the thymic tumours involved are usually benign but malignant tumours have been described.[13] In addition to thymoma, PRCA has been described with other non-haematological malignances although it is not clear whether the association is more than a chance occurrence.

Sideroblastic anaemia is occasionally found in patients with underlying cancer. A range of other forms of anaemia may be associated with malignancy such as megaloblastic anaemia due to a poor diet, marrow suppression secondary to drugs, hypersplenism and haemodilution. The causes of anaemia in malignant disease have been well reviewed elsewhere.[14,15]

Polycythaemia

In contrast to the frequency of anaemia as a complication of malignancy, polycythaemia is rare. Polycythaemia has been clearly documented in association with a number of tumours and remission of polycythaemia has followed their removal. It has been found in patients with renal tumours, hepatomas, hamartomas of the liver, uterine fibroids, vascular tumours and cystic adenomas of the cerebellum and carcinoma of the lung. The differentiation from polycythaemia rubra vera may be difficult, but the absence of associated leucocytosis, thrombocytosis and splenomegaly may help to distinguish secondary polycythaemia.

White cell abnormalities

Changes in the white cells of a non-specific nature may sometimes be a pointer to underlying malignant disease:

Neutrophilia may occur in patients with rapidly growing neoplasms, perhaps as a result of tumour necrosis. When the liver, gastrointestinal tract or bone marrow is involved the cell count may be sufficiently raised to warrant the description of a 'leukaemoid reaction' (see below). Eosinophilia has long been recognized as a feature of malignancy,[16] and was reported to occur in 0.5% of cases of malignant tumours in one large series.[16] It has been noted in tumours of various types, but can be particularly marked in Hodgkin's disease. The occurrence of eosinophilia often signifies widespread malignancy.

Lymphocytopenia may also occur in cases where malignancy is widespread, and again has been noted in Hodgkin's disease.[17] Monocytosis is also strongly associated with malignant disease; it occurs with high frequency in patients with malignant disease[18] and, conversely, malignancy is one of the commoner causes of monocytosis.[19]

Circulating malignant cells are rarely seen in peripheral blood films but can sometimes be demonstrated in buffy coat preparations.

Leukaemoid reactions (see below) occur most commonly in association with infection, but granulocytic leukaemoid reactions are not uncommon in disseminated malignancy.

Platelets

The first clue to an underlying malignancy may sometimes be an unexpected thrombocytosis. Whilst this is particularly common in association with chronic blood loss, it is important to be aware that other cancers may present in this way.

Bone marrow

The bones are often involved in metastatic spread of malignant disease. Carcinomas of the breast, lung, kidney, thyroid and prostate are the most frequently involved primary sites, but gastric, rectal and virtually any other malignant tumour may involve bone from time to time. The diagnosis may be made as a result of characteristic blood changes during the process of disease staging, or occasionally marrow deposits may be the first indication of malignant disease.

Carcinoma cells characteristically appear in clumps within bone marrow smears, but the marrow may be difficult to aspirate. Trephine biopsy is often necessary to obtain an adequate specimen to make the diagnosis. The use of immunocytochemistry[20] to demonstrate the presence of non-haemopoietic malignant cells in marrow material is sometimes of diagnostic value (Figs 1.5–1.7).

Childhood tumours, such as neuroblastoma, rhabdomyosarcoma, Ewing's tumour and medulloblastoma, not uncommonly involve the bone marrow.

On occasion these tumours may prove difficult to distinguish from leukaemic involvement, although some degree of cell clumping is usual. Immunocytochemistry may also be of value in these cases.

A less common result of marrow involvement by metastatic tumour is bone marrow necrosis. This condition may occur as a consequence of both primary haematological malignancy and secondary involvement of the marrow. There is usually a pancytopenia, severe bone pain is often present, marrow aspirate produces watery brown material with few identifiable cells and the trephine biopsy shows necrotic material. The prognosis is grave in these circumstances, most patients being dead within a few weeks.[21]

BACTERIAL INFECTION

Responses to infection produce some of the most frequently seen changes in the blood film and bone marrow. The responses seen depend to some extent on the nature of the organism responsible, and only the major points can be described here.

Neutrophil responses

A neutrophil leucocytosis is a common accompaniment of acute bacterial infection. There is a rough relationship between the severity of the infection and the neutrophil count: counts of $10–15 \times 10^9$ per litre may be seen with a mild or localized infection, whilst counts of $50–75 \times 10^9$ per litre may occur in severe systemic infections, although these are generalizations and the individual's response may vary widely. Both host factors and the nature of the infection can affect the response, for example suppurative infections such as deep-seated abscesses, empyema and meningitis tend to produce a more marked neutrophilia than an uncomplicated urinary tract infection; infections with 'cocci' (staphylococci, streptococci, pneumococci, gonococci) and some bacilli (*E.coli, Pseudomonas, C.diptheriae* and others) may be expected to produce neutrophilia whilst infections due to *Salmonella, Chlamydia, Rickettsia* and *Mycobacteria* are not usually associated with a granulocyte response. Occasionally no significant granulocyte response occurs in situations where it might be expected. Often this may reflect underlying problems such as alcohol abuse or malnutrition, but a transient neutropenia in the face of severe infection is sometimes seen in patients who appear haematologically normal in other respects, and whose blood returns to normal following recovery. A poor granulocyte response to infection is often the case in premature infants.

As neutrophilia develops there is frequently a release from the marrow of myeloid precursors resulting in a so-called 'left shift'. Band forms, metamyelocytes, myelocytes and even occasional myeloblasts may appear in the peripheral blood giving rise to leukaemoid reactions (see below).

In severe bacterial infection it is common to see *changes in neutrophil morphology*. Toxic granulation, cytoplasmic vacuoles, diffuse cytoplasmic basophilia, pyknotic areas in the nucleus and Döhle bodies have long been recognized as important markers of severity in infection.[22,23] Toxic granulation refers to deeply staining, metachromatic primary granules which arise in stimulated neutrophils[24] (Fig. 1.8).

Döhle bodies are lamellar aggregates of rough endoplasmic reticulum which appear by light microscopy as discrete round or oval sky-blue cytoplasmic inclusions in the periphery of Romanosky stained neutrophils. A close relationship between cytoplasmic vacuolation (Fig. 1.9) and the presence of bacteraemia has been described.[25]

Neutropenia

Neutropenia can occur during the course of almost any bacterial infection but is particularly common in certain types of infection (e.g. *Salmonella*, brucellosis, pertussis and some rickettsial infections). Certain other infections such as malaria, Kala-azar, trypanosomiasis, histoplasmosis and psittacosis are also associated with neutropenia. Disseminated tuberculosis has been associated with a range of haematological changes from neutropenia or pancytopenia on one hand to leukaemoid reactions and atypical myeloproliferative disorders on the other. It is not clear whether the reports of haematological states associated with tuberculosis represent superimposition of mycobacterial infections on an underlying blood disorder or whether disseminated tuberculosis can produce a leukaemia-like condition.

Lymphocyte response

Lymphocytosis occurs frequently in children with pertussis but is otherwise an uncommon response to bacterial or fungal infections. Lymphocyte counts of $15–25 \times 10^9$ per litre are typical but much higher counts do occur and may produce a so-called lymphoid leukaemoid reaction (see below). Lymphocytosis has also been found frequently in some forms of rickettsial infection.[26] Whilst lymphocytosis is reported to be a feature of tuberculosis, brucellosis and syphilis, this association appears to be of low frequency.

Monocyte response

Monocytosis is reported in association with a variety of infections particularly those with a chronic or subacute course, such as tuberculosis or bacterial endocarditis, although this response actually occurs in a minority of cases with these disorders.[24] A low-grade monocytosis may be quite a common feature in the convalescent phase of acute bacterial infection.

Other blood film changes in bacterial infections

Anaemia frequently occurs in chronic bacterial infection and may also arise in severe acute infections. Generally this takes the form of the 'anaemia of chronic disorders' (see below) but in certain circumstances haemolytic anaemia may accompany infections. Whilst in patients with sickle cell anaemia or glucose-6-phosphate dehydrogenase (G6PD) deficiency haemolytic episodes may be triggered by infections, this rarely occurs in other patients.

A dramatic intravascular haemorrhage may be caused by *Clostridium perfringens* septicaemia in some patients. Blood films show striking microspherocytosis, and leucocytosis with a left shift is often present. Hemoglobinuria, haemoglobinaemia and renal failure commonly occur. It is worth noting that this syndrome is distinctly uncommon, and in the majority of patients with *C.perfringens* septicaemia it does not occur.[27] Many other bacterial infections have been reported to cause haemolysis, but the frequency of these associations is low and haemolytic disease would seem to be a rare complication of infection.

Mycoplasma pneumoniae infection is frequently associated with the production of cold agglutinins but an overt haemolytic anaemia is uncommon.[28,29]

In contrast to other bacteria, *Bartonella bacilliformis* is regularly associated with haemolytic anaemia. This organism is the causative agent of Oroya fever, an endemic disease of Peru, Equador and Columbia. Haemolysis is common in Oroya fever and may be severe – the organisms may be visible in the blood film both within and closely adherent to erythrocytes.

Thrombocytopenia commonly accompanies severe infections, particularly those involving bacteraemia.[30] In contrast it is not uncommon for thrombocytosis to be found in patients with chronic infections such as tuberculosis, osteomyelitis and bacterial endocarditis.

VIRAL INFECTIONS

The whole topic of the haematological effects of viral infections is discussed elsewhere (Chapter 11) and therefore only a few points will be made here. Viruses may produce relatively non-specific changes in the blood or they may lead to specific haematological syndromes.

Leucocyte changes

Leucopenia is commonly associated with viral infections. Classically influenza,[31] parainfluenza, measles,[32] rubella[33] and mumps are associated with this response. Adenovirus and coxsackie virus infections have also been implicated.[31] Infective hepatitis may produce a neutropenia[34] but a neutrophil leucocytosis often arises in more severe cases.

The leucocyte response to viral illness is actually quite variable. In one study[31] lymphopenia occurred early in the illness, followed by a moderate granulocytosis and culminating in a mild neutropenia late in the course of the illness. Many viral illnesses are associated with an increase in total lymphocyte count and changes in the morphology of blood lymphocytes is common.

'Atypical lymphocytes', similar in appearance to those seen in infectious mononucleosis,[35] are commonly found in the blood of patients with viral infections (Fig. 1.10) (Table 1.5). These cells represent a T-'suppressor' cell response to infection and can be shown to be activated 'T8' cells.[36] Another morphological type of reactive lymphocyte frequently seen in the blood of patients with viral illnesses (and sometimes with bacterial sepsis) is the 'Turk cell'. These cells have an appearance intermediate between lymphocyte and plasma cells and are often termed 'lymphoplasmacytoid'.

Platelets

Thrombocytopenia is another non-specific feature of viral infection which occurs quite frequently. In some cases the bone marrow shows reduced numbers of megakaryocytes,[37,38] whilst in other cases typical immune (idiopathic) thrombocytopenia follows shortly after a viral illness.

A more severe form of bone marrow failure has been associated with viral infections, particularly in the immunosuppressed patient. The *virus associated haemophagocytic syndrome* is characterized by fever, hepatomegaly, splenomegaly, lymphadenopathy, skin rashes and pancytopenia. The bone marrow shows prominent haemophagocytosis with depression of normal haemopoietic activity (Fig. 1.11). Infections with Epstein–Barr virus (EBV), cytomegalovirus (CMV), herpes simplex, herpes zoster and adenoviruses have all been implicated.[39]

Many more specific haematological responses to virus infections are described. Aplastic anaemia has been associated with viral hepatitis[40] and it is probable that non-A non-B hepatitis is the usual culprit.[41] Parvovirus has been implicated as a cause of pure red cell aplasia in the immunocompromised[42] and of transient aplastic crises in those with chronic haemolytic anaemias.[43] EBV infections are of particular importance to the haematologist because of the variety of haematological changes they can produce. EBV infections may be asymptomatic, or may produce typical infectious mononucleosis. In addition they may be associated with some cases of lymphoma and with bone marrow failure in certain susceptible families. The human lymphotropic viruses, including HTLV-1, associated with the adult T-cell leukaemia/lymphoma syndrome, and HIV-1 (formerly known as

Table 1.5 Viral Causes of 'Atypical Lymphocytes'

Herpes viruses	EB virus
	Cytomegalovirus
	Herpes zoster
	Herpes simplex
Hepatitis	
Mumps	
Rubella	
Influenza	
Roseola infantum	
Rubeola	
HIV	

Based on data from Ref. 73.

HTLV III), the virus associated with the acquired immunodeficiency syndrome, are clearly of haematological importance. They are described elsewhere in this volume (Chapter 11) and have been reviewed in detail recently.[44,45]

PARASITIC DISEASE

Parasitic diseases may produce very dramatic haematological changes, only the more important of which can be summarized here.

Protozoal infections

Toxoplasmosis

In adults toxoplasmosis may produce an illness closely resembling infectious mononucleosis. The blood film shows 'atypical lymphocytes' and there is often an associated eosinophilia. A more severe form of the illness, particularly in the immunosuppressed patient, may be manifest as encephalitis, chorioretinitis and generalized disease.[46] Congenital toxoplasmosis may lead to severe anaemia, thrombocytopenia and leucocytosis in the infant. The blood film in these cases shows erythroblastosis, neutrophil leucocytosis with a left shift and eosinophilia. Plasma cells and reactive lymphocytes may also be present.

Malaria

On a world scale malaria is probably the most important protozoal infection, and it is regularly associated with profound haematological effects. The changes described are those which follow *Plasmodium falciparum* infections; the consequences of *P.vivax*, *P.malariae* and *P.ovale* infections are generally milder. In the acute attack in the non-immune individual there may be no anaemia at the outset, with a falling haemoglobin in the following 2–3 weeks. Chronically infected, partially immune individuals may have a severe anaemia with reticulocytopenia and bone marrow evidence of dyserythropoiesis.[47] Folate deficiency frequently complicates the situation in areas where malaria is endemic.[48]

Thrombocytopenia is extremely common in patients with acute malaria, without disturbance of other haemostatic parameters. Bone marrow megakaryocytes are normal or increased in number with active budding of platelets.[49]

White cell changes in malaria include dramatic changes in lymphocytes, monocytes and granulocyutes as summarized in Table 1.6.

Kala-azar

Visceral leishmaniasis or Kala-azar is associated with progressive pancytopenia, massive splenomegaly, hepatomegaly and lymphadenopathy.

Table 1.6   Blood Film Features of Malaria

Red cells	Parasites Anisocytosis, microspherocytosis (during second week), macrocytosis, polychromasia
Neutrophils	Neutrophil leucocytosis (first 2 days) Moderate neutropenia Marked leucocytosis with left shift (during recovery) + toxic granulation
Eosinophils	Reduced initially, sometimes increased during recovery
Monocytes	Increased, vacuolation, malarial pig- ment, erythrophagocytosis
Lymphocytes	Reactive transformed lymphocytes Plasma cells
Platelets	Moderate to severe reduction

After ref. 48.

The severity of pancytopenia is closely related to splenic size.[50] The bone marrow is generally hypercellular and there is a marked increase in macrophages, many of which contain numerous Leishman–Donovan bodies.

Helminthic infections

A wide variety of pathology may result from helminthic infections but there are only two characteristic features in the blood.[48]

1. Eosinophilia. This arises when infection of blood, lymphatics, lungs and solid tissues occurs. When these tissues are involved transiently during the invasive phase the eosinophilia is transient. When infection is established in tissue the eosinophilia may be persistent. Extremely marked eosinophilia may occur particularly in visceral larva migrans and in filarial infections. Occult filarial infections are associated with 'tropical eosinophilia' where eosinophil counts of 30–80×10^9 per litre are recorded.[51] Those infestations associated with eosinophilia are listed in Ref. 48.

2. Established infestations of the gastrointestinal tract leading to impaired host nutrition.

Hookworm infestation is one of the commonest causes of iron deficiency anaemia in the world. Chronic blood loss of the order of 0.03–0.05 ml per day per worm for *Necator americanus* and 0.16–0.34 ml per day per worm for *Ancylostoma duodenale* has been estimated.[52] This can result in a daily loss of blood of over 200 ml with heavy infestation. Severe infestations with whipworm (*Trichuris trichiura*) may occasionally cause iron deficiency.

The fish tapeworm *Diphyllobothrium latum* may interfere with vitamin B_{12}

absorption in the host, however, this rarely produces megaloblastic anaemia.

Leukaemoid reactions

Extremely high leucocyte counts may sometimes occur in non-leukaemic conditions, particularly in severe infections. In these cases the leucocyte count may exceed 50×10^9 per litre and many immature forms, suggestive of leukaemia, may appear in the blood. Most frequently such reactions are 'granulocytic' and the blood may show blast cells, myelocytes and metamyelocytes in addition to many neutrophils. 'Lymphocytic' reactions may also occur, particularly in children with pertussis.

The distinction between leukaemoid reactions and leukaemia may be difficult. The presence of toxic granulation, elevated leucocyte alkaline phosphatase and Döhle bodies is good evidence in favour of a reactive condition.

In addition to bacterial infection, leukaemoid reactions may accompany severe viral infections, metastatic malignancy, severe haemorrhage or haemolysis, eclampsia and burns. These reactions are seen most frequently in children.

CONNECTIVE TISSUE DISEASES

Rheumatoid arthritis

The majority of patients with active rheumatoid arthiritis will be anaemic to some degree. Characteristically the picture is of the *'anaemia of chronic disorders'*. This type of anaemia, which is also a frequent accompaniment of infection and malignant disease, is typically mild or moderate, the haemoglobin rarely falling below 8–9 g/dl unless there are other factors present. Anaemia tends to develop in the first month or two of illness and is usually non-progressive thereafter. The blood film is typically normochromic and normocytic with moderate anisocytosis, although a degree of hypochromasia may be seen in up to half of patients. Microcytosis is seen less often than hypochromasia and is generally less pronounced than that seen in iron deficiency. Polychromasia and nucleated red cells are absent and the reticulocyte count normal or reduced.

The bone marrow appearances in the anaemia of chronic disorders are characteristic. Erythropoiesis is normoblastic or micronormoblastic, but iron stores are generally plentiful with reduced or absent siderotic granules in the developing erythroblasts.

In patients with rheumatoid arthritis it is not uncommon for iron deficiency to complicate the haematological picture. This may result from long-term ingestion of non-steroidal anti-inflammatory agents, aspirin or corticosteroids leading to gastrointestinal blood loss. In the investigation of anaemia in these patients the serum iron and iron-binding capacity may be misleading because of the presence of inflammation and serum ferritin levels also may be raised as part of the acute phase response. Examination of the bone marrow iron stores is occasionally needed to determine the iron status.

A common accompaniment of active rheumatoid disease is a moderate thrombocytosis which tends to parallel disease activity. In uncomplicated rheumatoid disease there are no specific leucocyte changes but in *Felty's syndrome* marked neutropenia, often with thrombocytopenia and anaemia, is characteristic. The triad of neutropenia, splenomegaly and rheumatoid arthritis, which constitutes Felty's syndrome occurs in about 1% of patients with rheumatoid disease.[53] The bone marrow generally shows normal or increased cellularity with normal myeloid precursors but absence of mature neutrophils. The exact mechanism of the neutropenia of Felty's syndrome is not known, but immune destruction of neutrophils is believed to be a major feature.[54]

Another important aspect of the haematological complications of rheumatoid arthritis is the frequency of adverse reactions to the drugs used in its therapy. These will be discussed below with drug reactions in general.

SYSTEMIC LUPUS ERYTHEMATOSUS AND OTHER COLLAGEN DISORDERS

Systemic lupus erythematosus (SLE) has a particular propensity to produce haematological changes (Table 1.7) and it is not uncommon for these to be the presenting features. A degree of anaemia is present in the majority of cases and this is typically of the 'anaemia of chronic disorders' pattern as described above. Drug-induced chronic blood loss, intercurrent infections and renal impairment can all further exacerbate this anaemia. Autoimmune haemolytic anaemia, with its characteristic blood film appearances (spherocytosis, polychromasia, reticulocytosis) occurs in around 10% of patients with SLE at some time during their illness and may occasionally be the presenting feature. The direct Coombs test (DCT) is normally positive in these cases for both complement components and IgG. An isolated positive DCT may also occur in SLE without evidence of active haemolysis.

Leucopenia is a common feature of SLE, reported in 17% of cases[55] in one series but considered by others to appear in the majority of cases at some

Table 1.7   Haematological Changes in Systemic Lupus Erythematosus

Anaemia
  Anaemia of chronic disorders
  Autoimmune haemolytic anaemia
  Anaemia of renal impairment
  Iron deficiency (drug-induced chronic blood loss)
Leucopenia
Leucocytosis
Thrombocytopenia
Pancytopenia
Lupus anticoagulant
Functional hyposplenism
Bone marrow necrosis

stage in their disease. A moderate neutropenia in association with a moderate lymphopenia is the usual finding. Leucocytosis may occur in response to infection, corticosteroid therapy or rarely due to disease activity itself.

Thrombocytopenia, with platelet counts of less than 100×10^9 per litre can occur in up to 20% of cases. Severe thrombocytopenia, virtually indistinguishable from idiopathic thrombocytopenic purpura occurs in a smaller number of patients and may be the presenting feature of SLE in 1–2% of cases.[56] Another interesting feature of SLE is the occasional occurrence of *functional hyposplenism*. The blood film shows the characteristic changes of target cells, acanthocytes, spherocytes, Howell–Jolly bodies and Papenheimer bodies (Fig. 1.12). This association has been well-recognized in rheumatological circles[57,58] but is less widely appreciated among haematologists.

The other collagen diseases are less closely associated with haematological disorders. The anaemia of chronic disorders is commonly present, and the ESR may be elevated.

Polymyalgia rheumatica is often associated with quite marked anaemia and in conjunction with very high ESR this may raise suspicions of a diagnosis of myeloma. It is not uncommon for patients with this condition to appear in the haematology clinic.

RENAL DISEASE

Renal failure is associated with a variety of haematological changes including anaemia, abnormalities of platelet and leucocyte function, and disturbed coagulation. Erythrocytosis may accompany certain renal disorders.

Anaemia

Anaemia is a consistent feature of chronic renal failure which until recently has proved intractable. The aetiology of anemia is complex although it has now become clear that impaired erythropoietin production is the principal factor. Recent clinical trials with recombinant human erythropoietin have shown that the anaemia of renal failure can be improved or corrected by this means alone[59,60] and it would appear therefore that the other mechanisms of anaemia in chronic renal failure (Table 1.8) are of significantly less importance. The anaemia of chronic renal failure is normochromic and normocytic in the uncomplicated case. The severity of anaemia is highly variable and the correlation between blood urea and haemoglobin is inconsistent; in general the haemoglobin ranges from 5 to 10 g/dl. A characteristic morphological change in the red cells is the presence of numerous surface spicules (Fig. 1.13). These 'burr' cells or echinocytes are seen in greatest numbers in the more severely anaemic patient. The presence of spherocytes suggests haemolysis or hypersplenism and schistocytes are characteristic of the microangiopathic haemolysis which can accompany such conditions as accelerated hypertension.

Table 1.8   Causes of Anaemia in Renal Failure

Major factors
  Inadequate erythropoietin production
  Uraemic inhibitors of erythropoiesis
  Reduced red cell lifespan

Minor factors
  Expanded plasma volume
  Iron deficiency
  Folate deficiency
  Blood loss
  Infection
  Hypersplenism
  Aluminium toxicity
  Hyperparathyroidism with osteitis fibrosa

The bone marrow in renal failure usually shows normoblastic erythropoiesis but fails to show the degree of erythroid hyperplasia one would expect for a given severity of anaemia. Bone marrow biopsy may show a variety of changes in the bones including osteitis fibrosa, osteosclerosis, osteomalacia and secondary myelofibrosis.

Leucocyte changes

Leucocyte changes are usually unremarkable, both the total and differential white cell count being normal in most patients with renal disease. Hypersplenism occasionally arises in chronic renal failure patients undergoing dialysis and in these cases both leucopenia and thrombocytopenia are seen.[61] Temporary granulocytopenia during haemodialysis may occur as a result of stasis of leucocytes in the pulmonary circulation. Neutrophil hypersegmentation in the absence of bone marrow megaloblastic change may occur in renal failure.[62]

Haemostatic defects are a characteristic feature of renal failure, acute renal failure in particuilar is often associated with a serious bleeding diathesis. The main cause of this bleeding tendency is platelet dysfunction which is believed to be due to the accumulation of toxic substances in the plasma.[63]

Mild thrombocytopenia is a common feature of chronic renal failure and this may exacerbate the bleeding tendency. More severe thrombocytopenia may be associated with many of the conditions leading to renal failure. For example, the disseminated intravascular coagulation which may accompany acute renal failure produces a marked thrombocytopenia. The platelet count may fall as a consequence of circulating immune complexes in polyarteritis nodosa or acute glomerulonephritis. In acute renal allograft rejection increased platelet consumption is usually present and thrombocytopenia frequently results.[64]

Erythrocytosis

Erythrocytosis or 'secondary polycythaemia' may arise in association with a variety of renal diseases. This physiologically inappropriate response results from either ectopic erythropoietin production by renal tumours or from increased erythropoietin production in response to regional renal hypoxia. Renal carcinomas, Wilms' tumour and a variety of benign renal disorders have been associated with erythrocytosis (Table 1.9).

Haemolytic uraemic syndrome and thrombotic thrombocytopenic purpura

The haemolytic uraemic syndrome (HUS) and thrombotic thrombocytopenic purpura (TTP) are both characterized by microangiopathic haemolytic anaemia and thrombocytopenia. There are significant clinical differences between the two syndromes but there is a wide area of overlap. In HUS, acute renal failure is a major feature, whilst in TTP uraemia is usually mild and neurological problems are often a major feature. In both conditions the blood film shows the characteristic features of microangiopathic haemolysis (red cell fragmentation, spherocyte formation, and polychromasia) and thrombocytopenia is seen in virtually all patients. Laboratory tests of coagulation may show some evidence of disseminated intravascular coagulation but are usually normal. The underlying mechanisms of both TTP and HUS are uncertain although a clear association between HUS and infection with certain toxin-producing strains of *E.coli* has been described[65,66] and other associations are recognized.[67]

GASTROINTESTINAL DISEASES

The blood may be affected in many ways by gastrointestinal diseases, and it is not uncommon for haematological changes to be the initial manifestation of serious underlying disease of the gut (Table 1.10).

Table 1.9 Renal Lesions Associated with Erythrocytosis

Renal cell carcinoma
Wilms' tunmour
Renal cysts
Hydronephrosis
Nephrotic syndrome
Diffuse parenchymal renal disease
Bartter's syndrome
Renal transplantation
Renal artery stenosis

Table 1.10   Haematological Associations of Gastrointestinal Diseases

Gastrointestinal disorder	Haematological changes
Cancer	Iron deficiency
Peptic ulceration	Iron deficiency
Hiatus hernia/gastro-oesophageal reflux	Iron deficiency
Chronic gastritis	Iron deficiency
	B_{12} deficiency
Gastrectomy	Iron deficiency
	B_{12} deficiency
Coeliac disease	Folate deficiency
	Iron deficiency
	Hyposplenism
	B_{12} deficiency (rarely)
Bacterial overgrowth syndrome	B_{12} deficiency
	Iron deficiency
Inflammatory bowel disease	Anaemia of chronic disorders
	Iron deficiency
	B_{12} deficiency (ileal disease or resection)
	Haemolysis (drug-induced)
	Haemolysis (autoimmune)

Gastrointestinal blood loss

The loss of blood from the gastrointestinal tract is the commonest cause of iron deficiency anaemia in men and post-menopausal women. Whatever the source of blood loss the principal haematological features of hypochromasia and microcytosis (Fig. 1.14) will be the same. In cases of chronic blood loss a moderate thrombocytosis is common and when iron deficiency is partly treated a dimorphic red cell picture may be seen. Cancer of any part of the gastrointestinal tract, peptic ulceration, ingestion of aspirin or non-steroidal anti-inflammatory drugs and inflammatory bowel disease are the commonest causes of gastrointestinal blood loss producing anaemia. It cannot be reiterated too frequently that iron deficiency anaemia should be considered as a symptom rather than a diagnosis in its own right, and it is incumbent on the clinician to seek an explanation for it.

Structural abnormalities of the gastrointestinal tract

Anaemia is a common complication of both partial and total gastrectomy. Total gastrectomy is most commonly carried out in patients with gastric carcinoma and in those relatively few patients who survive long enough, vitamin B_{12} deficiency is bound to arise unless prophylactic supplementation is used. Anaemia is a frequent late complication of partial gastrectomy, with a reported incidence of 40% after 10–15 years.[60] In the majority of cases the anaemia is due to iron deficiency, whilst in a small proportion of patients vitamin B_{12} deficiency may be either a contributory or sole cause. A mixed deficiency of both iron and B_{12} may lead to a dimorphic red cell picture in the peripheral blood and can occasionally produce diagnostic difficulty. In the bone marrow the characteristic megaloblastic changes can be masked by iron deficiency, but the presence of giant metamyelocytes and megakaryocyte abnormalities may reveal the true diagnosis.

Megaloblastic anaemia may be the presenting feature of anatomical and functional abnormalities of the small bowel. Vitamin B_{12} deficiency can be produced by the overgrowth of intestinal bacteria which are able to utilize this vitamin. This syndrome can arise from anatomical abnormalities such as intestinal diverticulum, strictures, anastomoses, fistulae, blind loops and in situations where there is altered gut motility such as scleroderma. The syndrome can also follow vagotomy, partial gastrectomy and malfunctioning gastroenterostomies. Vitamin B_{12} deficiency can also arise following resection of the terminal ileum as this is the site at which its active absorption normally occurs.

Impaired absorption of haematologically important substances can occur in a variety of conditions which impair small bowel function. Coeliac disease, tropical sprue, Whipple's disease, radiation damage to the small intestine, Crohn's disease and certain neoplasms can all produce such malabsorption.

Coeliac disease is a good example of a gastrointestinal disorder which frequently presents to the haematologist. Once again megaloblastic anaemia is the usual result although in this condition folate deficiency is the prime cause. Folic acid is normally absorbed in the jejunum, and this is the area most severely affected in coeliac disease. Vitamin B_{12} deficiency can occur, but is uncommon except in severe and extensive disease which involves the terminal ileum. Iron deficiency frequently coexists and may produce a dimorphic blood picture. In childhood, iron deficiency anaemia is a more common presentation than megaloblastic anaemia.

Hyposplenism occurs quite frequently in coeliac disease, and the characteristic appearances described above (Fig. 1.12) may be superimposed on a dimorphic blood film. The incidence of functional hyposplenism in untreated patients has been reported to be as high as 76%.[69] Hyposplenism may partly account for the thrombocytosis which occurs in over half of coeliac patients.[70]

Inflammatory bowel diseases

The anaemia of chronic disorders is a common feature of inflammatory bowel disease. Chronic gastroinestinal blood loss frequently produces iron deficiency which contributes to this anaemia.

In Crohn's disease, involvement or resection of more than 90 cm of the terminal ileum produces vitamin B_{12} malabsorption which may lead to clinically significant B_{12} deficiency.[71] Folate deficiency may arise when there is very extensive disease or poor nutrition and it is not uncommon for patients with Crohn's disease to develop bacterial overgrowth syndromes.

In contrast to patients with Crohn's disease the anaemia in ulcerative colitis is rarely megaloblastic and the main cause of anaemia is chronic blood loss. An autoimmune haemolytic anaemia has been described in association with ulcerative colitis on occasions.[10,72]

There is a well-recognized association between intestinal disorders, particularly coeliac disease, and hyposplenism. Hyposplenism is recognized as a complication of both Crohn's disease and ulcerative colitis,[73] and has also been reported in tropical sprue, Whipple's disease and non-specific ulcerative jejunitis.

The drugs used in the management of inflammatory bowel disease may cause anaemia in their own right. Salazopyrin is an oxidative drug which can produce an acute haemolytic anaemia of Heinz body type. The blood film in these cases can be characteristic (Fig. 1.15) with the appearance of irregularly contracted cells, spherocytes, cells with 'bites' out of the membrane, red cell 'hemighosts', some fragmentation and, of course, polychromasia. Heinz bodies may be demonstrated by supravital staining with methyl violet, but these are rarely numerous except in splenectomized individuals.

LIVER DISEASES

Diseases of the liver frequently have a profound effect on blood coagulation, whilst the changes to the formed elements of the blood are usually less severe (Table 1.11).

In chronic liver failure from whatever cause there is usually a moderate degree of anaemia. Target cells, burr cells and macrocytosis are frequently present. Slight polychromasia may be apparent. The anaemia is of multifactorial aetiology and contributing factors include nutritional deficiency of folic acid, iron deficiency secondary to GI blood loss, hypersplenism, and changes to the red cell membrane resulting from disordered lipid metabolism.

Table 1.11   Haematological Associations of Liver Disease

Disease	Haematological changes
Viral hepatitis	Shortened red cell survival Haemolytic anaemia (rare) Aplastic anaemia (rare)
Chronic active hepatitis	Autoimmune haemolytic anaemia
Chronic liver failure/cirrhosis	Target cells, burr cells, macrocytosis Iron deficiency (2° to GI blood loss) Folate deficiency Hypersplenism Acute haemolysis (Zieve's) Hypersplenism

Haemolytic anaemias of various types may arise in association with liver disease. Autoimmune haemolysis occurs in association with chronic active hepatitis; oxidative haemolysis has been described in association with viral hepatitis (particularly in G6PD-deficient individuals);[74,75] Wilson's disease may present with acute haemolysis in association with acute liver failure.[76,77]

Changes in the lipid content of the red cell membrane are associated with a shortened red cell survival and this has its most dramatic manifestation as 'spur cell' anaemia.[78] In this condition the red cell membrane cholesterol content is greatly increased as a result of disordered plasma lipoprotein metabolism. The blood film shows bizarre spiculated red cells with marked reticulocytosis. The spur cells are morphologically indistinguishable from the acanthocytes which are seen in the rare condition of abetalipoproteinaemia.

Zieve described in 1958 a triad of acute haemolysis in association with alcohol-induced fatty liver and hypertriglyceridaemia.[79] This syndrome characteristically follows acute alcoholic excess and the mechanism of haemolysis, which appears to be self-limiting, is unknown.

RESPIRATORY DISEASES

Changes in the blood film and bone marrow are not often considered a prominent feature of chest disease, but those changes discussed above in association with infections and malignancy may, of course, arise.

Chronic hypoxia resulting from lung disease is the major cause of secondary polycythaemia (or more correctly erythrocytosis), the degree of polycythaemia corresponding roughly with the severity of the hypoxia. The condition can usually be differentiated from primary polycythaemia by the absence of an associated leucocytosis or thrombocytosis. An interesting but unexplained feature of chronic obstructive airway disease is a moderate macrocytosis.[80]

Acute infections of the lung generally produce a neutrophil leucocytosis but other responses may arise in associations with certain organisms. Tuberculosis, as mentioned earlier, may be associated with a variety of haematological reactions; mycoplasma pneumoniae infections are frequently associated with the production of cold agglutinins which may occasionally precipitate significant haemolysis. Pulmonary eosinophilia describes those disorders in which peripheral blood eosinophilia coexists with pulmonary infiltrates seen on chest X-ray. In Britain probably the commonest cause of this condition is hypersensitivity to *Aspergillus fumigatus*. A similar clinical picture arises in allergic alveolitis including farmer's lung, bird fancier's lung and a number of lesser known occupational lung diseases.[81] A variety of parasitic disorders may cause transient respiratory distress with eosinophilia (e.g. *Ascaris, Ankylostoma, Filaria, Trichuris, Taenia*). A similar clinical picture may occur in association with drug hypersensitivity reactions, and polyarteritis nodosa can produce a more severe clinical illness.

In all these various conditions, the major change in the blood film is a raised eosinophil count, which may be very marked. There is also, of course, quite frequently an eosinophilia associated with atopic asthma.

ENDOCRINE AND METABOLIC DISORDERS

The haematological manifestations of endocrine disease are rarely severe and are usually self-limiting. Serious haematological disorders in patients with such disease can usually be attributed to associated or coincident abnormalities rather than to the endocrine disorder.

Hypothyroidism is associated with mild anaemia in about one quarter to one third of patients.[82] In the majority of cases the anaemia is normochromic and normocytic although even in this group the MCV may be towards the upper limit of the normal range, and may fall when thyroid replacement therapy is introduced. In a small group of patients iron deficiency may produce a hypochromic microcytic anaemia (most frequently as a result of the menorrhagia which may be associated with myxoedema) which responds to iron without treatment of the underlying hypothyroidism.

A larger group of patients present a macrocytic blood picture. When this is marked it is usually a result of coexistent B_{12} or folate deficiency, and it is important to be aware of the association between pernicious anaemia and immune diseases of the thyroid. When patients with B_{12} or folate deficiency are excluded there remain a proportion of cases with macrocytosis which appears to be a direct result of hypothyroidism and which is responsive to thyroid hormone replacement. In these cases there is usually less marked macrocytosis, less ovalocytosis and absence of associated changes in the leucocytes when compared to the true megaloblastic anaemias.

The presence of a small number of acanthocytes in the blood film of up to 20% of cases has been described.[82]

The red cell mass is characteristically increased in patients with *hyperthyroidism*,[83] but the haematocrit is usually unchanged as there is a corresponding increase in plasma volume. Anaemia occurs rarely in severe cases of thyrotoxicosis.[84]

There are no consistent leucocyte abnormalities associated with thyroid disease, but for the haematologist it is most important to be aware of the propensity of antithyroid drugs to produce leucopenia and agranulocytosis. As many as one in 200 patients treated with antithyroid drugs have been reported to develop agranulocytosis, and a transient leucopenia is even more common.[85]

Hypopituitarism is well-recognized as a cause of a moderately severe non-progressive anaemia which is characteristically normochromic and normocytic. The mechanism is not entirely clear though failure of production of hormones from target glands, particularly the thyroid and adrenal glands, seems to be important.

A variety of haematological changes occur in patients with *Cushing's syndrome*. A 1–2 g/dl increase in haemoglobin concentration may occur and occasionally frankly increased red cell mass is seen. The most prominent effects of glucocorticoids are on the leucocytes. A significant neutrophilia may occur, whilst in contrast eosinophils, basophils and monocyte numbers may all be decreased.[86]

In *Addison's disease*, a mild normochromic normocytic anaemia may occur, although in the untreated dehydrated patient this may be masked by haemoconcentration.

Hyperparathyroidism has been associated on rare occasions with a normochromic normocytic anaemia.[87] Bone marrow biopsy in these patients frequently reveals fibrotic marrow but the characteristic changes seen in the blood of patients with idiopathic myelofibrosis are lacking.

Diabetes mellitus is associated with structural and functional changes in haemoglobin,[88] but is not generally directly responsible for changes in the blood film or bone marrow. A neutrophil leucocytosis often occurs in severe diabetic ketoacidosis even when there is no underlying infection.

SKIN DISEASE

Whilst there are frequent skin manifestations of haematological disease, the converse is not well-defined.

Eosinophilia is the commonest haematological association of skin diseases and may be particularly marked in pemphigus and in dermatitis herpetiformis. It has also been reported in association with exfoliative dermatitis, psoriasis, pruritus, prurigo, eczema, dermatitis venenata, icthyosis, mycosis fungoides, pityriasis rubra, facial granuloma, scabies, urticaria and angioneurotic oedema.[24]

Dermatitis herpetiformis is strongly associated with coeliac disease and as a result both folate deficiency and hyposplenism may occur along with their characteristic blood film appearances.

Diffuse fasciitis is an uncommon disorder characterized by thickening and induration of the skin, usually involving the limbs and trunk, which can be distinguished from classical scleroderma on clinical grounds. There is frequently an associated eosinophilia (indeed the condition is often known as 'eosinophilic fasciitis'), a raised ESR and hypergammaglobulinaemia. There is an interesting but unexplained association between this condition and severe aplastic anaemia. In addition various malignant and pre-malignant blood disorders have been recorded in these patients.[89,90,91]

EFFECTS OF DRUGS AND TOXINS

Alcohol

Alcohol is perhaps pre-eminent as a cause of toxic haematological effects, and it is important that both clinicians and haematologist are aware of the diverse changes it can produce. It is very common for chronic alcoholics to be anaemic. Many factors are involved in the aetiology, including direct toxicity of alcohol, chronic blood loss, dietary deficiencies and hepatic dysfunction.[92]

Macrocytosis is an extremely common finding in alcoholics, and can be attributed to at least four potential causes: (a) folate deficiency, (b) reticulocyte response to bleeding or haemorrhages, (c) liver disease, or (d) direct toxicity of alcohol. The macrocytosis of alcohol is usually mild, with MCV in the 100–110 range in most patients, and anaemia either absent or very slight. So frequent is this change, that the MCV has been proposed as useful screening test for alcoholism.[93] This macrocytosis may exist in the absence of folate deficiency or liver disease and will slowly correct over 2–4 months of alcohol abstension. Folate deficiency is common in severe alcoholics who are malnourished and probably represents both dietary deficiency and a direct effect of ethanol upon folate metabolism. Megaloblastic haematopoiesis is manifest in these cases by ovalocytosis, anisocytosis and neutrophil hypersegmentation features which are not seen in the 'macrocytosis of alcoholism'.

Alcohol may lead to sideroblastic anaemia and in these cases the blood film may be dimorphic with a macrocytosis.

The bone marrow in alcoholism may demonstrate iron deficiency, megaloblastic changes, sideroblastic changes or no specific changes whatever. A particularly characteristic feature is vacuolation of early normoblasts[94] which appears to be both one of the earliest changes to appear following alcohol ingestion and one of the first to disappear following abstinence.[95]

Neutropenia and thrombocytopenia may also occur in alcoholics, and once again both direct toxicity and folate deficiency may be implicated. Platelets and neutrophil numbers usually recover within a few days of alcohol withdrawal.[96,97]

Poisons

Lead poisoning is associated with a wide range of clinical effects, including haematological manifestations. Chronic lead poisoning produces a hypochromic microcytic anaemia with prominent basophilic stippling[98] (Fig. 1.16). The bone marrow usually shows erythroid hyperplasia with many ring sideroblasts. The basophilic stippling of lead poisoning is a prominent, but not specific finding. It is believed to be to be a result of acquired pyrimidine-5'-nucleotidase deficiency[99] leading to accumulation of incompletely degraded ribosomal RNA within the reticulocyte.[100]

Several other chemical compounds, including arsine and inorganic copper, most frequently encountered in industrial settings, may be associated with severe haemolytic anaemias.[101] The characteristic features of intravascular haemolysis (spherocytosis, polychromasia, haemoglobinaemia and haemoglobinuria) will be present. Snake venoms, spider bites and occasionally multiple bee stings may also produce episodes of intravascular haemolysis.[102]

Drug reactions

When considering the haematological effects of systemic disease it is important to be aware that drugs rather than disease may be the prime cause of the changes (although a full discussion of this is outside the remit of this review). The major drug-induced haematological changes are listed in Table 1.12. Neutropenia is the most commonly described drug-induced blood dyscrasia and an extensive list of offending drugs can be found in Ref. 19. The same reference contains an extensive list of drugs incriminated in causing thrombocytopenia, which is probably second only to neutropenia in its frequency. This topic is discussed fully in Chapter 10.

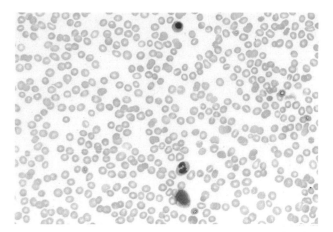

Fig.1.1 Blood film: leucoerythroblastic change (p.2).

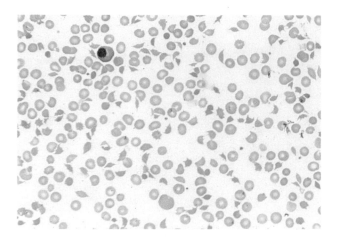

Fig.1.2 Blood film: microangiopathic haemolysis (p.2).

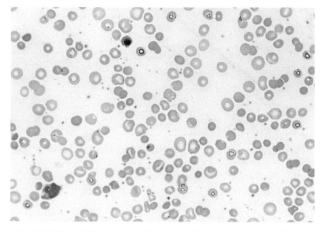

Fig.1.3 Blood film: autoimmune haemolysis (p.4).

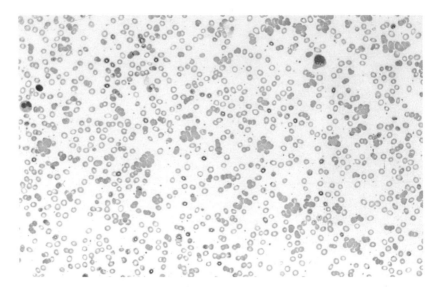

Fig.1.4 Blood film: cold agglutinins (p.5).

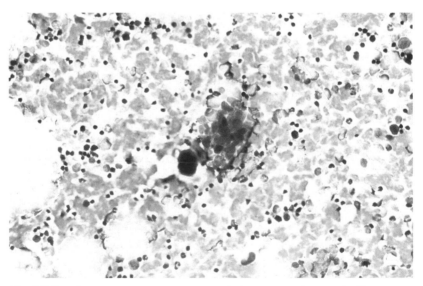

Fig.1.5 Bone marrow smear: metastatic breast carcinoma (p.6).

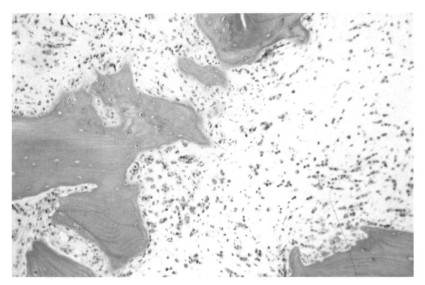

Fig.1.6 Bone marrow trephine: metastatic carcinoma (p.6).

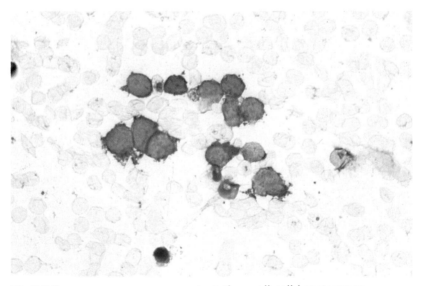

Fig.1.7 Bone marrow smear: metastatic small cell lung cancer.
Immunoalkaline phosphatase technique using UJ13A (antibody to
neural antigens) primary antibody (p.6).

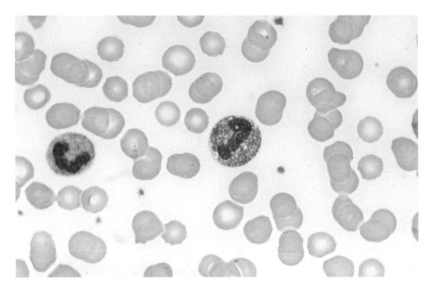

Fig.1.8 Blood film: toxic granulation of neutrophils (p.8).

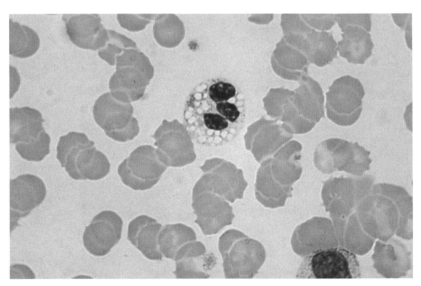

Fig.1.9 Blood film: neutrophil cytoplasmic vacuolation (p.8).

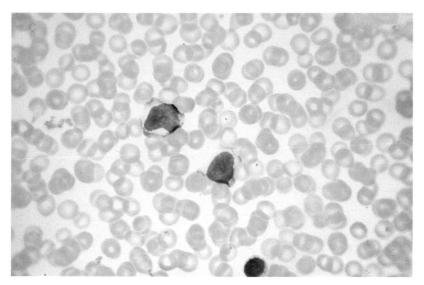

Fig.1.10 Blood film: infectious mononucleosis (p.10).

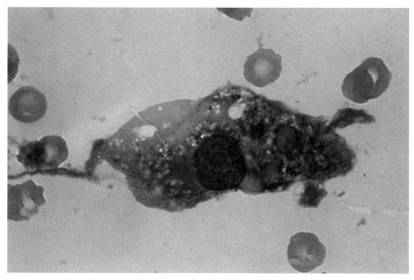

Fig.1.11 Marrow smear: viral-associated haemophagocytic syndrome (p.10).

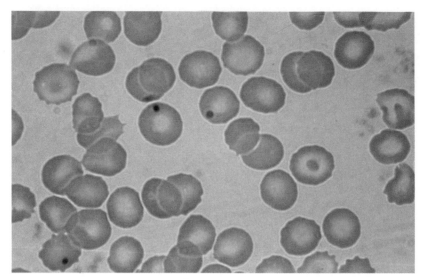
Fig.1.12 Blood film: hyposplenism (p.15).

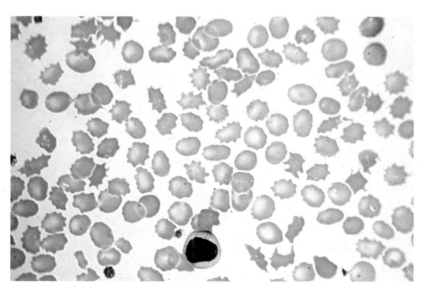
Fig.1.13 Blood film: renal failure (p.15).

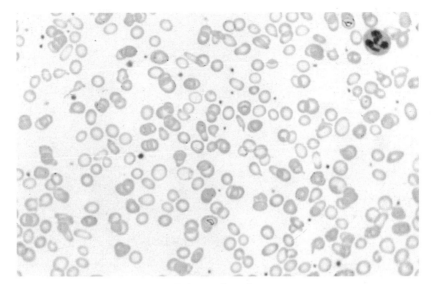

Fig.1.14 Blood film: iron deficiency (p.18).

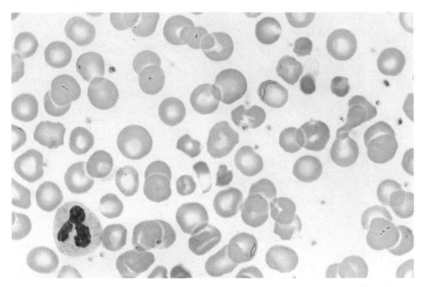

Fig.1.15 Blood film: oxidative haemolysis due to Salazopyrin (p.20).

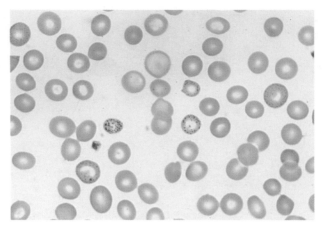

Fig.1.16 Blood film: lead poisoning (p.24).

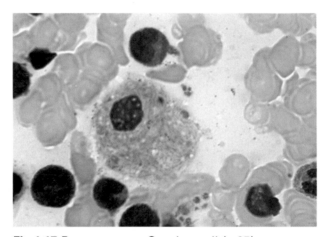

Fig.1.17 Bone marrow: Gaucher cell (p.25).

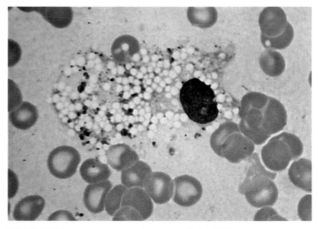

Fig.1.18 Bone marrow: foam cell (p.25).

Table 1.12 Effects of Drugs on the Formed Elements of the Blood

Red cells	Example drugs
Iron deficiency (GI blood loss)	Aspirin, non-steroidal anti-inflammatory agents
Immunohaemolysis	α-Methyl DOPA, penicillin
Oxidative haemolysis (particularly in G6PD deficient individuals)	Dapsone, salazopyrin
Megaloblastic (folate deficiency	Phenytoin
Aplastic anaemia	Chloramphenicol, phenylbutazone
Sideroblastic anaemia	Isoniazid
White cells	
Neutropenia/agranulocytosis	Sulphonamides, anti-thyroid drugs
Neutrophilia	Corticosteroids
Eosinophilia	Sulphonamides, gold salts
Platelets	
Thrombocytopenia	Thiazides, quinine, sulphonamides

MISCELLANEOUS

Inborn errors of metabolism

In many lipid-storage disorders and in mucopolysaccharidoses there are characteristic changes in the blood and/or bone marrow. The haematological changes are usually overshadowed by the other clinical features, but they may be of great diagnostic importance. Abnormal storage histiocytes seen in the marrow are the commonest finding. In Gaucher's disease these have a very characteristic lamellar or onion-skin appearance (Fig. 1.17), whilst in Niemann–Pick disease and other lipidoses 'foam' cells are more usual (Fig. 1.18) (Table 1.13).

In the mucopolysaccharidoses the presence of vacuolated lymphocytes in the peripheral blood is a distinctive feature. Similar vacuolation may be seen in Wolman's disease, Niemann–Pick disease, Batten's disease and mannosidosis.

Non-specific inflammatory responses in bone marrow biopsies

Bone marrow biopsies may reveal various stromal reactions in patients with a wide range of underlying disease; infections, malignancies (without overt marrow involvement), collagen diseases and sarcoidosis are all prone to produce such effects. According to Burkhardt, Bartl and others these reactions can be roughly divided[103] into six types:

1. Acute inflammation 'exudative' or 'necrotic' types: There may be necrosis of haemopoietic cells, oedema and increase in mature granulocytes.

Table 1.13 Storage Disorders Associated With Marrow 'Foam Cells'

Niemann–Pick

Gaucher's[a]

GM, gangliosidosis

Lactosyl ceramidosis

Fabry's disease

Wolman's disease

Cholesterol ester storage disease

Cerebrotendinous xanthomatosis

Hyperlipoproteinaemia
  Type I
  Type II
  Type III
  Type IV
  Type V

Tangier disease

Lecithin: cholesterol acyltransferase deficiency

---

[a] Usually characteristic 'Gaucher' cells rather than 'foam cells'.

Considerable residual haematopoiesis may be present.
2. Chronic inflammation 'atrophic' types: Little haematopoiesis remains and there is oedema with an infiltrate of lymphocytes, plasma cells and mast cells.
3. Chronic inflammation 'fibrotic' type: There is reduction in both haematopoiesis and fat cells. Reticulin is increased, collagen fibrosis and possibly new bone formation is present. A variable chronic inflammatory cell infiltrate may be present.
4. Chronic inflammation 'proliferative' type: normocellular to hypocellular marrow with increases in plasma cells, mast cells, lymphocytes and eosinophils.
5. Chronic inflammation 'leukaemoid' type: hypercellular marrow with increases in neutrophils, eosinophils and megakaryocytes.
6. Chronic inflammation 'granulomatous' type: Characterized by the presence of granulomata.

Granulomata are not uncommon in the bone marrow. They appear as nodular aggregates composed primarily of modified macrophages with variable numbers of fibroblasts, plasma cells, lymphocytes and neutrophils. Giant cells may be produced when macrophages fuse or coalesce. Granulomata may be single or multiple, large or small and may contain a variety of cell types. They may be found in association with infections, particularly histoplasmosis or tuberculosis, malignancy including Hodgkin's disease, various autoimmune disorders and may arise as part of a drug reaction.

It is important to realize that the presence of granulomata in the marrow in a patient with malignant disease is a non-specific reaction which does not imply bone marrow involvement. (See Refs 103 and 104 for a full discussion of marrow granulomata.)

CONCLUSION

Haematological changes can arise in association with almost the whole spectrum of human disease. The changes are rarely specific for a single condition but are frequently of diagnostic importance. It behoves both the haematologist and the clinician to be aware of the importance of these associations.

REFERENCES

1. Bentley, D.P. Anaemia and chronic disease. *Clin. Haematol.* **ii**: 465–74, 1982.
2. Antman, K.H., Skarin, A.T., Mayer, R.J. *et al.* Microangiopathic haemolytic anaemia and cancer: A review. *Medicine (Baltimore)* **58**: 377–84, 1979.
3. Doll, D.C. & Weiss, R.B. Chemotherapeutic agents and the erythron. *Cancer Treat. Rev.* **10**: 185–200, 1983.
4. Pirofsky, B. When autoimmune haemolytic anaemia complicates chronic lymphocytic leukaemia. *Geriatrics* **33**: 71–9, 1978.
5. Eisner, E., Ley, A.B. & Mayer, K. Coombs positive haemolytic anaemia in Hodgkin's disease. *Ann. Intern. Med.* **66**: 258–73, 1967.
6. Jones, S.E. Autoimmune disorders and malignant lymphoma. *Cancer* **31**: 1092–8, 1973.
7. Spira, M. & Lynch, E.C. Autoimmune haemolytic anaemia and carcinoma: An unusual association. *Am. J. Med.* **67**: 753–8, 1979.
8. Bernstein, D., Shiman, M., Rikover, M. *et al.* Haemolytic anaemia related to ovarian tumour. *Obstet. Gynaecol.* **43**: 276–80, 1974.
9. Wortman, J., Rosse, W. & Logne, G. Cold agglutinin autoimmune haemolytic anaemia in non haematological malignancies. *Am. J. Hematol.* **6**: 275–83, 1979.
10. Sokol, R.J., Hewitt, S. & Stamps, B.K. Autoimmune haemolysis: An 18 year study of 865 cases referred to a regional transfusion centre. *Br. Med. J.* **282**: 2023–6, 1981.
11. Jacobs, E.M., Hutter, R.U.P., Pool, J.L., *et al.* Benign thymoma and selective erythroid aplasia of the bone marrow. *Cancer* **12**: 47–57, 1959.
12. Hirst, E. & Robertson, T.F. The syndrome of thymoma and erythroblastopenic anemia. A review of 56 cases. *Medicine (Baltimore)* **46**: 225–64, 1967.
13. Desevilla, E., Forrest, J.V., Zirnuska, F.R. *et al.* Metastatic thymoma with myasthenia gravis and pure red cell aplasia. *Cancer* **36**: 1154–7, 1975.
14. Crowther, D. & Bateman, C.J.T. Malignant disease. *Clin. Haematol.* **1**: 447–73, 1972.
15. Doll, D.C. & Weiss, R.B. Neoplasia and the erythron. *J. Clin. Oncol.* **3**, 429–46, 1985.
16. Isaacson, N.H. & Rapoport, P. Eosinophilia in malignant tumours. Its significance. *Ann. Intern. Med.* **25**: 893–902, 1946.
17. Aisenberg, A. Lymphocytopenia in Hodgkin's disease. *Blood* **25**: 1037–42, 1965.
18. Barret, O' N. Jr. Monocytosis in malignant disease. *Ann. Intern. Med.* **73**: 991–2, 1970.
19. Maldonada, J.E. & Hanlon, D.G. Monocytosis: A current appraisal. *Mayo Clin. Proc.* **40**: 248–59, 1965.

20. Ghosh, A.K., Erber, W.N. & Hatton, C. Detection of metastatic tumour cells in routine bone marrow smears by immunoalkaline phosphatase labelling with monoclonal antibodies. *Br. J. Haematol.* **61**: 21–30, 1985.
21. Kiraly, J.R. & Wheby, M.S. Bone marrow necrosis. *Am. J. Med.* **60**: 361–8, 1976.
22. Ponder, E. & Ponder, R.V. The cytology of the polymorphonuclear leucocyte in toxic condition. *J. Lab. Clin. Med.* **28**: 316–22, 1942.
23. Sutro, C.J. Cytoplasmic changes in circulating leukocytes in infection. *Arch. Intern. Med.* **51**: 747–53, 1933.
24. Wintrobe, M.M., Lee, G.R., Boggs, D.R. *et al.* (Eds) Variations of leukocytes in disease. In *Clinical Haematology*, pp. 1284–323. Lee & Febiger, Philadelphia, 1981.
25. Zieve, P.D., Hagashenass, M. & Blank, S.M. *et al.* Vacuolization of the neutrophil. *Arch. Intern. Med.* **118**: 356–7, 1966.
26. Berman, S.J. & Kunein, W.B. Scrub typhus in South Vietnam. A study of 87 cases. *Ann. Intern. Med.* **79**: 26–30, 1973.
27. Gorbach, S.L. & Thadepalli, H. Isolation of clostridium in human infections. Evaluation of 114 cases. *J. Infect. Dis.* **131**: Suppl: 581–5, 1975.
28. Murray, H.N., Masur, H., Senterfit, L.B. *et al.* The protean manifestations of *Mycoplasma pneumoniae* infections in adults. *Am. J. Med.* **58**: 229–42, 1975.
29. Tanowitz, H.B., Robbins, N. & Leidich, N. Hemolytic anemia associated with severe *Mycoplasma pneumoniae* pneumonia. *N.Y. State J. Med.* **78**: 2231–2, 1978.
30. Wilson, J.J., Neame, P.B. & Kelton, J.G. Infection induced thrombocytopenia. *Semin. Thromb. Haemost.* **8**: 217–33, 1982.
31. Pouglas, R.G., Alford, R.H., Cate, T.R. *et al.* The leukocyte response during viral respiratory illness in man. *Ann. Intern. Med.* **64**: 521–30, 1965.
32. Katz, S.L. & Enders, J.F. Measles virus. In *Viral and Rickettsial Disease of Man*, 4th Edn (eds J.F. Horshall & I. Tamm). Lipincott, Philadelphia, 1965.
33. Hillenbrand, F.K.M. The blood picture in rubella. *Lancet* **ii**: 66–8, 1956.
34. Kivel, R.M. Hematologic aspects of acute viral hepatitis. *Am. J. Diag. Dis.* **6**: 1017–31, 1961.
35. Wood, T.A. & Frenkel, E.P. The atypical lymphocyte. *Am. J. Med.* **42**: 923–36, 1967.
36. Tosato, G., Magrath, I., Koski, I. *et al.* Activation of suppressor T cells during Epstein Barr virus induced infectious mononucleosis. *N. Engl. J. Med.* **301**: 1133–7, 1979.
37. Halstead, S.B. Dengue, Hematologic aspects. *Semin. Hematol.* **19**: 116–31, 1982.
38. Oski, F.A. & Naiman, J.L. Effects of live measles vaccine on the platelet count. *N. Engl. J. Med.* **275**: 352–6, 1966.
39. Risdall, R.J., McKenna, R.W., Nesbit, M.E. *et al.* Virus associated haemophagocytic syndrome. A benign histiocytic proliferation distinct from malignant histiocytosis. *Cancer* **44**: 993–1002, 1979.
40. Young, N.S. & Mortimer, P.P. Viruses and bone marrow failure. *Blood* **63**: 729–37, 1984.
41. Zeldis, J.B., Dienstag, J.L. & Gale, R.P. Aplastic anaemia and non A non B hepatitis. *Am. J. Med.* **74**: 64–8, 1983.
42. Van Horn, D.K., Mortimer, P.P., Young, N. *et al.* Human parvovirus associated red cell aplasia in the absence of underlying haemolytic anaemia. *Am. J. Pediatr. Haematol./Oncol.* **8**: 235–8, 1986.
43. Pattision, J.R., Jones, S.E., Hodgson, J. *et al.* Parvovirus infections and hypoplastic crises in sickle cell anaemia. *Lancet* **i**: 664–5, 1981.
44. Wong-Staal, F. & Gallo, R.C. The family of human T-lymphotrophic viruses: HTLV-1 as the cause of adult T-cell leukaemia and HTLV III as the cause of the acquired immuno deficiency syndrome. *Blood* **65**: 253–63, 1985.
45. Wong-Staal, F. & Gallo, R.C. Human T-lymphotrophic viruses. *Nature* **317**:

395–403, 1985.
46. Krick, J.A. & Remington, J.S. Toxoplasmosis in the adult. An overview. *N. Engl. J. Med.* **289**: 550–3, 1978.
47. Abdalla, S., Weatherall, D.J., Wickramasinghe, S.N. & Hughes, M. The anaemia of falciparum malaria. *Br. J. Haematol.* **46**: 171–83, 1980.
48. Fleming, A.F. Haematological manifestations of malaria and other parasitic diseases. *Clin. Haematol.* **10**: 983–1011, 1981.
49. Beale, P.J., Cormack, J.D. & Oldrey, T.B.N.Thrombocytopenia in malaria with immunoglobulin (IgM) changes. *Br. Med. J.* **1**: 345–9, 1972.
50. Cartwright, G.E., Chung, H.L. & Chang, A. Studies on the pancytopenia of Kala-Azar. *Blood* **3**: 249–75, 1948.
51. Neva, F.A. & Otteson, E.A. Current concepts in parasitology. Tropical (filarial) eosinophilia. *N. Engl. J. Med.* **298**: 1129–31, 1978.
52. Eddington, G.M. & Gilles, H.M. *Pathology in the Tropics*, 2nd Edn. Edward Arnold, London, 1976.
53. Bishop, C.R. The neutropenia of Felty's syndrome. *Am. J. Hematol.* **2**: 203–7, 1977.
54. Richert-Boe, K. Hematologic complications of rheumatic disease. *Hematol. Oncol. Clin. North. Am.* **1**: 301–20, 1987.
55. Roughfield, N. Clinical features of systemic lupus erythematosus. In *Textbook of Rheumatology* (eds W.N. Kelley, E.D. Harris, J.S. Ruddy & C.B. Sledge), pp. 1106–32. W.B. Saunders, Philadelphia, 1981.
56. Estes, D. & Christian, C.L. The natural history of systemic lupus erythematosus by prospective analysis. *Medicine (Baltimore)* **50**: 85–95, 1971.
57. Dillon, A., Stein, H.B. & English, R.A. Splenic atrophy in systemic lupus erythematosus. *Ann. Intern. Med.* **96**: 40–3, 1982.
58. Dillon, A., Stein, H.B., Kassen, B.O. & Ibbot, J.W. Hyposplenia in a patient with systemic lupus erythematosus. *Rheumatology* **7**: 196–8, 1980.
59. Winearls, C.G., Oliver, D.O., Pippard, M.J. *et al.* Effect of human erythropoietin derived from recombinant DNA on the anaemia of patients maintained by chronic haemodialysis. *Lancet* **ii**: 1175–8, 1986.
60. Eschbach, J.W., Egrie, J.C., Downing, M.R. *et al.* Correction of anemia of end-stage renal disease with recombinant human erythropoietin. *N. Engl. J. Med.* **316**: 73–8, 1987.
61. Neiman, R.S., Bischel, M.D. & Lukes, R.J. Hypersplenism in the uremic hemodialysed patient. *Am. J. Clin. Pathol.* **60**: 502–11, 1973.
62. Hattersley, P.G. & Engels, J.L. Neutrophilic hypersegmentation without macrocytic anaemia. *West. J. Med.* **121**: 179–84, 1974.
63. Hocking, W.G. Hematologic abnormalities in patients with renal disease. *Hematol. Oncol. Clin. North Am.* **1**: 229–60, 1987.
64. Rodriguez-Erdmann, F. & Guttmann, R.D. Coagulation in renal allograft rejection. *N. Engl. J. Med.* **281**: 1428, 1969.
65. Karmali, A.M., Steele, B.T., Petric, M. & Lim, C. Sporadic cases of haemolytic uraemic syndrome associated with faecal cytotoxin and cytotoxin producing *Escherichia coli* in stools. *Lancet* **i**: 619–20, 1983.
66. Karmali, M.A., Petric, M., Lim, C., Felming, P.C. & Steele, B.T. *Escherichia coli* cytotoxin, haemolytic uraemic syndrome and haemorrhagic colitis. *Lancet* **ii**: 1299–300, 1983.
67. Drummond, K.N. Haemolytic uraemic syndrome – then and now (editorial). *N. Engl. J. Med.* **312**: 116–18, 1985.
68. Tovey, Fi & Clark, C.G. Anaemia after partial gastrectomy. A neglected curable condition. *Lancet* **i**: 956–8, 1980.
69. O'Grady, J.G., Stevens, F.M., Harding, B. *et al.*. Hyposplenism in gluten sensitive enteropathy. Maternal history, incidence and relationship to diet and small bowel morphology. *Gastroenterology* **87**: 1327–31, 1984.

70. Nelson, E.W., Ertan, A., Brooks, F.P. *et al.* Thrombocytosis in patients with coeliac sprue. *Gastroenterology* **70**: 1042–4, 1976.
71. Gerson, C.D., Cohen, N. & Janowitz, H.D. Small intestinal absorptive function in regional enteritis. *Gastroenterology* **64**: 907–12, 1973.
72. Gorst, D.W., Leyland, M.J. & Delamore, I.W. Autoimmune haemolytic anaemia and ulcerative colitis. *Postgrad. Med. J.* **51**: 409–11, 1975.
73. Palmer, K.R., Sherriff, S.B., Holdsworth, C.D. & Ryan, F.P. Further experience of hyposplenism in inflammatory bowel disease. *Q.J. Med.* **50**: 463–71, 1981.
74. Clearfield, H.R., Brody, J.I. & Tumen, H.T. Acute viral hepatitis, glucose-6-phosphate dehydrogenase deficiency and hemolytic anemia. *Arch. Intern. Med.* **123**: 689–91, 1969.
75. Chan, T.K. & Todd, D. Haemolysis complicating viral hepatitis in patients with glucose-6-phosphate dehydrogenase deficiency. *Br. Med. J.* **1**: 131–3, 1975.
76. McIntyre, N., Clink, H.M., Levi, A.J. *et al.* Hemolytic anemia in Wilson's Disease. *N. Engl. J. Med.* **276**: 439–44, 1967.
77. Roche-Sicot, J. & Benhamon, J. Acute intravascular haemolysis and acute liver failure associated as first manifestation of Wilson's Disease. *Ann. Intern. Med.* **86**: 301–3, 1977.
78. Cooper, R.A. Hemolytic syndromes and red cell membrane abnormalities in liver disease. *Semin. Haematol.* **17**: 103–12, 1980.
79. Zieve, L. Jaundice, hyperlipaemia and haemolytic anaemia: A heretofore unrecognised syndrome associated with alcoholic fatty liver and cirrhosis. *Ann. Intern. Med.* **48**: 471–96, 1958.
80. O'Neill, B.J., Marlin, G.E. & Streeter, A.M. Red cell macrocytosis in chronic obstructive airways disease. *Med. J. Aust.* **1**: 283, 1972.
81. Stretton, T.B. & Lee, H.Y. Respiratory disease. *Clin. Haematol.* **1**: 645–70, 1972.
82. Horton, L., Coburn, R.J., England, J.M. & Hinsworth, R.L. The haematology of hypothyroidism. *Q. J. Med.* **45**: 101–24, 1976.
83. Muldowney, F.P., Crooks, J. & Wayne, E.J. The total red cell mass in thyrotoxicosis and myxoedema. *Clin. Sci.* **16**: 309–14, 1957.
84. Rivlin, R.S. & Wagner, H.N. Anaemia in hyperthyroidism. *Ann. Intern. Med.* **79**: 507–15, 1969.
85. Cooper, D.S. Anti thyroid drugs. *N. Engl. J. Med.* **311**: 1353–62, 1984.
86. Ross, E.J., Marshall Jones, P. & Friedman, M. Cushings syndrome: Diagnostic criteria. *Q. J. Med.* **35**: 149–92, 1966.
87. Mallette, L.E. Anemia in hypercalcemic hyperparathyroidism. *Arch. Intern. Med.* **137**: 572–3, 1977.
88. Schwartz, J.S. & Clancy, C.M. Glycosylated hemoglobin assays in the management and diagnosis of diabetes mellitus. *Ann. Intern. Med.* **101**: 710–13, 1984.
89. Hoffman, R. Hematological sequelae of diffuse fasciitis. In *Aplastic Anemia: Stem Cell Histology and Advances in Treatment*, pp. 185–96. Alan R. Liss, New York, 1984.
90. Doyle, J.A., Connolly, S.M. & Hoagland, H.C. Hematologic disease in scleroderma syndromes. *Arch. Derm. Venereol. (Stockh.)* **65**: 521–5, 1985.
91. Hoffman, R., Young, N., Eshler, W.B., Mazur, E. & Gewirtz, A. Diffuse fasciitis and aplastic anemia: A report of four cases revealing an unusual association between rheumatologic and haematologic disorders. *Medicine (Baltimore)* **61**: 373–81, 1982.
92. Herbert, V. & Colman, N. The multifactorial causes of hematologic problems seen with alcoholism. *Semin. Haematol.* **17**: 83–4, 1980.
93. Lindenbaum, J. Folate and vitamin B_{12} deficiency in alcoholism. *Semin Haematol.* **17**: 119–29, 1980.
94. McCurdy, P.R., Pierce, L.E. & Rath, C.E. Abnormal marrow morphology in acute alcoholism. *N. Engl. J. Med.* **266**: 505–7, 1962.

95. McCurdy, P.R. & Rath, C.E. Vacuolated nucleated bone marrow cells in alcoholism. *Semin. Haematol.* **17**: 100–2, 1980.
96. Cowan, D.H. Effects of alcoholism on haemostasis. *Semin. Haematol.* **17**: 137–47, 1980.
97. Lia, Y.K. Effects of alcohol on granulocytes and lymphocytes. *Semin. Haematol.* **17**: 130–6, 1980.
98. White, J.M. & Selhi, I.I.S. Lead and the red cell. *Br. J. Haematol.* **30**: 133–8, 1975.
99. Paglia, D.E., Valentine, W.N. & Dahlgren, J.G. Effects of low level lead exposure on pyrimidine 5' nucleotidase and other erythrocyte enzymes. *J. Clin. Invest.* **56**: 1164–9, 1975.
100. Valentine, W.N., Paglia, D.E., Frik, K. & Madokora, G. Lead poisoning-association with hemolytic anemia, basophilic stippling, erythrocyte pyrimidine 5' nucleotidase deficiency and intra erythrocytic accumulation of pyrimidines. *J. Clin. Invest.* **58**: 926–32, 1976.
101. Wintrobe, M.M. Acquired hemolytic anaemia due to direct effects of infections, chemical or physical agents. In *Clinical Hematology*, 8th Edn (eds M.M. Wintrobe *et al.*) pp. 949–57, Lea & Febiger, Philadelphia, 1981.
102. Santer, D. & Goldfrank, L. Hematologic aspects of toxicology. *Hematol. Oncol. Clin. North Am.* **1**: 335–49, 1987.
103. Frisch, B., Lewis, S.M., Burkhardt, R. & Bartl, R. The cytopenias: non haemopoietic components. In *Biopsy Pathology of Bone and Bone Marrow* (eds B. Frisch, S.M. Lewis, R. Burkhardt & R. Bartl), pp. 47–56. Chapman & Hall, London, 1985.
104. Bodem, C.R., Hamory, B.H., Taylor, H.M. & Kloepfer, L. Granulomatous bone marrow disease. A review of the literature and a clinico-pathological analysis of 58 cases. *Medicine (Baltimore)* **62**: 372–83, 1983.

2

Anaemia in systemic disease

N.T.J. O'Connor
Consultant Haematologist, Royal Shrewsbury Hospital, Shropshire, UK

A.V. Hoffbrand
Professor of Haematology, Royal Free Hospital, London, UK

Patients with systemic disease are commonly anaemic. This may be due to coincidental haematological disease which has been previously unrecognized and needs further investigation. More frequently, however, the anaemia occurs as a complication of the disease or its treatment. Since abnormalities in the blood count or film, including anaemia, may be identified before the underlying disorder has been diagnosed, the haematologist may often be referred patients with a range of clinical conditions, or be of help to other clinicians in establishing a diagnosis.

The normal haemoglobin concentration (Hb) for a healthy male is 135–175 g/litre and for a healthy female 120–160 g/litre. As these values are concentrations, they depend on both the red cell mass and the plasma volume, alterations in the plasma volume will change the Hb. Thus an increase in the plasma volume gives rise to an apparent anaemia. For example, trained athletes have a red cell mass elevated by up to 20%,[1,2] but the plasma volume is usually increased by 25%.[1,3] As plasma volume changes occur more rapidly there is frequently an apparent anaemia, especially seen during training. This anaemia is physiological rather than pathological as some have erroneously suggested.[4] Similarly in pregnant women there is usually an increase in both plasma volume and red cell mass,[5] but the former is usually more marked, resulting in apparent anaemia. In contrast, smoking,[6] dehydration and Addison's disease[7] are all associated with a low plasma volume which may mask an anaemia or even give rise to a 'pseudopolycythaemia'. In these circumstances anaemia, if present, is only discovered if the plasma volume is restored to normal.

It is important to identify the mechanism causing anaemias seen in association with systemic disease so that appropriate investigations for the underlying disease may be undertaken and correct treatment given. This chapter will review the anaemias which occur in patients with systemic disease and describe them from the aspect of the pathological mechanisms responsible for the anaemia. Haematological malignancy will not be considered, and haemolytic anaemias complicating systemic disease are discussed elsewhere.

IRON DEFICIENCY

Deficiency of iron is the commonest cause of anaemia throughout the world. This arises because most of the body iron (about two-thirds) is contained in the blood as haemoglobin and haemorrhage is a major source of iron loss. Each litre of blood contains about 0.5 g iron and total body iron is 3–4 g. Daily iron absorption from a normal diet, in normal iron replete subjects is about 1 mg,[8] equivalent to normal losses of iron, and thus appropriate to maintain iron balance.

The normal Western mixed diet contains around 15 mg of iron each day, from which 5–10% is absorbed. The availability of food iron depends partly on the form of the iron: inorganic iron in the ferrous form is best absorbed partly due to the presence of associated compounds in the diet. Low molecular weight chelating compounds such as vitamin C, some sugars and amino acids, may enhance absorption of inorganic iron by making it more soluble in the lumen of the small intestine. In contrast phytates and phosphates inhibit iron absorption, and a vegetarian diet is a less good source of iron than a normal mixed diet.[9]

Iron stores, consisting mainly of haemosiderin and ferritin in the macrophages of the reticulo-endothelial system and in some parenchymal cells (e.g. hepatic) are about 0.5–1.5 g in an average Western adult, being greater in males than females. Given normal daily iron losses it takes several years for iron deficiency anaemia to develop on the basis of inadequate intake or malabsorption alone. These stores tend to be reduced in countries where the quality of the diet is poor and protein intake is low. Also demands for iron are relatively high in premature infants, growing children, menstruating females and in pregnancy, and these groups therefore tend to have low iron stores. Thus, any additional demand for iron is more likely to lead to anaemia. Although absorption from the diet is increased to 3–4 mg in iron deficiency, this cannot make up for the losses that occur with haemorrhage of more than 10 ml of blood daily.

Haematological changes and diagnosis

When a negative iron balance occurs, iron is transferred from macrophages to the marrow erythroblasts to be incorporated into haemoglobin and thus tissue stores become depleted.[9] During this phase, the serum ferritin and serum iron levels fall and the serum transferrin (or iron-binding capacity) and red-cell-free protoporphyrin rise. If the negative iron balance continues, anaemia develops and the red cells are reduced in size (measured as MCV), haemoglobin content (MCH) and in haemoglobin concentration (MCHC). The more severe the anaemia, the lower these indices. The indices may become subnormal even before the haemoglobin is below the accepted lower limit of normal.

In iron deficiency the peripheral blood film shows hypochromic, microcytic red cells with considerable poikilocytosis, 'pencil' cells and target cells. The platelet count tends to rise to levels between 400 and 900×10^9 per litre. As well as anaemia, patients may show koilonychia, ridged and brittle nails, thinning of the hair, atrophy of the oral mucosa and glossitis. The

Patterson–Brown–Kelly syndrome, post-cricoid obstruction with dysphagia, is an unusual pre-malignant complication. Superficial gastritis or gastric atrophy are also more common, and in children there may be stunting of the duodenal villi. There is considerable debate about whether latent iron deficiency (absence of iron stores without anaemia) causes symptoms, such as poor exercise tolerance, work capacity and difficulty concentrating, although these are all associated with iron deficiency.

Aetiology (Table 2.1)

Females are more at risk of developing iron deficiency because of menstrual blood loss and pregnancy (in which adequate iron supplementation is needed). In both sexes bleeding from the gastrointestinal tract is also a common cause of iron deficiency. The lesions may be anywhere from the oesophagus to the anus, and include inflammatory or malignant conditions. In some countries hookworm is a dominant cause of gastrointestinal blood loss. In Britain piles, salicylate ingestion, peptic ulceration, hiatus hernia, malignancy and diverticulosis have been estimated as most common.[10] In many cases, symptoms of the anaemia are the first presenting features.

Inadequate intake of iron may give reduced iron stores, but in Western countries a poor diet is rarely the sole cause of anaemia. Malabsorption (e.g. due to gluten enteropathy) may cause combined iron and folate deficiency but must be present for several years before iron deficiency anaemia develops.[11]

Table 2.1 Causes of Iron Deficiency[10]

Blood loss
  Menstrual
  GI tract, e.g. hiatus hernia, oesophageal varices, peptic ulcer, aspirin, ulcerative colitis, caecal and colonic carcinoma, diverticulosis, angiodysplasia, piles, hookworm
  Renal tract
  Pulmonary

Dietary

Malabsorption
  Coeliac disease
  Gastrectomy

Pregnancy

Unusual
  Paroxysmal nocturnal haemoglobinuria
  Factitious, i.e. self-bleeding

Treatment

The aims of treatment are to correct the underlying cause of the deficiency, to restore the haemoglobin level to normal, and to replenish iron stores. Correction of the underlying cause may involve treatment of a gynaeco-logical or gastrointestinal disorder. In some cases the cause is difficult to find, for example in angiodysplasia of the intestine when coeliac axis angiography may be needed, and in self-bleeding (particularly common among emotionally disturbed female paramedical staff).

Treatment of iron deficiency is usually with oral iron as anhydrous ferrous sulphate 200 mg (= 67 mg iron) tablets. Since the intestine is refractory to iron absorption for about 6 h following a single dose, the tablets are given spaced out during the day. Iron absorption is reduced by food so maximum iron absorption occurs if the tablets are given about an hour before meals. Side-effects of iron therapy occur in some individuals, and may consist of constipation, diarrhoea, flatulence or abdominal pain. These effects can be reduced by taking ferrous sulphate with food, or by taking an alternative preparation of lower iron content, for instance ferrous gluconate 300 mg (= 37 mg iron). Other iron preparations include those combined with vitamins and slow-release formulations. These are all more expensive and, for the slow-release preparations, less effective. The rise in haemoglobin with adequate iron therapy occurs at about the rate of 20 g/litre every 3 weeks. Therapy needs to be continued for 3 months after the haemoglobin is normal in order to replenish stores, although one study showed that the serum ferritin may become normal within 1–2 months. Failure to respond may be due to continued haemorrhage, non-compliance, incorrect diag-nosis, additional causes for anaemia or to gross malabsorption.

Parenteral iron (e.g. total dose infusion of iron dextran or iron sorbitol citrate) is reserved for patients who cannot or will not swallow tablets, or in whom it is difficult to keep pace with iron loss, as in haemorrhage which cannot be prevented (e.g. hereditary telangiectasia). It may also be needed in patients with malabsorption.

FOLATE DEFICIENCY

Adult body levels of folate are about 10–15 mg and normal daily requirements are 100–200 µg.[12,13] Thus stores are sufficient for only about 4 months. The normal Western diet contains 500–700 µg, depending on the type of food but also on the method of preparation, since folate is easily destroyed by high temperatures and large volumes of water. It is partly protected by vitamin C, which is itself easily destroyed by heat in cooking. Folate in food consists of many different derivatives at various levels of reduction, with various 1-carbon units (CH_3, CH_2, CH, CHO, CH-NH_2) attached and a glutamate chain of length 1–8. About 80% of folate monoglutamates are absorbed, whatever the size of the dose, but absorption of the polyglutamate forms is more restricted, particularly when large doses are given. On average, 50–60% of dietary folate is absorbed. The compounds are converted during absorption through the duodenum and jejunum to the single monoglutamate compound 5-methyltetrahydrofolate (methyl THF), a fully reduced monoglutamate which enters portal blood. Folic acid (pteroylglutamic acid) does not occur in natural materials, but when given in therapeutic doses, most of it is absorbed unchanged and is carried to the liver where it displaces methyl THF.

Folate is only loosely bound to protein in plasma, so when the plasma folate level is high, it is filtered by the kidneys, the reabsorptive mechanism is overloaded and unchanged folate is lost in the urine. An enterohepatic circulation of folate is also present with about 60–90 µg folate, as methyl and formyl derivatives, being reabsorbed. Folate coenzymes are involved in the transfer of single carbon units, and are concerned in three reactions in DNA synthesis: two in purine synthesis and one, thymidylate synthetase, in pyrimidine synthesis. The body is capable of degrading folate by splitting the molecule at the C_9–N_{10} bond. This degradation is increased when cell proliferation, and thus DNA synthesis, is increased, presumably due to incomplete recycling of folate coenzymes.[12,13]

Haematological features and diagnosis

Folate deficiency is diagnosed on the basis of the blood and bone marrow appearances, as well as measurement of serum and red cell folate. The haematological changes in severe cases consist of megaloblastic anaemia with oval macrocytes and hypersegmented neutrophils (more than five nuclear lobes) in the peripheral blood and a hypercellular marrow with megaloblastic erythroblasts, giant metamyelocytes and many dying cells.

The serum folate level falls within a few days on a folate-poor diet and is therefore the most sensitive test. If a negative balance continues, the red cell diameter (measured as MCV) increases and neutrophils with hyper-segmented nuclei appear in the blood. Recognizable megaloblastic changes in the marrow and subnormal red cell folate levels are relatively late changes. Therefore, the red cell folate is generally a better guide to tissue folate status than the serum folate. However, in three situations the red cell folate may be misleading: (i) the red cell folate is lowered in vitamin B_{12} deficiency because of the metabolic relations of the two vitamins, (ii) folate in transfused red cells remains until the cells die and so this may affect the red cell folate assay, and (iii) folate is higher in reticulocytes than mature red cells and thus in any patient with a reticulocytosis an artificially high concentration may be obtained. The deoxyuridine suppression test is a useful guide to the presence of B_{12} or folate deficiency and can be adapted to distinguish between them. The degree of abnormality corresponds to the severity of the marrow changes and anaemia. In severe megaloblastic anaemia the white cells and platelet counts are reduced.

When the anaemia develops rapidly and an infection supervenes there may be a 'megaloblastic arrest' of haemopoiesis with a rapidly developing pancytopenia. This has also been described in patients with pre-existing B_{12} or folate deficiency who are given cotrimoxazole. Folate deficiency may cause tissue changes, including a reversible skin pigmentation and folate-depleted mothers have an increased risk of delivering their babies prematurely. Neuropsychiatric disturbances have also been suggested but not fully documented.[14]

Aetiology (Table 2.2)

The incidence of folate deficiency in systemic diseases depends partly on the length, severity and nature of the disease and partly on the dietary intake of folate. Dietary deficiency as the sole cause of folate deficiency has been described in the poor taking a 'tea and toast' diet, the mentally ill, patients taking special diets and in infants fed goats' milk, which is of very low folate content. It may occur in association with protein calorie malnutrition or scurvy.

Malabsorption of folate is universal in untreated coeliac disease, either in children or adults, and all the patients show some degree of deficiency. Most frequently there is combined iron and folate deficiency and in 10–15% of adults the blood film shows the features of splenic atrophy (Howell–Jolly bodies, siderotic granules, fragmented and target cells).[11] Folate deficiency is also common in coeliac-disease-associated dermatitis herpetiformis. Tropical sprue in the early stage is complicated by severe folate malabsorption and megaloblastic anaemia, but in the more chronic forms B_{12} deficiency is often more important. Folate malabsorption occurs rarely as a congenital abnormality.

Chronic inflammation may lead to a deficiency because of anorexia, increased folate utilization and folate malabsorption. Folate deficiency has been described particularly in tuberculosis and malaria. Chronic inflammatory skin conditions (e.g. widespread eczema, exfoliative dermatitis and psoriasis) and rheumatoid arthritis may lead to folate deficiency. In Crohn's disease, poor dietary intake and excess consumption are factors and also occur if the upper small intestine is involved. In addition, the drug Salazopyrine, used in therapy of ulcerative colitis and Crohn's disease, may itself cause malabsorption of folate.[15] The intestinal blind loop syndrome, however, is a cause of high folate levels due to intestinal bacterial synthesis of folate and not of folate deficiency.

Table 2.2 Causes of Folate Deficiency[12,13]

Dietary, e.g. food faddists, old age, psychiatric patients, goats' milk

Malabsorption, e.g. coeliac disease, tropical sprue, jejunal resection, specific malabsorption

Excess utilization/loss
  Pregnancy
  Haemolytic anaemia, myelofibrosis
  Malignant disease
  Inflammation, e.g. tuberculosis, malaria
  Skin disease, e.g. psoriasis, eczema
  Right heart failure, dialysis
  Homocystinuria

Antifolate drugs, e.g. phenytoin

Mixed
  Alcohol abuse
  Liver disease

Malignant diseases are commonly associated with low serum folate lev which have been detected in up to 80% of patients with carcinom. However, severe folate deficiency with a low red cell folate and megalo-blastic anaemia is unusual, except in patients with tumours of the oesophagus or stomach, who may develop severe deficiency due to impaired folate intake. Severe folate deficiency has also been described in late stage myeloma. Unless severe megaloblastic anaemia is present, it is usually inadvisable to give folic acid therapy to patients with malignant diseases since it may 'feed' the tumour.

Mild degrees of folate deficiency may occur in all forms of liver disease but megaloblastic anaemia in Western countries is largely confined to alcoholics who drink spirits. Reduced dietary folate intake, poor storage and excess loss into plasma and urine are all factors. Anticonvulsant drugs may be associated with folate deficiency and a number of mechanisms have been proposed but none established. In cystathionase deficiency with homo-cystinuria, folate deficiency is common, probably due to increased con-version of homocysteine to methionine.

Increased urinary folate excretion has been described in right heart failure, due to loss of folate from the congested liver. Patients receiving haemodialy-sis or peritoneal dialysis may also become deficient, particularly if prolonged anorexia or vomiting occur. Most renal units now give these patients prophylactic folic acid, although its routine use has been questioned.[16]

Treatment

Treatment of folic acid deficiency is usually by oral folic acid given at 5 mg three times a day. The underlying cause of the deficiency should also be corrected. It is important to exclude B_{12} deficiency before starting folic acid therapy, since in B_{12} deficient patients, folic acid may precipitate a neurological deficit despite correcting the anaemia. It is usual to continue folic acid therapy for about 4 months after a single episode of deficiency, provided that the underlying cause has been corrected. In premature infants, pregnant women, haemolytic anaemias or in other marrow diseases with ineffective erythropoiesis (e.g. myelofibrosis or sideroblastic anaemia) folic acid is given prophylactically. In these situations 5 mg weekly is probably sufficient. Folinic acid (5-formyl THF) is used to prevent or reverse the effects of methotrexate which inhibits the enzyme dihydrofolate reductase responsible for keeping folate in the active tetrahydro state.

VITAMIN B_{12} DEFICIENCY

The normal Western diet contains about 15 µg vitamin B_{12} (B_{12}) daily and requirements are about 1–2 µg. B_{12} is synthesized in nature by microorganisms and is only present in foods of animal origin, so that a purely vegetarian diet, uncontaminated by bacteria, contains no B_{12}. B_{12} is absorbed through the ileum after it has been freed from protein binding in food, and bound to intrinsic factor (IF) secreted by the gastric parietal cells. The IF–B_{12} complex attaches to specific receptors for IF on the ileal enterocyte brush border; B_{12}

the portal blood after a delay of several hours while IF is
erocyte. The capacity of the ileum to absorb B_{12} is limited
ause of a limited number of ileal receptors for IF. An
ation exists, variously estimated at 1–43 µg B_{12} daily.[12]

Haematological changes and diagnosis

The appearances of the blood and bone marrow are identical to those seen
in folate deficient megaloblastic anaemia. In addition B_{12} deficiency may
cause a symmetrical neuropathy affecting mainly the long tracts of the spinal
cord as well as the posterior and lateral columns and the peripheral nerves.
It may also lead to dementia, optic atrophy and neuropsychiatric
disease.[14,17]

Vitamin B_{12} deficiency is diagnosed on the basis of the haematological
changes and a low serum B_{12} level. A fall in the serum B_{12} level is an early
feature of B_{12} deficiency. The serum B_{12} may also be low, however, in the
absence of B_{12} deficiency in pregnancy, severe folic acid deficiency and
possibly severe iron deficiency. B_{12} in serum is tightly bound to proteins,
largely to the glycoprotein transcobalamin TCI although it is the
polypeptide TCII which carries it to the marrow and other tissues but which
is largely unsaturated. A 'falsely' low B_{12} level has been described in TCI
deficiency, whereas in the more important congenital abnormality TCII
deficiency the serum B_{12} level is normal but megaloblastic anaemia
responding to large doses of B_{12} occurs through lack of TCII needed to
transport B_{12} to the marrow and other cells.[18] As for folate deficiency, the
deoxyuridine suppression test can be used to diagnose B_{12} deficiency.

Aetiology

Vitamin B_{12} deficiency usually arises because of malabsorption (Table 2.3),
most commonly adult (Addisonian) pernicious anaemia. Congenital IF
deficiency or abnormality and specific malabsorption of B_{12}[19] with proteinuria are important in infancy and early childhood. Veganism is
important in Hindus and some other communities,[20] although in many cases
low B_{12} levels are not accompanied by the anaemia. Whatever the cause, the
malabsorption must occur over 2–3 years before the megaloblastic anaemia
occurs because body stores are 2–3 mg. In patients who have had a
gastrectomy or ileal resection, this is the usual time to elapse before anaemia
or neuropathy develops. Increased utilization or degradation of vitamin B_{12}
is not a cause of B_{12} deficiency.

The anaesthetic gas nitrous oxide (N_2O) oxidizes body vitamin B_{12} from the
fully reduced Cob (I) state to the inactive Cob (II) or Cob (III) states. Both
coenzymes of B_{12}, methylcobalamin and deoxyadenosylcobalamin are in the
reduced Cob (I) form and so are inactivated. If the anaesthetic is prolonged,
as in intensive care units, acute megaloblastic anaemia may supervene.[21,22]
Reversal of this process occurs gradually over several days but can be
accelerated by large doses of hydroxycobalamin.

Table 2.3 Causes of B_{12} Deficiency

Dietary
  Vegan

Malabsorption
  Gastric
    Pernicious anaemia (congenital or acquired)
    Gastrectomy
  Ileal disease
    Resection
    Crohn's disease/tuberculosis
    Specific malabsorption with proteinuria
  Competition
    Jejunal diverticulosis
    Ileocolic fistulae
    Blind loop syndrome
    Fish tapeworm

Treatment

It is usual to replenish body stores of B_{12} in B_{12} deficient patients with six injections each of 1 mg hydroxycobalamin, given a few days apart. Subsequently patients are maintained with 1 mg injections given every 3 months for life. As cyanocobalamin is about one third less well-retained in the body than hydroxycobalamin, it is not used in therapy. Prophylactic maintenance B_{12} therapy can be given after a total (or subtotal) gastrectomy or ileal resection.

Oral vitamin B_{12} therapy can be used in vegans but, since B_{12} absorption by the IF mechanism is limited to a few micrograms daily, it has to be given daily and cannot be used to load stores. Some B_{12} (less than 1%) of an oral dose is absorbed passively through the buccal, gastric, duodenal and jejunal mucosa; very large doses can be used daily, for example in haemophiliacs who cannot take injections.

SIDEROBLASTIC ANAEMIA (SA)

This anaemia is characterized by ring sideroblasts in the marrow and hypochromic cells in the peripheral blood. The anaemia is classified as primary when no other disease is present and secondary if the anaemia is associated with other disease. In this condition iron accumulates in erythroblast mitochondria which assume a perinuclear position, and give rise to the ring appearance. In primary SA, at least 25% of bone marrow erythroblasts show complete or almost complete rings of iron, whereas in the secondary types only a few rings may be seen. Moreover, in the secondary types, the anaemia is usually reversible, whereas in primary SA some ring sideroblasts usually persist despite any response to therapy.[23,24]

The pathogenesis of SA probably results from defective haem synthesis,

Table 2.4   Causes of Acquired Sideroblastic Anaemia

Myeloproliferative disorder
  Myelodysplasia
  Myelofibrosis

Abnormal B$_6$ metabolism
  Antituberculous chemotherapy
  Coeliac disease
  Alcoholism
  Haemolytic anaemia
  Pregnancy

Disturbed haem synthesis
  Lead poisoning
  Alcohol
  Chloramphenicol
  Erythropoietic porphyria

Other
  Rheumatoid arthritis
  Megaloblastic anaemia
  Malignancy

although the exact mechanisms are unresolved.[23] Defective haem synthesis is thought to allow excess iron to enter mitochondria due to lack of the normal feedback inhibition. Several of the steps in haem synthesis occur in mitochondria, including two key enzymes, δ-amino laevulinic acid synthetase (ALA-S) and haem synthetase. ALA-S is a rate-limiting enzyme which catalyses the formation of ALA from glycine and succinyl-CoA and requires pyridoxal-phosphate as a coenzyme. Haem synthetase is the final enzyme which incorporates iron into protoporphyrin IX to form haem. Although defects in both enzymes and antagonists of pyridoxine may be associated with SA, it is not clear whether these defects are the primary causes of the anaemia or are secondary to mitochondrial damage.

Aetiology of acquired sideroblastic anaemia (Table 2.4)[24]

The congenital form, typically hypochromic microcytic, is likely to be due to an enzyme defect affecting haem synthesis or mitochondrial function. In primary acquired SA or in SA associated with other marrow defects (e.g. other types of myelodysplasia, myeloma or myeloproliferative diseases) a marrow stem cell defect underlies the condition, since defects occur in several haemopoietic cell lines. Moreover, the erythroblasts often show megaloblastic changes (not due to folate or B$_{12}$ deficiency) as well as rings of iron. The anaemia is usually macrocytic.

Alcohol is a recognized cause of SA, which occurs largely in association with a heavy intake, usually of spirits. The mechanism is probably alcohol inhibition of enzymes in haem and possibly globin synthesis. A specific effect on pyridoxal phosphorylation has also been suggested but not established. When alcohol intake is stopped, the ring sideroblasts disappear completely.

The antituberculous drugs isoniazid, cycloserine and pyrizinamide have all been associated with SA and are known to interfere with pyridoxine metabolism. The incidence is rare and there is some evidence that patients who develop the anaemia have a genetic tendency to ring sideroblastic formation and in some cases, ring sideroblasts may persist when the drug therapy is discontinued. More frequently a few ring sideroblasts which disappear with drug withdrawal occur in non-anaemic patients on antituberculous therapy.

Lead acts as a mitochondrial poison and inhibits synthesis of haem and globin. SA is one type of anaemia associated with chronic lead toxicity (haemolytic anaemia with basophilic stippling due to inhibition of pyrimidine-5-nucleotidase being typical). Chloramphenicol is another inhibitor of mitochondrial protein synthesis which may, in a few subjects, cause ring sideroblast formation.

Other systemic diseases in which sideroblastic anaemia have been described include rheumatoid arthritis, autoimmune diseases, carcinoma and gluten-induced enteropathy. In these conditions, as well as in cases of pregnancy and haemolytic anaemias in which ring sideroblasts occur, folate deficiency with megaloblastic changes are also frequently present. Ring sideroblasts have also been described in untreated pernicious anaemia, and other forms of megaloblastic anaemia. It appears likely that the combination of pyridoxine and folate (or B_{12}) deficiency is particularly likely to lead to ring sideroblastic formation. Megaloblastic anaemia is known to cause a rise in serum iron with an increase in coarse siderotic granules in marrow erythroblasts. It may be that, in the presence of mitochondrial dysfunction or pyridoxine deficiency or abnormality, the tendency to ring sideroblast formation is exaggerated. Although pure B_6 deficiency has not been proven to cause SA, the complete disappearance of ring sideroblasts in coeliac disease treated by a gluten-free diet is suggestive.

Treatment

Secondary SA may respond to withdrawal of the causative agent (e.g. drug or alcohol), vitamin B_6 (e.g. pyridoxine 100 mg daily) and folic acid, if folate deficiency is present. Where it is associated with an irreversible bone marrow disease it rarely responds to pyridoxine or folic acid, or indeed other therapy other than that aimed at the primary disease.

ERYTHROPOIETIN DEFICIENCY

Renal failure

Erythropoietin (Epo) is a 166 amino acid polypeptide which is heavily glycosylated so that it has a molecular weight of 34,000 Da. It is coded for by a gene on chromosome 7 and the hormone is principally produced by the kidney, although the liver is responsible for around 10% of all synthesis.

Epo acts as a growth factor stimulating production of erythroid progenitor cells from the late BFU_E stage (erythroid burst forming unit) and also acting as a differentiating agent;[25] the kidney senses tissue oxygenation and releases Epo into the circulation when there is renal hypoxia. This hypoxia may result from anaemia, cardiopulmonary disease, or a right shifted oxygen dissociation curve. There is therefore a feedback loop which acts to maintain a normal red cell mass and hence tissue oxygenation.

Aetiology of anaemia of renal failure

Although initial studies of Epo levels in disease were hampered by a bioassay[26] which was relatively cumbersome,[27] these assays convincingly demonstrated that Epo deficiency is the major cause of the anaemia of chronic renal failure (CRF).[28,29] More recently a radioimmunoassay has been developed which is much quicker to perform and the results correlate well with the bioassay.[27,30] Furthermore, to date there are no recorded cases in which the radioimmunoassay result has not been confirmed by a bioassay if this is carried out.[27] The anaemia of CRF is almost invariably normochromic normocytic, and, as might be expected, is more pronounced in patients who are anephric.[28]

Other factors which contribute to the anaemia of CRF are summarized in Table 2.5. Red cell survival studies using ^{51}Cr and other red cell labels have shown a shortening to around one-half normal.[29,31,32] This haemolysis is usually mild and cross-transfusion experiments have shown it to be caused by an extracorpuscular mechanism.[29,33] A normal marrow should be able to compensate, but in the presence of a marked Epo deficiency, the shortened red cell lifespan serves to worsen the degree of anaemia.

Inhibition of normal erythropoiesis has also been postulated as a contributory factor in the anaemia of CRF. One report described anaemia in patients with high Epo levels, and this implied that the marrow was unable to respond appropriately to this hormonal stimulus.[28] In many patients dialysis gives a small but definite improvement in the haematocrit and in a few cases this effect is dramatic.[34] However, several findings argue against the importance of such an inhibitory mechanism. Firstly, in vitro culture studies using a murine system and serum from patients with renal failure

Table 2.5   Factors Involved in the Anaemia of Renal Failure (see text)

Decreased red cell production
  Erythropoietin deficiency (primary mechanism)
  Inhibition of erythropoiesis by toxins
  Iron deficiency
  Folate deficiency
  Aluminium toxicity
  Osteitis fibrosa due to hyperparathyroidism

Increased red cell destruction
  Blood loss
  Haemolysis including mechanical destruction

---

have failed to show specific inhibition of erythropoiesis.[35] Secondly, patients with CRF have a predictable response to recombinant Epo. Thirdly, such an inhibitory effect, if present, is not mediated by parathyroid hormone,[36,37] or spermine[29] as was once believed. Lastly the anaemia is not always improved by dialysis,[29,34] and thus inhibition of erythropoiesis is usually of little significance in the anaemia of CRF.

The anaemia seen in patients on haemodialysis is more severe than that seen in similar patients on peritoneal dialysis[38,39] and this difference is corrected by changing from haemodialysis to peritoneal dialysis.[39] Blood loss during haemodialysis may play a role in explaining this difference and iron deficiency has also been shown to be commoner in patients on haemodialysis.[38] Other possible factors include the improved red cell survival observed in patients on peritoneal dialysis and the fact that these latter patients appear to control their plasma volume more efficiently.[40]

Many patients have plentiful iron stores at the time of starting dialysis because as renal failure progresses, a reduction in normal erythropoiesis causes iron to shift from circulating red cells to the reticulo-endothelial system.[29] However, patients on haemodialysis commonly develop iron deficiency due to recurrent dialyser blood loss, so that iron replacement may be needed if the serum ferritin level falls. In contrast, patients who are transfusion-dependent are at risk of haemosiderosis. Another factor which may contribute to the anaemia of CRF is folate deficiency, although most patients have adequate dietary intake.[16] Less frequent causes of haematological problems are osteitis fibrosa cystica due to hyperparathyroidism with a pancytopenia[41] and aluminium toxicity which may induce a reversible microcytic anaemia.[42]

Treatment

Purification of Epo in 1977[43] and the subsequent determination of its amino acid sequence led ultimately to the synthesis of recombinant Epo[44] which is now available for clinical use.

Trials of recombinant Epo have shown that thrice weekly injection reverses the anaemia of renal failure,[45,46] thus confirming that Epo deficiency is the major determinant of this anaemia. Such treatment is generally well-tolerated, although initially there may be problems with fluid balance, and hypertension is often exacerbated. Patients feel subjectively better and objectively they no longer require blood transfusions, which carry the risk of iron overload and transmission of infection, particularly non-A non-B hepatitis and human immunodeficiency virus. The elevated haematocrit also improves the bleeding tendency observed in renal failure.[47,48] Finally, no patient has yet developed antibodies to recombinant Epo and no increased immune elimination of Epo has been observed.[49]

Side-effects of Epo treatment include hypertension, and the increased haematocrit is accompanied by a higher incidence of clotting of the dialysis lines. There is also the risk of fistulae thrombosing and the anaemia seen in renal failure appears to be partly protective against the development of vascular thrombosis. There is therefore the danger that complete correction of anaemia could lead to an unacceptable increase in cardiovascular disease, which is already the principal cause of death in haemodialysis patients.[50] Although complete normalization of the Hb should probably not be undertaken, the beneficial effects of Epo are so great that a balance will need to be achieved and an optimal haematocrit defined. Epo clearly has great potential benefit and work is currently underway to establish the most appropriate replacement regimens.

Erythropoietin therapy will revolutionize the management of anaemia in CRF, since until now other therapies have had a minimal impact.[29] Prior to the introduction of Epo the only effective treatment for this anaemia was blood transfusion with the attendant risks outlined above. Androgens are of only limited benefit and are associated with unacceptable side-effects.[51] Another study has shown desferrioxamine to increase the Hb in renal failure.[52] This interesting finding is unexplained; postulated mechanisms include an increase in erythroid cell transferrin receptor levels or chelation of aluminium and possibly other inhibitors of erythropoiesis.[52]

Chronic disease

The significance of Epo levels in other disease states is less clear, although an inadequate Epo response has been postulated as contributing to the anaemia of chronic disease (ACD).[53] Some early studies, using bioassays of Epo, suggested that levels were not raised in proportion to the degree of anaemia in patients with chronic infection or inflammation.[54-57] In contrast, in the ACD secondary to solid tumours the Epo level was appropriately elevated,[56] and this raised the possibility that different mechanisms were responsible for the ACD in inflammation/infection as distinct from malignancy.[56] However more recent work, using a radioimmunoassay for Epo, has shown that Epo levels are appropriately raised in patients with infection and inflammation.[27,58] Thus Epo deficiency is not believed to contribute significantly to the aetiology of ACD.[59]

Previous reports have demonstrated that exogenous Epo may reverse anaemia induced in experimental animals by inflammation.[60,61] Trials of recombinant Epo therapy are being undertaken in ACD on an empirical basis, although the fact that Epo levels are not depressed in ACD suggests that recombinant Epo may be of limited use in these circumstances. It is possible, however, that Epo may have a pharmacological effect and accelerate red cell production in ACD, rather than acting as physiological replacement therapy as in chronic renal failure.[25] Even if its efficacy is less marked than in renal failure, or a larger dosage is required, a moderate rise in the Hb may be of great symptomatic benefit and avoid the need for blood transfusion in some patients.

Polycythaemia

A secondary polycythaemia may occur in patients with underlying disease, which may or may not be appropriate to tissue hypoxia. This inappropriate polycythaemia is caused by ectopic production of Epo and is rare. The diagnosis of ectopic Epo production should be suspected if the red cell mass is elevated in the presence of a normal arterial oxygen saturation but without the other features of primary proliferative polycythaemia (i.e. splenomegaly, elevation of the white cell and platelet counts and a high alkaline phosphatase score). The introduction of a radioimmunoassay for Epo is of value in the differentiation of these processes.[62] Causes of inappropriate polycythaemia include renal cysts and tumours, cerebellar haemangioma, hepatoma and uterine fibroids, and are considered in Chapter 3.

APLASIA

Red cell aplasia

The diagnosis of red cell aplasia rests on the finding of anaemia, reticulocytopenia and a marrow with markedly reduced red cell precursors, whilst the rest of the marrow and blood count are normal.[63]

Transient red cell aplasia is seen after primary infection with a human parvovirus (B19). In children, parvovirus gives rise to childhood erythema infectiosum (fifth disease)[64] whilst adults suffer a mild illness associated with small joint arthralgia.[65] It appears that infection invariably gives a transient erythroid hypoplasia with the marrow showing no erythroid precursors on day 10 despite a high erythropoietin level: the exact mechanism for this effect is unclear.[66] In normal individuals the red cell lifespan is 120 days, so although there may be a drop in Hb this is not clinically significant since the aplasia is short-lived.[67] However, in patients with a shortened red cell lifespan this transient erythroid hypoplasia may give rise to a severe anaemia, since the marrow hyperplasia is suppressed. Thus parvovirus-induced aplastic crisis is a worrying and potentially fatal complication in patients with sickle cell disease[68] or a severe haemolytic anaemia such as hereditary spherocytosis[69] and pyruvate kinase deficiency.[70] However, bacterial infections have also been shown to cause aplastic crises in patients with chronic haemolytic anaemia.[71] Finally the aetiology of transient erythroblastopenia of childhood,[72] in which children with normal marrow function develop a reversible red cell aplasia, has not been elucidated, but the picture does not match that of parvovirus infection.

Acquired pure red cell aplasia (PRCA) occurring as a chronic condition is rare but is often associated with an underlying disorder (see Table 2.6). Nearly half the cases are associated with a thymoma, which is usually benign, and around 5% of thymomas have coexistant PRCA.

The aetiology of PRCA is believed to be autoimmune[63,73] since it often occurs in association with other autoimmune diseases, may respond to immunosuppressive therapy and in some cases antibodies to erythroid precursors have been demonstrated.[74,75]

The mainstay of treatment is blood transfusion as needed. Drug-induced PRCA usually resolves on stopping the drug,[63] and in patients with thymoma, thymectomy gives disease remission in around 30% of cases.[76] Immunosuppression with steroids or cyclophosphamide may control the disease state,[77] as may plasmapheresis in occasional cases.[75]

Table 2.6 Causes of Red Cell Aplasia

Transient
  Parvovirus B19 infection
  Riboflavin deficiency
  Transient erythroblastopenia of childhood

Chronic
  Congenital
    Diamond Blackfan syndrome
  Acquired
    Idiopathic
    Immune
      Thymoma
      Non-Hodgkin's lymphoma
      Myasthenia gravis
      Systemic lupus erythematosus
    Drug related, e.g. phenytoin
    Erythropoietin deficiency

Aplastic anaemia

Many disorders may result in aplastic anaemia, and these are documented in Table 2.7. Aplastic anaemia is usually idiopathic but may occur as a rare but severe complication of viral infection. Post-viral aplasia is especially seen after non-B hepatitis and although serological tests for the causative virus have only recently been introduced it is believed that most cases follow non-A non-B hepatitis.[78] A togavirus designated hepatitis C has recently been implicated as a major cause of post-transfusion hepatitis,[79] but further studies are needed to determine whether this virus is responsible for post-hepatitis aplasia. Unfortunately the prognosis in post-hepatitis aplastic anaemia is bad.[80] The coexistence of thrombocytopenia may worsen the anaemia by leading to gastrointestinal blood loss.

A predictable pancytopenia may be induced by cancer chemotherapy, so that myelosuppression is often the dose-limiting consideration.[81] As this marrow hypoplasia is transient, this has led to the use of pulsed cycles of intensive cytotoxic therapy in the management of many high-grade malignancies. This allows the neutrophil and platelet counts to recover before the next cycle of cytotoxic agents. During such treatment anaemia is almost invariable and can be readily treated by red cell transfusion. Thrombocytopenia may require platelet transfusion and the possibility that occult blood loss is worsening any anaemia should be borne in mind.

MARROW REPLACEMENT

Tumours which metastasize to bone marrow may give rise to various cytopenias including anaemia, neutropenia and thrombocytopenia. The cytopenias result from 'crowding out' of normal marrow precursors, and the peripheral blood film shows a 'leucoerythroblastic picture' with nucleated

Table 2.7   Causes of Aplastic Anaemia[80]

Inevitable
  Cytoxic drugs
  Radiation

Idiopathic

Drug idiosyncrasy e.g. Chloramphenicol, phenylbutazone, sulphonamides, gold

Viral infection
  Hepatitis, especially non-A non-B
  Infectious mononucleosis

Associated with paroxysmal nocturnal haemoglobinuria

Congenital
  Fanconi's anaemia
  Dyskeratosis congenita

---

red cells and myelocytes. This blood picture should alert the clinician to the possibility of an underlying carcinoma (most commonly derived from lung, breast, kidney, prostate, or gastrointestinal tract) or a haematological/ lymphoid malignancy. These changes are, however, also seen in response to extreme stress and the diverse causes of a leucoerythroblastic anaemia are summarized in Table 2.8. Invasion of the marrow may also lead to a microangiopathic haemolytic anaemia.

The diagnosis of metastatic carcinoma is often established by examination of a stained marrow aspirate slide and it is of note that aspiration is often painless (Moir's sign). In disseminated carcinoma clumps of malignant cells may be identified, although if the cells are not forming syncytia the diagnosis may be more difficult. In these circumstances, monoclonal antibody studies using anti-epithelial markers and immunoalkaline phosphatase labelling may detect individual malignant cells.[82] or alternatively a trephine biopsy may reveal the true diagnosis.

Management of a patient with marrow failure secondary to carcinomatous invasion is difficult. Blood transfusion will control the anaemia and be helpful in the short term, but neutropenia and thrombocytopenia are very worrying complications which are frequently fatal. Treatment should be directed at controlling the underlying disease, but although endocrine therapy may be of value in prostatic carcinoma, other cancers generally

Table 2.8   Causes of Leucoerythroblastic Anaemia

Marrow infiltration
  Carcinoma
  Lymphoma/myeloma
  Myelofibrosis
  Tuberculosis

Acute stress, e.g. severe haemorrhage/haemolysis, overwhelming infection,
        severe burns, pre-eclampsia, gross megaloblastic anaemia

---

respond poorly to therapy. The possibility that iron or folate deficiency is contributing to such an anaemia should not, however, be forgotten as this may respond to haematinic therapy. High-dose chemoradiotherapy followed by autologous bone marrow transplant is not feasible in these patients, since the marrow is contaminated by malignant cells.[81]

ENDOCRINE DISEASE

Hormones exert control over many homeostatic mechanisms, so that deranged endocrine function is commonly associated with haematological abnormalities.

Hypothyroidism

A moderate anaemia is observed in around 25% of patients and its aetiology is variable. The anaemia may be due to an associated autoimmune pernicious anaemia which often coexists.[83,84] A low plasma iron is also observed, but although iron deficiency is seen, hypothyroidism is more often associated with a low iron-binding capacity. Folate deficiency is also described. However, in nearly half the cases of anaemia associated with hypothyroidism, assays of haematinic factors are normal,[83] thus hypothyroidism gives rise to an anaemia per se. The anaemia is typically macrocytic and even in the absence of anaemia, a macrocytosis is common although the MCV may be normal. The anaemia and macrocytosis both respond to replacement therapy. It has been postulated that the anaemia results from a reduction in erythropoiesis as there is reduced tissue oxygen demand, and there is some clinical evidence to support this thesis.[85]

Thyrotoxicosis

A mild anaemia occurs in up to 20% of thyrotoxic patients despite an increase in marrow erythroid activity.[86,87] In some patients the anaemia may be due to a deficiency of a haematinic; this is usually not the case and the anaemia responds to treatment of the thyrotoxicosis.[86] It is of note that patients who are not anaemic commonly have red cell microcytosis. The pathogenesis of this anaemia is unclear but it may be due to ineffective erythropoiesis and responds to treatment of the hyperthyroid state.[87] It is of note that some thyrotoxic patients develop polycythaemia, perhaps due to an increase in tissue oxygen demand.[85]

Diabetes mellitus

Anaemia is a frequent concomitant of diabetes but is usually attributable to unrelated pathology or a complication of the diabetes: for example renal failure.[88] Hyperglycaemia has been shown to impair erythropoiesis, and good diabetic control does enhance erythroid stem cell proliferation.[89] This effect is usually not clinically significant.

Adrenal cortical hormones

Cushing's syndrome is frequently associated with a moderate polycythaemia (Hb elevated by 10–20 g/litre).[90] The cause of this is unclear but gluco-corticoids do potentiate erythroid colony formation *in vitro*.[91] In contrast, adrenal insufficiency is usually accompanied by a normochromic normocytic anaemia, although this may be masked by a reduction in the plasma volume and only become apparent after the patient has been rehydrated.[7] This anaemia responds well to steroid replacement therapy.

Sex hormones

Androgens stimulate erythropoeisis[92] by direct stimulation of erythroid colony forming units[93] and possibly by increasing erythropoietin production. Thus males have a higher Hb than females and this only becomes apparent after puberty.[90] Administration of androgens causes a rise in Hb which is more marked in females.[94] Furthermore, castrated males commonly have a mild anaemia which reverses if replacement therapy is provided.[90] Androgen therapy may be of value in the treatment of aplastic anaemia or pure red cell aplasia, occasionally being associated with a dramatic response.[94]

HYPERSPLENISM

The diagnosis of hypersplenism rests on the finding of a peripheral blood cytopenia coupled with splenomegaly and in the presence of a normocellular/hypercellular bone marrow.[95] It is conventional to exclude those conditions where the major defect is found in the circulating red cells and not in the spleen itself (e.g. beta thalassaemia major). Although splenomegaly may complicate many haematological or non-haematological diseases (see Table 2.9) and contribute to a pancytopenia, the cause of the anaemia is usually multifactorial.[96] Therefore, other causes of peripheral blood cytopenia should be excluded before a diagnosis of hypersplenism is accepted. It is also imperative to establish the cause of splenomegaly, so if hypersplenism is suspected examination of the bone marrow is mandatory.

Hypersplenism often causes moderate pancytopenia and the Hb is commonly in the range 80–100 g/litre. The pathogenesis of the anaemia is principally increased red cell destruction,[95,97] but blood pooling within the splanchnic circulation and an elevation of the plasma volume also serve to worsen the blood count.[97] (See Chapter 14.)

The anaemia of hypersplenism can initially be readily controlled by blood transfusion. Thus although splenectomy is obviously of value in alleviating the moderate pancytopenia, the operation is most often performed because of thrombocytopenia, neutropenia or local symptoms. Splenectomy is of particular value when hypersplenism compounds a cytopenia occurring in conjunction with haematological disease. In experienced hands splenectomy, even for massive splenomegaly (>1.5 kg), is a relatively safe procedure,[98] but rarely resolves the pancytopenia completely.

Table 2.9   Disorders Associated with Hypersplenism[95]

Primary hypersplenism

Hematological
  Myeloproliferative
    Myelofibrosis[a]
  Malignant
    Chronic lymphocytic leukaemia[a]
    Lymphoma[a]
  Haemoglobinopathies
    Sickle cell syndromes
    Thalassaemia syndromes[a]
  Reactive
    Chronic haemolytic anaemia

Infectious
  Bacterial, e.g. brucellosis
  Parasitic, e.g. malaria,[a] tropical spenomegaly,[a] Leishmaniasis[a]
  (Viral)

Congestive splenomegaly
  Portal hypertension

Infiltrative/storage disorders
  Lipid storage diseases
  Gaucher's disease[a]
  Amyloid

Inflammatory
  Felty's syndrome/SLE/sarcoidosis

---

[a] May be massive splenomegaly.

ANAEMIA OF CHRONIC DISEASE (ACD)

This term defines a specific refractory anaemia seen in association with underlying disease. The anaemia may be seen in patients with chronic infection, inflammation or malignancy, and is often associated with other causes of anaemia, since these patients may become anaemic for a variety of causes (see Table 2.10). The common laboratory features of this anaemia, especially those relating to iron status and utilization, give rise to the belief that the pathogenesis of the anaemia in each of these disorders is the same.[53,59,99]

The anaemia is usually mild with Hb 85–120 g/litre and develops within 2 months of the underlying disorder, the degree of anaemia generally reflecting disease activity. It is usually normochromic and normocytic although it may be hypochromic and microcytic; red cell morphology is unremarkable.[100,101] The reticulocyte count is low for the degree of anaemia. There is plentiful iron demonstrable on marrow smears, which show an increase in reticulo-endothelial haemosiderin but a marked reduction in the number of iron-containing erythroblasts to 5–20% as compared to the normal 30–50%.[99] ACD is further characterized by a reduced serum iron in

Table 2.10   Diseases which May Lead to the Anaemia of Chronic Disease

Chronic infection

Malignancy

Chronic inflammation
   Rheumatoid arthritis, juvenile chronic arthritis
   Systemic lupus erythematosus, polyarteritis nodosum
   Giant cell arteritis/polymyalgia rheumatica

the presence of normal or increased iron stores,[53] and this low serum iron is associated with a low iron-binding capacity; in contrast to patients with iron deficiency in whom there is decreased plasma iron and a high total iron-binding capacity.[59]

The distinction between ACD and iron deficiency is important, especially as the two conditions may coexist, and the latter will respond to iron replacement therapy. Differentiating between ACD and iron deficiency on the basis of the haematological indices and the serum iron and transferrin levels is often difficult. In normal situations the serum ferritin is considered the most useful means of assessing iron stores since it is in equilibrium with tissue ferritin and correlates well with stainable marrow iron.[102] It might therefore be expected to be of value in this situation, especially as there is considerable observer error in assessing marrow iron levels.[103] Ferritin, however, acts as an acute phase protein, so serum levels are often elevated in inflammation[101,102] and malignancy.[99,104] A serum ferritin of less than 12 µg/litre may be taken to indicate definite iron deficiency,[105] but in patients with ACD a serum ferritin in the low normal range (13–100 µg/litre) may be seen in the presence of iron deficiency and no stainable marrow iron.[101,103] Therefore, in patients with ACD and a serum ferritin of less than 100 µg/litre,[105] it may be necessary to perform a bone marrow aspiration to look for stainable iron and thus uncover the cause of the anaemia. Alternatively a short diagnostic trial of oral iron replacement may clarify the situation.

A recent study has shown that red cell ferritin may help to accurately determine the iron status of patients with rheumatoid arthritis.[106] If this holds true for other diseases which cause ACD, this measurement would avoid the necessity of performing a bone marrow aspirate. An alternative problem is a patient who presents with an unexplained moderate anaemia, and a low iron and iron-binding capacity. In these circumstances an underlying disease should be suspected, possibly an occult infection, especially tuberculosis, or an underlying malignancy.

Pathogenesis of ACD

This is unclear, despite the considerable published data on the subject, since many of the findings are either inconclusive or contradictory. It is likely that the anaemia results from a combination of causes and as yet the relative importance of each has not been determined. In ACD there is a modest reduction in the red cell lifespan and blood transfused into patients with rhematoid arthritis (RA) has a shortened lifespan of 80–90 days. Cross-transfusion experiments show that blood from patients with RA has a normal lifespan in healthy subjects,[107,108] and therefore this effect is due to an extracorpuscular mechanism.[100] Red cell survival studies using ^{51}Cr as a red cell label, or cohort labelling using ferrokinetics, have confirmed this finding in patients with RA[109] but not in those with Hodgkin's disease.[104] The reason for the reduced red cell survival is unclear, although it may be related to stimulation of the reticulo-endothelial system with concomitant increase in phagocytic activity.[100] However, the shortened red cell lifespan is probably not a major determinant of ACD since a normal marrow would easily compensate for this mild degree of haemolysis.[59] Indeed, there is little biochemical evidence of increased red cell destruction (hyperbilirubinaemia or urobilinogenuria) in ACD, but there is reticulocytopenia out of proportion to the anaemia and so the anaemia is principally due to an impaired marrow response.

A defect in iron metabolism such that iron is unavailable to developing erythroblasts is probably the most important factor in the genesis of ACD. This postulate follows from the finding of normal marrow iron stores in the context of a low plasma iron. Various mechanisms which might explain this apparently defective supply of iron to developing erythroblasts have been put forward and they will be considered separately.

It has been established that acute inflammation may be associated with a reduction in iron absorption,[110,111] but in ACD total body iron absorption is normal,[112] although the transfer of iron from intestinal mucosal cells to the plasma is reduced.[110] Furthermore, in experimentally induced inflammation, hypoferraemia and a fall in the iron-binding capacity precedes the onset of fever or other symptoms.[113] In RA there has been a suggestion that iron is deposited in the synovial membrane, where it causes local damage and is unavailable for erythropoiesis.[114]

Ferrokinetic studies show a normal or slight increase in plasma iron turnover in patients with ACD.[99,107,109] In animal studies red cell utilization of iron bound to transferrin has also been shown to be normal.[115] More recent analyses have enabled the distinction to be made between erythroid and non-erythroid iron turnover,[110] and these studies have not shown an association between hypoferraemia and depression of marrow iron turnover in patients with inflammatory or neoplastic disease.[104,109,116] In fact, marrow iron turnover studies are unremarkable in RA unless there is a super-imposed iron deficiency.[109]

As the supply of iron to erythroblasts is defective in ACD the next mechanism which should be considered is the possibility of a block in the release of iron by the reticulo-endothelial system (RES). Normal erythro-poiesis requires up to 800 µmol iron per day and this is almost entirely derived from breakdown of senescent red cells by the RES. A block in RES iron release would explain the low serum iron and increased macrophage iron deposits seen in ACD[100,107] and there is some animal data to support this concept.[111,117] These experiments also showed that in the presence of inflammation hepatocyte and intestinal mucosal cells do not release iron normally.[111] Early studies in patients with inflammation, renal failure and

Hodgkin's disease showed reduced RES iron release using heat-damaged red cells[118] and iron dextran.[119,120] However, later work has challenged this explanation by showing normal iron release and utilization in most patients with rheumatoid arthritis.[121,122] Thus it appears that even though iron release may be normal, it is unavailable to erythroid precursors,[59] thus giving rise to an iron-deficient type of erythropoiesis, reduction in marrow sideroblasts, and accumulation of free red cell protoporphyrin.[100]

A second mechanism proposed to explain the anaemia in ACD is an inadequate erythropoietin response as has been discussed earlier. Recent evidence of erythropoietin levels in non-uraemic patients with ACD does not support this contention.[27,58] The results of erythropoietin therapy in the ACD are also not yet available.

Thirdly, a defective marrow response to erythropoietin has been proposed as an important factor in the pathogenesis of ACD, especially in RA.[59] One ferrokinetic study suggested that ineffective iron utilization contributed to the anaemia in RA;[123] however, this finding has been contra-dicted.[104,109,116,124] An alternative method for assessing ineffective erythro-poiesis has been developed and relies on *in vitro* marrow culture. In anaemic patients with RA there was an increase in the release of ^{59}Fe-haem from erythroblasts, which was not seen in other causes of ACD.[125] This finding suggests that ineffective erythropoiesis may make a contribution to the chronic anaemia seen in RA, but that it is unlikely to be significant in the genesis of ACD in other situations.[59,99]

The possibility of abnormal erythroid colony growth has been implicated as a fourth possible mechanism in ACD. Using *in vitro* marrow culture techniques two types of erythroid precursor can be grown: colony forming units (CFU_E), and the more primitive blast forming units (BFU_E).[59] Results of such studies in patients with systemic lupus erythematosus,[126] RA[127] and juvenile chronic arthritis[128] show that in some situations a humoral factor may inhibit erythropoiesis. These studies show that serum from anaemic patients (with systemic lupus erythematosus or RA) may suppress CFU_E proliferation. Interestingly, in two patients, plasmapheresis was associated with clinical improvement and an improvement in the *in vitro* culture tests.[126] Although the nature of the factor(s) involved was not fully characterized, it may have been an immunoglobulin. Thus auto-antibodies may play a role in ACD associated with certain autoimmune diseases, but are unlikely to be relevant to the anaemia seen in chronic infection or malignancy. Similar studies have been carried out in patients with systemic fungal infection and macrophages from these patients inhibited the growth

Table 2.11 Factors which May Contribute to the Anaemia of Chronic Disease

Non-availability of iron to erythroblasts ?mechanism

Shortened red cell lifespan

Ineffective erythropoieis

Humoral inhibition of erythropoiesis

(Erythropoietin deficiency – disputed)

of CFU_E and BFU_E from both autologous and normal marrow.[129] Again it was postulated that this effect was mediated by a soluble factor.

In conclusion the pathogenesis of ACD is unclear but represents an inadequate marrow response to anaemia mediated through a combination of factors (Table 2.11). The most important of these is inadequate availability of iron to developing erythroblasts, but there is also some degree of dyserythropoiesis and a shortening of the red cell lifespan. The possible role of inadequate erythropoietin production is unclear.

Biochemical mediators of ACD

Despite the fact that the exact mechanisms behind the development of ACD are uncertain, various biochemical factors have been proposed as being responsible for this effect, including interleukin-1 (IL-1: previously named leucocyte endogenous mediator). Many infectious agents induce monocytes to produce IL-1 which is responsible for an acute-phase reaction, causing fever, leucocytosis, lactoferrin release and decreased transferrin synthesis.[61,130] This leads to hypoferraemia and has been proposed as the cause of ACD.[61] It is also possible that IL-1 suppresses erythropoietin production.[53] Purification of IL-1 has been difficult and so studies of its exact mode of action are limited. The effect of IL-1 may possibly be mediated via lactoferrin, an iron-binding glycoprotein with molecular weight 80,000 Da, which is found in the secondary granules of neutrophils.[131] Lactoferrin is released during neutrophil phagocytosis and has a higher affinity for iron than transferrin, and it has been shown that the development of hypoferraemia in inflammation depends on the presence of neutrophils. Once formed, iron–lactoferrin complexes are taken up by macrophages and iron is not released to erythroblasts.[131] The lactoferrin hypothesis does explain many of the features of ACD, particularly the ferrokinetic findings and the role of IL-1. Criticisms of the theory include the fact that it does not explain the retention of iron by liver and intestinal mucosal cells and the lactoferrin dosages used in the experiments were not physiological.[53] An alternative hypothesis is that apoferritin synthesis may be enhanced sufficiently to give rise to hypoferraemia and there is some experimental evidence to support this contention.[132] Tumour necrosis factor-α has also been proposed as a substance which might cause these effects.[133]

These hypotheses all suggest that ACD is an appropriate response to bacterial or fungal infection. Since iron utilization is crucial to many infectious agents, a host response which starves the microorganism of available iron may be rational: so called 'nutritional immunity'.[53] Most bacteria require an iron concentration of around 10^{-6} M and plasma iron is around 10^{-15} M due to transferrin binding. *In vitro* studies show that both transferrin and lactoferrin inhibit bacterial growth and that this effect is blocked by adding iron to the system.[53] In clinical practice hypoferraemia may act to ameliorate the effects of many infections,[134] and patients with iron overload (haemochromatosis and beta thalassaemia major) appear more prone to bacterial infection. The moderate anaemia observed during acute infections is probably caused by a similar mechanism,[133] although in these circumstances haemolysis may also be important.

Treatment

Treatment of ACD is not usually needed since the anaemia is mild and the patient's complaints are attributable to the underlying disorder. Treatment should be directed at the underlying disorder and if this responds to therapy the anaemia will also improve. It should be recognized that the effect of ACD is ameliorated by an increase in red cell 2,3-DPG levels so that haemoglobin oxygen affinity is reduced, thereby improving oxygen delivery to the tissues.[124] It is also important to remember that other anaemias may supervene on ACD, especially iron or folate deficiency. Occasionally blood transfusion may be needed to alleviate the symptoms should the anaemia be severe.

Oral iron is generally ineffective in ACD but it is of interest that parenteral iron will partially correct the anaemia, although the effect is short lived.[53,135] This finding supports the thesis that a defect in iron metabolism is central to the causation of ACD. Trials of erythropoietin in ACD are currently underway, and this hormone may prove useful at elevating the Hb. If the erythropoietin level is appropriate to the degree of anaemia then any effect will be pharmacological rather than physiological.[27] Clearly it is important that any trial of Epo in ACD should critically assess the patients' symptoms rather than merely measuring the Hb level.

INFECTIOUS DISEASE

Anaemia is an infrequent finding in acute infection, because the normal red cell lifespan is 120 days. However, autoimmune haemolysis can follow acute viral infection (see Chapter 11). In contrast, chronic bacterial or fungal infection is usually associated with a moderate anaemia which is often present at diagnosis and does not require specific treatment. This anaemia is primarily attributable to impaired red cell production, the anaemia of chronic disease.[133] Anaemia is a very common feature of malarial infection, although the aetiology of this anaemia is complex. Table 2.12 lists the mechanisms which are believed to be important in producing the anaemia.[136,137] In some circumstances blood loss and/or haemolysis may contribute to the anaemia. Treatment of the underlying infection will lead to a clinical improvement and usually blood transfusion is not needed.

Table 2.12 Contributory Factors to the Anaemia Seen in Malaria

Increased red cell destruction
  Haemolysis by parasites
  Hypersplenism
  Drugs: blackwater fever

Decreased red cell production
  Dyserythropoiesis
  Anaemia of chronic disease
  Folate deficiency
  Pre-existing factors, e.g. iron deficiency, protein calorie malnutrition

ALCOHOL ABUSE

Alcohol is toxic to all organs so that alcohol abuse is associated with multiple metabolic effects, which frequently coexist, Anaemia is seen in up to 50% of chronic alcoholics[138] and is usually multifactorial.

Macrocytosis is a common feature of alcohol abuse, being observed in 90% of chronic alcoholics.[139] This macrocytosis occurs in the absence of liver disease or folate deficiency,[139,140] and the majority of patients with macrocytosis have a normal serum folate.[138] Ethanol has a directly toxic effect on red cell precursors: it causes decreased marrow cellularity, vacuolization of erythroblasts and macronormoblastic erythro- poiesis.[139,141-143] This effect may persist for up to 4 months after abstaining from alcohol, and occurs in the absence of folate or B_{12} deficiency.[139] *In vitro* studies have shown that erythropoiesis is suppressed by alcohol or acetaldehyde and that this effect is much more marked on the erythroid than myeloid precursors.[144] This explains the predominant effect of alcohol on the red cell rather than the white cell series.[140]

Other problems seen in alcoholics include folate deficiency and liver disease. Folate deficiency is common in spirit-drinking alcoholics and should be suspected if an anaemia develops with the blood film showing oval macrocytosis and hypersegmented neutrophils.[142,145] This effect is princip- ally attributable to poor dietary intake since megaloblastic anaemia is rare in well-nourished beer drinkers. It is of note that poor diet appears to be commoner in American rather than British alcoholics,[141] and also that beer is rich in folate compared to wine and spirits which are not.[145] However, alcohol also potentiates the effect of a folate-depleted diet. In normal individuals it takes about 19 weeks for megaloblastic change to occur on a low folate diet, but if alcohol is added to the diet these changes occur within 2 weeks.[143] The effect is probably mainly due to an impairment of the enterohepatic circulation of folate and may be due to the fact that the hepatocytes do not release folate normally.[145] Vitamin B_{12} levels are usually

Table 2.13   Possible Causes of Anaemia in Alcohol Abuse[138,141]

Acute blood loss

Iron metabolism
  Deficiency due to blood loss
  Sideroblastic anaemia
  Anaemia of chronic disease

Megaloblastic erythropoiesis
  Folate deficiency
  Direct alcohol toxicity

Poor diet

Hypersplenism

Haemolysis
  Zieve's syndrome
  Spur cell

elevated in alcoholics because of liver damage; however, the possibility of an unrelated B_{12} deficiency must be remembered since the neurological consequences of treating such a deficiency with folic acid may be tragic.

Various abnormalities of iron metabolism are also observed in alcohol abuse, including the anaemia of chronic disease.[143] Iron deficiency is common and is usually caused by gastrointestinal bleeding, particularly from peptic ulceration or varices. Concurrent clotting abnormalities and moderate thrombocytopenia are common in alcohol abuse and will tend to worsen these bleeding episodes. However, the assessment of iron status in alcoholics may be difficult for various reasons. Firstly, the microcytosis seen in iron deficiency may be masked by the macrocytosis. Secondly, although the serum ferritin appears the best indicator of iron deficiency, this level may be elevated in liver disease and give a false normal reading. Sideroblastic change may also be observed, usually in an acute episode associated with megaloblastic anaemia due to folate deficiency. The cause of the sideroblastosis is unknown although the effect reverses when the patient stops drinking. Lastly, iron overload is commonly seen in alcoholics and may contribute to the hepatic impairment.

In summary, the anaemia occurring in the context of alcohol abuse may be due to many mechanisms, which have been extensively studied (Table 2.13).

REFERENCES

1. Brotherhood, J., Brozovic, B. & Pugh, L.G.C. Haematological status of middle- and long-distance runners. *Clin. Sci. Mol. Med.* **48**: 139–45, 1975.
2. Holmgren, A., Mossfeldt, F., Sjorstrand, T. & Strom, G. Effect of training on work capacity, total haemoglobin, blood volume, heart volume and pulse rate in recumbent and upright positions. *Acta Physiol. Scand.* **50**: 72–83, 1960.
3. Oscai, L.B., Williams, B.T. & Hertig, B.A. Effect of exercise on blood volume. *J. Appl. Physiol.* **24**: 622–4, 1968.
4. Bell, J. & Cowan, G.S.M. Low blood hematocrits in male army volunteers during basic training. *N. Engl. J. Med.* **299**: 491, 1978.
5. Chesley, L.C. Plasma and red cell volumes during pregnancy. *Am. J. Obs. Gynae.* **112**: 440–50, 1972.
6. Smith, J.R. & Landlaw, S.A. Smokers' polycythaemia. *N. Engl. J. Med.* **298**: 5–10, 1978.
7. Orwoll, E.S. & Orwoll, R.L. Haematologic abnormalities in patients with endocrine and metabolic disorders. *Haem/Oncology Clin. N. America* **I**: 261–79, 1987.
8. Charlton, R.W. & Bothwell, T.H. Definition, prevalence and prevention of iron deficiency. *Clin. Haematol.* **11**: 309–25, 1982.
9. Jacobs, A. & Worwood, M. Iron metabolism, iron deficiency and iron overload. In *Blood and its Disorders* (eds R.M. Hardisty & D.J. Weatherall), pp. 149–68. Blackwell Scientific, Oxford, 1982.
10. Beveridge, B.R., Bannerman, R.M., Evanson, J.M. & Witts, L.J. Hypochromic anaemia: a retrospective study and follow up of 378 in-patients. *Quart. J. Med.* **34**: 145–61, 1965.
11. Hoffbrand, A.V. Anaemia in adult coeliac disease. *Clin. Gastroenterology* **3**: 71–89, 1974.
12. Chanarin, I. *The Megaloblastic Anaemias*, 2nd Edn. Blackwell Scientific, Oxford, 1979.

13. Hoffbrand, A.V. Vitamin B_{12} and folate metabolism, the megaloblastic anaemias and other nutritional anaemias. In *Blood and its Disorders* (eds R.M. Hardisty & D.J. Weatherall), pp. 199–264. Blackwell Scientific, Oxford, 1982.

14. Shorvon, S.D., Carney, M.W.P., Chanarin, I. & Reynolds, E.H. The neuropsychiatry of megaloblastic anaemia. *Br. Med. J.* **281**: 1036–8, 1980.

15. Prouse, P.J., Shawe, D. & Gumpel, J.M. Macrocytic anaemia in patients treated with sulphasalazine for rheumatoid arthritis. *Br. Med. J.* **293**: 1407, 1986.

16. Sharman, V.L., Cunningham, J., Goodwin, F.J. *et al.* Do patients receiving regular haemodialysis need folic acid supplements? *Br. Med. J.* **285**: 96–7, 1982.

17. Lindenbaum, J., Healton, E.B., Savage, D.G. *et al.* Neuropsychiatric disorders caused by cobalamin deficiency in the absence of anemia or macrocytosis. *N. Engl. J. Med.* **318**: 1720–8, 1988.

18. Zeitlin, H.C., Sheppard, K., Baum, J.D., Bolton, F.G. & Hall, C.A. Homozygous transcobalamin II deficiency maintained on oral hydroxycobalamin. *Blood* **66**: 1022–7, 1985.

19. Cooper, B.A. & Rosenblatt, D.S. Inherited defects of vitamin B_{12} metabolism. *Ann. Rev. Nutri.* **7**: 291–320, 1987.

20. Chanarin, I., Malakowska, V., O'Hea, A.-M. *et al.* Megaloblastic anaemia in a vegetarian Hindu community. *Lancet* **II**: 1168–72. 1985.

21. Amos, R.J., Amess, J.A.L., Hinds, C.J. & Mollin, D.L. Incidence and pathogenesis of acute megaloblastic bone marrow change in patients receiving intensive care. *Lancet* **II**: 835–8, 1982.

22. Editorial. Nitrous oxide and acute marrow failure. *Lancet* **II**: 856–7, 1982.

23. White, J.M. & Nicholson, D.C. Haem and pyridoxine metabolism. The sideroblastic and other related refractory anaemias. In *Blood and its Disorders* (eds R.M. Hardisty & D.T. Weatherall), pp. 545–76. Blackwell Scientific, Oxford, 1982.

24. Bottomley, S.S. Sideroblastic anaemia. *Clin. Haematol.* **11**: 389–409, 1982.

25. Erslev, A. Erythropoietin coming of age. *N. Eng. J. Med.* **316**: 101–3, 1987.

26. Cotes, P.M. & Bangham, D.R. Bioassay of erythropoietin in mice made polycythaemic by exposure to air at a reduced pressure. *Nature* **191**: 1065–7, 1961.

27. Erslev, A.J., Wilson, J. and Caro, J. Erythropoietin titers in anemic, nonuremic patients. *J. Lab. Clin. Med.* **109**: 429–33. 1987.

28. Caro, J., Brown, S., Miller, O., Murphy, T. & Erslev, A. Erythropoietin levels in uremic nephric and anephric patients. *J. Lab. Clin. Med.* **93**: 445–55, 1979.

29. Eschbach, J.W. & Adamson, J.W. Anemia of end-stage renal disease. *Kid. Int.* **28**: 1–5, 1985.

30. Cohen, R.A., Clemons, G. & Ebbe, S. Correlation between bioassay and radioimmune assay for erythropoietin in human serum and urine concentrates. *Proc. Soc. Exp. Biol. Med.* **179**: 269–78, 1985.

31. Shaw, A.B. Haemolysis in chronic renal failure. *Br. Med. J.* **2**: 213–5, 1967.

32. Kock, K.M., Patyna, W.D., Shaldon, S. & Werner, E. Anemia of the regular hemodialysis patients and its treatment. *Nephron* **12**: 405–19, 1974.

33. Joske, R.A., McAlister, J.M. & Prankerd, T.A.J. Isotope investigations of red cell production and destruction in chronic renal disease. *Clin. Sci.* **15**: 511–22, 1956.

34. Eschbach, J.W., Adamson, J.W. & Cook, J.D. Disorders of red cell production in uremia. *Arc. Intern. Med.* **126**: 812–5, 1970.

35. Delwiche, F., Eschbach, J.W. & Adamson, J.W. The anemia of chronic renal failure (CRF): lack of *in vitro* specificity of serum inhibitors. *Blood* **62**: 45A (abstract), 1983.

36. Delwiche, F. Garrity, M.J., Powell, J.S., Robertson, R.P. & Adamson, J.W. High levels of the circulating form of parathyroid hormone do not inhibit in vitro erythropoiesis. *J. Lab. Clin. Med.* **102**: 613–20, 1983.

37. McGonigle, R.J.S., Wallin, J.D., Husserl, F. *et al.* Potential role of parathyroid hormone as an inhibitor of erythropoiesis in the anemia of renal failure. *J. Lab. Clin. Med.* **104**: 1016–26, 1984.
38. Winearls, C.G., Savage, C.O.S., Oliviera, D.B.G. & Midgley, K. Anaemia in CAPD and haemodialysis. *Lancet* **II**: 1488, 1983.
39. Cantaluppi, A., Scalamonga, A., Castelnovo, L., Graziani, G. & Ponticelli, C. Anaemia in CAPD and haemodialysis. *Lancet* **II**: 1489, 1983.
40. Summerfield, G.P., Bellingham, A.J. & Goldsmith, H.J. Anaemia in CAPD and haemodialysis. *Lancet* **II**: 1489, 1983.
41. Weinberg, S.G., Lubin, A., Wiener, S., Deoras, M.P., Ghose, M.K. & Kopelman, R.C. Myelofibrosis and renal osteodystrophy. *Am. J. Med.* **63**: 755–64, 1977.
42. Short, A.I.K., Winney, R.J. & Robson, J.S. Reversible microcytic hypochromic anaemia in dialysis patients due to aluminium intoxication. *Proc. Eur. Dial. Transplant. Assoc.* **17**: 226–33, 1980.
43. Miyake, T., Kung, C.K.H. & Goldwasser, E. Purification of human erythropoietin. *J. Biol. Chem.* **252**: 5558–64, 1977.
44. Jacobs, K., Shoemaker, C., Rudersdorf, R. *et al.* Isolation and characterisation of genomic and cDNA clones of human erythropoietin. *Nature* **313**: 806–10, 1985.
45. Winearls, C.G., Oliver, D.O., Pippard, M.J., Reid, C., Downing, M.R. & Cotes, P.M. Effect of human erythropoietin derived from recombinant DNA on the anaemia of patients maintained by chronic haemodialysis. *Lancet* **II**: 1175–7, 1986.
46. Eschbach, J.W., Egrie, J.C., Downing, M.R., Browne, J.K. & Adamson, J.W. Correction of the anemia of end-stage renal disease with recombinant human erythropoietin. *N. Engl. J. Med.* **316**: 73–8, 1987.
47. Moia, M., Mannucci, P.M., Vizzotto, L., Casati, S., Cattaneo, M. & Ponticelli, C. Improvement in the haemostatic defect of uraemia after treatment with recombinant human erythropoietin. *Lancet* **II**: 1227–9, 1987.
48. Remuzzi, G. Bleeding in renal failure. *Lancet* **I**: 1205–7, 1988.
49. Editorial. Cotes, P.M. Erythropoietin: the developing story. *Br. Med. J.* **296**: 805–6, 1988.
50. Editorial. Erythropoietin. *Lancet* **I**: 781–2, 1987.
51. Eschbach, J.W. & Adamson, J.W. Improvement in the anaemia of chronic renal failure with fluoxymesterone. *Ann. Intern. Med.* **78**: 527–34, 1973.
52. Javier De La Serna, F., Praga, M., Gilsanz, F. *et al.* Improvement in the erythropoiesis of chronic haemodialysis patients with desferrioxamine. *Lancet* **I**: 1009–11, 1988.
53. Lee, G.R. The anemia of chronic disease. *Semin. Hematol.* **20**: 61–80, 1983.
54. Ward, H.P., Kurnick, J.E. & Pisarczyk, M.J. Serum levels of erythropoietin in anaemias associated with chronic infection, malignancy and primary haemopoietic disease. *J. Clin. Invest.* **50**: 332–5, 1971.
55. Mahmood, T., Robinson, W.A., Kurnick, J.E. & Vautrin, R. Granulopoietic and erythropoietic activity in patients with anaemias of iron deficiency and chronic disease. *Blood* **50**: 449–55, 1977.
56. Zucker, S., Friedman, S. & Lysik, R. Bone marrow erythropoiesis in the anaemia of infection, inflammation and malignancy. *J. Clin. Invest.* **53**: 1132–8, 1974.
57. Ward, H.P., Gordon, B. & Pickett, B. Serum levels of erythropoietin in rheumatoid arthritis. *J. Lab. Clin. Med.* **74**: 93–7, 1969.
58. Birgegard, G., Hallgren, R. & Caro, J. Serum erythropoietin in rheumatoid arthritis and other inflammatory arthritides: relationship to anaemia and the effect of anti-inflammatory treatment. *Br. J. Haematol.* **65**: 479–83, 1987.
59. Samson, D. The anaemia of chronic disorders. *Postgrad. Med. J.* **59**: 543–50, 1983.
60. Gutnisky, A. & van Dyke, D. Normal response to erythropoietin or hypoxia in

rats made anaemic with turpentine abscess. *Proc. Soc. Exp. Biol. Med.* **112**: 75–8, 1963.

61. Lukens, J.N. Control of erythropoiesis in rats with adjuvant-induced chronic inflammation. *Blood* **41**: 37–44, 1973.
62. Cotes, P.M., Dore, C.J., Yin, J.A.L. *et al.* Determination of serum immunoreactive erythropoietin in the investigation of erythrocytosis. *N. Engl. J. Med.* **315**: 283–7, 1986.
63. Editorial. Pure red cell aplasia. *Lancet* **II**: 546–7, 1982.
64. Plummer, F.A., Hammond, G.W., Forward, K. *et al.* An erythema infectiosum-like illness caused by human parvovirus infection. *N. Engl. J. Med.* **313**: 74–9, 1985.
65. Reid, D.M., Reid, T.M.S., Brown, T., Rennie, J.A.N. & Eastmond, C.J. Human parvovirus-associated arthritis: a clinical and laboratory description. *Lancet* **I**: 422–5, 1985.
66. Potter, C.G., Potter, A.C., Hatton, C.S.R. *et al.* Variation of erythroid and myeloid precursors in the marrow and peripheral blood of volunteer subjects infected with human parvovirus (B19). *J. Clin. Invest.* **79**: 1486–92, 1987.
67. Editorial. Bentley, D.P. Hypoplastic anaemia and parvovirus infection. *Br. Med. J.* **293**: 836–7, 1986.
68. Serjeant, G.R., Mason, K., Topley, J.M. *et al.* Outbreak of aplastic crises in sickle cell anaemia associated with parvovirus-like agent. *Lancet* **II**: 595–7, 1981.
69. Kelleher, J.F., Luban, N.L.C., Mortimer, P.P. & Kamimura, T. Human serum parvovirus. A specific cause of aplastic crisis in children with hereditary spherocytosis. *J. Pediatr.* **102**: 720–2, 1983.
70. Duncan, J.R., Potter, C.G., Cappelini, M.D., Kurtz, J.B., Anderson, M.J. & Weatherall, D.J. Aplastic crisis due to parvovirus in pyruvate kinase deficiency. *Lancet* **II**: 14–16, 1983.
71. Davis, L.R. Annotation: Aplastic crisis in haemolytic anaemias: the role of a parvovirus like agent. *Br. J. Haematol.* **55**: 391–3, 1983.
72. Wranne, L. Transient erythroblastopenia in infancy and childhood. *Scand. J. Haematol.* **7**: 76–81, 1970.
73. Krantz, S.B. Pure red cell aplasia. In *Current Therapy in Hematology–Oncology 1983–4* (eds M.C. Brian & P.B. McCulloch). BC Decker Inc, Ontario, 1984.
74. Marmont, A., Peschle, C., Sanguineti, M. & Condorelli, M. Pure red cell aplasia. Response of three patients to cyclophosphamide and/or anti-lymphocyte globulin and demonstration of two types of serum IgG inhibitors to erythropoiesis. *Blood* **45**: 247–61, 1975.
75. Messner, H.A., Fauser, A.A. Curtis, J.E. & Dotten, D. Control of antibody mediated pure red cell aplasia by plasmapaheresis. *N. Engl. J. Med.* **304**: 1334–8, 1981.
76. Roland, A.S. The syndrome of benign thymoma and primary aregenerative anemia: an analysis of 43 cases. *Am. J. Med. Sci.* **247**: 719–31, 1964.
77. Beard, M.E.J., Krantz, S.B., Johnson, S.A.N., Bateman, C.J.T. & Whitehouse, J.M.A. Pure red cell aplasia. *Quart. J. Med.* **47**: 339–48, 1978.
78. Zeldis, J.B., Dienstag, J.L. & Gale, R.P. Aplastic anemia and non-A, non-B hepatitis. *Am. J. Med.* **74**: 64–8, 1983.
79. Kuo, G., Choo, Q.L. Alter, H.J. *et al.* An assay for circulating antibodies to a major etiologic virus of human non-A non-B hepatitis. *Science* **244**: 362–4, 1989.
80. Camitta, B.M., Storb, R. & Thomas, E.D. Aplastic anaemia: pathogenesis, diagnosis, treatment and prognosis (part I). *N. Engl. J. Med.* **306**: 645–52, 1982.
81. Editorial. Autologous bone marrow transplantation. *Lancet* **I**: 303–4, 1987.
82. Ghosh, A.K., Erber, W.N., Hatton, C.S.R. *et al.* Detection of metastatic tumour cells in routine bone marrow smears by immuno-alkaline phosphatase labelling with monoclonal antibodies. *Br. J. Haematol.* **61**: 21–30, 1985.
83. Horton, L., Coburn, R.J., England, J.M. *et al.* The haematology of hypo-

thyroidism. *Quart. J. Med.* **46**: 101–23.

84. Volpe, R. The role of autoimmunity in hypoendocrine and hyperendocrine function: with special emphasis on autoimmune thyroid disease. *Ann. Int. Med.* **87**: 86–99, 1977.
85. Muldowney, F.P., Crooks, J. & Wayne, F.J. The total red cell mass in thyrotoxicosis and myxoedema. *Clin. Sci.* **16**: 309–14, 1957.
86. Perlman, J.A. & Sternthal, P.M. Effect of ^{131}I on the anemia of hyperthyroidism. *J. Chronic Dis.* **36**: 405–12, 1983.
87. Rivlin, R.S. & Wagner, H.N. Anemia in hyperthyroidism. *Ann. Intern. Med.* **70**: 507–16, 1969.
88. Bern, M.M. & Busick, E.J. Disorders of the blood and diabetes. In *Joslins' Diabetes Mellitus*, Vol. 12, pp. 748–56. Lee & Febiger, Philadelphia, 1985.
89. Ritchey, A.K., Tamborlane, W.V. & Gertner, J. Improved diabetic control enhances erythroid stem cell proliferation *in vitro*. *J. Clin. Endocrinol. Metab.* **60**: 1257–60, 1985.
90. Shahidi, N.T. Androgens and erythropoiesis. *N. Engl. J. Med.* **289**: 72–80, 1973.
91. Golde, D.W., Berchu, N. & Cline, M.J. Potentiation of erythropoiesis *in vitro* by dexamethasone. *J. Clin. Invest.* **57**: 57–62, 1976.
92. Kennedy, B.J. & Gilbertsen, A.S. Increased erythropoiesis induced by androgenic-hormone therapy. *N. Engl. J. Med.* **256**: 719–26, 1957.
93. Singer, J.W., Samuels, A.I. & Adamson, J.W. The effect of steroids on *in vitro* erythroid colony growth: structure/activity relationships. *J. Cell. Physiol.* **88**: 127–33, 1976.
94. Wilson, J.D. & Griffin, J.E. The use and misuse of androgens. *Metabolism* **29**: 1278–95, 1980.
95. Bowdler, A.J. Splenomegaly and hypersplenism. *Clin. Haematol.* **12**: 467–88, 1983.
96. Bowdler, A.J. The spleen in disorders of the blood. In *Blood and its Disorders* (eds. R.M. Hardisty & D.J. Weatherall) pp. 763–6. Blackwell Scientific, Oxford, 1982.
97. McFadzean, A.J.S., Todd, D. & Tsang, K.C. Observations on the anaemia of cryptogenic splenomegaly II: expansion of the plasma volume. *Blood* **13**: 524–32, 1958.
98. Bickerstaff, K.I. & Morris, P.J. Splenectomy for massive splenomegaly. *Br. J. Surg.* **74**: 346–9, 1987.
99. Bentley, D.P. Anaemia and chronic disease. *Clin. Haematol.* **11**: 465–79, 1982.
100. Cartwright, G.E. & Lee, G.R. The anaemia of chronic disorders. *Br. J. Haematol.* **21**: 147–52, 1971.
101. Baynes, R.D., Bothwell, T.H., Bezwoda, W.R., Gear, A.J. & Atkinson, P. Hematologic and iron-related measurements in rheumatoid arthritis. *Am. J. Clin. Pathol.* **87**: 196–200, 1987.
102. Lipschitz, D.A., Cook, J.D. & Finch, C.A. A clinical evaluation of serum ferritin as an index of iron stores. *N. Engl. J. Med.* **290**: 1213–6, 1974.
103. Bentley, D.P. & Williams, P. Serum ferritin concentration as an index of storage iron in rheumatoid arthritis. *J. Clin. Pathol.* **27**: 786–8, 1974.
104. Al-Ismail, S., Cavill, I., Evans, I.H. *et al.* Erythropoiesis in Hodgkin's disease. *Br. J. Cancer* **40**: 365–70, 1979.
105. Blake, D.R., Scott, D.G., Eastham, E.J. & Rashid, J. Assessment of iron deficiency in rheumatoid arthritis. *Br. Med. J.* **280**: 527, 1980.
106. Davidson, A., van Der Weyden, M.B., Fong, H., Breidahl, M.J. & Ryan, P.F.J. Red cell ferritin content: a re-evaluation of indices for iron deficiency in the anaemia of rheumatoid arthritis. *Br. Med. J.* **289**: 648–50, 1984.
107. Freireich, E.J., Ross, J.F., Bayles, T.B., Emerson, C.P. & Finch, S.C. Radioactive iron metabolism and erythrocyte survival studies of the mechanism of the anemia associated with rheumatoid arthritis. *J. Clin. Invest.* **36**: 1043–58, 1957.

108. Lee, G.R. The anemia of chronic disorders. In *Clinical Haematology* (eds M. Wintrobe, G.R. Lee, D.R. Boggs *et al.*) pp. 646–53, 1981.
109. Cavill, I. & Bentley, D.P. Erythropoiesis in the anaemia of rheumatoid arthritis. *Br. J. Haematol.* **50**: 583–90, 1982.
110. Cavill, I. & Ricketts, C. Human iron kinetics. In *Iron in Biochemistry and Medicine* (eds A. Jacobs & M. Worwood) Vol. II, pp. 573–604. Academic Press, London and New York, 1980.
111. Hershko, C., Cook J.D. & Finch, C.A. Storage iron kinetics VI. The effect of inflammation on iron exchange in the rat. *Br. J. Haematol.* **28**: 67–75, 1974.
112. Boddy, K. & Will, G. Iron absorption in rheumatoid arthritis. *Ann. Rheum. Dis.* **28**: 537–40, 1969.
113. Pekarek, R.S., Bostian, K.A., Bartonelli, P.J., Calia, F.M. & Beisel, W.R. The effects of *Francisella tularensis* infection on iron metabolism in man. *Am. J. Med. Sci.* **258**: 14–25, 1969.
114. Giordano, N., Fioravanti, A., Sancasciani, S., Marcolongo, R. & Borghi, C. Increased storage of iron and anaemia in rheumatoid arthritis: usefulness of desferrioxamine. *Br. Med. J.* **289**: 961–2, 1984.
115. Freireich, E.J., Miller, A., Emerson, C.P. & Ross, J.F. The effect of inflammation on the utilization of erythrocyte and transferrin bound radioiron for red cell production. *Blood* **12**: 972–83, 1957.
116. Cavill, I., Ricketts, C. & Napier, J.A.F. Erythropoiesis in the anaemia of chronic disease. *Scand. J. Haematol.* **19**: 509–12, 1977.
117. Fillet, G., Cook J.D. & Finch, C.A. Storage iron kinetics VII. A biological model for reticuloendothelial iron transport. *J. Clin. Invest.* **53**: 1527–33, 1974.
118. Noyes, W.D., Bothwell, T.H. & Finch, C.A. The role of the reticuloendothelial cell in iron metabolism. *Br. J. Haematol.* **6**: 43–55, 1960.
119. Beamish, M.R., Davies, A.G., Eakins, J.D., Jacobs, A. & Trevett, D. The measurement of reticuloendothelial iron release using iron dextran. *Br. J. Haematol.* **21**: 617–22, 1971.
120. Davies, A.G., Beamish, M.R. & Jacobs, A. Utilisation of iron dextran. *Br. Med. J.* **1**: 146–7, 1971.
121. Williams, P., Cavill, I. & Kanakakorn, K. Iron kinetics and the anaemia of rheumatoid arthritis. *Rheumatol. Rehabilitation* **13**: 17–20, 1974.
122. Bentley, D.P., Cavill, I., Ricketts, C. & Peake, S. A method for the investigation of reticuloendothelial iron kinetics in man. *Br. J. Haematol.* **43**: 619–24, 1979.
123. Dinant, H.J. & de Maat, C.E.M. Erythropoiesis and mean red cell lifespan in normal subjects and in patients with the anaemia of active rheumatoid arthritis. *Br. J. Haematol.* **39**: 437–44, 1978.
124. Douglas, S.W. & Adamson, J.W. The anemia of chronic disorders: studies of marrow regulation and iron metabolism. *Blood* **45**: 55–65, 1975.
125. Williams, R.A., Samson, D., Tikerpae, J., Crowne, H. & Gumpel, J.M. *In vitro* studies of ineffective erythropoiesis in rheumatoid arthritis. *Ann. Rheum. Dis.* **41**: 502–7, 1982.
126. Dainiak, N., Hardin, J., Floyd, V., Callahan, M. & Hoffman, R. Humoral suppression of erythropoiesis in systemic lupus erythematosus (SLE) and rheumatoid arthritis. *Am. J. Med.* **69**: 537–44, 1980.
127. Reid, C.D.L., Prowse, P., Gumpel, J.M. & Chanarin, I. Suppression of *in vitro* erythropoiesis by serum in the anaemia of rheumatoid arthritis. *Br. J. Haematol.* **58**, 607–15, 1984.
128. Prouse, P.J., Harvey, A.R., Bonner, B., Reid, C.D.L., Ansell, B.M. & Gumpel, M. Anaemia in juvenile chronic arthritis: serum inhibition of normal erythropoiesis *in vitro*. *Ann. Rheum. Dis.* **46**: 127–34, 1987.
129. Zanjani, E.D., McGlave, P.B., Davies, S.F. *et al.* *In vitro* suppression of erythropoiesis by bone marrow adherent cells from some patients with fungal infection. *Br. J. Haematol.* **50**: 479–90, 1982.

130. Neta, R. & Oppenheim, J.J. (Editorial). Why should internists be interested in interleukin 1. *Ann. Int. Med.* **109**: 1–3, 1988.
131. Van Snick, J.L., Masson, P.L. & Heremans, J.F. The involvement of lactoferrin in the hyposideremia of acute inflammation. *J. Exp. Med.* **140**. 1068–84, 1974.
132. Konijn, A.M. & Hershko, C. Ferritin synthesis in inflammation I. Pathogenesis of impaired iron release. *Br. J. Haematol.* **37**: 7–16, 1977.
133. Stransbough, L.J. Haematologic manifestations of bacterial and fungal infections. *Haem./Oncology Clin. North Am.* **I**: 185–205, 1987.
134. Hershko, C., Peto, T.E.A., Weatherall, D.J. Iron and infection. *Br. Med. J.* **296**: 660–4, 1988.
135. Bentley, D.P. & Williams, P. Parenteral iron therapy in the anaemia of rheumatoid arthritis. *Rheumatol. Rehabilitation* **21**: 88–92, 1982.
136. Perrin, L.J., Mackey, L.J. & Miescher, P.A. The hematology of malaria in man. *Semin. Haematol.* **19**: 70–82, 1982.
137. Weatherall, D.J. & Abdalla, S. The anaemia of *Plasmodium falciparum* malaria. *Br. Med. Bull.* **38**: 147–51, 1982.
138. Savage D. & Lindenbaum, J. Anaemia in alcoholics. *Medicine* **65**: 322–38, 1986.
139. Wu, A., Chanarin, I. & Levi, A.J. Macrocytosis of chronic alcoholism. *Lancet* **I**: 829–30, 1974.
140. Editorial. Blood and alcohol. *Lancet* **I**: 397, 1983.
141. Chanarin, I. Haemopoiesis and alcohol. *Br. Med. Bull.* **38**: 81–6, 1982.
142. Larkin, E.C. & Watson-Williams, E.J. Alcohol and the blood. *Med. Clin. North Am.* **68**: 105–20, 1984.
143. Girard, D.E., Kumar, K.L. & McAfee, J.H. Hematologic effects of acute and chronic alcohol abuse. *Haematology/Oncology Clin.* **1**: 321–34, 1987.
144. Meagher, R.C., Sieber, F. & Spivak, J.L. Suppression of hematopoietic-progenitor-cell proliferation by ethanol and acetaldehyde. *N. Engl. J. Med.* **307**: 845–9, 1982.
145. Hillman, R.S. & Steinberg, J. The effects of alcohol on folate metabolism. *Ann. Rev. Med.* **33**: 345–54, 1982.

3

Polycythaemia in systemic disease

T.C. Pearson
Reader, United Medical and Dental Schools of Guy's and St Thomas's Hospitals, London, UK

D.F. Treacher
Consultant Physician, St Thomas's Hospital, London, UK

INTRODUCTION

The term polycythaemia may be used to apply to all patients who have a raised packed cell volume (PCV) demonstrated on two consecutive occasions on samples taken without venous occlusion. Since changes in PCV in the order of 0.02 occur as a result of diurnal, postural and post-prandial changes, samples should be taken under standard conditions – in the morning after a light breakfast with the patient in a sitting position.[1] Although there are some discrepancies in published normal PCV values, a PCV for a male above 0.51 and for a female above 0.48 may be regarded as raised. It must be appreciated, however, that these values represent the upper end of the 95% confidence limits and that by definition 2.5% of the normal population will have results above this level.

The definition of polycythaemia in terms of haemoglobin (Hb) value is inappropriate, since occasionally iron deficiency and its associated red cell changes of microcytosis and hypochromia may accompany the poly-cythaemia and under these circumstances the Hb value is disproportionately lower than the PCV. In this situation, the method of measurement of PCV is also important. Some electronic cell counters underestimate the true PCV when the mean corpuscular haemoglobin (MCH) is low. For this reason, the microhaematocrit has been suggested as the most reliable method when screening for polycythaemia and monitoring progress during treatment.[2] Although the trapped plasma in the microhaematocrit red cell column is higher at low MCH compared with normal red cell indices the difference is very small and for clinical practice the difference can be ignored.[3]

Measurement of red cell mass (RCM) and plasma volume (PV) should be performed in all patients with elevated PCV values to determine the changes in RCM and PV causing the raised PCV. In patients with palpable splenomegaly, significant splenic red cell pooling and PV expansion may occur. Hence an increase in RCM may be demonstrated when their peripheral blood PCV is within the normal range. Therefore, in patients with splenomegaly measurement of RCM and PV may be indicated at normal PCV values.

There are standard, well-established methods for measuring RCM and

PV,[4] although duplicate measurements in a single patient may show a variation of up to 5%.[5] The interpretation of the measured RCM and PV values is less standardized, although there is agreement about the limitations of expressing predicted normal and measured values in terms of millilitres per kilogram body weight. This particularly applies in obese individuals.[6,7] The use of both height and weight in predicting normal values improves precision, and for RCM gives estimates similar to those based on lean body mass.[7] Various formulae using both height and weight have been proposed and comparison of them has been made.[8] For RCM the 95% confidence limits have been given as 25% above and below the mean normal value for each height/weight combination. Thus, patients with a measured RCM greater than 25% above their mean predicted normal value may be regarded as having a raised RCM – an absolute polycythaemia.[8,9]

These patients may be further sub-divided on the basis of clinical and other laboratory findings. Those patients with a measured RCM falling within their normal range may be termed as having an 'apparent polycythaemia' with reservation of the term, 'relative polycythaemia', for those with a low measured PV. Unfortunately, the various prediction methods for PV give different mean normal values[8] and the lower limit of normal has been taken to be 12.5–20%[9,10] below the predicted mean value. Thus at the present time no precise definition of relative polycythaemia in terms of PV reduction can be given.

The general classification for patients with raised PCV values is given in Table 3.1. While this may provide a useful framework, the limitations of the measurements and their interpretation should not be overlooked and the clinician should retain a flexible approach, and an awareness of the possible evolution of a pathological process, in his investigation and management of the patient with a raised PCV.

Table 3.1   The Classification of Patients with Raised PCV Values

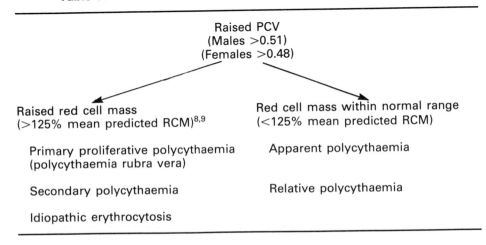

Raised PCV
(Males >0.51)
(Females >0.48)

Raised red cell mass
(>125% mean predicted RCM)[8,9]

Red cell mass within normal range
(<125% mean predicted RCM)

Primary proliferative polycythaemia
(polycythaemia rubra vera)

Apparent polycythaemia

Secondary polycythaemia

Relative polycythaemia

Idiopathic erythrocytosis

THE INVESTIGATION AND CLASSIFICATION OF THE ABSOLUTE POLYCYTHAEMIAS

A standard approach should be used when investigating patients with a raised RCM. Various algorithms have been published[11] but unless the cause of the polycythaemia is obvious, such an approach detracts from 'clinical' judgement. In addition, no allowance is given for the occasional finding of two completely different causes of an absolute polycythaemia in the same patient, or two contributory factors being responsible for the increased RCM.

From the history an underlying cause may be revealed. However, symptoms may arise from the primary pathology as well as from the polycythaemia. The particular features to enquire about include a history of vascular occlusion, bruising, bleeding, pruritus, gout, urinary tract and neurological symptoms. Special attention should be given to exercise tolerance, smoking history, alcohol intake and drug therapy. On examination any abnormal physical sign may be important but splenomegaly has particular relevance. Table 3.2 gives a list of investigations that may be performed. Stage 1 gives those which are non-invasive apart from a single

Table 3.2 Proposed Scheme for the Investigation of a Patient with an Absolute Polycythaemia

---

Stage 1: Initial investigations

  WBC and differential
  Neutrophil alkaline phosphatase
  Platelet count and morphology
  Serum iron and iron-binding capacity
  B_{12} (B_{12}-binding capacity)
  Serum/red cell folate
  Urea, creatinine and electrolytes
  Liver function tests
  Carboxyhaemoglobin level
  Arterial oxygen saturation
  Chest X-ray
  Renal ultrasound
  Urinalysis

Stage 2: Further investigations

  Intravenous urogram
  Oxygen dissociation curve
  Arterial oxygen saturation during sleep
  Isotopic spleen scan
  Liver scan
  Serum erythropoietin
  Erythroid colony growth from peripheral blood or marrow
  Abdominal CT scan
  CT scan of head
  Methaemoglobin level

---

venepuncture and should be performed in all patients. The oxygen saturation may be measured using an ear oximeter and the carboxy-haemoglobin level from a venous blood or an alveolar gas sample. Stage 2 gives further tests which are either less widely available or would only be performed if an indication to do them emerged from Stage 1.

The aim of the investigations is to establish whether in the first instance one of the many causes of secondary polycythaemia is present. These are listed in Table 3.3. In some cases it will be obvious that the patient has a secondary polycythaemia, for example due to a very low arterial oxygen sarturation (SaO_2) or due to a renal tumour. In many patients, however, the findings are less clear-cut. This particularly applies to the diagnosis of secondary hypoxic polycythaemia. A value for SaO_2 of 92% has been given as the value below which secondary hypoxic polycythaemia can be entertained.[12] Unfortunately, SaO_2 is not a steady value and a daytime saturation just above the lower limit of normal may be accompanied by significant desaturation during sleep. In addition, there are other factors influencing oxygen delivery to the renal oxygen sensor, such as raised carboxyhaemoglobin levels in smokers and renal blood flow. This is further discussed under the heading of 'Chronic lung disease' later in this chapter. In patients with symptoms suggestive of nocturnal oxygen desaturation, such as snoring, nocturnal restlessness and polyuria, early morning headache and daytime somnolence, a sleep study is indicated (Table 3.2; Stage 2). Some patients, who otherwise would have an unexplained absolute polycythaemia, will be found to have significant nocturnal arterial oxygen desaturation.[13]

Apart from the problems of the interpretation of individual investigations, another problem occasionally arises. This is where definite pathology is established, but its causal relationship to the polycythaemia cannot be confirmed. Examples of this problem would be the discovery of a renal cyst or mild renal impairment as the only abnormality emerging from the thorough investigation of an elderly patient with an absolute polycythaemia. This emphasizes the problems that may arise from the use of algorithms and the importance of careful evaluation of all the information available for each patient.

In patients without secondary polycythaemia clinical and laboratory features are examined to see whether they meet the criteria for a diagnosis of primary proliferative polycythaemia.[11] These are listed in Table 3.4. It has been argued that the term 'primary proliferative polycythaemia' (PPP) is preferable for these patients since it has greater descriptive validity than the term 'polycythaemia rubra vera', since it is now established that PPP is a clonal marrow proliferation involving the megakaryocytes as well as the granulopoietic and erythropoietic precursors.[14] Examination of Table 3.4 reveals the importance of the finding of splenomegaly. This has led some workers[15] to use isotopic scanning methods to complement clinical examination (Table 3.2; Stage 2). If there is experience in the interpretation of these scans, there is no doubt that this helps in the evaluation of polycythaemic patients. In the absence of splenomegaly (Table 3.4), other haematological findings are examined to lend support to the diagnosis of PPP. The limitation of using these parameters is that occasionally in secondary polycythaemia, for example in hypernephroma, reactive increases

Table 3.3   The Causes of Secondary Polycythaemia

Arterial hypoxaemia
  High altitude
  Cyanotic congenital heart disease
  Chronic lung disease
  Alveolar hypoventilation
  Pulmonary arterio-venous malformations

Other causes of impaired tissue oxygen delivery
  Smoking
  Congenital methaemoglobinaemia
  Congestive cardiac failure
  Increased Hb oxygen affinity
    Abnormal haemoglobin
    Congenital low 2,3-DPG
    Hereditary persistence of foetal Hb

Renal lesions
  Hypernephroma
  Wilms' tumour
  Cysts
  Diffuse renal parenchymal disease
  Hydronephrosis
  Bartter's syndrome
  Renal artery stenosis
  Renal transplantation

Hepatic lesions
  Hepatoma
  Cirrhosis
  Hepatitis
  Hepatic haemangiomata

Endocrine lesions
  Adrenal tumours
    Cushing's syndrome
    Conn's syndrome
    Phaeochromocytoma
    Thyroid disease

Miscellaneous tumours
  Cerebellar haemangioblastoma
  Uterine fibroids
  Ovarian tumours
  Cutaneous leiomyomata
  Bronchial carcinoma
  Argentaffinoma
  Parotid tumour
  Lymphoma

Drugs and chemicals
  Androgens
  Cobalt
  Nickel

Autonomous high erythropoietin production

Neonatal polycythaemia

in both white cells and platelets may be found. In addition, in a heavy smoker with alcoholic cirrhosis, an absolute polycythaemia may complicate the smoking and/or liver disease, and splenomegaly and raised B_{12} levels may be caused by the cirrhosis. Given the criteria in Table 3.4, a mistaken diagnosis of PPP may be reached.[11] On the other hand, patients in the early phase of evolution of PPP may not meet the requisite criteria. Initially these patients will be classified as idiopathic erythrocytosis, while the true nature of the underlying pathology will only emerge from a period of observation of the haematological parameters.[16]

One might expect that the measurement of serum erythropoietin levels would always be helpful in the differentiation of the various forms of polycythaemia. Unfortunately, there are two drawbacks: the measurement is not widely available at present and there is not always a clear distinction between the values obtained in PPP and those in secondary polycythaemia. In patients with PPP serum erythropoietin levels lie below or in the low normal range. Although some patients with secondary polycythaemia have raised or high values, many have normal results.[17] Despite these limitations, the measurement of serum erythropoietin is valuable in the evaluation of the individual patient with an absolute polycythaemia and in the small group of patients with autonomous high erythropoietin production it is essential for their diagnosis.

Although not widely available, another investigation that undoubtedly has a place in the characterization of polycythaemic patients is in the *in vitro* culture of erythroid colonies.[18] It has been shown that the red cell precursors of the clonal abnormality of PPP are hypersensitive to very small amounts of erythropoietin. Culture of the peripheral blood and bone marrow from patients with PPP has shown that in serum containing media, so-called endogenous or spontaneous erythroid colonies grow without any additional erythropoietin.[19-22] This observation has recently been extended to serum-free media.[23,24] Although more widespread experience needs to be gained in the use of these cultures, it currently appears that endogenous erythroid colony growth is found in nearly all patients who meet the more routine

Table 3.4   Criteria for the Establishment of a Diagnosis of Primary Proliferative Polycythaemia in Patients Without Secondary Polycythaemia

---

Increased RCM + splenomegaly

In the absence of splenomegaly, two of the following three criteria must be met:

1. Platelet count $> 400 \times 10^9$ per litre

2. Leucocytosis $> 12.0 \times 10^9$ per litre
     (no fever or infection)

3. Raised neutrophil alkaline phosphatase score
     (no fever or infection)
     or Raised serum B_{12} (> 900 ng/litre)
     or Unbound B_{12}-binding capacity (> 2200 ng/litre)

Adapted from Ref. 11

criteria of PPP but not in patients with secondary polycythaemia. This investigation is therefore useful in distinguishing between the two forms of polycythaemia, particularly in doubtful cases.[18]

Following detailed investigation, a group of patients emerge where a cause of polycythaemia cannot be established but neither do they have features to fulfil the criteria of PPP. These account for up to one-third of patients presenting with an absolute polycythaemia.[10] The term 'idiopathic erythrocytosis' may be used for this group, although the terms 'benign'[25] and 'pure'[26] erythrocytosis have also been used. The patients within the group are undoubtedly heterogenous. Up to a quarter of them will develop additional haematological features to enable a diagnosis of PPP to be made during the years of follow-up.[16] In some, a cause of secondary poly-cythaemia is found or becomes clinically overt later, while the majority remain for the time being a group with unexplained erythrocytosis. In a few individuals with a measured RCM just above the upper limit of normal, it must be appreciated that they may represent the end of the normal RCM distribution curve.

THE CLASSIFICATION OF INDIVIDUALS WITH A RAISED PCV AND NORMAL RCM: APPARENT AND RELATIVE POLYCYTHAEMIA

As described previously, the typical features of these patients are an increased PCV with a normal measured RCM. The other terms that have been used to describe these patients include 'Geisbock's syndrome', 'spurious', 'pseudo-' and 'stress polycythaemia'.[27–30] While some members of the group probably represent individuals at one extreme of the normal distribution curve, others have a PCV significantly above their normal value. The assumption that all these patients have a low PV that was made when simple millilitre per kilogram expressions were used is certainly untrue. Using height/weight predictions, it has been shown that some patients have a measured RCM in the high normal range, others have a low PV, while the remainder have a normal PV with a RCM well within the normal range.[10]

All patients who develop an absolute polycythaemia must pass through a phase where their measured RCM is raised compared with their normal value but still within the wide normal range for each height–weight combination. In these patients any of the causes of secondary polycythaemia may be found. This is an important concept since it underlines the value of thorough investigation of all patients with raised PCV values even if the measured RCM falls within their normal range. There are no published studies of the incidence of positive findings in these patients and the safe approach is to complete as a minimum the investigations given in Table 3.2 Stage 1 in all patients.

Some patients with a raised PCV and normal RCM definitely have a reduced PV, although as discussed earlier the normal range for PV is poorly defined; for these patients the term 'relative polycythaemia' should be reserved. In many clinical situations a cause of a low PV will be obvious from the clinical setting, such as dehydration from diarrhoea, vomiting or excess diuretic therapy, but in most cases the cause will remain obscure.[31]

CONSIDERATIONS OF OXYGEN DELIVERY AND RHEOLOGY IN THE POLYCYTHAEMIAS

Overall oxygen delivery to the tissues (OD) will vary with changes in cardiac output (Qt), haemoglobin concentration (Hb) and arterial oxygen saturation (SaO_2), which in turn will be determined by arterial oxygen tension (PaO_2) and the position/shape of the oxygen dissociation curve.

$$\begin{array}{ccccc} \text{OD} & = SaO_2 \times \dot{Q}t & & \times \text{ Hb concentration} \times 1.39^* \times 10^{-2} \\ \text{(ml/min)} & \text{(\%)} & \text{(litres/min)} & \text{(g/litre)} & \text{(ml/g)} \end{array}$$

* 1.39 represents the theoretical volume of oxygen in millilitres that would combine with 1 g of Hb when 100% saturated with oxygen.

In conditions that affect any one of these variables, compensatory changes will occur in the others to maintain an adequate oxygen delivery. Regional variations in blood flow and oxygen delivery may result from changes in vasomotor tone, induced centrally or by local factors (hypoxia, metabolites) or arise due to other local influences such as atheroma.

Interrelationship between OD and PaO_2/SaO_2

The shape of the oxyhaemoglobin dissociation curve dictates that an increase in PaO_2 above 60 mm Hg (8 kPa) cannot achieve any significant improvement in arterial oxygen content although a fall below these levels will lead to a significant reduction in oxygen saturation and hence OD. A shift in the oxyhaemoglobin dissociation curve has mixed benefits in terms of oxygen delivery to the tissues as a response to hypoxaemia. Although a rightward shift in the curve results in a lower SaO_2 for a given PaO_2 and favours oxygen unloading in the non-pulmonary tissues, oxygen loading in the pulmonary capillaries will be reduced. A leftward shift will enhance oxygen uptake in the lungs in the presence of alveolar hypoxaemia but tissue OD will be impaired. Therefore, the overall effect on oxygen availability to the tissues resulting from a change in P_{50} will depend on the precise shape of the oxygen dissociation curve and the relative alveolar and tissue oxygen tensions. This point is illustrated by the differing responses of different groups of high-altitude dwellers discussed later.

Interrelationship between OD and cardiac output

An increase in cardiac output occurs with reduction of SaO_2, as demonstrated following ascent to high altitude[32] and in patients with severe lung disease.[33] However, the response of increasing cardiac output to compensate for the effects of arterial hypoxaemia is limited. Despite the small fall in systemic vascular resistance observed with hypoxaemia, any significant increase in flow requires increased left ventricular work in the presence of a reduced oxygen content of the coronary arterial blood. There will be an even greater increase in right ventricular work, since unlike the systemic vascular bed, pulmonary vascular resistance (PVR) increases with hypoxaemia. Expansion of the blood volume, as found in the absolute polycythaemias, will increase both cardiac output and OD due to the passive dilatation of the arteriolar beds reducing systemic and pulmonary vascular resistances.

Interrelationships between OD and Hb concentration

An increase in Hb is the predominant long-term adaptation to maintain OD in hypoxaemia since the increase in cardiac output is generally a short-term adaptation, except when increased erythropoiesis is not possible as in chronic anaemia. Although beneficial in terms of increased oxygen-carrying capacity, an increase in Hb and PCV may have a deleterious effect on overall and particularly regional OD due to the increase in viscosity limiting blood flow. In deciding on the appropriate balance it must be remembered that oxygen content rises linearly with Hb concentration while blood viscosity increases exponentially with the rise in PCV.

Interrelationship between OD and blood viscosity

As a non-Newtonian fluid, the viscosity of blood depends on the shearing forces applied to it. Blood viscosity is lowest at high shear rates (greater than 100/s), and as shear rate falls below this level there is an exponential increase in viscosity. For a constant perfusion pressure, the flow achieved is given by Poiseuille's law:

$$\text{Flow} \propto \frac{\pi r^4}{\eta l}$$

where r = vessel radius, l = vessel length, η = viscosity. For *in vitro* situations, this relationship predicts a reduction in flow with increasing viscosity. However, *in vivo* under physiological conditions, blood viscosity is lower than that found *in vitro* and flow is not determined by viscosity. The reasons for these observations are many. In larger arteries flow is determined by inertial (product of mean flow velocity and vessel diameter) not viscous forces. Axial migration of red cells occurring during flow gives a relatively cell-free plasma zone with low viscosity at the walls and a lower PCV in the smaller vessels. *In vivo*, flow can readily be improved by vasodilation as predicted by Poiseuille's formula, and thereby compensate for any increased blood viscosity. However, in pathological conditions when the vasodilator response is maximal or limited by vessel disease, flow may be determined by the blood viscosity, particularly in situations when the perfusion pressure is globally or locally reduced. The level of blood viscosity may then become the critical factor in determining flow and oxygen delivery.[34–36] In addition, in the hypoxic polycythaemias, pulmonary vasoconstriction and the increased blood viscosity further increase PVR.[37,38]

Studies on the cerebral circulation in the different forms of polycythaemia illustrate that flow is determined by OD rather than viscosity. In untreated patients with PPP, idiopathic erythrocytosis and both apparent and relative polycythaemia cerebral blood flow (CBF) is low but returns to normal on reduction of the PCV to normal.[39,40] In patients with a mutant high oxygen affinity Hb, CBF is very high despite increased PCV and blood viscosity.[41] Thus changes in CBF occur to maintain a constant cerebral oxygen transport.[42] However, as suggested earlier, cerebral ischaemia may occur in untreated polycythaemic patients due to local vessel disease and in this situation an improvement in symptoms often occurs on PCV reduction.[40,43]

The clinical impact of a raised PCV depends not only on the level of the PCV but also on the underlying cause, any associated conditions and the particular region of the body under consideration. Nonetheless the cardiovascular implications and the definite increase in the incidence of vascular occlusive events with increasing PCV[44-47] provide the rationale for the investigation and treatment of such patients.

CONTROL OF BLOOD VOLUME, PLASMA VOLUME AND RED CELL MASS

The blood volume may be regarded as a volume of fluid contained in an essentially closed pumping system with elastic pipes. The contained volume influences every facet of circulatory performance. The flows around the circuit depend ultimately upon the balance between the work generated by each side of the heart and the resistance faced by each ventricle; volume is a major determinant of both the work generated and resistance.

The work generated is a function of the active muscle mass of the heart and its inotropic state on the one hand, and the filling pressure to which it is charged during diastole on the other. The filling pressure of each side of the heart is the resultant of the wall tone of the systemic or pulmonary capacity vessels and their contained volume.

The resistance to flow offered by the systemic and pulmonary vascular beds depends upon viscosity and vessel diameter. Vessel diameter depends not only on vascular tone, but also and most importantly upon the volume of the incompressible fluid within the vessels.

A variety of homeostatic mechanisms control the body's fluid intake and output and hence the volume of fluid contained within the circulation. The neuro-endocrine system, acting through the vasomotor centre in the brainstem and the autonomic nervous system, controls sympathetic and parasympathetic tone and adrenaline and noradrenaline release, thereby regulating myocardial contractility and arteriolar and venular tone. Control of salt and water balance is achieved by the renin–angiotensin–aldosterone system, antidiuretic hormone (ADH) released from the posterior pituitary and the recently identified atrial natriuretic peptide (ANP) released from the right and left cardiac atria. The sensors in this system are the aortic and carotid baroreceptors, osmoreceptors in the hypothalamus, the juxta-glomerular apparatus in the kidney and the cardiac atria responding to changes in atrial filling pressures. The position of these sensors in the high and low pressure systems of the cardiovascular system, in the central nervous system and in the kidney permits a delicate control to be achieved. In concert this system represents a series of interacting negative feedback loops which controls blood volume, cardiac output, arterial perfusion pressure and renal blood flow. Supratentorial influences such as stress/anxiety may interact with this control system.

The recent demonstration of ANP in granules in the walls of the cardiac atria and its release in response to volume loading[48] has provided the explanation of the natriuretic response to intravenous saline infusion that occurs without change in renal haemodynamics or aldosterone level. ANP increases renal blood flow despite reducing systemic vascular resistance and mean arterial pressure[49] and has an inhibitory effect on the renin/aldosterone system causing a significant reduction in aldosterone levels.[50]

Many physiological and pathological factors affect this control mechanism. Blood volume is increased in pregnancy, following prolonged exercise, in cirrhosis, congestive cardiac failure and in PPP, whereas changing position from lying to standing, long-term recumbency and short-term exercise will reduce blood volume. Acute changes in blood volume other than that caused by acute haemorrhage or transfusion must result from changes in PV and hence PCV, since humans cannot acutely alter the circulating RCM.

A reduced PV may result from dehydration (increased fluid loss, reduced intake, excess diuretic therapy), increase in capillary leakage (septicaemia, anaphylaxis, severe burns), reduced osmotic pressure (nephrotic syndrome, liver disease) or due to loss to an extracellular extra vascular space (ascites, peripheral oedema). In addition, PV reduction may be due to a primary contraction of the vascular space as is found with the hypoxaemia of high altitude and phaeochromocytoma where the persistent high levels of catecholamines produce a small volume circulation with increased peripheral resistance and the initially increased filling pressures, arterial pressures, cardiac output and renal blood flow secondarily reduce PV.

Much remains to be discovered about the factors that determine and maintain RCM within close limits. In the adult, the majority of erythropoietin (Epo) is released from the kidney but small amounts are found in the liver, which is the major site of foetal production. Epo acts on committed erythroid precursors to increase protein synthesis, the rate of cell division and the speed of cell transit through the marrow. Other hormones, including corticosteroids, androgens, growth hormone and thyroxine may all affect erythropoiesis, but the central role of Epo and its major site of origin is emphasized by the anaemia found in anephric patients and the use of recombinant Epo to treat the anaemia of chronic renal failure.[51]

Tissue hypoxia appears to be the stimulus for Epo production and release. The precise site of the renal sensor is unknown although recent work suggests the peritubular capillary endothelial cells of the cortex or outer medulla.[52] With its high oxygen delivery (up to 25% of cardiac output) which is considerably in excess of its own requirements, the kidney is an ideal site for a sensor mechanism since it will be sensitive to relatively small changes in oxygen delivery without being influenced by fluctuations in its own metabolism and oxygen consumption. The exact mechanism by which tissue hypoxia acts on the renal sensor is uncertain, but it seems to be unrelated to mitochondrial energy metabolism, since unlike the carotid body, the response of the renal sensor to hypoxia is not cyanide-sensitive. The current postulate is that the tissue hypoxia results in ATP depletion leading to loss of the intracellular ionic homeostasis, in particular for calcium, and this in turn leads to an increase in prostacyclin with subsequent activation of protein kinase, leading to erythropoietin biosynthesis and release.[53,54]

It seems probable that the control mechanisms described would be adequate to adjust PV, RCM and hence overall blood volume to achieve an optimum tissue oxygen delivery in the face of various physiological and pathological conditions. It is clearly important that any interpretation of RCM and in particular of PV should be made with a clear understanding of the various integrated homeostatic mechanisms that operate, and with due consideration to the effects of drug therapy and any coexisting disease processes on these control mechanisms.

THE CLINICAL FEATURES OF PRIMARY PROLIFERATIVE POLYCYTHAEMIA AND IDIOPATHIC ERYTHROCYTOSIS

Primary proliferative polycythaemia

Only a summary of the clinical features and treatment of primary proliferative polycythaemia (PPP) will be given. PPP is a clonal myeloproliferative disorder,[14] which presents at a median age of approximately 60 years with a slight male predominance. Between one-third and one-half of the patients present with vascular complications – equally divided between the venous and arterial parts of the circulation.[55] The arterial occlusive lesions may be divided into two types – larger vessel and microvascular. Although the larger vessel occlusion may occur anywhere in the circulation, the cerebral vessels appear to be at particular risk.[45,56] The microvascular occlusive lesions and symptoms, which are almost certainly due to the thrombocythaemic component of PPP, occur in the digits, typically the toes, but may affect the cerebral circulation.[55,57] Venous occlusion is more common in the superficial veins but may occur in 'deep' veins, with pulmonary embolization being an occasional further complication.[55]

The cause of the high incidence of vascular occlusive episodes in PPP is certainly multifactorial. Factors involved include the increased blood viscosity, quantitative and qualitative platelet changes, reduction in blood flow and increased platelet–vessel wall interactions at raised PCV values.[39,58,59]

Excessive bruising or bleeding following trauma, but rarely spontaneously may occur[60] and is due mostly to abnormal platelet function. Haemorrhage from peptic ulceration may paradoxically lead to presentation with an iron-deficiency anaemia, although peptic ulceration per se is probably no more common than in an age-matched population.[61]

Other symptoms and methods of presentation include pruritus, characteristically induced by contact with water and heat and gout.

The median survival of patients with PPP is in the order of 9–14 years.[11,62] Management is aimed at adequate control of the peripheral blood count to minimize the vascular occlusive risk.[45,63] The therapeutic measures include venesection, low- or high-dose intermittent chemotherapy, and [32]P. There is a higher incidence of acute leukaemia in PPP than the normal population, but this risk is further increased by the use of ^{32}P and high-dose chemotherapy.[11,64] Myelofibrosis may be regarded as the 'natural' haemato-logical end-stage of PPP and usually takes a considerable time to develop and thus is only seen in some 15% of patients.[62]

Idiopathic erythrocytosis

As for primary proliferative polycythaemia (PPP) only a brief outline of the clinical features of idiopathic erythrocytosis (IE) will be given. These patients probably do not represent a single pathological entity. The age distribution is similar to PPP with a male predominance.[16,25,26] Presentation with larger vessel occlusion of either arteries or veins is most common. Haemorrhagic manifestations are not found and up to 20% of patients are asymptomatic at presentation.[16] The precise indications for treatment in patients with IE have not been established. However, high PCV values are associated with an increased incidence of vascular occlusion.[16,26,61]

Thus the limited evidence would suggest that patients with PCV >0.51, should be treated to reduce their PCV to 0.45. Other risk factors such as hypertension should also be treated. Venesection is the treatment of choice since acute leukaemic transformation has been observed in these patients when either ^{32}P or chemotherapeutic agents have been used.[25,26] To establish the precise role of venesection in the management of patients with IE, they have been included in a prospective trial which also involves patients with relative and apparent polycythaemia.[65] The length of survival of patients with IE has not been satisfactorily established but is likely to be similar to PPP. During the first few years of follow-up, up to 25% of them develop additional haematological features, which enable them to be re-classified as PPP.[16]

PATHOGENESIS AND CLINICAL FEATURES OF THE SECONDARY, APPARENT AND RELATIVE POLYCYTHAEMIAS

Arterial hypoxaemia

High altitude

High altitude is usually regarded as 3000 m or more above sea-level since ascent to these levels produces physiological changes and characteristic symptoms and signs in the majority of sea-level dwellers.[66] The physio-logical changes that occur with the ascent to high altitude are a response to the progressive fall in the partial pressure of oxygen in the ambient air (Table 3.5), but the nature and extent of these changes depend on the rate of ascent and the length of time the subject stays at high altitudes. Furthermore there are important differences between the sea-level dweller who ascends to high altitude and the chronic mountain dweller who was born and lived all his life at high altitude.

For the normal subject it will only be at altitudes above 3000 m that the fall in alveolar oxygen tension will produce a fall in PaO_2 to less than 60 mm Hg and hence result in significant oxygen desaturation. Arterial

Table 3.5 Relationship Between Altitude, Barometric Pressure and Partial Pressures of Oxygen in Ambient Air and Alveolar Gas Saturated With Water Vapour (47 mm Hg; 6.3 kPa) With Assumed Values for Alveolar CO_2 Pressure

Altitude	Barometric pressure mm Hg (kPa)	Oxygen pressure mm Hg (kPa)		Assumed alveolar CO_2 pressure mm Hg (kPa)
		Ambient air	Alveolar	
Sea-level	760	159	116	40
	(101)	(21.2)	(15.5)	(5.3)
3000 m	530	111	75	34
(10,000 ft)	(71)	(14.8)	(10.0)	(4.5)
6000 m	340	71	40	30
(20,000 ft)	(45)	(9.5)	(5.3)	(4.0)

Adapted from Ref. 67.

hypoxaemia results in increased pulmonary ventilation due to a rise in both respiratory rate and tidal volume. The resulting respiratory alkalosis causes a shift in the oxygen dissociation curve to the left, producing a higher arterial oxygen saturation for any given value of arterial oxygen tension. The extent of this shift is limited by an increase in 2,3-DPG which occurs within 24 h.[68,69]

Initially there is an increase in cardiac output and basal oxygen uptake increases due to the increased energy requirements for ventilation.[70] If the individual remains at high altitude pulmonary ventilation falls somewhat but remains higher than at sea-level. The cardiac output, however, gradually falls to a level below that at sea-level.[71] After prolonged exposure to altitude and hypoxia, the maximal oxygen uptake is reduced due to a limit in cardiac output possibly related to the increase in pulmonary vascular resistance.[72]

The changes in haemoglobin (Hb) and PCV that occur on ascent to high altitude are due to changes in both RCM and PV. The early increase in Hb level which stabilizes early is mainly due to a reduction in PV. There is evidence[73] that this change in PV is at least in part mediated by changes in ANP level by the mechanism discussed earlier. However, the continued hypoxic stimulus to erythropoiesis leads to an increase in RCM and an increase in blood volume.[74]

The increase in oxygen-carrying capacity that is achieved by the increased Hb value is greater than the reduction in maximum cardiac output. Thus a rise in Hb is advantageous in terms of oxygen delivery and hence in increasing work capacity at high altitude.[75] However, in a small group of mountaineers the effect of isovolaemic haemodilution with reduction of the PCV from 0.58 to 0.51 was shown not to influence the maximum work level, although a small improvement in mental performance was observed.[62] As in the polycythaemia of chronic lung disease discussed later, it may be that an excessive increase in Hb and PCV occurs in certain individuals and is disadvantageous.

The increased PCV, dehydration, and, in bad weather, enforced inactivity are predisposing factors to thrombosis[66] and both cerebral thrombosis and venous thrombosis with pulmonary embolization have been recorded in mountaineers.[74]

Chronic mountain dwellers.   The Amerindians of Peru and the Sherpas of Tibet are two groups of chronic mountain dwellers that have been fairly extensively studied. Interestingly both groups probably originate from mongoloid stock.[66] Characteristic changes occur in the heart, lungs and carotid bodies of these individuals. The vital capacity of the lungs is increased due to an increase in alveolar space. The changes in the internal surface area of the lung with increased pulmonary capillary volume account for the improved pulmonary diffusion with reduced alveolar–arterial O_2 gradient that is observed.[67] Arterial hypoxaemia will initially produce pulmonary vasoconstriction but subsequently thickening of the muscular layer of the pulmonary arteries and arterioles occurs. Together with the increase in PCV this results in an increased pulmonary vascular resistance and right ventricular hypertrophy.

It is of note that the changes in Hb and PCV values are different in the Sherpas and Amerindians. While the latter develop a marked increase in Hb and PCV values (up to 20 g/dl and 0.60 respectively) and a right-shifted dissociation curve (P_{50} approximately 33 mm Hg, 4.4 kPa), the Sherpas have only a modest increase in the haemoglobin (16 g/dl) and a left-shifted oxygen dissociation curve (P_{50} approximately 22 mm Hg, 2.9 kPa) due to slightly reduced 2,3-DPG levels.[66,77,78] Since chronic mountain sickness does not seem to occur in Sherpas, it has been suggested that their haematological adaptation is more beneficial than that seen in the Amerindians. This may be explained by the fact that the Sherpas have spent several hundred thousand years longer at high altitude and that evolutionary, genetic changes have occurred over that period.[78] This is supported by the fact that haematological changes seen in the Sherpas are similar to those observed in animals such as the llamas and vicunas that live at high altitude.[66] The fact that a left shift in oxygen dissociation curve is beneficial at high altitudes is supported by the observation that individuals with Hb Andrew–Minneapolis, a high oxygen affinity Hb (P_{50} 17 mm Hg, 2.3 kPa), could exercise with less cardiovascular disturbance at low oxygen pressures than their siblings with HbA.[79]

Another additional adaptation found in animals indigenous to high altitude is an increase in the capillary bed, with an almost 50% increase in the number of open muscle capillaries compared to the number seen at low altitude.[80] This both increases the blood perfusion to a given volume of tissue and reduces the mean distance for oxygen to diffuse from the capillary to the mitochondria in the cells, and results in an increased rate of oxygen diffusion to the tissues despite the lower oxygen tension of the arterial blood.[81] Among natives to high altitude there is also an increase in muscle myoglobin concentration and this further enhances oxygen diffusion.[82]

Chronic mountain disase (Monge's disease).   A small number of people living in the Andes develop chronic mountain sickness.[84,85] Affected individuals are typically males between 25 and 45 years and they complain of headaches, somnolence, dizziness and reduced exercise tolerance. Examination reveals cyanosis, clubbing, conjunctival congestion, nail haemorrhages and evidence of pulmonary hypertension.[66] These Amerindians have excessive polycythaemia with PCV values in the order of 0.80 with a greatly increased blood volume. Their SaO_2 is significantly lower than unaffected colleagues (69% compared to 81%[84]) and the pulmonary hypertension is more severe. Marked right ventricular hypertrophy with the development of right ventricular overload and peripheral oedema occurs in a manner analogous to the patient with irreversible obstructive airways disease and associated chronic hypoxaemia who develops the clinical picture of cor pulmonale.

The cause of chronic mountain sickness is thought to be alveolar hypoventilation although the precise cause is not fully established. A loss of sensitivity of the respiratory centre to carbon dioxide[83] or reduced sensitivity of the peripheral chemoreceptors to hypoxia,[66] both resulting in a reduction of respiratory drive, have been proposed. Nocturnal hypoventilation with exacerbation of pulmonary hypertension as well as smoking and additional underlying lung pathology such as pneumoconiosis may also be factors in certain individuals.[85,86]

The treatment of chronic mountain sickness is relatively simple. Affected individuals should be moved to a lower altitude and after a couple of months the haematological changes reverse and the pulmonary artery pressure falls.[84,87] For the individual that stays at high altitude, two other therapeutic measures have been tried. Isovolaemic venesection does seem to be effective and increases SaO_2 apparently by improving the matching of ventilation to perfusion.[88,89] The stimulation of respiration during sleep using medroxyprogesterone has also been demonstrated to improve SaO_2.[85]

Cyanotic congenital heart disease

In cyanotic congenital heart disease (CCHD) an abnormal structure or connection between right- and left-sided cardiac structures results in the admixture of desaturated systemic venous blood with fully saturated pulmonary venous blood. The degree of arterial hypoxaemia resulting from such extra-pulmonary 'shunting' will be determined by the relative flows through the normal pulmonary vasculature and the abnormal right to left shunt. The direction of flow through such an abnormal connection will depend on the pressures in the relevant structures and this will frequently result in a left to right shunt initially (acyanotic CHD, e.g. atrial or ventricular septal defects). However, with the development of secondary pulmonary vascular disease (Eisenmenger reaction) or in the presence of pulmonary arterial or valvular stenosis (e.g. Fallot's tetralogy), the right-sided pressures exceed the left-sided pressures resulting in a right to left shunt and the development of arterial hypoxaemia. Obviously the patients involved are usually children and lengthy survival into adulthood is unusual in lesions that are not corrected surgically.

The most severely affected patients have markedly increased haemoglobin and PCV values (up to 0.80) and very high levels of Epo have been recorded.[90] Overall a significant negative correlation exists between SaO_2 and RCM. Although the PV remains normal or even falls as the RCM rises, the total blood volume increases due to the rise in RCM and values of blood volume up to twice normal have been reported.[91]

Patients with CCHD may complain of headache, 'muzziness' and impaired concentration; these symptoms may be attributable to the polycythaemia since marked improvement may occur when the PCV is reduced.[92]

In view of the extremely high blood viscosity resulting from the high PCV levels found in these patients, it is not surprising that thromboembolic and ischaemic complications are relatively common. The cerebral and pulmonary circulations are the commonest sites for thrombosis, and one study showed that at post mortem, 20% of patients had a thrombosis of a cerebral vessel.[93] Cerebral arterial occlusion may occur due to in situ thrombosis or as a result of paradoxical embolization from the systemic venous circulation.[93,94] Spontaneous cerebral venous thrombosis also occurs and appears to be as common as arterial thrombosis.[95] The high blood viscosity and low pulmonary blood flow predispose to pulmonary thrombosis which is frequently found at post-mortem examination, particularly in cases of Fallot's tetralogy.[96]

The level of PCV at which the benefits of an increased oxygen-carrying capacity are off-set by the increased blood viscosity is debated. Isovolaemic reduction of PCV from 0.73 to 0.62[97] and from 0.66 to 0.58[92] reduced pulmonary vascular resistance and increased stroke volume and cardiac output, with no change in PaO_2. Exercise tests performed several days later showed an increased oxygen uptake and reduced oxygen debt compared to the baseline results.[92] A reduction in PCV may also improve regional flow in these patients if cerebral ischaemic symptoms occur.[98,99] The overall evidence would suggest that in cases of severe polycythaemia, reduction of PCV is beneficial but the optimum level of PCV cannot be precisely stated since the individual circumstances often vary significantly.

Venesection prior to surgery has been shown to improve the reduced platelet counts and coagulation factor levels found in some patients, and results in significantly lower peri-operative blood loss.[100] Operations on patients with CCHD may be performed with the heart arrested under hypothermic conditions. In this situation the marked rise in viscosity that occurs at low temperatures, particularly at high PCV values, may contribute to the surgical morbidity and mortality.[101–103]

During venesection in these patients it is important to maintain the blood volume since any significant fall may seriously compromise cardiac output and oxygen delivery. No more than 300 ml should be removed as an outpatient procedure, and when volumes over 500 ml are removed the replacement fluid should have a suitable oncotic pressure, e.g. PPF, dextran.

With chronic venesection, and occasionally even before therapeutic intervention, the red cell changes of iron deficiency occur and it is important to monitor PCV rather than Hb in these patients.[104] Provided the PCV is appropriately measured, blood with microcytic hypochromic red cells has the same viscosity at the same PCV as blood with normal red cells.[105,106] Microhaematocrit measurement of the PCV should be used since some electronic counters underestimate the true PCV at reduced MCH values.[2]

The fall in MCHC/MCH occurring with iron deficiency will reduce the Hb and oxygen-carrying capacity.[106] Iron therapy combined with venesection can increase Hb for the same PCV and blood viscosity and this may improve cerebral symptoms in some patients.[107] However, only small doses of iron should be used and the PCV monitored carefully since it may rise quite steeply.

Chronic lung disease

A wide variety of pulmonary conditions may cause arterial hypoxaemia and result in the development of secondary polycythaemia. The commonest and most widely studied condition is chronic irreversible obstructive airways disease (COAD), embracing both chronic bronchitis and emphysema, which frequently coexist since smoking is almost invariably the predominant aetiological factor. However, advanced forms of restrictive lung disease such as pulmonary fibrosis and kyphoscoliosis may result in hypoxia and an increased drive to erythropoiesis.

To exclude hypoxaemia as a cause of polycythaemia it is important to measure oxygen saturation (SaO_2) directly as well as arterial oxygen tension (PaO_2),[108] particularly in subjects who may be smokers where an oxygen saturation derived from the oxygen tension would be inaccurate. Furthermore, a single daytime assessment may be misleading since the desaturation may be far more severe with exercise and during sleep. A level of SaO_2 below 92% has been suggested as the critical level below which secondary polycythaemia develops.[12] This corresponds to a PaO_2 of between 60 and 65 mm Hg, and lies at the top of the steep part of the oxygen dissociation curve.

Taking a large group of patients an inverse relationship can be shown between RCM and SaO_2,[109-111] but there is a very wide scatter and some individuals do not show the expected erythropoietic response.[112-114] It is also important to consider influences on the plasma volume rather than examining the RCM alone when considering the cause of a raised PCV in these patients. Normally the PV is within the normal range or slightly reduced in these patients[110] but occasionally the plasma volume is expanded,[109] particularly in the presence of cardiac failure.[110] Very occasionally the RCM may be normal and a raised PCV is due to a significant reduction in PV even in the absence of diuretic therapy. Therefore, the patient with hypoxic chronic lung disease may develop absolute, apparent and very occasionally relative polycythaemia due to the variety of influences on both RCM and PV.

The factors involved in the erythropoietic response to the reduced SaO_2 include variation in SaO_2 within the individual patient, other influences on arterial oxygen carriage and delivery, renal blood flow and the response of the renal sensor, and finally the erythropoietic response of the marrow. Attention has focused on the diurnal variation of SaO_2, particularly the reduction that may occur during sleep.[111,114,115] At the low PaO_2 of these patients the observed scatter in P_{50} values probably does not influence oxygen delivery.[116] Smoking increases the carbon monoxide level of the blood, and since carbon monoxide has a higher affinity for Hb than oxygen, a proportion of the Hb becomes unavailable for oxygen transport. Carboxyhaemoglobin also shifts the oxygen dissociation curve to the left and alters its shape.[117] The severity of secondary polycythaemia in chronic lung disease has been shown to be related to smoking.[118] Renal blood flow is influenced by polycythaemia[119,120] and intracellular changes occur as a result of hypoxia.[121] Relative changes in these factors may influence the response of the renal sensor to the hypoxaemia in the individual patient. The serum erythropoietin (Epo) levels are variable and some patients do not have levels outside the normal range.[115]

Significant reduction of the PCV results in an increase in Epo levels even in those patients with values falling within the normal range before treatment.[115] Failure of the marrow erythropoietic response has been shown despite increased Epo.[112] The reason for this is not clear but chronic infection suppressing erythropoietic activity,[122] reduced testosterone levels, which may be seen in severely hypoxic male patients,[123] as well as iron and folate deficiency, may play a part.

Chronic arterial hypoxaemia, particularly when associated with hypercapnia, increases the cardiac output and reduces systemic vascular resistance. The pulmonary vascular bed, however, responds to hypoxaemia by vasoconstriction, resulting in an increased pulmonary vascular resistance and pulmonary hypertension which may in turn lead to right ventricular hypertrophy and the development of right ventricular overload and a clinical picture of cor pulmonale. Structural changes in the pulmonary vascular bed with muscularization of the pulmonary arterioles and destruction of part of the vasculature, especially in emphysema, also occurs.[124] Additionally, an increased blood viscosity due to polycythaemia also contributes to the increase in pulmonary vascular resistance.[38,125]

Drug therapy designed to exert a primary influence on the pulmonary vasculature might, as a secondary effect ameliorate the polycythaemia. Various drugs, including almitrine, nifedipine and verapamil, have been used to reduce pulmonary vasconstriction and do so by 15–20%.[126,127] In the rat hypoxic model, verapamil has also been shown to reduce the PCV and RCM[128] but the limited human experiments have not shown a consistent fall in RCM.[129]

Domiciliary long-term oxygen therapy given for up to two-thirds of the day for some months has been shown to improve the morbidity and prognosis.[130,131] Unfortunately patients with severe respiratory failure (PaO_2 < 45 mm Hg, < 6.0 kPa) are the least likely to benefit.[126] However, in patients with less severe lung disease, oxygen therapy has been shown to lower the PCV and whole-blood viscosity. In individual patients there is a fall in pulmonary vascular resistance[132] and overall, treated patients do not show the rise seen in the control subjects.[131]

Reduction of the PCV can be achieved by venesection, erythrapheresis or drug therapy. Although the latter is virtually never used, successful PCV reduction has been claimed with dapsone, phenylhydrazine and pyrimethamine.[133,134] Venesection and, more recently, erythrapheresis have been widely reported in the literature, and nearly all have addressed the problem of whether PCV reduction is of overall benefit. Although it is difficult to make strict comparison between studies because of different patient selection, methods and amount of blood removed, a general consensus emerges. PCV reduction reduces pulmonary vascular resistance and possibly pulmonary artery pressure and right ventricular work, particularly on exercise[135–138] but generally without any significant effect on the arterial blood gases. The reduction in pulmonary vascular resistance is brought about by the fall in PCV and blood viscosity.[37] The amount the PCV should be reduced is suggested in a study where two stages of PCV reduction were performed.[137] The first, with reduction of the PCV to 0.50, demonstrated cardiovascular improvement, but no further improvement occurred in the second stage with PCV reduction to 0.44. The evidence suggests that the optimal PCV in terms of oxygen delivery in these patients is in the range of 0.50–0.55.

The improvement in exercise tolerance that has been reported following venesection and PCV reduction[136,139] has been suggested to be no more than a placebo effect. However, a genuine influence on exercise tolerance has been confirmed by comparison of the effects of real and dummy erythraphenesis[140] or venesection.[141]

The effect of the secondary polycythaemia in COAD on cerebral and renal flow has been reported. Before treatment the cerebral blood flow (CBF) is variable, with some authors finding values as low as in primary poly-cythaemia,[142] while other studies have shown higher values.[143] The observed differences probably reflect differences in arterial PCO_2, which when elevated causes cerebral vessel dilatation and increases CBF. PCV reduction is accompanied by a rise in CBF but not in such a consistent way as seen in primary polycythaemia.[39,142,143] Objective assessment of mental alertness has shown improvement with PCV reduction.[144,145] Sometimes the rather non-specific subjective symptoms of, for example, headache and lethargy are similarly improved but not necessarily in those showing an increase in CBF on venesection,[143] suggesting other influences such as pH on these symptoms.

Studies of renal function have been performed before and after PCV reduction. At the raised PCV, effective renal plasma flow (ERPF) is reduced but glomerular filtration rate (GFR) is maintained due to a rise in filtration fraction (FF)[119,120] possibly from a passive increase in glomerular efferent arteriolar resistance due to the increased blood viscosity.[146] Reduction in PCV increases ERPF and reduces FF.[119,120] Reduction in body weight occurred on PCV reduction and thus the increase in FF, which would tend to increase water and sodium excretion, would be an advantage in those with cor pulmonale and fluid retention.[119] Renal oxygen delivery is preserved by the increased Hb before therapy but falls following PCV reduction.[120] This change in renal oxygen delivery may be responsible for the increase in erythropoietin which is observed on PCV reduction in these patients.[115,147]

The method of PCV reduction has been debated. Simple venesection of 500 ml has been compared with a similar procedure plus a dextran infusion to maintain blood volume.[148] Although there was no difference at 48 h, before that time cardiac output and systemic oxygen transport fell in the simple venesection group. Simple venesection, however, should never exceed 200–250 ml initially and in patients who show untoward effects, have prior ischaemic symptoms or evidence of myocardial ischaemia, volume replacement should always be performed since the very rare fatality has been reported in such patients undergoing venesection.[149] Erythrapheresis has the merit of rapid isovolaemic PCV reduction but requires expensive equipment and trained staff. Its use is rarely required but is indicated when PCV reduction could be required as an emergency, for example, in patients with ischaemic signs or symptoms.

As discussed under cyanotic congenital heart disease, chronic venesection may lead to iron deficiency and microcytic hypochromic red cell changes. To monitor the blood viscosity it is essential to measure the PCV accurately. As long as this is done[2] blood viscosity is no higher in the presence of iron-deficient red cell changes than with normochromic normocytic cells.[106] The reduced Hb and hence oxygen-carrying capacity in the presence of hypochromic red cells at any given PCV might, however, be a disadvantage in patients in whom oxygen carriage should be maximized. Cautious iron therapy is occasionally effective at improving symptoms, as long as the PCV is closely monitored and it is appreciated that an increased venesection rate will be required.[150] Normal therapeutic doses of iron may be associated with a rapid rise in PCV and if not controlled may precipitate a vascular occlusive event.

Alveolar hypoventilation

Factors such as anatomical and neurological defects, obesity and sleep apnoea, of which more than one may be present in a single patient, can cause alveolar hypoventilation. Additional factors such as primary lung pathology, smoking and sedative drug treatment may also be involved. If a sufficient reduction in SaO_2 and oxygen carriage occurs either intermittently or continuously, a rise in red cell mass and PCV may be induced. The observed increase in RCM may be such as to cause an absolute polycythaemia, while in other patients, although the PCV is raised, the measured RCM still falls within the patient's normal range: an apparent polycythaemia. The possible causes of hypoventilation will be discussed separately although, as explained, they may be interrelated.

Anatomical and neurological defects. There are a number of anatomical changes to the spine and/or chest wall which may cause alveolar hypoventilation. These include advanced kyphoscoliosis and severe ankylosing spondylitis.[151] Neurological defects are either peripheral or central. Peripheral lesions include poliomyelitis, myasthenia gravis and certain myopathies.[152] Central lesions include infarction of the respiratory centre[153,154] and reduced sensitivity of the respiratory centre to reduced PaO_2 or increased $PaCO_2$.[151,155]

Obesity. Alveolar hypoventilation may arise in approximately 10% of adults with uncomplicated extreme obesity.[156] The condition can occasionally be found in children[157] and has been observed in the congenitally obese mouse.[158] The term 'Pickwickian syndrome' has been coined following the observations of Dickens of the fat boy in *Pickwick Papers*. Features of the syndrome included marked obesity, somnolence, cyanosis and secondary polycythaemia.[159] The patho-physiology of the condition is complex and includes reduced lung function, cardiomegaly, left as well as right heart failure, increased nocturnal arterial oxygen desaturation, nocturnal obstruction to the airway and reduced hypoxic and hypercapnic ventilatory drive.[160–162] The condition is reversible on weight reduction.[157]

Sleep apnoea syndromes.   Any cause of arterial hypoxaemia in the waking state will be associated with worse desaturation in the sleeping patient.[152] In addition, the adoption of the supine position, even in the occasional waking subject, may give rise to hypoxaemia from airway closure leading to the 'closing volume' significantly overlapping the tidal volume.[163,164] The effect is more marked in smokers.[165]

Sleep apnoea syndromes are characterized by cessation of breathing for more than 10 s, many times per hour during sleep.[166] Sleep apnoea most commonly develops in the deeper stages of sleep and rapid eye movement sleep. The causes can be divided into central and obstructive.[152] In any one patient both elements may be present. Short episodes of central apnoea may occur in the normal population with advancing age, particularly in males[161] and more commonly in hypertensive patients.[162] Other causes of central apnoea include brainstem disease, myxoedema and congestive cardic failure. Obstruction to the air passage can occur at nasal, pharyngeal and laryngeal levels.[152] The extent of arterial oxygen desaturation during sleep may be quite severe, sufficient to lead to cardiopulmonary effects and stimulate erythropoiesis. The condition should be considered in patients with unexplained polycythaemia[13] particularly in those who smoke, have restless disturbed sleep, awake unrefreshed and have daytime somnolence.

Pulmonary arterio-venous malformations

Hereditary haemorrhagic telangiectasia or Rendu–Osler–Weber syndrome, an autosomal dominant condition, is an unusual cause of secondary polycythaemia due to the presence of pulmonary arterio-venous fistulae leading to reduced SaO_2. Pulmonary lesions, which are usually multiple, occur in approximately 10% of these patients. More commonly, lesions are present in the skin, mouth, upper respiratory and gastrointestinal tracts. Symptoms and signs in patients with significant pulmonary lesions include dyspnoea, haemoptysis, cyanosis and clubbing. Usually, but not always, other telangiectasia are present. Since these lesions bleed, iron deficiency is common and may ameliorate the degree of polycythaemia.[168]

Other causes of impaired tissue oxygen delivery

Smoking

It is well-recognized that smokers have higher Hb and PCV values than non-smokers.[169,170] An absolute polycythaemia resulting solely from cigarette smoking is uncommon but small numbers of cases have been reported.[171–173] More commonly some increase in RCM occurs within the normal range. A reduction in PV from smoking per se may occur as a result of increased venous tone;[174] alternatively the reduced PV may occur as a homeostatic mechanism to maintain a normal blood volume at increased RCM levels.[171] Therefore, the RCM/PV findings in smokers with elevated PCV levels without any complicating factors might reveal an absolute polycythaemia, most commonly an apparent polycythaemia or, rarely, a relative (low PV) polycythaemia. The role of smoking, combined often with alcohol consumption, should not be forgotten when investigating patients with elevated PCV values.[175] Smoking is frequently additive to other factors which decrease the arterial oxygen content, such as lung disease, sleep apnoea syndromes and obesity.

The principal effect of smoking on arterial oxygen content is an increase in carbon monoxide (CO) level in the blood. Carbon monoxide has a higher affinity for Hb than oxygen and hence reduces the amount of Hb available for oxygen carriage. In non-smokers, carboxyhaemoglobin (COHb) levels are generally not above 2.5% whereas in cigarette smokers values up to 10% are found with higher values in occasional patients.[171–173] Cigar smokers have higher COHb levels than cigarette smokers.[171,177] Apart from the influence of CO on reducing the available Hb for oxygen carriage, the presence of COHb shifts the oxygen dissociation curve to the left and alters its shape, reducing the amount of oxygen released at any given PO_2.[117,178,179] Thus tissue oxygen delivery is further compromised.[180]

Another effect of cigarette smoking, in addition to increasing the incidence of chronic bronchitis, is on the small airways. This leads to an increase in 'closing volume' and impaired ventilation distribution to the dependent lung zones in the supine position.[163,165,181]

The reversibility of the effects of smoking on PCV, RCM and PV has been demonstrated.[117,171,182] On the other hand, in a study of patients with hypoxic polycythaemia due to COAD, oxygen therapy produced a satisfactory response, with marked PCV reduction in non-smokers, but failed to produce a similar response in smokers, presumably due to continuing high COHb levels.[183] Reduction in the number of cigarettes smoked, however, is not necessarily effective in reducing COHb levels, since subjects respond by inhaling more deeply.[182]

Congenital methaemoglobinaemia

Congenital methaemoglobinaemia due to methaemoglobin reductase deficiency is an autosomal recessive condition. The usual clinical manifestation is cyanosis with methaemoglobin levels up to 40% (normally less than 1%). Severely affected patients may have high normal or slightly raised Hb and PCV values due to the reduced oxygen-carrying capacity of the blood and left shift of the oxygen dissociation curve. Either ascorbic acid or methylene blue may be used in treatment.

Congestive cardiac failure

Normally, in congestive cardiac heart failure the PCV is normal and the total blood volume is increased due particularly to an increase in PV although the RCM may also rise. The RCM may be significantly increased to produce an absolute polycythaemia. In the few patients who have raised PCV values,[184,185] treatment and resolution of the heart failure leads to a fall in PCV, RCM and PV.[186]

Increased haemoglobin oxygen affinity

Abnormal haemoglobins.   Over 30 different α and β chain variants with markedly increased oxygen affinity have been described. Patients with the same Hb variant do not exhibit uniform *in vivo* adaptations to the very low P_{50}, which is usually in the order of 12–13 mm Hg (1.67 kPa). The observed changes include an increase in Hb, PCV, cardiac output and cerebral blood flow.[41,187] PCV values are usually between 0.52 and 0.60 although occasionally higher values are found. Individual patients experiencing vascular occlusive episodes have been recorded,[188–190] but there is an impression that the incidence of these episodes is not as high in these patients as might be expected given the increased PCV and blood viscosity. The increased blood flow might explain the relative reduction in risk.[59] Very high PCV values (0.60) have been associated with non-specific symptoms such as headache and dizziness. These have been relieved by modest PCV reduction by venesection.[188,189] In general, however, PCV reduction is not indicated since this might carry cardiovascular disadvantages.[191] Limited exchange transfusion has been shown to be effective in those patients with unrelated coronary vessel disease or myocardial pathology.[192]

Congenital low 2,3-diphosphoglycerate.   A patient with complete absence of activity of diphosphoglycerate mutase has been described. He had very low levels of 2,3-diphosphoglycerate with a consequent left shift in the oxygen dissociation curve (P_{50} 17.3 mm Hg; 2.30 kPa). His Hb and PCV were 17.4 g/dl and 0.54 respectively.[193]

Hereditary persistence of foetal haemoglobin.   There are a number of genetic mutations that give rise to hereditary persistence of foetal haemoglobin. Homozygotes produce 100% HbF. Since HbF has a slightly left-shifted oxygen dissociation curve compared with HbA, these individuals may have high normal Hb and PCV values but not as high as one might expect from the P_{50} value since they probably have a mild thalassaemic syndrome.[194]

Renal lesions

It is not surprising to find that polycythaemia often accompanies renal pathology, since the kidney is the major source of erythropoietin (Epo) production. Lesions causing local or generalized renal ischaemia may be responsible for polycythaemia as well as tumours of renal origin.

Renal tumours

Hypernephroma.   Hypernephroma, or adenocarcinoma of the kidney, gives rise to polycythaemia in 2–10% of patients.[195,196] However, a renal tumour is found in only 1% of patients investigated for an absolute polycythaemia.[196] Anaemia is much more common in hypernephroma and occurs in one-third of patients.[197] Extracts of the renal tumour may have a high concentration of Epo but not invariably, and serum Epo levels are usually within the normal range.[198–200] Pressure from the tumour may cause ischaemia of the normal renal tissue and may be an additional or sole factor in some polycythaemic patients.[196,201] Occasionally an increase in RCM may occur without the RCM being sufficiently elevated to be classified as an absolute polycythaemia. Thus, a renal ultrasound scan is advisable in patients with raised Hb and PCV even when the RCM measurement does not reveal an absolute polycythaemia. Another diagnostic difficulty might arise if it is not appreciated that between 5 and 30% of patients have a reactive thrombocytosis and/or neutrophilia.[196] The association of these haematological changes with polycythaemia might incorrectly lead to a diagnosis of PPP unless the renal tract is examined.

The treatment of this form of polycythaemia should obviously be directed at the primary cause. The haematological abnormalities disappear on successful removal of the tumour[201] but may recur with relapse. It would be reasonable to reduce the PCV to normal values by venesection pre-operatively or in patients with inoperable lesions to reduce the thromboembolic risk.

Wilms' tumour.   Wilms' tumour or nephroblastoma, arises from embryonic renal tissues. Patients are usually under 3 years of age but may be older. Polycythaemia is an occasional complication.[202] Increased serum Epo levels have been found in some patients and the tumour may be shown to contain Epo.[203,204]

Renal cysts

Polycythaemia has been described in patients with simple renal cysts, polycystic disease and medullary cystic kidney.[205–208] Serum Epo levels are elevated in some of the polycythaemic patients.[209] Erythropoietic activity in the fluid from approximately half of the aspirated single cysts is increased but there is no simple relationship between the size of the cyst, the erythopoietic activity of the fluid and the presence or absence of polycythaemia.[198,207,210] Increased pressure producing ischaemia of the tissue surrounding a cyst may cause increased Epo production in some patients.

The incidence of simple cysts of the kidney increases with age. Over the age of 40 years about 20% of individuals have one or more renal cysts. This increases to about 45% in those over 60 years. Obviously the presence of a renal cyst in an elderly polycythaemic patient may cause diagnostic difficulty. As discussed earlier, aspiration of the cyst and the examination of the erythropoietic activity of the fluid is not helpful. However, aspiration and cytological examination of the cyst fluid is essential if the ultrasound examination suggests anything but a simple benign cyst. The only real way of being certain that a benign cyst is causing the polycythaemia is to remove it and show that the blood count returns to normal. Although this has been done and demonstrated[207] such a procedure is rarely indicated. Generally, having established the presence of a simple renal cyst, it is safer to complete the other investigations and manage the patient without renal intervention. The finding of PPP and a renal cyst in the same patient has been described.[207,211,212] The association is almost certainly coincidental since both conditions affect the elderly.

Diffuse renal parenchymal disease

Renal disease of sufficient severity to impair renal function usually leads to a normochromic normocytic anaemia. However, a variety of diffuse renal parenchymal diseases are very occasionally associated with polycythaemia presumably due to an increased Epo output. The lesions involved include focal glomerulosclerosis,[213,214] nephrotic syndrome[215,216] and renal tuberculosis.[209] A case of Wegener's granulomatosis with renal involvement has been described but almost certainly the patient had coincidental PPP.[217] A study of the RCM and PV values in a selected group of patients with raised PCV values and with different forms of diffuse renal disease showed that the RCM was between 118 and 154% of the predicted mean normal value while the PV ranged between 73 and 110% of the predicted value. Obviously the PV reduction would enhance any effect of an increased RCM on the PCV.[216]

Hydronephrosis

In the experimental animal, a relationship between the degree of unilateral hydronephrotic pressure and RCM increase has been described. Moderately increased pressure, even if intermittent, induced polycythaemia while high pressure did not produce any haematological effect, presumably due to rapidly progressive renal atrophy.[218] In man, the rare association between hydronephrosis and polycythaemia has been described. It occurs in either segmental or total collecting system obstruction and intrapelvic and intraparenchymal pressure leads to cortical and medullary ischaemia with increased Epo secretion. Remission of the polycythaemia has been demonstrated on removal of the obstruction, or by partial or total removal of the affected kidney.[219] Obviously, as shown in the experimental animal, there is a balance between moderate hydronephrotic pressure ischaemia and polycythaemia and high pressure with total destruction of the renal parenchyma and no polycythaemia.

Bartter's syndrome

This is an uncommon, probably autosomal recessive condition with considerable heterogeneity of the clinical and biochemical features. These include hypokalaemic alkalosis, a normal or low arterial pressure, hyponatraemia and hypercalcaemia. There are probably a number of different causes of Bartter's syndrome but a primary defect of renal tubular resorption of chloride and occasionally sodium and potassium has been proposed. The original cases showed hypertrophy of the juxta-glomerular apparatus but other histological features may also be present. Polycythaemia has been described occasionally in these patients.[220,221] This finding and the increased granularity of the juxta-glomerular cells in the polycythaemia of experimental hydronephrosis in animals[222] suggests that these cells may be responsible for Epo production although this is probably not the only production site in the kidney.

Renal artery stenosis

Stenosis of the renal artery has been associated with hypertension and polycythaemia, presumably due to renal ischaemia.[223,224] In a case report of a young adult male, ischaemia due to thickening of the interlobular and afferent arteries was suggested to be the cause of polycythaemia. The PCV returned to normal following nephrectomy.[225]

Renal transplantation

Polycythaemia is a well-recognized complication of renal allo-transplantation, occurring in 15–20% of cases.[226–228] PCV values may rise up to 0.66 but usually not above 0.58.[226] The rise in PCV usually occurs between 3 and 90 months after transplantation and may persist from 1 to 84 months. The haematological change is usually self-limiting. The RCM is not always raised above the upper limit of normal and apparent or relative polycythaemia with a low PV is seen in some patients.[227–230] The mechanism of the polycythaemia is probably multifactorial although a single mechanism may apply in the individual patient. Initially it was proposed that acute or chronic rejection of the transplanted kidney, renal artery stenosis or hydronephrosis were the most likely causes, resulting in increased Epo production by the ischaemic transplanted kidney.[231–234] In patients with impaired hepatic function, reduced Epo clearance may be an additional mechanism.[227,228,235] A single patient with polycythaemia, increased amounts of Epo arising from the native kidneys and haematological improvement following removal of the kidneys has been described.[236,237] In a large series of patients it was established that smoking, diabetes and a rejection-free course were most likely 'risk' factors related to the development of polycythaemia.[226] The interesting association with a rejection-free course was also shown in another series.[228] The mechanism in these patients may relate to removal of plasma factors that normally inhibit the marrow in the dialysis-dependent patient and an increased sensitivity of the erythropoietic compartment of the marrow to the Epo arising from the transplanted kidney.[228,238] Whatever the cause of the raised PCV, there is evidence of an increased thromboembolic risk in these patients compared with non-polycythaemic transplanted patients.[226,229] Regular venesection to control the PCV at normal values should be performed while awaiting the usual amelioration of the haematological manifestation.

Hepatic lesions

Evidence from both anephric animals[239] and man[235] has shown that the adult liver is capable of producing Epo. Normally, the hepatic contribution is only a few per cent of the total production. The observation that the Epo produced in nephrectomized animals is biologically functional suggests that an intact kidney is not necessary for its activation, although renal transformation of an hepatic precursor substance had been proposed.[240] Since the liver removes Epo from the circulation, reduced clearance may be another explanation of increased plasma erythropoietic activity in diffuse liver disease. Diminished clearance of other erythropoietic factors, such as androgen, may also be relevant.[241]

Hepatoma

This tumour is particularly common in Negroes, the Bantu and Chinese.[242,243] The mean age at presentation is 60 years although childhood cases have been reported.[242] The incidence of proven cirrhosis before development of the tumour varies between 50 and 100% in different series.[242,243]

The incidence of polycythaemia in patients with hepatoma is between 3 and 12%.[243–246] The criteria used for defining polycythaemia have varied in different series although the majority have used only raised Hb and/or PCV values. RCM and PV measurement in patients with hepatoma following cirrhosis, show that when the PCV is above 0.48, the RCM is invariably raised. Many patients have an increased PV and this can mask the effect of the increase in RCM.[244]

The cause of the polycythaemia is almost certainly due to Epo production by the tumour. However, increased Epo in the tumour extract or serum are not always found.[241,247–250] Increased hormone production by ischaemic normal liver around the tumour has also been proposed.[251] An Epo response of normal liver tissue to hypoxaemia has been shown in nephrectomized rats.[239] Successful removal of the hepatoma followed by chemotherapy has been shown to relieve the polycythaemia.[252]

Cirrhosis

Polycythaemia has been found in some patients with cirrhosis. This has been shown to be due to arterial hypoxaemia, resulting from the development of pulmonary arterio-venous anastomoses.[253,254] Reduced hepatic clearance of Epo might enhance the erythropoietic effect. A sudden rise in PCV in a patient with cirrhosis should arouse suspicion of the development of a hepatoma.[244,255]

Hepatitis

Regenerating hepatic tissue following hepatitis probably elaborates increased amounts of Epo. A rise in Hb and PCV has been shown in patients receiving renal dialysis, some of whom were anephric, following the development of hepatitis.[235,256,257] Although these patients did not become polycythaemic due to the initial anaemia, an increased PCV might be expected in patients developing hepatitis without preceding renal impairment.

Hepatic haemangiomata

A patient with raised Hb and PCV values and diffuse hepatic haemangiomata has been described.[258] Epo production by the tumour or increased levels resulting from renal ischaemia due to pressure on the right renal artery were postulated.

Endocrine lesions

Adrenal tumours

Cushing's syndrome.   Cortisol overproduction may be due to a pituitary basophilic adenoma associated with adrenal hyperplasia (Cushing's disease) or to an adenoma or carcinoma of the adrenal or arise from ectopic ACTH production, such as found in lung carcinoma.[259] In addition to high cortisol levels, increased secretion of androgens may also occur and be important in some patients. The classical features include central obesity, plethora, hypertension and proximal muscle wasting. A review of 33 patients with Cushing's syndrome[259] showed that approximately half had red cell counts within the normal range but some had counts up to 6.9 × 10^9 per litre (Hb and PCV values were not recorded). Detailed measurements of RCM and PV findings in Cushing's syndrome are not to be found in the literature. Some animal experiments have been performed to examine the effects of steroid hormones and some of the results are contradictory. While one study showed an increase in RCM following hydrocortisone and cortisone administration,[260] this was not confirmed in later studies.[261,262] *In vivo* animal experiments have shown an increase in RCM following testosterone administration.[261,262] *In vitro*, erythroid colony growth has been shown to be inhibited by cortisol[263] but in different reports a variable response to testosterone has been demonstrated.[263,264] In addition to these direct effects of steroid hormones on erythropoiesis, other influences should be considered. These include modification of lymphocyte sub-populations and other erythropoietic growth factors.[265] Furthermore, excessive obesity, which may occur in Cushing's syndrome may also influence erythropoiesis due to hypoventilation and arterial hypoxaemia.

Conn's syndrome.   Increased erythropoietic activity has been demonstrated in the plasma of a patient with polycythaemia and primary aldosteronism. Although aldosterone has not been shown to have any direct effect on erythropoiesis, following removal of the adrenal tumour in this patient the blood count returned to normal.[266]

Phaeochromocytoma.   Phaeochromocytomas arise in chromaffin cells of neuro-ectodermal origin. They are usually situated in the adrenal medulla but extra-adrenal tumours are found. Since these tumours secrete catecholamines their usual presentation is with episodic hypertension. Polycythaemia is an uncommon complication. In a study of 15 patients with phaeochromocytoma,[267] two were found to have a raised RCM and a further four had a reduced PV. Increased serum Epo levels and increased erythropoietin activity of tumour extracts have been documented in patients with associated polycythaemia which resolves following removal of the tumour.[267-269] Measurement of blood volume prior to surgery can be helpful since blood volume replacement at surgery is necessary to correct the small volume circulation and avoid the circulatory instability associated with it.[267]

Thyroid disease

In thyrotoxicosis a rise in RCM occurs while in myxoedema there is a fall. However, the PCV is usually within the normal range in thyrotoxicosis[270] except for an occasional patient with an absolute polycythaemia.[271] A patient with a high Hb (22.1 g/dl) and PCV (0.627) presumed to be due to a thyroid papillary carcinoma has been described.[272]

Miscellaneous tumours

Cerebellar haemangioblastoma

These benign posterior fossa tumours probably arise from the endothelium of the primitive blood vessels of the developing choroid plexus.[273] They present at any age, usually between 4 and 60 years with symptoms of headache and vomiting and with papilloedema and cerebellar signs. Very occasionally a cerebellar haemangioblastoma (Lindau's syndrome) is associated with an angiomatous malformation of the retina (von Hippel's syndrome).[274] Polycythaemia has been observed in 10–18% of patients with cerebellar haemangioblastoma.[273-275] A single case with polycythaemia and a supratentorial lesion of similar histology has also been described.[276] There is some evidence that the more differentiated the tumour the more likely it is to be complicated by polycythaemia.[273] Extracts from the tumour have been shown to possess erythropoietic activity.[277-279]

Successful treatment results in amelioration of the polycythaemia while relapse can be heralded by a rise in Hb and PCV above normal.[274,280]

Uterine fibroids

Although the total number of cases recorded in the literature is relatively small, uterine fibromyomata may be associated with an absolute poly-cythaemia. Cases with haematological improvement following removal of the tumour have been documented.[281–283] Extracts from the tumour have been shown to contain erythropoietic activity.[284–286] The risk associated with the secondary polycythaemia is suggested by a patient with a large uterine mass and Hb of 19 g/dl who presented with a myocardial infarction.[288]

Ovarian tumours

Individual case descriptions have been recorded of an absolute poly-cythaemia associated with a dermoid cyst[289] and virilizing tumours of the ovary.[290]

Cutaneous leiomyomata

A single case of polycythaemia in a patient with leiomyomata of the skin has been reported.[291] The RCM fell to normal following removal of several of the largest tumours, which provided extracts with erythropoietic activity.

Bronchial carcinoma

A very few cases of carcinoma of the bronchus and polycythaemia have been described.[247,292] Presumably this tumour, which may elaborate a variety of different hormones, may very occasionally produce Epo.

Argentiffinoma

A patient with a caecal tumour, hepatic metastases and carcinoid syndrome with polycythaemia has been recorded. The patient had profound arterial hypoxaemia which, in the authors' opinion, was due to microscopic pulmonary fistulae with right to left shunting.[293]

Parotid tumour

A single patient with a malignant parotid fibrous histiocytoma and an Hb of 20.2 g/dl, and PCV of 0.64 has been reported.[294] These haematological values returned to normal following removal of the tumour.

Lymphoma

An absolute polycythaemia has been shown in a patient with a diffuse B-cell 'large cell' lymphoma. The Hb and PCV fell following combination chemotherapy. However, a primary myeloproliferative disorder cannot be excluded although no other haematological manifestations of it were present.[295]

Drugs and chemicals

Androgens

An increase in erythropoietic activity following administration of androgen has been well-documented in both animals[262] and man,[296] even in anephric individuals.[297] This has led to the use of androgenic preparations in the treatment of various anaemias.[298] An absolute polycythaemia has been induced in patients with metastatic breast cancer[299] and elderly males[296] following androgen therapy.

It is thought that the erythropoietic effect of androgen is due to two biologically active metabolites with differing molecular configurations. The first stimulates Epo secretion; the second increases the number of pluripotent stem cells of the marrow in the erythropoietic 'compartment'.[298]

Cobalt

Increased erythropoietic activity has been observed in animals and patients receiving cobalt chloride.[300,301] The compound is no longer used following the demonstration that its erythropoietic effects are produced by inhibiting oxidative metabolism.[302]

Nickel

A marked increase in RCM has been shown in experimental animals treated with nickel subsulphide caused either by a direct effect on renal mesangial cells or by widespread renal arteriosclerotic changes leading to renal ischaemia.[303]

Autonomous high erythropoietin

A number of patients with an absolute polycythaemia and PCV values between 0.50 and 0.77 associated with unexplained high Epo levels have been described. Many reports have related to children or young adults. Autosomal recessive[304] and dominant[305,306] inheritance has been demonstrated. Where there is a clear genetic basis the term 'familial polycythaemia' has been used. This should not be confused with other forms of 'inherited' polycythaemia, such as that related to the high oxygen affinity haemoglobins. In the individual patient, the increased Epo level is either strictly autonomous[304,305] or rises after the Hb and PCV have been reduced by venesection, suggesting some retention of physiological control.[307,308] *In vitro* culture of erythropoietic cells from these patients shows that they demonstrate normal sensitivity to erythropoietin.[306] The risk of vascular occlusion at the high PCV levels often observed in this condition has been well-documented[304] and the PCV should be adequately controlled by venesection.

Autonomous high Epo will be recognized more frequently when serum

Epo measurements become widely available. This probably applies to some of the patients currently placed in the idiopathic erythrocytosis group.[7] Similarly, in the occasional young patient with an autonomous high Epo value splenomegaly is present[306] and this could lead to an incorrect diagnosis of PPP if the Epo levels are not measured.

Neonatal polycythaemia

Definition

In the neonate Hb and PCV values are higher than at any other time of life, reflecting the physiological adaptation to the relative hypoxia of intra-uterine existence. Venous Hb or PCV values above 20 g/dl and 0.65 have been given as the definition of neonatal polycythaemia.[309] Higher values should be taken if capillary samples are used.[310] The effect of the elevated PCV on blood viscosity in the newborn is not as marked as in an adult sample with a similar PCV due to lower plasma proteins and plasma viscosity in the newborn period.[311,312]

Causes

There are a variety of causes of neonatal polycythaemia and these are listed in Table 3.6. Delayed clamping of the cord leads to a significant transfusion from the placenta. Babies with late clamping of the cord have mean venous PCV values 0.09 higher at 3–5 days of life than those with early clamping.[313] Foetus–foetus transfusion occurs in 15% of multiple pregnancies with a single placenta and may lead to marked polycythaemia associated with a

Table 3.6 Causes of Neonatal Polycythaemia

Placental transfusion
  Delayed clamping of the cord
  Twin-to-twin
  Mother–foetus

Intra-uterine hypoxia
  Placental insufficiency

Endocrine disorders
  Maternal diabetes
  Thyrotoxicosis[322]
  Adrenal hyperplasia[323]

Congenital anomalies and other causes
  Trisomy 13–15, 18, 21[321,324,325]
  Beckwith's syndrome[326]
  Myeloid metaplasia, erythroderma ichthyosiforme congenitum[327]

Adapted from Ref. 310.

significantly increased mortality.[314] Very occasionally mother–foetus transfusions may be sufficient to raise the foetal PCV above normal.[315] Placental
insufficiency leading to foetal hypoxia may also produce polycythaemia.
Half of the small-for-gestational-age infants have venous PCV values in
excess of 0.60.[316]

Endocrine disorders may be associated with neonatal polycythaemia. In
particular, a PCV above 0.64 was found in approximately 40% of infants
born to diabetic mothers.[317] The mechanism of the polycythaemia in these
offspring is possibly related to hypoxia, reduced plasma volume[318] and/or
increased sensitivity of foetal red cell precursors to insulin.[319]

A significantly higher incidence of polycythaemia is found in infants with
Down's syndrome than in normal babies.[320,321] The mechanism remains
unclear although abnormal marrow proliferation may occur in Down's
syndrome. In addition, other chromosomal or neonatal abnormalities have
rarely been associated with polycythaemia as listed in Table 3.6.

Clinical manifestations

There is difficulty in separating the features, which can be ascribed to
hyperviscosity, from those due to the primary underlying pathology. The
incidence of clinical manifestations of neonatal polycythaemia has been
given as high as 85%[325] but is usually lower.[328] Manifestations include
respiratory distress, seizures, hypotonia, diminished renal function, peripheral gangrene, priapism and necrotizing colitis. Laboratory changes
include hypoglycaemia, hypocalcaemia, hyperbilirubinaemia and thrombocytopenia.[309,310,325] The pathophysiology of these changes has been well
summarized by Mentzer.[310] The central problem is hyperviscosity causing
reduced cardiac output, reduced peripheral blood flow and increased
pulmonary pressure producing right to left shunting with cyanosis.

Treatment and prognosis

It is widely agreed that exchange transfusion to lower the PCV is appropriate
in symptomatic infants. A randomized study of plasma exchange transfusion
or symptomatic treatment only showed that at 2 years, the group receiving
exchange transfusion had less neurological impairment than the control
group.[328] On the other hand, follow-up of children with neonatal
polycythaemia associated with no or only minor manifestations, showed
that there were no significant associated neurological sequelae.[329] Thus the
decision to use haemodilution must be decided on clinical grounds in the
individual patient.

Other factors in the pathogenesis of polycythaemia

Dehydration

As discussed earlier (page 77) there are a great variety of conditions where 'dehydration' occurs, resulting in a sufficient reduction in PV to cause a relative polycythaemia.

Diuretics

High-dose diuretic therapy can lead to a significant reduction in PV and rise in PCV. Chronic low-dose diuretic therapy with thiazides has been shown to reduce the PV by about 5% equivalent to a rise in PCV of 0.02–0.03.[330,331] Although small, this rise could be sufficient to increase the PCV above the normal range in an occasional patient.

Alcohol

Chronic alcohol ingestion has been proposed as a cause of relative (low PV) polycythaemia since alcohol is a diuretic. Although single cases have been described,[332] in large studies, patients with regular heavy consumption have not been found to have lower PV values than abstainers.[30] Other factors that increase RCM may be responsible for the raised PCV: these include hepatocellular damage causing increased production or reduced clearance of erythropoietin, as seen in vital hepatitis[256] and a direct effect on the respiratory centre[333] resulting in a reduced respiratory drive, particularly during sleep.[175]

Hypertension

There are some interesting possible relationships between hypertension and polycythaemia. Originally it was suggested that the incidence of hypertension in PPP was more common than in the normal population. However, these studies lacked age-matched controls and the association is probably coincidental.[334] On the other hand, hypertension is an established risk factor in cerebrovascular occlusive events and these are particularly common in PPP.[56] However, the incidence of cerebrovascular occlusion is as common in normotensive as hypertensive PPP patients. In apparent and relative polycythaemia, those patients who additionally have hypertension have a much higher incidence of vascular occlusive disease.[30]

In large surveys of hypertensive patients it has been found that the PCV is higher than for normotensive individuals but the PCV is usually well within the normal range.[335] In a small percentage of hypertensive patients the PCV is above normal. The patients with raised PCV values are more likely to have renal arterial disease.[336] Renal ischaemia with the increased elaboration of Epo has been proposed as the cause.[337] An entirely different mechanism for increased erythropoiesis in these patients could be suggested on the basis of the high incidence of sleep apnoea in hypertensive patients.[167] Studies of PV in hypertension have revealed rather inconsistent reuslts,[331,338] with some patients showing a reduced and some an increased PV.

In only a small number of highly selected patients, has a fall in a raised PCV and a rise in a low PV been documented with the introduction of hypotensive therapy (methyldopa or guanethidine).[339] Conversely, reduction in PV and control of hypertension by the introducton of diuretics (frusemide and thiazides) has been shown in hypertensive patients.[338]

Diabetes

In 'controlled' diabetes, particularly in those with diabetic complications, some authors have shown marginally higher PCV values or red cell counts than in control subjects[340,341] while other studies have not confirmed these findings.[342-344] A positive correlation has been shown between HbA_1 values and red cell count and PCV.[341,344]

Stress

The term 'stress polycythaemia' was introduced by Lawrence & Berlin in 1952.[28] They described a small selected group of males with raised PCV values and normal RCM. They felt this group had features in common, namely obesity and emotional stress. The only evidence that emotional stress might be involved in lowering the PV is from a study of two patients with reduced rapid eye movement sleep and reduced nocturnal ADH secretion.[345]

High venous tone

A study of a small group of males with relative polycythaemia demonstrated that they had elevated resting venous tone and reduced venous distensibility compared with normal subjects.[174] These findings were found to be made worse by smoking, which in part was thought to be responsible for the low PV.

COURSE AND MANAGEMENT OF APPARENT AND RELATIVE POLYCYTHAEMIA

In patients where the raised PCV is due to acute fluid loss treatment is obvious. However, in the majority of patients one or more possible factors relating to changes in RCM/PV are found. These include hypertension, diuretic therapy, smoking, obesity and alcohol. Where possible, modification of these factors should be performed. Observation over time has shown that the PCV falls in some patients while a smaller number show a progressive rise with the development of an absolute polycythaemia. In the majority, however, the PCV, RCM and PV remain unchanged for some years.[29]

There are two retrospective studies which examine the clinical course of these patients. The study of Burge *et al.* (1975)[29] showed a mortality rate, particularly from cardiovascular complications, that was six times greater than expected for an age- and sex-matched population. These authors concluded that PCV reduction was the appropriate management. The study of Weinreb & Shih[30] also showed an increased incidence of cardiovascular complications, but particularly in those with hypertension. These authors suggested that the hypertension required energetic treatment but that PCV reduction was not indicated. These two studies indicate that in these patients controversy exists about the importance of PCV reduction although the importance of controlling established risk factors is not disputed. A prospective study, which has already been initiated,[65] is required to resolve the controversy.

While awaiting the outcome of this study, it is suggested that patients with PCV values above 0.550 should be venesected, since there is evidence that such high values are associated with vascular occlusive risk.[45,46] Patients with PCV values between 0.510 and 0.549 should only be venesected if there is evidence of a previous vascular occlusive episode or if they have ischaemic symptoms. The remaining patients should be seen at regular intervals of 3–4 months to follow the haematological course and monitor the occurrence of any symptoms/signs.

Venesection is proposed as the method of PCV control since it has been shown that long-term control could not be achieved with either dextran or fludrocortisone in relative polycythaemia[346] and that venesection was both safe and effective in the long-term. It also improves ischaemic symptoms and increases cerebral blood flow in both apparent and relative polycythaemia.[40]

REFERENCES

1. Mayer, G.A. Diurnal, postural and postprandial variations of hematocrit. *Can. Med. Assoc. J.* **93**: 1006–8, 1965.
2. Guthrie, D.L. & Pearson, T.C. PCV measurement in the management of polycythaemic patients. *Clin. Lab. Haematol.* **4**: 257–65, 1982.
3. Pearson, T.C. & Guthrie, D.L. Trapped plasma in the microhaematocrit. *Am. J. Clin. Pathol.* **78**: 770–2, 1982.
4. International Committee for Standardization in Haematology: Recommended methods for measurement of red-cell and plasma volume. *J. Nucl. Med.* **21**: 793–800, 1980.
5. Mollison, P.L. In *Blood Transfusion in Clinical Medicine*, p. 102. Blackwell Scientific Publications, Oxford, 1972.
6. Najean, Y. & Cacchione, R. Blood volume in health and disease. *Clin. Haematol.* **6**: 543–66, 1977.
7. Pearson, T.C., Glass, U.H. & Wetherley-Mein, G. Interpretation of measured red cell mass in the diagnosis of polycythaemia. *Scand. J. Haematol.* **21**: 153–62, 1978.
8. Pearson, T.C. & Guthrie, D.L. The interpretation of measured red cell mass and plasma volume in patients with elevated PCV values. *Clin. Lab. Haematol.* **6**: 207–17, 1984.
9. Hurley, P.J. Red cell and plasma volumes in normal adults. *J. Nucl. Med.* **16**: 46–52, 1975.

10. Pearson, T.C., Botteril, C.A., Glass, U.H. & Wetherley-Mein, G. Interpretation of measured red cell mass and plasma volume in males with elevated venous PCV values. *Scand. J. Haematol.* **33**: 68–74, 1984.
11. Berk, P.D., Goldberg, J.D., Donovan, P.B., Fruchtman, S.M., Berlin, N.I. & Wasserman, L.R. Therapeutic recommendations in polycythemia vera based on Polycythemia Vera Study Group protocols. *Semin. Hematol.* **23**: 132–43, 1986.
12. Berlin, N.I. Diagnosis and classification of polycythaemia. *Semin. Hematol.* **12**: 339–51, 1975.
13. Moore-Gillon, J.C., Treacher, D.F., Gaminara, E.J., Pearson, T.C. & Cameron, I.C. Intermittent hypoxia in patients with unexplained polycythaemia. *Br. Med. J.* **293**: 588–90, 1986.
14. Adamson, J.W. & Fialkow, P.J. The pathogenesis of myeloproliferative syndromes. *Br. J. Haematol.* **38**: 299–303, 1978.
15. Bateman, S., Lewis, S.M., Nicholas, A. & Zaafran, A. Splenic red cell pooling: a diagnostic feature in polycythaemia. *Br. J. Haematol.* **40**: 389–96, 1978.
16. Pearson, T.C. & Wetherley-Mein, G. The course and complications of idiopathic erythrocytosis. *Clin. Lab. Haematol.* **1**: 189–96, 1979.
17. Cotes, P.M., Doré, C.J., Liu Yin, J.A., Lewis, S.M., Messinezy, M., Pearson, T.C. & Reid, C. Determination of serum immunoreactive erythropoietin in the investigation of erythrocytosis. *N. Engl. J. Med.* **315**: 283–7, 1986.
18. Reid, C.D.L. The significance of endogenous erythroid colonies (EEC) in haematological disorders. *Blood Rev.* **1**: 133–40, 1987.
19. Golde, D.W., Bersche, N. & Cline, M.J. Polycythemia vera: hormonal modulation of erythropoiesis *in vitro*. *Blood* **49**: 399–405, 1977.
20. Lacombe, C., Casadevall, N. & Varet, B. Polycythaemia vera: *in vitro* studies of circulating erythroid progenitors. *Br. J. Haematol.* **44**: 189–99, 1980.
21. Eridani, S., Pearson, T.C., Sawyer, B., Batten, E. & Wetherley-Mein, G. Erythroid colony formation in primary proliferative polycythaemia, idiopathic erythrocytosis and secondary polycythaemia. *Clin. Lab. Hematol.* **5**: 121–9, 1983.
22. Lemoine, F., Najman, A., Baillou, C., Stachowiak, J., Bofa, G., Aegerter, P., Ouay, L., Laporte, J., Gorin, N. & Duhamel, G. A prospective study of the value of bone marrow erythroid progenitor cultures in polycythemia. *Blood* **68**: 996–1002, 1986.
23. Casadevall, N., Vainchenker, W., Lacombe, C., Vinci, G., Chapman, J., Breton-Gorius, J. & Varet, B. Erythroid progenitors in polycythemia vera: demonstration of their hypersensitivity to erythropoietin using serum free cultures. *Blood* **59**: 447–51, 1982.
24. Eridani, S., Dudley, J.M., Sawyer, B.M. & Pearson, T.C. Erythropoietic colonies in a serum-free system: results in primary proliferative polycythaemia and thrombocythaemia. *Br. J. Haematol.* **67**: 387–91, 1987.
25. Modan, B. & Modan, M. Benign erythrocytosis. *Br. J. Haematol.* **14**: 375–81, 1968.
26. Najean, Y., Triebel, F. & Dresch, C. Pure erythrocytosis: Reappraisal of a study of 51 cases. *Am. J. Hematol.* **10**: 129–36, 1981.
27. Geisbock, F. Die bedentung der blutdricknessung für die artzliche praxis. *Dt Arch. Klin. Med.* **83**: 363, 1905.
28. Lawrence, J.H. & Berlin, N.I. Relative polycythemia – the polycythemia of stress. *Yale J. Biol. Med.* **24**: 498–505, 1952.
29. Burge, P.S., Johnson, W.S. & Prankerd, T.A.J. Morbidity and mortality in pseudopolycythaemia. *Lancet* **i**: 1266–9, 1975.
30. Weinreb, N.J. & Shih, C.-F. Spurious polycythemia. *Semin. Hematol.* **12**: 397–407, 1975.
31. Pearson, T.C. Stress polycythaemia. In *Advanced Medicine* (eds R.E. Pounder & P.L. Chiodini), Vol. 23, pp. 263–74. Baillière Tindall, London, 1987.
32. Vogel, J.A. & Harris, C.W. Cardiopulmonary responses of resting man during

early exposure to high altitude. *J. Appl. Physiol.* **2**: 1124–8, 1967.

33. Finlay, M., Middleton, H.L., Peake, M.D. & Howard, P. Cardiac output, pulmonary hypertension, hypoxaemia and survival in patients with chronic obstructive airway disease. *Eur. J. Respir. Dis.* **64**: 252–63, 1983.
34. Ring, C.P., Pearson, T.C., Sanders, M.D. & Wetherley-Mein, G. Viscosity and retinal vein thrombosis. *Br. J. Ophthalmol.* **60**: 397–410, 1976.
35. Harrison, M.J.G., Kendall, B.E., Pollock, S. & Marshall, F. Effect of haematocrit on carotid stenosis and cerebral infarction. *Lancet* **ii**: 114–15, 1981.
36. Pollock, S., Tsitsopoulos, P. & Harrison, M.J.G. The effect of haematocrit on cerebral perfusion and clinical status following carotid occlusion in the gerbil. *Stroke* **13**: 167–70, 1982.
37. Harrison, B.D.W. & Stokes, T.C. Secondary polycythaemia: its causes, effects and treatment. *Br. J. Dis. Chest.* **76**: 313–40.
38. Barer, G., Bee, D. & Wach, R.A. Contribution of polycythaemia to pulmonary hypertension in simulated high altitude rats. *J. Physiol.* **336**: 27–8, 1983.
39. Thomas, D.J., du Boulay, G.H., Marshall, J., Pearson, T.C., Ross Russell, R.W., Symon, L., Wetherley-Mein, G. & Zilkha, E. Cerebral blood flow in polycythaemia. *Lancet* **ii**: 161–3, 1977.
40. Humphrey, P.R.D., du Boulay, G.H., Marshall, J., Pearson, T.C., Ross Russell, R.W., Symon, L., Wetherley-Mein, G. & Zilkha, E. Cerebral blood-flow and viscosity in relative polycythaemia. *Lancet* **ii**: 873–7, 1979.
41. Wade, J.P.H., du Boulay, G.H., Marshall, J., Pearson, T.C., Ross Russell, R.W., Shirley, J.A., Symon, L., Wetherley-Mein, G. & Zilkha, E. Cerebral blood flow, haematocrit and viscosity in subjects with a high oxygen affinity haemoglobin variant. *Acta Neurol. Scand.* **61**: 210–15, 1980.
42. Brown, M.M., Wade, J.P.H. & Marshall, J. Fundamental importance of arterial oxygen content in the regulation of cerebral blood flow in man. *Brain* **108**: 81–93, 1985.
43. Millikan, C.J., Siekert, R.G. & Whisnant, J.P. Intermittent carotid and vertebral-basilar insufficiency associated with polycythemia. *Neurology* **10**: 188–95, 1960.
44. Elwood, P.C., Benjamin, I.T., Waters, W.E. & Sweetnam, P.M. Mortality and anaemia in women. *Lancet* **i**: 891–4, 1974.
45. Pearson, T.C. & Wetherley-Mein, G. Vascular occlusive episodes and venous haematocrit in primary proliferative polycythaemia. *Lancet* **ii**: 1219–22, 1978.
46. Tohgi, H., Yamanouchi, H., Murakami, M. & Kameyama, M. Importance of the hematocrit as a risk factor in cerebral infarction. *Stroke* **9**: 369–74, 1978.
47. Lowe, G.D.O. Blood rheology in arterial disease. *Clin. Sci.* **71**: 137–46, 1986.
48. Anderson, J.V., Donckier, J., McKenna, W.J. & Bloom, S.R. The plasma release of atrial natriuretic peptide in man. *Clin. Sci.* **71**: 151–5, 1986.
49. Caramelo, L., Fernandez-Cruz, A., Villamediana, L.M., Sanz, E., Rodriguez-Puyol, D., Hernando, L., Lopez-Novoa, J.M. Systemic and regional haemodynamic effects of a synthetic atrial natriuretic peptide in conscious rats. *Clin. Sci.* **71**: 322–5, 1986.
50. Hirata, Y., Ishii, M., Sugimoto, T., Matsuoka, H., Ishimitsu, T., Atarashi, K., Sugimoto, T., Miyata, A., Kangawa, K. & Matsuo, H. Relationship between the renin–aldosterone system and atrial natriuretic polypeptide in rats. *Clin. Sci.* **72**: 165–70, 1987.
51. Winearls, C.G., Oliver, D.O., Pippard, M.J., Reid, C., Downing, M.R. & Cotes, P.M. Effect of human erythropoietin derived from recombinant DNA on the anaemia of patients maintained by chronic haemodialysis. *Lancet* **ii**: 1175–8, 1986.
52. Bruneval, P., da Silva, J.L., Lacombe, C., Fournier, J.G., Belair, M.F., Tambourin, P., Varet, B., Camilleri, J.P. & Bariety, J. Detection and localization of erythropoietin messenger-RNA in vascular endothelial cells of mouse kidney using in-situ hybridisation. *10th International Congress on Nephrology*, Satellite

Workshop on Erythropoietin, 1987.
53. Nathan, D.G. & Sykkowski, A. Editorial: Erythropoietin and the regulation of erythropoiesis. *N. Eng. J. Med.* **308**: 502–2, 1983.
54. Fisher, J.W. Control of erythropoietic production. *Proc. Soc. Exp. Biol. Med.* **173**: 289–305, 1983.
55. Barabas, A.P., Offen, D.N. & Meinhard, E.A. The arterial complication of polycythaemia vera. *Br. J. Surg.* **60**: 183–7, 1973.
56. Chievitz, E. & Thiede, T. Complications and causes of death in polycythaemia. *Acta. Med. Scand.* **172**: 513–23, 1962.
57. Preston, F.E., Marlin, J.F., Stewart, R.M. & Davies-Jones, G.A.B.: Thrombocytosis, circulating platelet aggregates and neurological dysfunction. *Br. Med. J.* **2**: 1561–3, 1979.
58. Schmid-Schönbein, H. Interaction of vasomotion and blood rheology in haemodynamics. In *Clinical Aspects of Blood Viscosity and Cell Deformability* (eds G.D.O. Lowe, J.D. Barbenel & C.D. Forbes), pp. 49–66. Springer, Berlin, 1981.
59. Pearson, T.C. Rheology of the absolute polycythaemias. *Clin. Haematol.* **1**: 637–64, 1987.
60. Schafer, A.I. Bleeding and thrombosis in the myeloproliferative disorders. *Blood* **64**: 1–12, 1984.
61. Pearson, T.C. Clinical and laboratory studies in the polycythaemias. MD. thesis, London University, 1977.
62. Messinezy, M., Pearson, T.C., Prockazka, A. & Wetherley-Mein, G. Treatment of primary proliferative polycythaemia by venesection and low dose busulphan: retrospective study from one centre. *Br. J. Haematol.* **61**: 657–66, 1985.
63. Dawson, A.A. & Ogston, D. The influence of the platelet count on the incidence of thrombotic and haemorrhagic complications in polycythaemia vera. *Postgrad. Med. J.* **46**: 76–8, 1970.
64. Berk, P.D., Goldberg, J.D., Silverstein, M.N., Weinfeld, A., Donovon, P.B., Ellis, J.T., Landow, S.A., Laszlo, J., Najean, Y., Pisciotta, A.V. & Wasserman, L.R. Increased incidence of acute leukaemia in polycythemia vera associated with chlorambucil therapy. *N. Engl. J. Med.* **304**: 441–7, 1981.
65. Wetherley-Mein, G., Pearson, T.C., Burney, P.G.J. & Morris, R.W. The Royal College of Physicians Research Unit, Polycythaemia Study. 1. Objective, background and design. *J. R. Coll. Physicians Lond.* **21**: 7–16, 1987.
66. Heath, D. & Williams, D.R. *Man at High Altitude*, 2nd Edn. Churchill Livingstone, Edinburgh, 1981.
67. Frisancho, A.R. Functional adaptation to high altitude hypoxia. *Science* **187**: 313–19, 1975.
68. Eaton, J.W., Brewer, G.J. & Grover, R.F. Role of red cell 2,3-diphosphoglycerate in the adaptation of man to altitude. *J. Lab. Clin. Med.* **73**: 603–9, 1969.
69. Moore, L.G. & Brewer, G.J. Beneficial effect of rightward hemoglobin-oxygen dissociation curve shift for short term high altitude adaptation. *J. Lab. Clin. Med.* **98**: 145–54, 1981.
70. Grover, R.F. Basal oxygen uptake of man at high altitude. *J. Appl. Physiol.* **18**: 909–12, 1963.
71. Klausen, K. Cardiac output in man in rest and work during and after acclimatization to 3800 m. *J. Appl. Physiol.* **21**: 609–16, 1966.
72. Rennie, D. Diseases of high terrestrial altitudes. In *Oxford Textbook of Medicine* (eds D.J. Weatherall, J.G.G. Ledingham & D.A. Warrell), pp. 6.57–6.64. Oxford University Press, Oxford, 1983.
73. Henry, J.P. & Pearce, J.W. Possible role of cardiac atrial stretch receptors in induction of change in urine flow. *J. Physiol.* **131**: 572–85, 1956.
74. Pugh, L.G.C.E. Physiological and medical aspects of the Himalayan scientific and mountaineering expedition, 1960–61. *Br. Med. J.* **2**: 621–7, 1962.
75. Horstman, D., Weiskopf, R. & Jackson, R.E. Work capacity during 3-week

sojourn at 4,300 m: effects of relative polycythemia. *J. Appl. Physiol.* **49**: 311–18, 1980.

76. Sarnquist, F.H., Schoene, R.B., Hackett, P.H. & Townes, B.D. Hemodilution of polycythemic mountaineers: effects of exercise and mental function. *Aviat. Space Environ. Med.* **57**: 313–17, 1986.

77. Adams, W.H. & Strang, L.J. Hemoglobin levels in persons of Tibetan ancestry living at high altitude. *Proc. Soc. Exp. Biol. Med.* **149**: 1036–9, 1975.

78. Morpurgo, G., Arese, P., Bosia, A., Pescarmona, G.P., Luzzana, M., Modiano, G. & Ranjit, S.K. Sherpas living permanently at high altitude: a new pattern of adaptation. *Proc. Natl. Acad. Sci. U.S.A* **73**: 747–51, 1976.

79. Hebbel, R.P., Eaton, J.W., Kronenberg, R.S., Zanjani, E.D., Moore, L.G. & Berger, E.M. Human llamas: adaptation to altitude in subjects with high hemoglobin oxygen affinity. *J. Clin. Invest.* **62**: 593–600, 1978.

80. Tenney, S.M. & Ou, L.C. Physiological evidence for increased tissue capillarity in rats acclimatized to high altitude. *Resp. Physiol.* **8**: 137–50, 1970.

81. Rahn, H. & Otis, A.B. Man's respiratory response during and after acclimatization to high altitude. *Am. J. Physiol.* **157**: 445–53, 1949.

82. Reynafarse, B. Myoglobin content and enzymatic activity of muscle and altitude adaptation. *J. Appl. Physiol.* **17**: 301–5, 1962.

83. Hurtado, A. Some clinical aspects of life at high altitudes. *Ann. Intern. Med.* **53**: 247–58, 1960.

84. Peñaloza, D., Sime, F. & Ruiz, L. Cor pulmonale in chronic mountain sickness: present concept of Monge's disease. In *High Altitude Physiology: Cardiac and Respiratory Aspects.* Ciba Foundation Symposium (eds. R. Porter & J. Knight), pp. 41–60. Churchill Livingstone, London, 1971.

85. Kryger, M., Glas, R., Jackson, D., McCullough, R.E., Scoggin, C., Grover, R.F. & Weil, J.V. Impaired oxygenation during sleep in excessive polycythemia of high altitude: improvement with sleep stimulation. *Sleep* **1**: 3–17, 1978.

86. Arias-Stella, J., Krüger, H. & Recavarren, S. Pathology of chronic mountain sickness. *Thorax* **28**: 701–8, 1973.

87. Gronbeck, C. Chronic Mountain Sickness at an elevation of 2000 metres. *Chest* **85**: 577–8, 1984.

88. Cruz, J.C., Diaz, C., Marticorena, E. & Hilario, V. Phlebotomy improves gas exchange in chronic mountain polycythemia. *Respiration* **38**: 305–13, 1979.

89. Winslow, R.M., Monge, C.C., Brown, E.G., Klein, H.G., Sarnquist, F., Winslow, N.J. & McKneally, S.S. Effect of hemodilution on O₂ transport in high-altitude polycythemia. *J. Appl Physiol.* **59**: 1495–502, 1985.

90. Koeffler, H.P. & Goldwasser, E. Erythropoietin radioimmunoassay in evaluating patients with polycythemia. *Ann. Intern. Med.* **94**: 44–7, 1981.

91. Rosenthal, A., Button, L.N., Nathan, D.G., Miettinen, O.S. & Nadas, A.S. Blood volume changes in cyanotic congenital heart disease. *Am. J. Cardiol.* **27**: 162–7, 1971.

92. Oldershaw, P.J. & St.John Sutton, M.G. Haemodynamic effects of haematocrit reduction in patient with polycythaemia secondary to cyanotic congenital heart disease. *Br. Heart J.* **44**: 584–8, 1980.

93. Bethrong, M. & Sabiston, D.C. Cerebral lesions in congenital heart disease. *Bull. Johns Hopkins Hosp.* **89**: 384–401, 1951.

94. Shapiro, E.P., Al-Sadir, J., Campbell, N.P.S., Thilenius, O.G. Anagnostopoulos, C.E. & Hays, P. Drainage of right superior vena cava into both atria. Review of the literature and description of a case presenting with polycythemia and paradoxical embolization. *Circulation* **63**: 712–17, 1981.

95. Cottrill, C.M. & Kaplan, S. Cerebral vascular accidents in cyanotic congenital heart disease. *Am. J. Dis. Childh.* **125**: 484–7, 1973.

96. Rich, A.R. A hitherto unrecognised tendency to the development of widespread pulmonary vascular obstruction in patients with congenital pulmonary stenosis

(tetralogy of Fallot). *Bull. Johns Hopkins Hosp.* **82**: 389–95, 1948.
97. Rosenthal, A., Nathan, D.G., Marty, T.L., Button, L.N., Mietinen, O.S. & Nadas, A.S. Acute hemodynamic effects of red cell volume reduction in polycythemia of cyanotic congenital heart disease. *Circulation* **42**: 297–307, 1970.
98. Edwards, P.D., Prosser, R. & Wells, C.E.C. Chorea, polycythaemia and cyanotic heart disease. *J. Neurol. Neurosurg. Psychiat.* **39**: 729–39, 1975.
99. Kontras, S.B., Bodenbender, J.G., Craenen, J. & Hosier, D.M. Hyperviscosity in congenital heart disease. *J. Pediatr.* **76**: 214–20, 1970.
100. Wedemeyer, A.L. & Lewis, J.H. Improvement in haemostasis following phlebotomy in cyanotic patients with heart disease. *J. Pediatr.* **83**: 46–50, 1973.
101. Rand, P.W., Lacombe, E., Hunt, H.E. & Austin, W.H. Viscosity of normal human blood under normothermic and hypothermic conditions. *J. Appl. Physiol.* **19**: 117–22, 1964.
102. Marath, A. Personal communication, 1987.
103. Settergren, G., Öhqvist, G., Lundberg, S., Henze, A., Björk, V.O. & Persson, B. Cerebral blood flow and cerebral metabolism in children following cardiac surgery with deep hypothermia and circulatory arrest. Clinical course and follow-up pyschomotor development. *Scand. J. Thorac. Cardiovasc. Surg.* **16**: 209–15, 1982.
104. Cottril, C.M. & Kaplan, S. Cerebral vascular accidents in cyanotic congenital heart disease. *Am. J. Dis. Childh.* **125**: 484–7, 1973.
105. Pearson, T.C., Guthrie, D.L., Slater, N.G.P. & Wetherley-Mein, G. Method of PCV measurement and the effect of iron deficiency on whole blood viscosity. *Br. J. Haematol.* **52**: 166–9, 1982.
106. Van de Pette, J.E.W., Guthrie, D.L. & Pearson, T.C. Whole blood viscosity in polycythaemia: the effect of iron deficiency at a range of haemoglobin and packed cell volumes. *Br. J. Haematol.* **63**: 369–75, 1986.
107. Smith, C.M., McClain, K.L., Tukey, D.F. & Moller, J.H. Relationship of cerebrovascular symptoms to blood viscosity in a patient with iron deficiency and cyanotic heart disease. *Clin. Hemorheol.* **6**: 257–69, 1986.
108. Weil, J.V., Jamieson, G., Brown, D.W. & Grover, R.F. The red cell mass-arterial oxygen relationship in normal man. *J. Clin. Invest.* **47**: 1627–39, 1968.
109. Shaw, D.B. & Simpson, T. Polycythaemia in emphysema. *Q. J. Med.* **30**: 135–52, 1961.
110. Hume, R. Blood volume changes in chronic bronchitis and emphysema. *Br. J. Haematol.* **15**: 131–9, 1968.
111. Stradling, J.R. & Lane, D.J. Development of secondary polycythaemia in chronic airways obstruction. *Thorax* **36**: 321–5, 1981.
112. Gallo, R.C., Fraimow, W., Cathcart, R. & Erslev, A.J. Erythropoietic response in chronic pulmonary disease. *Arch. Intern. Med.* **113**: 559–68, 1964.
113. Harrison, B.D.W. Polycythaemia in a selected group of patients with chronic airways obstruction. *Clin. Sci.* **44**: 563–70, 1973.
114. Flenley, D.C. Oxygen transport in chronic hypoxic lung disease. *J. Clin. Pathol.* **35**: 797–9, 1982.
115. Wedzicha, J.A., Cotes, P.M., Empey, D.W., Newland, A.C., Royston, J.P. & Tam, R.C. Serum immunoreactive erythropoietin in hypoxic lung disease with and without polycythaemia. *Clin. Sci.* **69**: 413–22, 1985.
116. Flenley, D.C., Fairweather, L.J., Cooke, N.J. & Kirby, B.J. Change in haemoglobin binding curve and oxygen transport in chronic hypoxic lung disease. *Br. Med. J.* **1**: 602–4, 1975.
117. Sagone, A.L., Lawrence, T. & Balcerzak, S. Effect of smoking on tissue oxygen supply. *Blood* **41**: 845–51, 1973.
118. Calverley, P.M.A., Leggett, R.J., McElderry, L. & Flenley, D.C. Cigarette smoking and secondary polycythemia in hypoxic cor pulmonale. *Am. Rev. Respir. Dis.* **125**: 507–10, 1982.

119. Wilcox, C.S., Payne, J. & Harrison, D.B.W. Renal function in patients with chronic hypoxaemia and cor pulmonale following reversal of polycythaemia. *Nephron* **30**: 173–7, 1982.
120. Wallis, P.J.W., Cunningham, J., Few, J.D., Newland, A.C. & Empey, D.W. Effects of packed cell volume reduction on renal haemodynamics and the renin-angiotensin-aldosterone system in patients with secondary polycythaemia and hypoxic cor pulmonale. *Clin. Sci.* **70**: 81–90.
121. Robin, E.D. Of men and mitochondria: coping with hypoxic dysoxia. *Am. Rev. Respir. Dis.* **122**: 517–31, 1980.
122. Vanier, T., Dulfano, M.J., Wu, C. & Desforges, J.F. Emphysema, hypoxia and polycythaemic response. *N. Engl. J. Med.* **269**: 169–78, 1963.
123. Semple, P.d'A., Beastall, G.H., Watson, W.S. & Hume, R. Serum testosterone depression associated with hypoxia in respiratory failure. *Clin. Sci.* **58**: 105–6, 1980.
124. Crofton, J. & Douglas, A. Respiratory failure. In *Respiratory Diseases* 3rd Edn, pp. 407–15. Blackwell Scientific Publications, Oxford, 1981.
125. Dintenfass, L. & Read, J. Pathogenesis of heart failure in acute-on-chronic respiratory failure. *Lancet* **i**: 570–2, 1968.
126. Howard, P. Drugs or oxygen for hypoxic cor pulmonale. *Br. Med. J.* **287**: 1159–60, 1983.
127. Treacher, D.F., Douglas, A., Jones, A., Bateman, N.T., Bradley, R.D. & Cameron, I.E. The acute haemodynamic effects of intravenous verapamil in patients with chronic obstructive airways disease. *Q. J. Med.* **66**: 941–52, 1987.
128. Douglas, A.R., Moore-Gillon, J.C., Sheldon, J.W.S. & Cameron, I.R. Effect of verapamil on polycythaemia secondary to hypoxia in rats. *Clin. Sci.* **73**: 665–7, 1987.
129. Treacher, D.F., Pearson, T.C. & Cameron, I.R. The effect of verapamil on polycythaemia in patients with chronic obstructive airways disease. *Clin. Sci.* **73**: 35p, 1987.
130. Neff, T.A. & Petty, T.L. Long-term continuous oxygen therapy in chronic airway obstruction. *Ann. Intern. Med.* **72**: 621–6, 1970.
131. Medical Research Council Working Party. Long term domiciliary oxygen therapy in chronic cor pulmonale complicating chronic bronchitis and emphysema. *Lancet* **i**: 681–6, 1981.
132. Gluskowski, J., Jedrzejewska-Makowska, M., Hawrylkiewicz, I., Vertun, B. & Zielinski, J. Effects of prolonged oxygen therapy on pulmonary hypertension and blood viscosity in patients with advanced cor pulmonale. *Respiration* **44**: 177–83, 1983.
133. Pengelly, C.D.R. Reduction of haematocrit and red-blood-cell volume in patients with polycythaemia secondary to hypoxic lung disease by dapsone and pyrimethamine. *Lancet* **ii**: 1381–6, 1966.
134. Pengelly, C.D.R. Reduction of excessive haematocrit levels in patients with polycythaemia due to hypoxic lung disease by phenylhydrazine hydrochloride and pyrimethanine. *Postgrad. Med.* **45**: 588–90, 1967.
135. Segel, N. & Bishop, J.M. Circulatory studies in polycythaemia vera at rest and during exercise. *Clin. Sci.* **32**: 527–49, 1967.
136. Harrison, B.D.W., Davis, J., Madgwick, R.G. & Evans, M. The effects of therapeutic decrease in packed cell volume on the responses to exercise of patients with polycythaemia secondary to lung disease. *Clin. Sci. Mol. Med.* **45**: 833–47, 1973.
137. Weisse, A.B., Moschos, C.B., Frank, M.J., Levinson, G.E., Cannilla, J.E. & Regan, T.J. Hemodynamic effects of staged hematocrit reduction in patients with stable cor pulmonale and severely elevated hematocrit levels. *Am. J. Med.* **58**: 92–8, 1975.
138. Erickson, A.D., Golden, W.A., Claunch, B.C., Donat, W.E. & Kaemmerlen, J.T.

Acute effects of phlebotomy on right ventricular size and performance in polycythemic patients with chronic obstructive pulmonary disease. *Am. J. Cardiol.* **52**: 183–6, 1983.

139. Chetty, K.G., Brown, S.E. & Light, R.W. Improved exercise tolerance of the polycythemic lung patient following phlebotomy. *Am. J. Med.* **74**: 415–20, 1983.

140. Wedzicha, J.A., Cotter, F.E., Rudd, R.M., Apps, M.C.P., Newland, A.C. & Empey, D.W. Erythrapheresis compared with placebo apheresis in patients with polycythaemia secondary to hypoxic lung disease. *Eur. J. Respir. Dis.* **65**: 579–85, 1984.

141. Hart, G., Stokes, T.C., Harrison, B.D.W. & Castell, D. Erythrapheresis in patients with polycythaemia secondary to hypoxic lung disease. *Br. Med. J.* **286**: 1284, 1983.

142. Semple, P.d'A., Lowe, G.D.O., Patterson, J., Beastall, G.H., Rowan, J.O., Forbes, C.D. & Hume, R. Comparison of cerebral blood flow after venesection of bronchitic secondary polycythaemia and primary polycythaemic patients. *Scott Med. J.* **28**: 332–7, 1983.

143. Wade, J.P.H., Pearson, T.C., Ross Russel, R.W. & Wetherley-Mein, G. Cerebral blood flow and blood viscosity in patients with polycythaemia secondary to hypoxic lung disease. *Br. Med. J.* **283**: 689–92, 1981.

144. Bornstein, R., Menon, D., York, E., Sproule, B. & Zak, C. Effect of venesection on cerebral function in chronic lung disease. *Can. J. Neurol. Sci.* **7**: 293–6, 1980.

145. Wedzicha, J.A., Rudd, R.M., Apps, M.C.F., Cotter, F.E., Newland, A.C. & Empey, D.W. Erythrapheresis in patients with polycythaemia secondary to hypoxic lung disease. *Br. Med. J.* **286**: 511–14, 1983.

146. Nashat, F.S., Scholefield, F.R., Tappin, J.W. & Wilcox, C.S. The effects of changes in PCV on the intrarenal distribution of blood flow in the dog's kidney. *J. Physiol.* **201**: 639–55, 1969.

147. Napier, J.A.F. & Janowska-Wieczorek, A. Erythropoietin measurements in the differential diagnosis of polycythaemia. *Br. J. Haematol.* **48**: 393–401, 1981.

148. Schaaning, J. & Sparr, S. Blood letting and exchange transfusion with Dextran 40 in polycythemia secondary to chronic obstructive lung disease. *Scand. J. Resp. Dis.* **55**: 237–44, 1974.

149. Constantinidis, K. Venesection fatalities in polycythaemia secondary to lung disease. *Practitioner* **222**: 89–91, 1979.

150. Sondel, P.M., Tripp, M.E., Ganick, D.J., Levy, J.M. & Shahidi, N.T. Phlebotomy with iron therapy to correct the microcytic polycythemia of chronic hypoxia. *Pediatrics* **67**: 667–70, 1981.

151. Fishman, A.P., Turno, G.M. & Bergofsky, E.H. The syndrome of alveolar hypoventilation. *Am. J. Med.* **23**: 333–9, 1957.

152. Apps, M.C.P. Sleep-disordered breathing. *Br. J. Hosp. Med.* **30**: 339–47, 1983.

153. Ratto, O., Briscoe, W.A., Morton, J.W. & Comroe, J.H. Anoxemia secondary to polycythemia and polycythemia secondary to Anoxemia. *Am. J. Med.* **19**: 958–65, 1955.

154. Neil, J.F., Reynolds, C.F., Spiker, D.G. & Kupfer, D.J. Polycythaemia vera and central sleep apnoea. *Br. Med. J.* **1**: 19, 1980.

155. Rodman, T. & Close, H.P. The primary hypoventilation syndrome. *Am. J. Med.* **26**: 808–17, 1959.

156. Alexander, J.K., Amad, K.H. & Cole, V.W. Observations on some clinical features of extreme obesity with particular reference to cardio-respiratory effects. *Am. J. Med.* **32**: 512–24, 1962.

157. Cayler, G., Mays, T. & Riley, H.D. Cardio-respiratory syndrome of obesity (Pickwickian syndrome) in children. *Pediatrics* **27**: 237–45, 1961.

158. Wittmers, L.E. & Haller, E.W. The onset and development of polycythaemia in the obese mouse. *J. Comp. Pathol.* **92**: 519–25, 1981.

159. Burwell, C.S., Robin, E.D., Whaley, R.D. & Bickelmann, A.G. Extreme obesity

associated with alveolar hypoventilation – a Pickwickian syndrome. *Am. J. Med.* **21**: 811–18, 1956.
160. Zwillich, C.W., Sutton, F.D., Pierson, D.J., Creagh, E.M. & Weil, J.V. Decreased hypoxic ventilatory drive in the obesity-hypoventilation syndrome. *Am. J. Med.* **59**: 343–8, 1975.
161. Block, A.J., Boysen, P.G., Wynne, J.W. & Hunt, L.A. Sleep apnea, hypopnea and oxygen desaturation in normal subjects. *N. Engl. J. Med.* **300**: 513–17, 1979.
162. Flenley, D.C. Hypoxaemia during sleep. *Thorax* **35**: 81–4, 1980.
163. Ward, H.P., Bigelow, D.B. & Petty, T.L. Postural hypoxemia and erythrocytosis. *Am. J. Med.* **45**: 880–8, 1968.
164. Hamosh, P. & Da Silva, A.M.T. Supine hypoxaemia and erythrocytosis due to airway closure at low lung volumes. *Am. J. Med.* **55**: 80–5, 1973.
165. Strieder, D.J., Murphy, R. & Kazemi, H. Mechanism of postural hypoxemia in asymptomatic smokers. *Am. Rev. Respir. Dis.* **99**: 760–6, 1969.
166. Flenley, D.C. Disordered breathing during sleep: discussion paper. *J. R. Soc. Med.* **78**: 1031–3, 1985.
167. Kales, A., Cadieux, R.J., Shaw, L.C., Vela-Bueno, A., Bixler, E.O., Schneck, D.W., Locke, T.W. & Soldatos, C.R. Sleep apnoea in a hypersensitive population. *Lancet* **ii**: 1005–8, 1984.
168. Saunders, W.H. Hereditary hemorrhagic telangiectasia. *Arch. Otolaryngol.* **76**: 245–60, 1962.
169. Eisen, M.E. & Hammond, E.C. The effect of smoking on packed cell volume, red blood cell counts and platelet counts. *Can. Med. Assoc. J.* **75**: 520–3, 1956.
170. Isager, H. & Hagerup, L. Relationship between cigarette smoking and high packed cell volume and haemoglobin levels. *Scand. J. Haematol.* **8**: 241–4, 1971.
171. Smith, J.R. & Landaw, S.A. Smokers' polycythaemia. *N. Engl. J. Med.* **298**: 6–10, 1978.
172. Spiers, A.S.D. & Levine, M. Smokers' polycythaemia. *Lancet* **i**: 120, 1983.
173. Doll, D.C. & Greenberg, B.R. Cerebral thrombosis in smokers' polycythemia. *Ann. Intern. Med.* **102**: 786–7, 1985.
174. Velasquez, M.T., Schecter, G.P., McFarland, W. & Cohn, J.N. Relative Polycythemia: a state of high venous tone. *Clin. Res.* **22**: 409A, 1974.
175. Moore-Gillon, J. & Pearson, T.C. Smoking, drinking, and polycythaemia. *Br. Med. J.* **292**: 1617–18, 1986.
176. Stewart, R.D., Baretta, E.D., Platte, L.R., Stewart, E.B., Kalbfleisch, J.H., Yserloo, B.V. & Rimm, A.A. Carboxyhemoglobin levels in American blood donors. *J. Am. Med. Assoc.* **229**: 1187–95, 1974.
177. Goldman, A.L. Cigar inhaling. *Am. Rev. Respir. Dis.* **113**: 87–9, 1976.
178. Brody, J.S. & Coburn, R.F. Carbon monoxide-induced arterial hypoxemia. *Science* **164**: 1297–8, 1969.
179. Hlastala, M.P., McKenna, H.P., Franada, R.L. & Detter, J.C. Influence of carbon monoxide on hemoglobin-oxygen binding. *J. Appl. Phys.* **41**: 893–9, 1976.
180. Davies, J.M., Latto, I.P., Jones, J.G., Veale, A. & Wardrop, C.A.J. Effects of stopping smoking for 48 hours on oxygen availability from the blood: a study on pregnant women. *Br. Med. J.* **2**: 355–6, 1979.
181. Goldstein, R. Smokers' polycythemia. *N. Engl. J. Med.* **298**: 972, 1978.
182. Ho-Yen, D.O., Spence, V.A., Moody, J.P. & Walker, W.P. Why smoke fewer cigarettes? *Br. Med. J.* **1**: 1905–7, 1982.
183. Foster, L.J., Corrigan, K. & Goldman, A.L. Effectiveness of oxygen therapy in hypoxic polycythemic smokers. *Chest* **73**: 572–6, 1978.
184. Gunton, R.W. & Paul, W. Blood volume in congestive heart failure. *J. Clin. Invest.* **34**: 879–86, 1955.
185. Schreiber, S.S., Bauman, A., Yalow, R.S. & Berson, S.A. Blood volume alterations in congestive heart failure. *J. Clin. Invest.* **33**: 578–86, 1954.

186. Chodos, R.B., Wells, R. & Chaffee, W.R. A study of ferrokinetics and red cell survival in congestive heart failure. *Am. J. Med.* **36**: 553–60, 1964.
187. Charache, S., Achuff, S., Winslow, R., Adamson, J. & Chervenick, P. Variability of the homeostatic response to altered p_{50}. *Blood* **52**: 1156–62, 1978.
188. Fairbanks, V.F., Maldonado, J.E., Charache, S. & Boyer, S.H. Familial erythrocytosis due to electrophoretically undetectable hemoglobin with impaired oxygen dissociation (hemoglobin Malmö, $\alpha_2\beta_2^{97gln}$). *Mayo Clin. Proc.* **46**: 721–7, 1971.
189. White, J.M., Szur, L., Gillies, I.D.S., Lorkin, P.A. & Lehmann, H. Familial polycythaemia caused by a new haemoglobin variant. Hb Heathrow, β 103(G5) phenylalanine-leucine. *Br. Med. J.* **3**: 665–7, 1973.
190. Weatherall, D.J., Clegg, J.B., Callendar, S.T., Wells, R.M.G., Gale, R.E., Huehns, E.R., Perutz, M.F., Viggiano, G. & Ho, C. Haemoglobin Radcliffe: A high oxygen-affinity variant causing familial polycythaemia. *Br. J. Haematol.* **35**: 117–91, 1977.
191. Butler, W.M., Spratling, L., Kark, J.A. & Schoomaker, E.B. Hemoglobin Osler: Report of a new family with exercise studies before and after phlebotomy. *Am. J. Hematol.* **13**: 293–301, 1982.
192. Gau, T., Fairbanks, V.F., Maldonado, J.E., Bassingthwaighte, J.B. & Tanered, R.G. Cardiac dysfunction in a patient with hemoglobin Malmö treated with repeated transfusion. *Clin. Res.* **22**: 276A, 1974.
193. Rosa, R., Prehu, M-O., Beuza, Y. & Rosa, J. The first case of a complete deficiency of diphosphoglycerate mutase in human erythrocytes. *J. Clin. Invest.* **62**: 907–15, 1978.
194. Charache, S., Clegg, J.B. & Weatherall, D.J. The Negro variety of hereditary persistence of fetal haemoglobin is a mild form of thalassaemia. *Br. J. Haematol.* **34**: 527–34, 1976.
195. Smith, H. & Riches, E. Haemoglobin values in renal carcinoma. *Lancet* **i**: 1017–20, 1963.
196. Kazal, L.A. & Erslev, A.J. Erythropoietin production in renal tumours. *Ann. Clin. Lab. Sci.* **5**: 98–109, 1975.
197. von Knorring, J., Selroos, O. & Scheinin, T.M. Hematologic findings in patients with renal carcinoma. *Scand. J. Urol. Nephrol.* **15**: 279–83, 1981.
198. Murphy, G.P., Kenny, G.M. & Mirand, E.A. Erythropoietin levels in patients with renal tumours or cysts. *Cancer* **26**: 191–4, 1970.
199. Waldmann, T.A., Rosse, W.F., Swarm, R.L. The erythropoiesis-stimulating factors produced by tumours. *Ann. N.Y. Acad. Sci.* **149**: 509–15, 1968.
200. Erslev, A.J. & Caro, J. Pure erythrocytosis classified according to erythropoietin titers. *Am. J. Med.* **76**: 57–61, 1984.
201. Damon, A., Holub, D.A., Melicow, M.M. & Uson, A.C. Polycythemia and renal carcinoma: Report of 10 new cases, two with long hematologic remission following nephrectomy. *Am. J. Med.* **25**: 182–97,. 1958.
202. Thurman, W.G., Grabstald, H. & Lieberman, P.H. Elevation of erythropoietin levels in association with Wilms' Tumor. *Arch. Intern. Med.* **117**: 280–3, 1966.
203. Shalet, M.F., Holder, T.M. & Walters, T.R. Erythropoietin-producing Wilms' tumour. *J. Pediatr.* **70**: 615–17, 1967.
204. Kenny, G.M., Mirand, E.A., Stanbitz, W.J., Allen, J.E., Trudel, P.J. & Murphy, G.P. Erythropoietin levels in Wilms' tumour patients. *J. Urol.* **104**: 758–61, 1970.
205. Friend, D., Hoskins, R.G. & Kirkin, M.W. Relative erythrocythemia (polycythemia) and polycystic disease with uremia. Report of a case with comments on frequency of occurrence. *N. Engl. J. Med.* **264**: 17–19, 1961.
206. Ways, P., Huff, J.W., Kosmaler, C.H. & Young, L.E. Polycythemia and histologically proven renal disease. *Arch. Intern. Med.* **107**: 154–62, 1961.
207. Rosse, W.F., Waldmann, T.A. & Cohen, P. Renal cysts, erythropoietin and polycythemia. *Am. J. Med.* **34**: 76–81, 1963.

208. Fyhrquist, F.Y., Klockars, M., Gordin, A., Törnroth, T. & Kock, B. Hyperreninemia, lysozymuria, and erythrocytosis in Fanconi syndrome with medullary cystic kidney. *Acta Med. Scand.* **207**: 359–65, 1980.
209. Gallagher, N.I. & Donati, R.M. Inappropriate erythropoietin elaboration. *Ann. N.Y. Acad. Sci.* **149**: 528–38, 1968.
210. Plzak, L.F. Erythropoietin and renal cyst fluid. *Clin. Res.* **13**: 281, 1965.
211. Kaplan, J.P., Sprayregan, S., Ossias, A.L. & Zanjani, E.D. Erythropoietin-producing renal cyst and polycythaemia vera. *Am. J. Med.* **54**: 819–24, 1973.
212. Djaldetti, M., Bessler, H. & Kimche, D. Transformation of erythrocytosis associated with renal cyst to polycythemia vera. *Haematologica* **65**: 343–8, 1980.
213. Myers, D.I., Ciuffo, A.A. & Cooke, C.R. Focal glomerulosclerosis and erythrocytosis. *Johns Hopkins Med. J.* **145**: 192–5, 1979.
214. Walker, J.F., Dunn, J.M., Ryan, C.F., Carmody, M., Cronic, C., O'Dwyer, W.F., & Moher, M. Erythrocytosis associated with focal sclerosing glomerulonephritis. *Ir. Med. J.* **77**: 14–15, 1984.
215. Emmanuel, D.A. & Wenzel, F.J. Erythrocytosis associated with the nephrotic syndrome. *J. Am. Med. Assoc.* **181**; 788–90, 1962.
216. Hoppin, E.C., Depner, T., Yamuchi, H. & Hopper, J. Erythrocytosis associated with diffuse parenchymal lesions of the kidney, *Br. J. Haematol.* **32**: 557–63, 1976.
217. Frolick, H., Gourley, R.T. & Hansen, K.S. Wegener's granulomatosis with polycythemia. *West J. Med.* **136**: 350–3, 1982.
218. Toyama, F. & Mitus, W.J. Experimental renal erythrocytosis. *J. Lab. Clin. Med.* **68**: 740–52, 1966.
219. Hirsch, I. & Leiter, E. Hydronephrosis and polycythemia. *Urology* **21**: 345–50, 1983.
220. Jepson, J.H. & McGarry, E.E. Polycythemia and increased erythropoietin production by a patient with hypertrophy of the juxtaglomerular apparatus. *Blood* **32**: 370–5, 1968.
221. Erkelens, D.W. & Statius van Eps, L.W. Bartter's syndrome and erythrocytosis. *Am. J. Med.* **55**: 711–19, 1973.
222. Mitus, W.J., Toyama, K. & Braner, M.J. Erythrocytosis, juxtaglomerular apparatus and erythropoietin in the course of experimental unilateral hydronephrosis in rabbits. *Ann. N.Y. Acad. Sci.* **149**: 107–13, 1968.
223. Luke, R.G., Kennedy, A.C., Barr Stirling, W.B. & McDonald, G.A. Renal artery stenosis hypertension and polycythaemia. *Br. Med. J.* **1**: 164–6, 1965.
224. Hudgson, P., Pearce, J.M. & Yeates, W.K. Renal artery stenosis with hypertension and high hematocrit. *Br. Med. J.* **1**: 18–21, 1967.
225. Maezawa, M., Takaku, F., Muto, Y., Mizoguchi, H. & Miura, Y. A case of intrarenal artery stenosis associated with erythocytosis. *Scand. J. Haematol.* **21**: 278–82, 1978.
226. Wickre, C.G., Norman, D.J., Bennison, A., Barry, J.M. & Bennet, W.M. Postrenal transplant erythrocytosis: a review of 53 patients. *Kidney Int.* **23**: 731–7, 1983.
227. Saltissi, D., Chang, R. & Abomelha, M.S. Polycythaemia following renal transplantation at the Riyadh Armed Forces Hospital. In *Organ Transplantation* (ed. M.S. Abomelha). Medical Education Services, Oxford, 1986.
228. Davis, H.P. Polycythaemia following renal transplantation. *J. R. Soc. Med.* **80**: 475–6, 1987.
229. Swales, J.D. & Evans, D.B. Erythraemia in renal transplantation. *Br. Med. J.* **2**: 80–3, 1969.
230. Obermiller, L.E., Tzamaloukas, A.H., Avasthi, P.S., Halpern, J.A., Sterling, W.A. Decreased plasma volume in post-transplant erythrocytosis. *Clin. Nephrol.* **23**: 213–177, 1985.
231. Nies, B.A., Cohn, R. & Schrier, S.L. Erythremia after renal transplantation. *N.*

    Engl. J. Med. **273**: 785–8, 1965.
232. Westerman, M.P., Jenkins, J.L., Dekker, A., Kreutner, A. & Fisher, B. Significance of erythrocytosis and increased erythropoietin secretion after renal transplantation. *Lancet* **ii**: 755, 1967.
233. Nellans, R., Otis, P. & Martin, D.C. Polycythaemia following renal transplantation. *Urology* **6**: 158–63, 1975.
234. Bacon, B.R., Rothman, S.A., Ricanati, E.S. & Rashad, F.A. Renal artery stenosis with erythrocytosis after renal transplantation. *Arch. Intern. Med.* **140**: 1206–11, 1980.
235. Simon, P., Boffa, G., Ang, K.S. & Menault, M. Polycythaemia in a haemodialyzed anephric patient with hepatitis. Demonstration of erythropoietin secretion. *Nouv. Presse Med.* **11**: 1401–3, 1982.
236. Daghert, F.J., Ramos, E., Erslev, A.J., Alongi, S.V., Karmi, S.A. & Caro, J. Are the active kidneys responsible for erythrocytosis in renal allorecipients? *Transplantation* **28**: 496–8, 1979.
237. Dagher, F.J., Ramos, E., Karmi, S. & Alongi, S.V. Erythrocytosis after renal allotransplantation. Treatment by removal of the native kidneys. *South. Med. J.* **73**: 940–2, 1980.
238. Heilmann, E., Gottschalk, D., Gottschalk, I. & Lison, A.E. Studies in polycythemia after kidney transplantation. *Clin. Nephrol.* **20**: 94–7, 1983.
239. Fried, W. The liver as a source of renal erythropoietin production. *Blood* **40**: 671–7, 1972.
240. Gordon, A.S., Zanjani E.D. & Zavosky, R. A possible mechanism for the erythrocytosis associated with hepato-cellular carcinoma in man. *Blood* **5**: 151–7, 1970.
241. Davidson, C.S. Hepatocellular carcinoma and erythrocytosis. *Semin. Haematol.* **13**: 115–19, 1976.
242. Eppstein, S. Primary carcinoma of the liver. *Am. J. Med. Sci.* **247**: 137–44, 1964.
243. McFadzean, A.J.S., Todd, D. & Tsang, K.C. Polycythemia in primary carcinoma of the liver. *Blood* **8**: 427–35, 1958.
244. Kan, Y.W., McFadzean, A.J.S., Todd, D. & Tso, S.C. Further observations on polycythemia in hepatocellular carcinoma. *Blood* **18**: 592–8, 1961.
245. Browstein, M.H. & Ballard, H.S. Hepatoma associated with erythrocytosis: Report of eleven new cases. *Am. J. Med.* **40**: 204–10, 1966.
246. Mukiibi, J.M., Mwaungulu, G.S. & Wankya, B.M. Some haematological observations of Kenyan hepatocellular carcinoma patients. *East Afr. Med. J.* **59**: 118–26, 1982.
247. Donati, R.M., McCarthy, J.M., Lange, R.D. & Gallagher, N.J. Erythrocythemia and neoplastic tumors. *Ann. Intern. Med,.* **58**: 47–55, 1963.
248. Lehman, A.J., Erslev, A.J. & Myerson, R.M. Erythrocytosis associated with hepatocellular carcinoma. *Am. J. Med.* **35**: 439–42, 1963.
249. Nakao, K., Kimura, K., Miura, Y. & Takaku, F. Erythrocytosis associated with carcinoma of the liver (with erythropoietin assay of tumor extract). *Am. J. Med. Sci.* **251**: 161–5, 1966.
250. McFadzean, A.J.S., Todd, D. & Tso, S.C. Erythrocytosis associated with hepatocellular carcinoma. *Blood* **29**: 808–11, 1967.
251. Tso, S.C. & Hua, A.S.P. Erythrocytosis in hepatocellular carcinoma – a compensatory phenomenon. *Br. J. Haematol.* **28**: 497–503, 1974.
252. Okazaki, N., Ozaki, H., Arima, M., Hattori, N. & Kimura, K. Hepatocellular carcinoma associated with erythrocytosis and a nine year survival after successful left lateral hepatectomy. *Acta Hepato-Gastroenterol.* **26**: 248–52, 1979.
253. Hutchison, D.C.S., Sapru, R.P., Sumerling, M.D., Donaldson, G.W.K. & Richmond, J. Cirrhosis, cyanosis and polycythemia: multiple pulmonary arteriovenous anastomoses. *Am. J. Med.* **45**: 139–51, 1968.
254. Wolfe, J.D., Tashkin, D.P., Holly, F.E., Brachman, M.B. & Genovesi, M.G.

Hypoxemia of cirrhosis: Detection of abnormal small pulmonary vascular channels by a quantitative radionuclide method. *Am. J. Med.* **63**: 746–54, 1977.
255. Lizzi, F.A., Tartaglia, A.P. & Adamson, J.W. Hemachromatosis, hepatoma, erythrocytosis and erythropoietin. *N.Y. State J. Med.* **73**: 1098–1100, 1973.
256. Kolk-Vegter, A.J., Bosch, E. & van Leeuwen, A.M. Influence of serum hepatitis on haemoglobin levels in patients on regular haemodialysis. *Lancet* i: 526–8, 1971.
257. Simon, P., Meyer, A., Tanquerel, T. & Ang, K.-S. Improvement of anaemia in haemodialysis patients after viral or toxic hepatic cytolysis. *Br. Med. J.* **1**: 892–4, 1980.
258. Popa, G., Ambarus, V., Dolinescu, C., Daniil, C., Ungureanu, E. & Cosma, M. Diffuse hepatic hemangioma associated with polycythaemia. *Rev. Med. Chir. Soc. Med. Nat. Iasi.* **88**: 375–7, 1984.
259. Platz, C.M., Knowlton, A.J. & Ragan, C. The natural history of Cushing's syndrome. *Am. J. Med.* **13**: 597–614, 1952.
260. Fisher, J.W. Increase in circulatory red cell volume of normal rats after treatment with hydrocortisone or corticosterone. *Proc. Soc. Exp. Biol. Med.* **97**: 502–5, 1958.
261. Jepson, J.H. & Lowenstein, L. The effect of testosterone, adrenal steroids and prolactin on erythropoiesis. *Acta Haematol.* **38**: 292–9, 1967.
262. Glader, B.E., Rambach, W.A. & Alt, H.L. Observations on the effect of testosterone and hydrocortisone on erythropoiesis. *Ann. N.Y. Acad. Sci.* **149**: 383–8, 1968.
263. Singer, J.W., Samuels, A.I. & Adamson, J.W. Steroids and hematopoiesis. I. The effect of steroids on in vitro erythroid colony growth: structure/activity relationship. *J. Cell Physiol.* **88**: 127–34, 1976.
264. Reisner, E.H. Tissue culture of bone marrow. II. Effect of steroid hormones on hematopoiesis *in vitro*. *Blood* **27**: 460–9, 1966.
265. Eaves, A.C. & Eaves, C.J. Erythropoiesis in culture. *Clin. Haematol.* **13**: 371–91, 1984.
266. Mann, D.L., Gallagher, N.J. & Donati, R.M. Erythrocytosis and primary aldosteronism. *Ann. Intern. Med.* **66**: 335–40, 1967.
267. Sjoerdsma, A., Engelman, K., Waldmann, T.A., Cooperman, L.H. & Hammond, W.G. Phaechromocytoma: current concepts in diagnosis and treatment. *Ann. Intern. Med.* **65**: 1302–25, 1976.
268. Bradley, J.E., Young, J.D. & Lentz, G. Polycythemia secondary to phaeo-chromocytoma. *J. Urol.* **86**. 1–6, 1961.
269. Battle, J.D., Alfidi, R.J. & Straffon, F.A. Polycythaemia secondary to phaeo-chromocytoma. Report of a case. *Cleve. Clin. Q.* **38**: 121–4, 1971.
270. Muldowney, F.P., Crooks, J. & Wayne, E.J. The total red cell mass in thyrotoxicosis and myxoedema. *Clin. Sci.* **16**: 309–14, 1957.
271. Khojasteh, A. & Perry, M.C. Thyrotoxic erythrocytosis. *South Med. J.* **75**: 379–80, 1982.
272. Dallera, F. & Gamoletti, R. Erythrocytosis associated with thyroid tumor. *Tumori* **66**: 273–5, 1980.
273. Jeffreys, R. Pathological and haematological aspects of posterior fossa haemangioblastomata. *J. Neurol. Neurosurg. Psychiat.* **38**: 112–19, 1975.
274. Cramer, F. & Kimsey, W. The cerebellar hemangioblastoma. *Arch. Neurol. Psychiat.* **67**: 237–52, 1952.
275. Starr, G.F., Stroebel, C.F., Kearns, T.P. Polycythemia with papilledema and infratentorial vascular tumors. *Ann. Intern. Med.* **48**: 978–86, 1958.
276. Perks, W.H., Cross, J.N., Sivapragasam, S. & Johnson, P. Supratentorial haemangioblastoma with polycythaemia. *J. Neurol. Neurosurg. Psychiat.* **39**: 218–20, 1976.
277. Waldmann, T.A., Levin, E.H. & Baldwin, M. The association of polycythemia

with a cerebellar hemangioblastoma. *Ann. J. Med.* **31**: 318–24, 1961.

278. Boivin, P., Bousser, J., Brion, S. & Guiot, G. Polyglobulie et hémangiome du cervelet. Rapport de deux cas avec mise en évidence d'une substance erythropoièteque dans la tumeur et le plasma. *Presse Med.* **73**: 2799–803, 1965.
279. Hennessy, T.G., Stern, W.E. & Herrick, S.E. Cerebellar hemangioblastoma: erythropoietic activity by radio-iron assay. *J. Nucl. Med.* **8**: 601–6, 1967.
280. Brody, J.I. & Rodriguez, F. Cerebellar hemangioblastoma and polycythemia (erythrocythemia). *Am. J. Med. Sci.* **242**: 579–84, 1961.
281. Horwitz, A. & McKelway, W.P. Polycythemia associated with uterine myomas. *J. Am. Med. Assoc.* **158**: 1360–1, 1955.
282. Vanden Berg, A.R. & Vasu, C.M. Polycythemia associated with uterine fibroma. *J. Am. Med. Assoc.* **185**: 249–51, 1963.
283. Morton, E.D., Evans, E.F. & Daines, W.P. Polycythemia and uterine myomata. *J. Am. Med. Assoc.* **200**: 149, 1967.
284. Wrigley, P.F.M., Malpas, J.S., Turnbull, A.L., Jenkins, V. & McArt, A. Secondary polycythaemia due to a uterine fibromyoma producing erythropoietin. *Br. J. Haematol.* **21**: 551–5, 1971.
285. Ossias, A.L., Zanjani, E.D., Zalusky, R., Estren, S. & Wasserman, L.P. Case report – studies on the mechanism of erythrocytosis associated with a uterine fibromyoma. *Br. J. Haematol.* **25**: 179–85, 1973.
286. Wriss, D.B., Aldor, A. & Aboulafia, Y. Erythrocytosis due to erythropoietin – producing uterine fibromyomata. *Am. J. Obstet. Gynecol.* **122**: 358–60, 1975.
287. Naets, J.P., Wittek, M., Delwiche, F. & Kram, I. Polycythaemia and erythropoietin producing uterine fibromyoma. *Scand. J. Haematol.* **19**: 75–8, 1977.
288. Cundy, J. The perioperative management of patients with polycythemia. *Ann. R. Coll. Surg. Engl.* **62**: 470–5, 1980.
289. Ghio, R., Haupt, E., Ratti, M. & Boccaccio, P. Erythrocytosis associated with a dermoid cyst of the ovary and erythropoietic activity of the tumour fluid. *Scand. J. Hematol.* **27**: 70–4, 1981.
290. Thorling, E.B. Paraneoplastic erythrocytosis and inappropriate erythropoietin production. In *Inappropriate Erythrocytosis. Scand. J. Haematol.* Suppl. 17, 1972.
291. Eldor, A., Even-Paz, Z. & Polliack, A. Erythrocytosis associated with multiple cutaneous leiomyomata: report of a case with demonstration of erythropoietic activity in the tumour. *Scand. J. Haematol.* **16**: 245–9, 1976.
292. Shah, P.C., Patel, A.R., Dimaria, F., Raba, J. & Vohra, R.M. Polycythaemia in lung cancer. *Clin. Lab. Haematol.* **1**: 329–31, 1979.
293. Stewart, G.W., Freegard, S.P., Keeling, D.H. & Perrett, A.D. Cyanosis attributable to right to left shunt in the carcinoid syndrome. *Br. Med. J.* **292**: 589–90, 1986.
294. van Wingerden, J.J., van Rensburg, P.G. & Coetzee, B.P. Malignant fibrous histiocytoma of the parotid gland associated with polycythaemia. *Head Neck Surg.* **8**: 218–21, 1986.
295. Abdi, E.A., Ding, J.C. & Cooper, I.A. Secondary polycythaemia associated with large cell lymphoma. *Med. Pediatr. Oncol.* **13**: 363–5, 1985.
296. Gardner, F.H., Nathan, D.G., Piomelli, S., Cummins, J.F. The erythrocythaemic effects of androgens. *Br. J. Haematol.* **14**: 611–15, 1968.
297. Barton, I.K. & Mansell, M.A. Erythrocytosis induced by danazol in an anephric patient. *Br. Med. J.* **294**: 615, 1987.
298. Shahidi, N.T. Androgens and erythropoiesis. *N. Engl. J. Med.* **289**: 72–80, 1973.
299. Kennedy, B.J. & Gilbertson, A.S. Increased erythropoiesis induced by androgenic hormone therapy. *N. engl. J. Med.* **256**: 719–26, 1957.
300. Gardner, F.H. The use of cobaltous chloride in the anemia associated with chronic renal disease. *J. Lab. Clin. Med.* **41**: 56–64, 1953.
301. Goldwasser, E., Jacobson, L.O., Fried, W. & Plzak, L.F. Studies on erythropoiesis. V. The effects of cobalt on the production of erythropoietin.

Blood **13**: 55–60, 1958.
302. Thorling, E.B. & Erslev, A.J. The effect of some erythropoietic agents on the "tissue" tension of oxygen. *Br. J. Haematol.* **23**: 483–90, 1972.
303. McCully, K.S., Rinehimer, L.A., Gillies, C.G., Hopfer, S.M. & Sunderman, F.W. Erythrocytosis, glomerulomegaly, mesangial hyperplasia, sialyl hyperplasia and arteriosclerosis induced in rats by nickel sulphide. *Virchows Arch. [Pathol. Anat.]* **394**: 207–20, 1982.
304. Adamson, J.W., Stamatoyannopoulos, G., Kontras, S., Lascari, A. & Detter, J. Recessive familial erythrocytosis, aspects of marrow regulation in two families. *Blood* **41**: 641–52, 1973.
305. Distelhorst, C.W., Wagner, D.S., Goldwasser, E. & Adamson, J.W. Autosomal dominant familial erythrocytosis due to autonomous erythropoietin production. *Blood* **58**: 1155–8, 1981.
306. Hellmann, A., Rotoli, B., Cotes, P.M. & Luzzatto, L. Familial erythrocytosis with over-production of erythropoietin. *Clin. Lab. Haematol.* **5**: 335–42, 1983.
307. Whitcomb, W.H., Peschle, C., Moore, M., Nitschke, R. & Adamson, J.W. Congenital erythrocytosis: a new form associated with an erythropoietin dependent mechanism. *Br. J. Haematol.* **44**: 17–24, 1980.
308. Kulkarni, V., Ritchey, K., Howard, D. & Dainiak, N. Heterogeneity of erythropoietin-dependent erythrocytosis: case report in a child and synopsis of primary erythrocytosis syndromes. *Br. J. Haematol.* **60**: 751–8, 1985.
309. Kontras, S.B. Polycythemia and hyperviscosity syndromes in infants and children. *Pediatr. Clin. North Am.* **19**: 919–33, 1972.
310. Mentzer, W.C. Polycythaemia and the hyperviscosity syndrome in newborn infants. *Clin. Haematol.* **7**: 63–74, 1978.
311. Foley, M.E., Isherwood, D.M. & McNicol, G.P. Viscosity, haematocrit, fibrinogen and plasma proteins in maternal and cord blood. *Br. J. Obstet. Gynaecol.* **85**: 500–4, 1978.
312. Walker, C.H.M. Blood rheology in the newborn. In *Clinical Aspects of Blood Viscosity and Cell Deformability* (eds G.D.O. Lowe, J.C. Barbenel & C.D. Forbes), pp. 193–207. Springer-Verlag, Berlin, 1981.
313. Oh, W. & Lind, J. Venous and capillary hematocrit in newborn infants and placental transfusion. *Acta Paediatr. Scand.* **55**: 38–40, 1966.
314. Rausen, A.R., Seki, M. & Strauss, L. Twin transfusion syndrome. *J. Pediatr.* **66**: 613–28, 1965.
315. Michael, A.F., Mauer, A.M. Maternal–fetal transfusion as a cause of plethora in the neonatal period. *Pediatrics* **28**: 458–61, 1961.
316. Humbert, J.R., Abelson, H., Hathaway, W.E. & Battaglia, F.C. Polycythemia in small for gestational age infant. *J. Pediatr.* **75**: 812–19, 1969.
317. Warrner, R.A. & Cornblath, M. Infants of gestational diabetic mothers. *Am. J. Dis. Childh.* **117**: 678–83, 1969.
318. Klebe, J.G. & Ingomar, C.J. The fetoplacental circulation during parturition illustrated by the interfetal transfusion syndrome. *Pediatrics* **49**: 112–16, 1972.
319. Perrine, S.P., Greene, N.F., Lee, P.D.K., Cohen, R.A. & Faller, D.V. Insulin stimulates cord blood erythroid progenitor growth: evidence for an aetiological role in neonatal polycythaemia. *Br. J. Haematol.* **64**: 503–11, 1986.
320. Weinberger, M.M. & Oleinick, A. Congenital marrow dysfunction in Down's syndrome. *J. Pediatr.* **77**: 273–9, 1970.
321. Odievre, M., Gautier, M., Tchernia, G. & Abihssira, G. Les polyglobulies neonatales. *Arch. Fr. Pediatr.* **27**: 703–11, 1970.
322. Bussman, Y.L., Tillman, M.L. & Pagliava, A.S. Neonatal thyrotoxicosis associated with the hyperviscosity syndrome. *J. Pediatr.* **90**: 266–8, 1977.
323. Gold, A.P. & Michael, A.F. Congenital adrenal hyperplasia associated with polycythaemia. *Pediatrics* **23**: 727–30, 1959.

324. Baum, R.S. Hyperviscous blood and perinatal pathology. *Pediatr. Res.* **1**: 288–90, 1967.
325. Wiswell, T.E., Cornish, J.D. & Northam, R.S. Neonatal polycythaemia: frequency of clinical manifestations and other associated findings. *Pediatrics* **78**: 26–30, 1986.
326. Oski, F.A. & Naiman, J.L. Hematologic problems. In *The Newborn*. 3rd Edn, pp. 87–96. W.B. Saunders, Philadelphia, 1982.
327. de Seigneux, R., Humbert, J.R., Cox, J.N. & de Peyer, E. Metaplasie myeloide polycythemique chez un nouveau-né atteint d'erythrodermie icthyosiforme. *Helv. Paediatr. Acta* **28**: 51–60, 1973.
328. Black, C.D., Lubchenco, L.O., Luckey, D.W., Koops, B.L., McGuinness, G.A., Powell, D.P. & Tomlinson, A.L. Developmental and neurologic sequelae of neonatal hyperviscosity syndrome. *Pediatrics* **69**: 426–31, 1982.
329. Host, A. & Ulrich, M. Late prognosis in untreated neonatal polycythaemia with minor or no symptoms. *Acta Paediatr. Scand.* **71**: 629–33, 1982.
330. Leth, A. Changes in plasma and extracellular fluid volume in patients with essential hypertension during long-term treatment with hydrochlorthiazide. *Circulation* **42**: 479–85, 1970.
331. Tarazi, R.C., Dustan, H.P. & Frohlich, E.D. Long-term thiazide therapy in essential hypertension. *Circulation* **61**: 709–17, 1970.
332. Smith, J.F.B. & Lucie, N.P. Alcohol – a cause of stress erythrocytosis. *Lancet* **i**: 637, 1973.
333. Sahn, S.A., Lakshminarayan, S., Pierson, D.J. & Weil, J.V. Effect of ethanol on the ventilatory responses to oxygen and carbon dioxide in man. *Cli. Sci. Mol. Med.* **49**: 33–8, 1975.
334. Pearson, T.C. Haematological considerations. In the Proceedings of the Ciba workshop 'The treatment of hypertension and the treatment of stroke: a simple relationship'. In *International Medicine*, Suppl. 7, pp. 16–18. Franklin Scientific Publications, London, 1983.
335. Tibblin, G., Bergentz, S.-E., Bjure, J. & Wilhelmson, L. Hematocrit, plasma protein, plasma volume, and viscosity in early hypertensive disease. *Am. Heart J.* **72**: 165–76, 1966.
336. Tarazi, R.C., Frohlish, E.D., Dustan, H.P., Gifford, R.W., Page, I.H. Hypertension and high hematocrit. *Am. J. Cardiol.* **18**: 855–8, 1966.
337. Gaar, K.A. Renal disease and hypertension: the erythrocytosis factor. *Med. Hypotheses* **19**: 359–66, 1986.
338. Dustan, H.P., Tarazi, R.C. & Bravo, E.L. Dependence of arterial pressure on intravascular volume in treated hypertensive patients. *N. Engl. J. Med.* **286**: 861–6, 1972.
339. Emery, A.C., Whitcomb, W.H., Frohlich, E.D. "Stress" polycythemia and hypertension. *J. Am. Med. Assoc.* **229**: 159–62, 1974.
340. Lowe, G.D.O., Lowe, J.M., Drummond, M.M., Reith, S., Belch, J.J.F., Kesson, C.M., Wylie, A., Foulds, W.S., Forbes, C.D., MacCuish, A.C. & Mandersom, W.G. Blood viscosity in young male diabetics with and without retinopathy. *Diabetologia* **18**: 359–63, 1980.
341. Graham, J.J., Ryall, R.G. & Wise, P.H. Glycosylated haemoglobin and relative polycythaemia in diabetes mellitus. *Diabetologia* **18**: 205–7, 1980.
342. Bodansky, H.J., Cudworth, A.G., Swindlerhurst, C. & Welch, S.G. Haematocrit, glycosylated haemoglobin and diabetic microangiopathy. *Diabetologia* **19**: 163–4, 1980.
343. Barnes, A.J. Blood viscosity in diabetes mellitus. In *Clinical Aspects of Blood Viscosity and Cell Deformability* (eds G.D.O. Lowe, J.C. Barbenel & C.D. Forbes), pp. 151–62. Springer-Verlag, Berlin, 1981.
344. Ruben, L.A., Pearson, T.C., Shenouda, F., Sönksen, P.H. Packed cell volume in diabetes mellitus. *Practitioner* **230**: 649–51, 1986.

345. El-Yousef, M.K. & Bakewell, W.E. The Gaisböck syndrome. *J. Am. Med. Assoc.* **220**: 864, 1972.
346. Humphrey, P.R.D., Michael, J. & Pearson, T.C. Management of relative polycythaemia: studies of cerebral blood flow and viscosity. *Br. J. Haematol.* **46**: 427–33, 1980.

4

Granulocyte and monocyte abnormalities

J. Fletcher

Consultant Physician, Nottingham City Hospital and Clinical Teacher, Nottingham Medical School, Nottingham, UK

INTRODUCTION

Granulocytes and monocytes constitute the circulating phagocytes of the blood. They form an important part of the body's defence against invading microbes, as was summed up in George Bernard Shaw's famous aphorism 'There is, at bottom, only one genuinely scientific treatment of all diseases and that is to stimulate the phagocytes'. However, rather than stimulating it might be better to think of controlling the phagocytes as it is becoming clear that circulating phagocytic cells have both positive beneficial and negative harmful effects. They certainly have an antimicrobial function as is shown clearly by the increasing risk of infection in patients with neutropenia. Patients with low or absent granulocytes suffer with viral, bacterial and fungal infections of the mouth, skin and lungs. They are particuarly prone to invasion by organisms normally resident in their own gastointestinal tract and skin and this suggests that the phagocytes have a role in maintaining normal homeostasis by destroying bacteria which gain access to the tissues. On the other hand, activation of phagocytes leads to the release of various noxious substances which damage tissues and are probably important in a variety of pathological situations such as the lung damage of adult respiratory distress syndrome, the joint damage of rheumatoid arthritis and the vessel wall damage of arteritis.[1] Even in conditions which are not normally considered inflammatory, such as cerebrovascular accidents and myocardial infarction, phagocytes plugging small blood vessels and generating toxic products contribute to tissue damage and complications.[2] Consequently, the importance of understanding all aspects of circulating phagocyte biochemistry and physiology is beginning to be appreciated and the use of drugs aimed at modifying phagocyte behaviour is just beginning.

George Bernard Shaw obtained his insight into the phagocytes as a result of his friendship with Sir Almroth Wright. Wright was following the pioneering work of Eli Metchnikoff who discovered and named the phagocytic cells. In 1884 Metchnikoff demonstrated that cells in starfish larvae could ingest and destroy foreign substances or bacteria and could develop a granulomatous reaction. He hypothesized that because the leucocytes of vertebrates were also phagocytic they were the most important means of defence against infectious disease.[3] At that time his views were vigorously challenged as the prevailing concept was that the defence of an organism against bacterial infection was mediated by humoral factors. A century later the importance of circulating phagocytes in relation to infection is accepted without question but so is the importance of the humoral factors. Phagocytes, by their interaction with products of the complement and coagulation cascades, are the first cells attracted to an inflammatory site where they promote the inflammatory response and finally contribute to restraining that response. They not only ingest and kill microbes as described by Metchnikoff but also interact with the lymphoid system, vascular endothelium and fibroblasts.

MYELOPOIESIS

Polymorphonuclear neutrophils (PMN) and monocytes arise in the bone marrow from a common progenitor cell which has been described in *in vitro* culture systems as the granulocyte–monocyte colony forming unit (GM-CFU). The origin of GM-CFU is the pluripotent stem cell. In the normal bone marrow most of these stem cells are not in cycle, but the small proportion which are in cycle give rise to progenitor cells of progressively more restricted lineage until the GM-CFU is formed which is committed to only PMN and monocytes. This restriction of potential from the pluripotent to the committed cell takes place at the same time as expansion in the numbers of progenitor cells and requires the presence of a family of factors known as colony stimulating factors (CSF). These are elaborated by a variety of cells including macrophages, lymphocytes, endothelial cells and fibroblasts and are an important part of the micro-environment required for the normal production of phagocytes.[4] This micro-environment must be influenced by factors released from sites of inflammation but as yet this is not understood. The progenitor cells for eosinophilic and basophilic granules appear to be separate from GM-CFU and while under the influence of colony stmulating factors their production is, at least partly, independent of the factors influencing PMN and monocytes.

Following commitment there is a phase of intense proliferation which can be regarded as the engine of myelopoiesis, producing the enormous numbers of cells required to be released into the peripheral circulation. Consequently, when sampling the bone marrow it is these rapidly proliferating cells and their products which are recognized and are described according to their morphological characteristics as promyelocytes, myelocytes, metamyelocytes, band forms and morphologically mature granulocytes. It is important to understand the distinction between, on the one hand, stem cells and progenitor cells, most of which are not dividing and on the other the rapidly proliferating compartment which is sensitive to the effects of systemic diseases and their treatment. Proliferation actually ceases at the stage of myelocytes and is then followed by further maturation of cells which are not dividing. Following this final phase of maturation the cells are ready to be released into the peripheral circulation, but 90% of the PMN are retained in the bone marrow and constitute a reserve storage pool. Production of monocytes is similar to PMN but intermediate steps of maturation are not morphologically identified and therefore lumped together as monoblasts which give rise directly to monocytes. A proportion of monocytes are temporarily retained in the marrow as a reserve pool but this is smaller than the PMN marrow reserve. The factors which control release of cells from the marrow are not yet understood but probably involve the expression of receptors which are able to interact with the stroma, including the vascular endothelium. The numbers involved are enormous, particularly for PMN with a turnover calculated as approximately 1.6×10^9 cells per kg per day.[5]

PERIPHERAL BLOOD PHAGOCYTES

Granulocytes and monocytes together form the phagocytic cells in the circulation. Their morphology and function will be discussed separately but in the blood they both form two pools which continually interchange; approximately half are circulating while half are attached to the endothelium of small blood vessels, mainly post-capillary venules. This marginated pool is rapidly mobilized in response to any stress. In the absence of inflammation, phagocytic cells appear to leave the circulation at random with a half-life for both monocytes and PMN of approximately 6.5 h. Subsets can be identified but it is not known whether this affects their behaviour. The fate of PMN is a mystery although it seems likely that they survive for 24–48 h in the tissues and large numbers are excreted in the faeces. Monocytes migrate into the tissues where they form distinct populations of macrophages.

POLYMORPHONUCLEAR NEUTROPHILS (PMN)

As already indicated, PMN are concerned with host defence and inflammation and therefore their structure and function will be discussed from this point of view. The normal PMN is 10–14 µm in diameter and has the characteristics of an end-stage cell, not replicating and with only limited capacity for protein synthesis as shown by condensed heterochromatin, no nucleolus, and small numbers of mitochondria and ribosomes. The cytoplasm contains various granules upon which the PMN's function largely depends. The granule contents are summarized in Table 4.1.

Table 4.1 Contents of PMN Granules

Primary	Secondary	Tertiary
Myeloperoxidase	Lactoferrin	Gelatinase
Lysozyme	Vitamin B_{12}-binding protein	Acid hydrolases
Acid hydrolases	Collagenase	CR3 receptor
Neutral proteases	Histaminase	
Cationic proteins	CR3 receptor	
Elastase	fMLP receptor	
Cathepsin	Cytochrome-B_{245}	
β-Glucuronidase		

Primary (azurophil) granules

These are discrete structures which develop during the promyelocyte stage of PMN maturation and may be either elliptical or spherical in shape.[6] The primary granules are lysozomes containing hydrolytic enzymes involved in the killing and digestion of ingested organisms and other particles. The enzymes include myeloperoxidase, lysozyme, acid hydrolases, neutral proteases, cationic proteins, elastase, cathepsin and β-glucuronidase. They are surrounded by a membrane of similar composition to the plasma membrane and since the latter forms the membrane of the phagocytic vacuole it is not surprising that primary granules fuse with the phagosome membrane during phagocytosis and so discharge their enzymes into the phagocytic vacuole. Only small quantities of primary granule enzymes are normally discharged outside the cell. Their function appears to be entirely concerned with the killing and digestion of phagocytosed organisms and other material.

Secondary (specific) granules

Secondary granules appear at a later stage, the myelocyte, in the maturation of the PMN and after this PMN division ceases so that the secondary granules come to outnumber primary granules by a ratio of approximately 2:1.[6] They are smaller than primary granules and can be spherical or rod-shaped. Like primary granules they are contained in a discrete package and are discharged during phagocytosis. However, discharge of secondary granules occurs prior to discharge of the primary granules and can be caused by stimuli which do not affect degranulation of primary granules and do not result in formation of a phagocytic vacuole. The secondary granules contain some lysozyme, collagenase, lactoferrin, vitamin B_{12} binding protein, histaminase, and an activator of complement. During phagocytosis more than 60% of these substances are released outside the cell and this suggests that their function is extracellular and concerned with the control of inflammation.[7] Recently it has been suggested that the secondary granules are the source of various receptors which are translocated to the cell's surface during activation of PMN. These receptors include CR3, the receptor for the complement component C3bi and the receptor for the bacterial peptide N–formyl–methionyl–leucyl–phenylalanine (fMLP).[8] The cytochrome-B_{245} component of the NADPH oxidase system may also be in the secondary granules.

Tertiary granules

Zonal centrifugation of PMN has shown the existence of a third population of cellular storage particles smaller than the other particles but of the same density as the secondary granules.[9] These tertiary granules are thought to contain acid hydrolases, a proteinase and gelatinase. Like the secondary granules they may be a major intracellular storage site for the CR3 receptor and for the cytochrome-B_{245}.[10,11] It is at present difficult to know whether these tertiary granules should be distinguished from secondary granules as there is considerable overlap in the components which each is claimed to contain. However, it certainly seems that there is a population of granules which is released very rapidly and extensively as a result of mild stimuli such as warming cells from 0°C to 37°C or by very low concentrations of regulatory molecules such as fMLP.[12] It seems likely that release of tertiary granules or at least a sub-population of the secondary granules occurs early in cell activation and primes the cell for further activity by increasing the number of receptors on the cell's surface and bringing components of the respiratory burst to the cell surface.

Microtubules and microfilaments

These structures are thought to be concerned in cell mobility and maintenance of shape. The microtubules formed of tubulin are found radiating from the centriole and appear to form a cytoskeleton for the PMN. The microfilaments are composed of myosin and actin and play an essential role in cell movement required for chemotaxis and also for the flow of membrane around a particle which is being ingested.

Glycogen

Glycogen particles are randomly distributed throughout the cytoplasm and appear to provide the energy source for anaerobic metabolism producing ATP required for phagocytosis.

PMN function

PMN are among the first cells to arrive at a site of inflammation and to achieve this they must respond to a series of signals. These signals result in mobilization of the marginated pool and the marrow reserve pool together with an increase in myelopoiesis and PMN production. As a result the number of PMN in the peripheral circulation rises. These increased numbers of PMN are then delivered to the site of inflammation as a result of vasodilation which is the first sign of inflammation and may itself be, at least partly, dependent upon PMN. Increased vascular permeability to protein-rich fluid leading to local swelling is also dependent upon PMN as is the microvascular thrombosis and local haemorrhage which accompanies more severe inflammation.[13,14] The next requirement is for the PMN to attach to the vascular endothelium, migrate through the vessel wall and then by directed migration or chemotaxis to move towards microbes and particles which require ingestion. These particles are identified by interaction between their coating of opsonins and specific receptors on the surface of the PMN. They are then phagocytosed, killed and digested. Finally the PMN may be involved in reining back the inflammatory reaction.

Regulatory molecules

The complicated sequence outlined above is controlled by a series of regulatory molecules which are listed in Table 4.2. They act as ligands for which there are specific receptors on the surface of PMN. The result of their binding is stimulation of cell adherence, aggregation, movement, degranulation and the respiratory burst. These ligands include products from the activation of complement, from the coagulation cascade, from bacteria, from the oxidation of arachidonic acid and cytokines from mononuclear cells.

Table 4.2   Soluble Regulatory Molecules

Direct stimuli	Stimulus response modifiers
C5a and C5a des-Arg	Adenosine
Fibronectin	Histamine
LTB_4	Adrenalin
fMLP	
TNF (IL-1, CSF, γ-IFN)	

The complement component C5a is produced by both the classical and alternative pathways of complement activation which means by both immune complexes and by gram-negative bacterial cell wall components. In plasma C5a is rapidly converted to its des-Arg form but both C5a and C5a des-Arg are chemoattractants and activators of neutrophils. C5a may also be produced by proteolytic splitting of C5 and this seems to be the mechanism of activation of complement by PMN themselves via an enzyme released from secondary granules.

Plasma not only contains products of the complement cascade but also of the coagulation cascade which can activate PMN through their receptor for the peptide sequence arginine, glycine, aspartate and serine. This is contained within fibrinectin and fibrinogen and is unmasked by partial proteolysis as occurs following surface activation of Factor XII or release of proteolytic enzymes, such as elastase, from PMN themselves.[15]

Leukotriene-B_4 (LTB_4) is produced by lipoxygenase-catalysed oxidation of arachidonic acid when PMN and T-lymphocytes are stimulated. It is the most potent stimulus of PMN among the large range of products of arachidonic acid oxidation.

The N-formyl peptide (fMLP) is a product of mitochondrial activity of growing gram-negative bacteria. However, it may have a wider role in regulation of inflammation than simply in infections, as similar chemotactic peptides are produced by mammalian cells.[17]

The cytokines interleukin 1 (IL-1) and tumor necrosis factor (TNF) are products of monocytes and macrophages while γ-interferon (γ-IFN) and colony stimulating factors (CSF) are products of T-lymphocytes. Of these, TNF in particular is a potent stimulus of PMN. The role of the other cytokines is not clear as many of the functions originally attributed to IL-1 are now thought to be due to TNF. Now that recombinant IL-1 and TNF are available their separate roles are being defined.[18]

A list of regulatory factors includes a wide range of molecules which are orchestrated to produce the PMN response to inflammation. There are several different mechanisms to stimulus–response coupling within the cell and therefore there may be qualitative differences in the effect of different stimuli.[19] At present quantitative differences seem more important. TNF is a considerably more potent stimulus on a molar basis than the other factors. However, the response to all these stimuli appears to be graded and increase with increasing concentration and receptor occupancy. They all depend upon receptors which are only expressed in small numbers on the surface of circulating unstimulated PMN but receptor expression is increased by translocation from intracellular pools as the result of stimulation. As already described, these pools are either in the more labile of the secondary granules or in tertiary granules. Low concentrations of stimuli are chemotactic and cause partial degranulation with increased expression of receptors for C3bi, fMLP, LTB$_4$ and probably C5a des-Arg. Higher concentrations lead to more extensive discharge of secondary granules with translocation of the cytochrome-B$_{245}$ to the cell surface and activation of the NADPH oxidase and the respiratory burst. The result is progressive up-regulation or priming of the cell with increased chemotatic responsiveness and oxygen radical production shown by exudate PMN compared with circulating PMN.[20]

The stimuli controlling PMN behaviour probably act in sequence with exposure to one increasing responsiveness to the next. There are also mechanisms for down-regulation as following exposure PMN show a reduced response towards the same stimulus. This chemotactic deactivation or tachyphylaxis means that a 'footprint' is left indicating previous exposure to the particular stimulus while response to a different stimulus is normal.[21] An example is the reduced response to C5a des-Arg of synovial PMN and monocytes from rheumatoid joints with normal responses to fMLP. Tachyphylaxis to C5a des-Arg and LTB$_4$ lasts for some hours, whereas a depressed responsiveness to low concentrations of fMLP is rapidly reversible. These differences may reflect the speed with which these bound receptors are internalized and returned to the cell surface.[22]

There is another way in which PMN function may be regulated involving another group of molecules well-recognized as inflammatory mediators. These include adenosine, histamine and adrenalin for which PMN express specific receptors A2, H2 and beta respectively. Binding of these ligands to their specific receptors has the effect of down-regulating the neutrophil's response to chemotactic and degranulating stimuli, including fMLP and C5a des-Arg, so that for a given concentration of stimulus the response is reduced. The physiological significance of this down-regulation is not clear and is complicated as PMN themselves produce adenosine and they also release enzymes which degrade both adenosine and histamine.[23] However, the presence of these receptors may indicate a way in which neutrophil behaviour can be manipulated by drugs.

Neutrophil response to inflammation

The function of neutrophils has to be considered in relation to this battery of regulatory molecules and a tentative scheme is shown in Fig. 4.1. Various

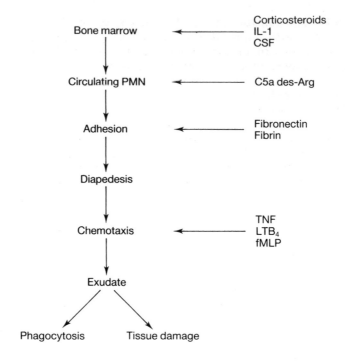

Fig. 4.1. PMN response to inflammation.

functions can be measured easily *in vitro* including changes in cell shape, random migration, directed migration or chemotaxis, adhesion and aggregation, degranulation, phagocytosis and microbial killing and the respiratory burst and its products. *In vivo* the first requirement is mobilization of neutrophils from the marginated and marrow pools and this can result from the action of corticosteroids, adrenalin and IL-1. IL-1 also has the effect of increasing myelopoiesis.[24] In the circulation it seems likely that the products of the complement and coagulation cascades are important. Factors including C5a des-Arg activate neutrophils and, as a result, there are changes in the cell surface charge and in the expression of receptors for adhesion proteins such as C3bi which lead to the cell becoming sticky with a tendency to adhere to inflamed endothelial surfaces. Attachment is associated with vasodilatation and an increase in vascular permeability. Following attachment of the PMN to the endothelial surface the cells migrate either between or actually through vascular endothelial cells by a process called diapedesis. By this stage the PMN have adopted a particular morphology with a blunt leading front and more attenuated body containing the nucleus and cytoplasmic structures including the granules. Release of granules appears to occur at the blunt front end resulting in the highest concentration of receptors and a gradient of receptors across the surface of the cell which explains the movement of the cell in a gradient of chemotactic factors resulting in directed movement of the cell towards a site of inflammation.[25] Bound receptors are probably internalized, the ligand digested and the receptor returned to the cell surface.[22] The factors important within an inflammatory focus are probably TNF, which is particularly stimulated by endotoxin from gram-negative bacteria, and LTB_4 which may be released from PMN to recruit more PMN and monocytes.

Phagocytosis

The PMN recognizes a particle to be phagocytosed as a result of an interaction between its surface receptors and opsonins on the surface of the particle. The most important opsonins are the Fc portion of immunoglobulin-G, particularly sub-clases IgG1 and IgG3. These immunoglobulins are capable of stimulating the whole range of neutrophil responses, including phagocytosis and the respiratory burst, and are a more potent stimulus than the soluble regulators already discussed. However, phagocytosis, at least in suspension, if not on a surface proceeds only slowly in the absence of the complement component C3. The neutrophil expresses receptors for two derivatives of C3, the CR1 receptor for C3b and the CR3 receptor for C3bi. The CR3 receptor, in particular, appears to be important in a number of neutrophil functions including adhesion and cell migration as well as phagocytosis. It appears that CR3 is part of a group of leucocyte adherence related glycoproteins which includes LFA-1 and p150, 95 and are known collectively as the Mac-1 complex.[26]

Ingestion depends upon the sequential reaction between opsonin and receptor as the blunt end of the neutrophil flows round the particle, binding of opsonin to its receptor leads to the release of actin-binding protein which causes actin filaments to form a solid gel which is then made to contract by myosin in the presence of ATP. Hence the pseudopod so formed will flow around the particle as sequential ligand binding activates further actin-binding protein.[19] The energy for this process is derived from glycolysis and does not require oxygen. Sequential binding between receptors and opsonins leads to a 'zipper effect' so that the particle becomes surrounded by a plasma membrane which forms the phagocytic vacuole.[27]

Microbial killing

If the ingested particle is a microorganism then it will be killed by products of the respiratory burst and granules which are discharged into the vacuole. The relative contribution of oxygen radicals and granule proteins varies with different organisms.[28]

The importance of oxygen radicals is shown by the human genetic disease, chronic granulomatous disease (CGD), characterized by a tendency to recurrent infection with catalase-positive bacteria.[1] This disease is due to lack of functioning NADPH oxidase which reduces oxygen to the superoxide radical O_2^-. The oxidase is an electron transport chain including a unique cytochrome-B_{245}, possibly a ubiquinone and a flavoprotein and it catalyses the reaction

$$O_2 + NADPH \rightarrow O_2^- + NADP^+ + H^+$$

Superoxide can then form other reactive oxygen radicals including hydroxyl and singlet oxygen. However, its most important product is hydrogen peroxide as a result of apparently spontaneous dismutation:

$$2O_2^- + 2H^+ \rightarrow H_2O_2 + O_2$$

Hydrogen peroxide is the substrate for myeloperoxidase, an enzyme delivered into the phagosome by discharge of the primary granules. Myeloperoxidase catalyses the reaction

$$H_2O_2 + Cl^- \rightarrow OCl^- + H_2O$$

and the hypochlorite ion can then react with amine groups to form chloramines thought to be a major cause of microbial damage:

$$OCl^- + NH_3 \rightarrow NH_2Cl + OH^-$$

The initial substrates for these reactions are O_2 and NADPH. O_2 consumption gives rise to the term 'respiratory burst', NADP requires recycling to NADPH through the hexose monophosphate shunt by oxidation of glucose-6-phosphate to pentose and CO_2 with concomitant reduction of NADP to NADPH.

The products of the respiratory burst are toxic not only to microbes but also to the cell and in the cytoplasm are a number of enzymes which can degrade oxygen radicals which may leak from the phagosome. Hydrogen peroxide is broken down to water through oxidation of glutathione which is then reduced by glutathione reductase and NADPH.[29] Catalase can also break down hydrogen peroxide but only appears to be important under conditions of exceptional oxidative stress.[30] Superoxide O_2^- dismutates within the phagosome but can be degraded by superoxide dismutase in both mitochondria and cytoplasm.

Catalase-negative organisms may produce sufficient hydrogen peroxide to contribute to their own destruction by the myeloperoxidase–halide–hydrogen peroxide system, but there are a variety of other microbicidal mechanisms not dependent upon oxygen. Immediately following ingestion the pH of the phagosome rises and provides the optimal conditions for the activity of cationic proteins.[31] These proteins appear to bind to anionic sites on the surface of bacteria, leading to irreversible loss of the ability to replicate but do not affect structural integrity. These actions may be synergistic with the myeloperoxidase–halide–hydrogen peroxide system.[28] Low molecular weight cationic proteins seem to be more active against gram-positive organisms such as staphylococci. High molecular weight cationic proteins, known as bactericidal permeability increasing proteins (BPI), bind to gram-negative bacteria, including *Escherichia*, *Salmonella* and *Pseudomonas*, increasing their permeability to hydrophobic molecules. After the initial rise in pH there is a fall and the resulting acid environment within the phagosome may cause damage to certain bacteria. The pH also becomes optimal for the activity of myeloperoxidase and hydrolases which are concerned with the digestion of phagocytosed particles.

PMN and control of inflammation

PMN, during activation and phagocytosis, release toxic products including oxygen radicals and proteolytic enzymes into the surrounding environment and this may be important in a number of diseases. Attachment to a surface increases release of primary granule enzymes so increasing local tissue damage.[32] However, oxygen radicals and myeloperoxidase can also denature enzymes and may serve to limit the extracellular damage and so restrain the inflammatory reaction. This may be the explanation for the development of chronic inflammation with granulomata and fibrous tissue formation in patients with CGD even after elimination of infection.[33] PMN also release into their environment the major part of their secondary granule proteins. The role of histaminase and the complement activating factor are understandable but the function of the B_{12}-binding protein, transcobalamin III, and the iron-binding protein, lactoferrin, are not clear. There is evidence that lactoferrin forms a feedback mechanism reducing cytokine production from macrophages and therefore also dampening down an inflammatory reaction.[34]

Systemic disease and acquired abnormalities of PMN function

Inflammation

In any inflammatory reaction whether the result of external insult such as burns, trauma, infection or surgery, or as part of systemic disease, PMN have only a limited repertoire of responses. Failure to understand this has led to descriptions in the literature as if the pattern of changes found in diseases including chronic liver inflammation or rheumatoid arthritis is specific to these conditions, which is not the case. There is a common pattern of changes detectable in circulating PMN which becomes more marked in exudate PMN and most marked following phagocytosis. The changes detectable in circulating PMN within 4 h of elective surgery are shown in Table 4.3.[35,36] The falls in vitamin B_{12}-binding protein and lactoferrin are accompanied by reciprocal rises in their plasma concentrations. The changes in these proteins indicate partial degranulation of the secondary granules and are associated with increased expression of CR3, the receptor for C3bi. Expression of this adhesion protein may account for increased stickiness to surfaces and increased phagocytic activity. Although myeloperoxidase is a primary granule constituent the fall in its activity is not accompanied by reduction in the level of other primary granule enzymes such as β-glucuronidase and may be due to interaction of the enzyme with oxygen radicals. Whatever the explanation, the change in its activity is quite marked and in the past has been used as a non-specific indicator of infection. Microbial killing indicated in Table 4.3 has been measured by using a yeast, *Candida*, which depends upon myeloperoxidase and therefore loss of this enzyme's activity may explain the loss of microbicidal activity. It is possible that there is increased microbicidal activity against some bacteria as a result of the increased oxygen radical production. Nitro-blue tetrazolium (NBT) is reduced to dark blue formazan deposits by superoxide

Table 4.3   Changes in Circulating PMN Following Elective Surgery

Number	↑	
Vitamin B$_{12}$-binding protein	↓	Constituents of secondary granules
Lactoferrin	↓	
Myeloperoxidase	↓	Constituents of primary granules
β-Glucuronidase	→	
Adhesion	↑	
Phagocytosis	↑	
Microbicidal killing (*Candida*)	↓	
Alkaline phosphatase	↑	

and this has been used as another non-specific test for infection. As well as the changes listed, which occur very rapidly, there is a rise in leucocyte alkaline phosphatase (LAP) but its kinetics are slower and probably reflect increasing numbers of young PMN released from the bone marrow reserve. In human PMN, alkaline phosphatase is a marker of vesicles associated with the cell's surface and not contained in the secondary granules.[37] If the inflammatory stimulus is severe, as with continuing infection, the staining characteristics of the primary granules change so that they become more obvious and this is called toxic granulation. Fused primary granules are recognized as Döhle bodies.

This pattern of changes indicates partial activation of circulating PMN and is probably due to their stimulation by products of the complement and coagulation cascades as the cells, when tested *in vitro* show reduced response to zymosan-activated serum which contains C5a des-Arg and 'activated' fibronectin. This tachyphylaxis is a 'footprint' indicating previous exposure to these agents and biological activity due to C5a cannot be detected in the plasma at the same time (J.M. Davies and J. Fletcher, unpublished).

Pregnancy

The foetus is antigenically foreign to the mother and although tolerated by the immune system, its presence is associated with changes in PMN. By the twelfth week of pregnancy there is the same pattern of PMN changes as in inflammatory diseases (Table 4.1) and these persist until term.[38] They suggest that the complement and coagulation cascades are being stimulated by the presence of the foreign body although other features of an inflammatory reaction are suppressed. It is possible that products of the PMN such as lactoferrin contribute to suppression of the normal immune response. The leucocyte alkaline phosphatase rises throughout pregnancy and this probably reflects changing hormonal levels. All of these changes disappear rapidly following delivery and the PMN have reverted to normal within 4 weeks.

PMN involvement in tissue damage

There are a number of conditions in which PMN appear to contribute to tissue damage listed in Table 4.4. This is not an exhaustive list as it is likely that whenever activated PMN accumulate there will be the potential for tissue damage by oxygen radicals and granule enzymes.

Adult respiratory distress syndrome (ARDS). The hallmark of ARDS is accumulation of protein-rich fluid in the alveoli as a result of an increase in microvascular permeability to plasma proteins. It seems that activated and therefore sticky PMN with platelet and protein microaggregates lodge in the pulmonary capillaries where they release toxic oxygen radicals and proteolytic enzymes and so injure the capillary and alveolar walls.[39] ARDS tends to complicate severe trauma or sepsis and may be an exaggeration and continuation of the normal activation of PMN which accompanies any inflammatory reaction. Furthermore, some temporary increase in pulmonary capillary permeability due to accumulation of sticky PMN may be a common feature of trauma and sepsis.

Conditions associated with local accumulation of PMN. There are a number of conditions listed in Table 4.4 which may all represent damage as a result of local accumulation of PMN. There is evidence for a connection between PMN accumulation and joint destruction in rheumatoid[40] and gouty arthritis[41] and a similar mechanism has been postulated in other diseases associated with deposition of immune complexes.[42] It must be presumed that generation of chemoattractants occurs in each of these. In gout, uric acid ingestion by macrophages can generate IL-1, in rheumatoid arthritis, immune vasculitis and glomerulonephritis complement components seem to be important, while in chronic bronchitis, psoriasis and ulcerative colitis the chemoattractant has not been defined.

Arterial obstruction. It is only recently that PMN have been implicated in the tissue damage resulting from arterial obstruction. The evidence is based upon experimental animals in which the extent of injury, complications and recovery from myocardial infarction is related to PMN infiltration.[2,34] As before, this seems to be due to release of oxygen radicals and

Table 4.4 Diseases in Which PMN Contribute to Tissue Damage

Adult respiratory distress syndrome
Chronic bronchitis and emphysema
Gout
Rheumatoid arthritis
Immune vasculitis
Glomerulonephritis
Psoriasis
Ulcerative colitis
Myocardial infarction
Cerebral thrombosis

tissue-damaging enzymes. It is also likely that activation, which causes PMN to become both sticky and stiff, leads to capillary blocking and contributes to the ischaemia. It is interesting that the drugs currently used to treat both myocardial and cerebral infarction, such as calcium channel antagonists, have the effect of reducing PMN responses to stimulatory molecules.

PMN involvement in infectious complications

The main cause of death in patients with ARDS and severe burns is infection. These two conditions are associated with massive stimulation of circulating PMN which may exhaust their potential microbicidal ability and interfere with tissue and wound healing. Patients with diabetes and chronic renal failure also suffer from a tendency to infection which contributes to morbidity and mortality but the mechanisms differ.

Diabetes mellitus.   Diabetic patients are susceptible to a variety of bacterial and fungal diseases and this has led to an interest in the possibility of abnormal neutrophil function. Much of the data in the literature are conflicting due to the use of inadequate techniques and it is probable that most of the abnormalities described in functions such as adherence, chemotaxis and microbicidal activity can be explained by keto-acidosis and hyperosmolar states which are not relevant to the majority of diabetics. However, if the initial rate of phagocytosis is measured then this is defective in insulin-dependent diabetics.[44] The mechanism is not known but it might relate to glycosylation of surface Fc receptors. There have also been reports of impaired killing of ingested organisms and an interesting speculation is whether this could be due to depletion of NADPH which is a required co-factor both for the oxidative burst and for the conversion of glucose to its alcohol, sorbitol in the aldose reductase pathway. The latter pathway is stimulated in diabetics by the high plasma glucose levels.[45]

Chronic renal failure.   Like diabetics, the PMN function abnormalities in renal failure are complex. There is a mild but measurable defect in opsonic activity in uraemic plasma. Perhaps more important is impairment of intracellular killing of staphylococci due to low molecular weight factors which have not been further characterized.[48]

Congenital abnormalities

A small number of congenital abnormalities of PMN with specific biochemical defects have been documented. These are important because of the insights they provide into particular aspects of normal function and some have been mentioned in the preceding review of function. A number of rare disorders including Chediak–Higashi syndrome, May–Hegglin and Pelger–Huet anomalies are not described as they do not, as yet, provide such insights.

Deficiency of adherence-related glycoproteins

There are a group of cell surface glycoproteins, including CR3, LFA1 and p150,95, known as the Mac-1 complex which are concerned with adhesion to other cells and surfaces.[26] Each consists of a different alpha sub-unit with a molecular weight of 150,000–180,000 Da and a common beta sub-unit of 95,000 Da. The function of these proteins has been defined partly as a result of monoclonal antibodies and partly by studying a rare autosomal recessive disorder in which there is a failure to synthesize normal beta sub-units.[47] The patients may present with a delayed separation of the umbilical cord followed by a tendency to skin infections, mucositis and otitis. More severe bacterial and fungal infections occur from time to time. There is a high peripheral blood neutrophil count, possibly due to lack of a marginated pool. There is a failure of adherence, diapedesis and chemotaxis so that neutrophils do not migrate to sites of infection and inflammation. *In vitro* there are defects in adhesion-related functions including aggregation of activated neutrophils, adherence to endothelial surfaces, chemotaxis and phagocytosis of opsonized particles. There are also abnormalities of monocyte and lymphocyte function. The defect has been mapped to chromosome 21.[47]

Chronic granulomatous disease (CGD)

This has been mentioned in the discussion of microbial killing. It is a defect of both the PMN and monocytes which are unable to mount the respiratory burst due to lack of the NADPH oxidase.[1] As a result the patients suffer with infections due to catalase-positive bacteria and fungi affecting skin, lungs, liver and bones. Furthermore, inflammation and fibrosis continue even after elimination of infection and may result in obstruction of the oesophagus or urinary tract.[33] The disease is rare (1 in 1,000,000) and has several forms of inheritance, two-thirds are X-linked and most of the other third are autosomal recessive. The NADPH oxidase is an electron transport chain containing cytochrome-B_{245}, possibly a ubiquinone, and a flavo-protein. The X-linked disease is due to a defective cytochrome-B_{245}. In the autosomal recessive form the cytochrome-B is usually normal but a cytosolic factor is missing. Both biochemical defects were corrected when monocytes from the two forms were fused to create a hybrid.

Myeloperoxidase deficiency

The myeloperoxidase–halide–hydrogen peroxide system is particularly important in fungal killing *in vitro* but lack of the enzyme is also associated with a moderate defect in bacterial killing. Hereditary myeloperoxidase deficiency is a relatively common autosomal recessive disorder, either total (1 in 4000) or partial (1 in 2000) and maps to chromosome 17. Some patients have been described with fungal infections, particularly due to *Candida*, but the majority do not suffer unduly with infections. The explanation is presumably that other microbicidal mechanisms can compensate. The condition is interesting because there is a prolonged respiratory burst in response to various stimuli which supports the hypothesis that myelo-peroxidase may be important in inactivating other enzymes and components of the inflammatory response.[48]

Secondary granule deficiency

Quite profound lack of secondary (specific granules) can be acquired, for example in severe burns and in myeloid metaplasia. However, another very rare congenital disorder has been described in which the PMN lack the specific granules but the abnormality is more general as it also affects some components of both the primary and tertiary granules.[49] The condition is important as the neutrophils are unable to increase surface expression of CR3 and fMLP receptors or to augment the respiratory burst. The patients suffer with recurrent bacterial infections of the skin and deep tissues associated with defective migration of PMN into inflammatory sites.

Abnormalities of PMN numbers

Neutrophilia

The number of PMN in the circulation rises as a result of mobilization from the marginated pool, from the marrow reserve and by increased myelopoiesis. The mediators involved include adrenalin, corticosteroids, IL-1 and colony stimulating factors. Stress, excitement and exertion are sufficient to mobilize at least part of the marginated pool and produce a temporary increase in PMN numbers. Pregnancy is associated with a persistent although mild neutrophilia. Any inflammatory stimulus, such as surgical trauma, will produce a rapid rise in circulating PMN, peaking at about 24 h and subsiding over the next 4 days. A similar pattern is seen following myocardial infarction and large cerebral infarcts when the increased numbers of stiff and sticky neutrophils may contribute to tissue damage by plugging capillaries and arterioles. It is also possible to speculate that neutrophilia from other causes may increase the risk of infarction and may be a factor in post-operative heart attacks and, perhaps, explain the association of myocardial infarction with stress.

A more persistent neutrophilia occurs with more persistent inflammation associated with release of mediators such as IL-1. Examples are any pyogenic infection, inflammatory arthritis including rheumatoid and gout, inflammatory conditions of the skin and intestine and diseases associated with immune complex formation. Neutrophilia may accompany neoplasia without direct involvement of the bone marrow, presumably because the tumour releases inflammatory mediators. The best known examples are Hodgkin's disease, T-cell lymphomas and renal carcinoma, when the neutrophilia is often associated with a swinging pyrexia suggesting release of IL-1. The common systemic causes of an increase in circulating PMN are listed in Table 4.5.

Occasionally the mobilization of PMN from the bone marrow is excessive and accompanied by circulating immature cells which raises the possibility

Table 4.5 Common Systemic Causes of Neutrophilia

Stress/exertion
Pregnancy
Trauma (including burns and surgery)
Pyogenic infections, particularly pneumonia, septicaemia, meningitis, pertussis
Neoplasms, particularly renal carcinoma, Hodgkin's disease, T-cell lymphomas
Myocardial infarction
Inflammation of joints, skin or bowel
Haemorrhage
Haemolysis

---

of leukaemia. Such 'leukaemoid' reactions can occur, particularly in children, with a variety of severe infections including pneumonia, septicaemia, meningococcal meningitis and pertussis. It can occur with neoplasia, especially with marrow infiltration and occasionally with severe haemorrhage or haemolysis. The diagnosis depends upon the clinical context but when due to infection is accompanied by high leucocyte alkaline phosphatase score and toxic granulation. The final proof depends upon resolution when the cause is treated.

Neutropenia

The number of circulating PMN depends upon the rate of entry from the marrow matched by the migration into the tissues. Therefore, neutropenia can be due to marrow failure or increased consumption in the tissues or a combination of both. Whatever the mechanism, neutropenia is associated with an increased tendency to infections of all sorts, viral, fungal and bacterial, but particularly to invasion of the tissues by the host's own bacterial flora. The danger of severe infection is minimal until the circulating PMN number falls below 0.8×10^9 per litre but then increases progressively and the patient is at considerable risk with a circulating count below 0.5×10^9 per litre. Table 4.6 gives a list of common systemic causes of neutropenia.

Table 4.6 Common Systemic Causes of Neutropenia

Drugs
   Cytotoxic by marrow depression
   Non-cytotoxic usually by marrow depression

Infections (usually by a combination of increased consumption and marrow depression)
   Viral (hepatitis, rubella)
   Bacterial (typhoid, brucellosis, miliary tuberculosis)

Malignant disease (usually associated with marrow infiltration)

Hypersplenism, systemic lupus erythematosus (increased consumption)

There are a number of rare congenital causes of neutropenia, one of which, cyclical neutropenia, is of particular interest. In this condition there is a more or less periodic oscillation in circulating PMN numbers; the period of oscillation varies but is usually about 21 days. The mechanism is a periodic reduction in the granulocyte mitotic compartment of the marrow. Interest in the condition was stimulated by finding that circulating PMN numbers are out of phase with monocyte numbers and this led to the suggestion that PMN production is dependent upon CSF from monocytes. However, it is now known that CSF comes from T-lymphocytes and vascular endothelium rather than monocytes.[50] Some normal individuals and patients with chronic myeloid leukaemia may show cyclical oscillations and this has led to the speculation that cyclical neutropenia is simply an exaggeration of a normal negative feedback control mechanism with an inherent time delay.

MONOCYTES

In the blood the monocyte is a relatively large cell (15 μm) with a single kidney-shaped nucleus. The cytoplasm is abundant and rich in endoplasmic reticulum, lysozomal granules and has a well-developed Golgi apparatus; all of which indicate a metabolically active cell which is actively producing and secreting proteins. Although derived from the same progenitor cell, unlike PMN, monocytes are not mature end-cells but rather immature cells which migrate into the tissues where they continue to differentiate under the influence of the local environment. Thus tissue macrophages form distinct populations including Kupffer cells, alveolar macrophages, peritoneal macrophages, connective tissue histiocytes, dendritic cells in lymph nodes and Langerhans cells in the skin. They are also related to bone osteoclasts and microglial cells in the central nervous system.

Monocytes and macrophages have a number of functional and histo-chemical properties in common. From the promonocyte stage in the marrow they are phagocytic and have the ability to adhere to surfaces. Pro-monocytes, monocytes, and macrophages all contain non-specific esterase in the cytoplasm. They all secrete lysozme independently of stimulation or activation so that diseases where monocytes are increased are characterized by high levels of lysozyme in blood and urine. Peroxidase is absent in promonocytes but develops in the rough endoplasmic reticulum of monocytes and then is lost again in tissue macrophages. Other enzymes change as the cells become activated, for example the ectoenzyme 5'-nucleotidase decreases while amino peptidase increases.

Monocyte macrophage function

Clearly the physiology of monocytes and macrophages is extraordinarily complex but can be considered in relation to four major functional activities. First they phagocytose and degrade all types of foreign material in their environment. Second they initiate inflammatory and immune responses and at the same time release cytokines active both locally and systemically. Thirdly, they are capable of destroying certain microorganisms associated with chronic infections. Finally, they can suppress the inflammatory reaction.

Phagocytic function

This is both non-specific for inert particles, such as latex beads, and specific for opsonized particles via Fc and CR3 receptors which are similar if not identical to those of PMN. Following ingestion, particles are digested by enzymes released from lysozomes. These enzymes include cathepsins, hyaluronidase and β-glucuronidase, and they are also released outside the cells where they may play a part in tissue damage in conditions associated with accumulations of macrophages such as in rheumatoid joints. Other enzymes, including elastase, collagenase and plasminogen activator, are not preformed but are synthesized following stimulation and therefore released later than lysozomal enzymes. Most ingested particles appear to be killed by the products of an NADPH oxidase which is identical to the PMN oxidase.

Initiation and control of inflammation

Not all material ingested by monocytes and macrophages is digested as, in some way, these cells present antigen to T-lymphocytes to initiate the immune response. This process is not understood but involves both the foreign antigen and self-recognition Ia antigens. At the same time monocytes synthesize and release cytokines, both IL-1 and TNF, which amplify the local inflammatory response by their effects on lymphocytes and by their chemotactic action on granulocytes. IL-1 and TNF have profound general effects as they are responsible for the pyrexia, acute-phase protein production and protein catabolism which are the systemic features of inflammation.[24,51]

Microbicidal activity

Chronic infections due to organisms able to survive intracellularly, including mycobacteria, listeria and unicellular parasites, are associated with accumulations of 'activated macrophages'.[53] Activation appears to be due to γ-interferon produced by T-lymphocytes. These macrophages show enhancement of the function already described as involved in phagocytosis and control of inflammation so that the cells synthesize and secret lysozomal enzymes, proteinases, oxygen radicals and, in particular, large amounts of hydrogen peroxide. In animal models such activated macrophages are also tumoricidal and are able to destroy both transplanted and spontaneous malignant cells without apparent damage to the host. Whether this tumoricidal ability is important in humans is not clear.

Suppression of inflammation

As already mentioned, activated macrophages secrete large amounts of enzymes and oxygen radicals capable of destroying inflammatory mediators. They also secrete prostaglandins, particularly PGE_2, which suppress lymphocyte proliferation. This is the suggested mechanism of the suppressed delayed immune response seen in miliary tuberculosis and Hodgkin's disease.

Monocyte response to inflammation

Monocyte development only diverges from PMN at a relatively late stage and consequently their response to inflammation is very similar. Monocytes respond to the same regulatory molecules leading to increased production and release from the bone marrow, attachment to and then diapedesis through the endothelium of post-capillary venules and directed migration towards inflammation. They arrive at inflammatory sites at the same time as PMN, rather than later as is often assumed. The difference in behaviour is their persistence and continuing differentiation into macrophages so that they become the major component of the infiltrate around chronic inflammation.

Just as exudate PMN are activated cells, the same is true of exudate macrophages when compared with monocytes. Morphologically they are larger, more spreading cells, with increased expression of the Mac-1 adhesion proteins including the CR3 receptor. They are metabolically more active with increased secretion of oxygen radicals, lysozomal hydrolases, proteinases and, particularly, plasminogen activator.[52]

Abnormalities of monocyte function

Like PMN, monocytes are affected by the congenital disorders chronic granulomatous disease and deficiency of adherence-related glycoproteins. As discussed, monocytes normally differentiate in response to inflammation and it is likely that, like PMN, they are affected by abnormalities of their environment in diabetes mellitus and chronic renal failure.

Abnormalities of monocyte numbers

As a result of their common origin monocytes and PMN tend to change together in the circulation. Thus a monocytosis is part of the leucocytosis of acute inflammation and a monocytopenia a part of the leucopenia caused by cytotoxic drugs. However, in some circumstances monocyte numbers are independent of PMN, for example when PMN numbers are reduced by specific mechanisms such as antibody-mediated consumption, monocytes are not affected. True monocytosis with an increase in the number of circulating cells is usually associated with chronic inflammation and the common causes are listed in Table 4.7. Sometimes the monocytosis is associated with morphological changes with the presence of larger spreading cells containing vacuoles or phagocytosed and partially degraded cells; in other words macrophages in the peripheral blood. This is particularly a feature of patients with sub-acute bacterial endocarditis.

Table 4.7 Systemic Causes of Monocytosis

Chronic bacterial infections
   Tuberculosis
   Sub-acute bacterial endocarditis
   Brucellosis

Parasitic infections
   Malaria
   Kala-azar
   Trypanosomiasis

Malignant disease
   Carcinoma
   Hodgkin's disease

Collagen disorders
   Rheumatoid arthritis
   Systemic lupus erythematosus

EOSINOPHIL GRANULOCYTES

Like PMN, eosinophils are end-cells with a condensed nuclear structure, a few mitochondria and small amounts of endoplasmic reticulum, indicating little ability to synthesize proteins. The characteristic granules are membrane-bound and contain a dense crystalloid core surrounded by a less-dense, enzyme-rich, homogeneous matrix. The core is almost entirely composed of major basic protein (MBP). Many of the enzymes are similar to those found in PMN but some are distinct. Peroxidase is abundant in the specific granules and is biochemically and antigenically unique to eosinophils. There is also a distinct eosinophilic cationic protein. Eosinophils are also rich in enzymes which break down inflammatory mediators, including histaminase, kininase and arysulphatase. Eosinophils do not contain lysozyme.[54]
   In the marrow eosinophils arise from a progenitor cell which is distinct from the GM-CFU and, although responsive to the same colony stimulating factors, can also respond to factors distinct from those affecting PMN and monocyte production. The first identifiable granules appear in promyelocytes which are followed by morphological stages in parallel with PMN. Again, like PMN, eosinophils have a short half-life in the circulation before migrating into the tissues, particularly gastrointestinal tract, skin and lungs.

Eosinophil function

Eosinophils are important in the immune response to parasites, particularly helminths, and they appear to modulate other inflammatory reactions, especially allergic reactions.
   Although phagocytic they have less capacity for phagocytosis and microbial killing than PMN but they appear to be unique in their ability to

kill or damage parasites. They bind tightly to the parasite, presumably by Fc and CR3 receptors, and they degranulate onto the surface of the parasite. Both MBP and eosinophil peroxidase, in association with hydrogen peroxide and halide, damage and kill the parasite.

The modulating role of eosinophils is suggested by their accumulation at the margins of inflammatory lesions. They are certainly effective phagocytes of antigen–antibody complexes. However, their particular relationship to allergic reactions appears to depend upon interaction with basophils and tissue mast cells. These cells are triggered by the reaction of IgE and antigen on their surface or by anaphylotoxic complement components, to release histamine, heparin, and small molecular weight eosinophil chemotactic factors. These, except heparin, are chemotactic for eosinophils and result in their accumulation at sites of allergic reactions. The eosinophils inactivate these, and other inflammatory mediators, through the action of histaminase, arylsulphatase and peroxidase; heparin is rapidly neutralized by MBP.

Abnormalities of eosinophil numbers

Eosinophilia

The common systemic causes of eosinophilia are listed in Table 4.8. The two commonest are immediate hypersensitivity reactions and parasitic diseases due to metazoan parasites invading tissues.

Idiopathic hyper-eosinophilic syndrome

This is defined as persistent eosinophilia of more than 1.5×10^9 per litre for at least 6 months, or death before 6 months, with no evidence for recognized causes of eosinophilia.[55] It is probably due to a variety of causes

Table 4.8 Systemic Causes of Eosinophilia

Allergic
  Asthma
  Pulmonary aspergillosis
  Drug reactions
  Atopic dermatitis

Parasitic
  Tissue invasive helminths, including strongyloides, trichinosis, schistosomiasis, filariasis

Vasculitic
  Associated with immune complexes in rheumatoid arthritis, systemic lupus erythematosus, arteritis nodosa

Neoplastic
  Hodgkin's disease
  T-cell lymphomas
  Metastatic adenocarcinoma

---

but forms a distinct syndrome because persistent eosinophilia leads to tissue damage as a result of cellular infiltration and discharge of toxic products including the major basic and cationic proteins. Any organ may be involved but particularly the central nervous system, heart, lungs and skin. The nervous system may show focal lesions or a symmetrical peripheral neuropathy. The heart develops a characteristic endocardial fibrosis complicated by thrombus formation and emboli. Lung involvement may be pulmonary infiltrates with or without broncho-spasm sometimes called Löffler's syndrome. The skin manifestations are various rashes due to eosinophil infiltrates and vasculitis. Treatment is to reduce the eosinophilia usually by giving hydroxyurea; corticosteroids have also been used.

BASOPHIL GRANULOCYTES

Basophils are the least numerous of the polymorphonuclear granulocytes in the blood. They appear as bags of large granules which stain intensely with metachromatic dyes. The granule contents and therefore function of basophils are almost identical to tissue mast cells but they are probably distinct populations, one in the circulation and the other in the tissues.[56]

Basophil function

The basophil granule staining characteristics are due to proteoglycans, chondroitin-sulphate and heparin, which form the granule matrix within which histamine is contained. Basophils also release lysozomal enzymes and produce oxygen radicals catalysed by an NADPH oxidase in common with PMN and monocytes. Both basophils and tissue mast cells express a high-affinity IgE receptor on their surface and are triggered by interaction of surface IgE with specific antigen. They are also triggered by the anaphylactic complement components C3a and C5a, for which they express distinct receptors. Triggering releases histamine which mediates the immediate hypersensitivty reaction. The wheel and flare in the skin subsides within 30–60 min and may be followed by a late-phase infiltration with PMN, eosinophils and mononuclear cells due to the attractive properties of histamine and a low molecular weight chemotatic factor released by basophils. A potent cause of IgE-mediated basophil granule discharge is invasion of tissues by parasites. Consequently the function of basophils appears to be the release of inflammatory mediators in response to tissue invasion by helminths.[56]

Abnormalities of basophil numbers

The numbers of basophils in the peripheral circulation are so low that obvious changes in numbers only occur in myeloproliferative disorders. However, the numbers probably do respond to systemic illness, as certainly they fall in patients receiving corticosteroids and they rise in parallel with eosinophils in patients with helminth infections.

REFERENCES

1. Malech, H.L. & Gallin, J.I. Neutrophils in human diseases. *N. Engl. J. Med.* **317**: 687–94, 1987.
2. Rowe, G.T., Eaton, L.R. & Hess, M.L. Neutrophil derived oxygen-free radical-mediated cardiovascular dysfunction. *J. Med. Cell. Cardiol.* **16**: 1075–9, 1984.
3. Metchinikoff, E. *Immunity in Infective Diseases.* Translated by F.A. Starling & E.J. Starling. Paul Trench, Trubner, London, 1970.
4. Metcalf, D. The granulocyte-macrophage colony stimulating factors. *Science* **229**: 16–22, 1985.
5. Athens, J.W, Haab, O.P., Raab, S.O., Mauer, A.M., Ahsenbrucker, H., Cartwright, G.E. & Wintrobe, M.M. Leukokinetic studies IV. The total blood circulating and granulocyte turnover rate in normal subjects. *J. Clin. Invest.* **40**: 989–95, 1961.
6. Bainton, D.F., Ullyot, J.L. & Farquhar, M.G. The development of neutrophilic polymorphonuclear leucocytes in human bone marrow. *J. Exp. Med.* **134**: 907–31, 1971.
7. Maallem, H., Sheppard, K. & Fletcher, J. The discharge of primary and secondary granules during immune phagocytosis by normal and chronic granulocytic leukaemia neutrophils. *Br. J. Haematol.* **51**: 201–10, 1982.
8. Gallin, J.I. Neutrophil specific granules: a fuse that ignites the inflammatory response. *Clin. Res.* **32**: 320–8, 1984.
9. Dewald, B., Bretz, U. & Baggiolini, M. Release of gelatinase from a novel secretory compartment of human neutrophils. *J. Clin. Invest.* **70**: 518–25, 1982.
10. Petrequin, P.R., Todd, R.F., Devall, L.J., Boxer, L.A. & Curnutte, J.T. Association between gelatinase release and increased plasma membrane expression of the MoI glycoprotein. *Blood* **69**: 605–10, 1987.
11. Mollinedo, F. & Schneider, D.L. Subcellular localisation of cytochrome b and ubiquinone to a tertiary granule of resting human neutrophils and evidence for a proton pump ATPase. *J. Biol. Chem.* **259**: 7143–50, 1984.
12. Baggiolini, M. & Dewald, B. The neutrophil. *Int. Archs. Allergy Appl. Immun.* **76**: Suppl. 1, 13–20, 1985.
13. Williamson, L.M., Sheppard, K, Davies, J.M. & Fletcher, J. Neutrophils are involved in the increased vascular permeability produced by activated complement in man. *Brit. J. Haematol.* **64**: 375–84, 1986.
14. Movat, H.Z., Cybulsky, M.I., Colditz, I.G., Chan, M.K.W. & Dinarello, C.A. Acute inflammation in gram-negative infection: endotoxin, interleukin 1, tumour necrosis factor and neutrophils. *Fedn. Proc.* **46**: 97–104, 1987.
15. Gustafson, E.J. & Colman, R.W. Interaction of polymorphonuclear cells with contact activation factors. *Semin. Thrombosis Haemostasis* **13**: 95–105, 1987.
16. Goetzel, E.J. & Sun, F.F. Generation of unique monohydroxyeicosatetraenoic acids from arachidonic acid by neutrophils. *J. Exp. Med.* **150**: 406–11, 1979.
17. Carp. H. Mitochondrial N-formylmethionyl proteins as chemoattractants for neutrophils. *J. Exp. Med.* **155**: 264–75, 1982.
18. Berger, M., Wetzler, E.M. & Wallis, R.S. Tumour necrosis factor is the major monocyte product that increases complement receptor expression on mature human neutrophils. *Blood* **71**: 151–8, 1988.
19. Smolen, J.E. & Boxer, L.A. Disorders of stimulus response coupling in neutrophils. *Clin. Lab. Med.* **3**: 779–800, 1983.
20. Zimmerli, W., Seligmann, B. & Gallin, J.I. Exudation primes human and guinea pig neutrophils for subsequent responsiveness to the chemotactic peptide N formylmethionylleucylphenylalanine and increases complement component C_3bi receptor expression. *J. Clin. Invest.* **77**: 925–33, 1986.
21. Ward, P.A. & Becker, E.L. The deactivation of rabbit neutrophils by chemotactic factor and the nature of the activatable esterase. *J. Exp. Med.* **127**: 693–709, 1968.

22. Nunoi, H., Endo, F., Chikazawa, S. & Matsuda, I. Regulation of receptors and digestive activity towards synthesised formyl-chemotactic peptide in human polymorphonuclear leukocytes. *Blood* **66**: 106–14, 1985.
23. Cronstein, B.N., Kramer, S.B., Weissmann, G. & Hirschhorn, R. Adenosine: a physiological modulator of superoxide anion generation by human neutrophils. *J. Exp. Med.* **158**, 1160–77, 1983.
24. Dinarello, L.A. Interleukin-1. *Rev. Infect. Dis.* **6**: 51–95, 1984.
25. Niedel, J.E., Kahane, I. & Cuatrecasas, P. Receptor mediated internalisation of fluorescent chemotactic peptide by human neutrophils. *Science* **205**: 1412–14, 1979.
26. Anderson, D.C., Miller, L.J., Schmalsteig, F.C., Rothlein, R. & Springer, T.A. Contributions of the Mac-1 glycoprotein family to adherence-dependent granulocyte functions: Structure–function assessments employing subunit specific monoclonal antibodies. *J. Immunol.* **137**: 15–27, 1986.
27. Wright, S.D. Cellular strategies in receptor-mediated phagocytosis. *Rev. Infect. Dis.* **7**: 395–7, 1985.
28. Elsbach, P. & Weiss, J. A re-evaluation of the roles of the O_2-dependent and O_2-independent microbicidal systems of phagocytes. *Rev. Infect. Dis.* **5**: 843–53, 1983.
29. Cohen, H.J., Tape, E.H., Novak, J., Chovaniec, M.E., Leigey, P. & Whitin, J.C. The role of glutathione reductase in maintaining human granulocyte function and sensitivity to exogenous H_2O_2. *Blood* **69**: 493–500, 1987.
30. Roos, D., Weening, R.S., Wyss, S.R. & Aebi, H.H. Protection of human neutrophils by endogenous catalase. Studies with cells from catalase deficient individuals. *J. Clin. Invest.* **65**: 1515–22, 1980.
31. Segal, A.W., Gaisow, M., Garcia, R., Harper, A. & Miller, R. The respiratory burst of phagocytic cells is associated with a rise in vacuolar pH. *Nature* **290**: 406–9, 1981.
32. Nathan, C.F. Neutrophil activation on biological surfaces. *J. Clin. Invest.* **80**: 1550–60, 1987.
33. Gallin, J.I. & Buescher, E.S. Abnormal regulation of inflammatory skin responses in male patients with chronic granulomatous disease. *Inflammation* **7**: 227–32, 1983.
34. Slater, K. & Fletcher, J. Lactoferrin derived from neutrophils inhibits the mixed lymphocyte reaction. *Blood* **69**: 1328–33, 1987.
35. EL-Maallem, H. & Fletcher, J. Effects of surgery on neutrophil granulocyte function. *Infect. Immun.* **32**: 38–41, 1981.
36. Davies, J.M., Sheppard, K. & Fletcher, J. The effect of surgery on the activity of neutrophil granule proteins. *Brit. J. Haematol.* **53**: 5–13, 1983.
37. Rustin, G.J.S., Wilson, P.D. & Peters, T.J. Studies on the subcellular localisation of human neutrophil alkaline phosphatase. *J. Cell Sci.* **36**: 401–12, 1979.
38. EL-Maallem, H. & Fletcher, J. Impaired neutrophil function and myeloperoxidase deficiency in pregnancy. *Br. J. Haematol.* **44**: 375–81, 1980.
39. Weinberg, P.F., Matthay, M.A., Webster, R.O., Roskos, K.V., Goldstein, I.M. & Murray, J.F. Biologically active products of complement and acute lung injury in patients with the sepsis syndrome. *Ann. Rev. Resp. Dis.* **130**, 792–6, 1984.
40. Weissmann, G. & Korchak, H. Rheumatoid arthritis: the role of neutrophil activation. *Inflammation* **8**: Suppl. 3–14, 1984.
41. Malawista, S.E. Gouty inflammation. *Arthr. Rheum.* **20**: Suppl. 241–8, 1977.
42. Fauci, A.S., Haynes, B.F. & Katz, P. The spectrum of vasculitis: clinical, pathologic immunologic and therapeutic considerations. *Ann. Intern. Med.* **89**: 660–76, 1978.
43. Bednar, M., Smith, B., Pinto, A. & Mullane, K.M. Nafazatrom-induced salvage of ischemic myocardium in anaesthetised dogs is mediated through inhibition of neutrophil function. *Circ. Res.* **57**: 131–41, 1985.
44. Davidson, N.J., Sowden, J.M. & Fletcher, J. Defective phagocytosis in insulin

controlled diabetics: evidence for a reaction between glucose and opsonising proteins. *J. Clin. Path.* **37**: 783–6, 1984.

45. Wilson, R.M. & Reeves, W.G. Neutrophil phagocytosis and killing. *Clin. Exp. Immunol.* **63**: 478–84, 1986.

46. Harvey, D.M., Sheppard, K.J., Morgan, A.G. & Fletcher, J. Neutrophil function in patients on continuous ambulatory peritoneal dialysis. *Br. J. Haematol.* **68**: 273–8, 1988.

47. Anderson, D.C. & Springer, T.A. Leukocyte adhesion deficiency: an inherited defect in the Mac-1 LFA-1 and p150, 95 glycoproteins. *Am. Rev. Med.* **38**: 175–94, 1987.

48. Clark, R.A. & Borregaard, N. Neutrophils autoinactivate secretory products by myeloperoxidase-catalysed oxidation. *Blood* **65**: 375–81, 1985.

49. Gallin, J.I. Neutrophil specific granule deficiency. *Am. Rev. Med.* **36**: 263–74, 1985.

50. Seiff, C.A., Tsai, S. & Faller, D.V. Interleukin-1 induces cultured human endothelial cell production of granulocyte-macrophage colony stimulating factor. *J. Clin. Invest.* **79**: 48–51, 1987.

51. Oppenheim, J.J., Kovacs, E.J., Matsushima, K. & Durum, S.K. There is more than one interleukin 1. *Immunology Today* **7**: 45–56, 1986.

52. North, R.J. The concept of the activated macrophage. *J. Immunol.* **121**: 806–9, 1978.

53. Allison, A.C. Mechanisms by which activated macrophages inhibit lymphocyte responses. *Immunol. Rev,* **40**: 3, 1978.

54. Mahmoud, A.A.F. & Austen, K.F. *The Eosinophil in Health and Disease.* Grune & Stratton, New York, 1980.

55. Fauci, A.S. Idiopathic eosinophilic syndrome: clinical, pathophysiologic and therapeutic considerations. *Ann. Intern. Med.* **97**: 78–92, 1982.

56. Galli, S.J., Dvorak, A.M. & Dvorak, H.F. Basophils and mast cells: morphologic insights into their biology, secretory patterns and function. *Progr. Allergy* **34**: 1–141, 1984.

5

Lymphocyte abnormalities

T.J. Hamblin
Professor of Immunohaematology, Southampton University,
Consultant Haematologist, Royal Victoria Hospital, Bournemouth,
UK

A. Kruger
Senior Registrar in Haematology, Southampton General Hospital,
Southampton, UK

It is hard to believe that as recently as 1956 a comprehensive textbook of immunology could have only one reference to the lymphocyte, and that to dismiss it as an antibody-producing cell in favour of the plasma cell.[1] Following the demonstration of lymphocyte recirculation by Gowans in 1957,[2] the lymphocyte has become the most studied of all cells and the model for most cellular physiology. Its pivotal role in the science of immunology and its relevance to almost all pathology has been revealed.

THE NORMAL LYMPHOCYTE

The majority of peripheral blood lymphocytes are small cells with an average volume of 180 fl and a diameter in stained films of 7–12 μm. Romanowsky stained preparations demonstrate a round or slightly indented nucleus, containing very condensed chromatin, surrounded by scanty bluish cytoplasm. Smaller numbers of large lymphocytes, 12–16 μm in diameter, with less condensed chromatin and more cytoplasm, are usually seen. The cytoplasm of both small and large lymphocytes may contain a few azurophil granules. Ultrastructural examination demonstrates a small nucleolus, but few cytoplasmic organelles. Small numbers of mitochondria, scattered monoribosomes and an inactive Golgi apparatus are usually seen.

Sub-populations of lymphocytes cannot easily be recognized on morphological grounds, but cytochemical, immunological and functional assays will easily distinguish B-cells, T-cells and null cells.

B-Lymphocytes

The role of B-cells is to produce specific antibody in response to antigenic stimulation. Quintessential 'B'ness is conferred by the immunoglobulin molecule which, for much of the B-cell's lifespan, is carried on the surface membrane and there acts as a receptor for antigen. Each particular B-lymphocyte is committed to a specific immunoglobulin molecule known as its idiotype. The enormous conformational variety of immunoglobulins is pre-programmed in the genome and is developed in two main ways. First, the gene coding for the antibody combining site (or variable region) has two or three segments: V, D and J for the heavy chains and V and J for the light chains. Within the genome there are hundreds of copies of the V segment, each slightly different, and several copies of both D and J. For each immunoglobulin molecule, one copy each of the V, D and J (or V and J) segments is selected and recombined to form the template for mRNA. Secondly, somatic point mutations occur in the DNA sequence at the time of class switching from IgM to IgG or IgA. These mutations allow for the selection of antibody molecules which fit best to antigen, and explain the refinement in specificity that occurs during a secondary immune response.

B-Cells are produced initially by the foetal liver, but after birth that duty is subsumed by the bone marrow. Commitment to the B lineage is accompanied by recombination of the V, D and J genes of the immuno-globulin heavy chain, and slightly later by the expression of small amounts of free μ chains in the cytoplasm. At this stage of development, which continues in the bone marrow, the B-cell has a blast-like conformation, and is often designated a pre-B-cell. Recombination of light-chain genes is followed by the expression of surface IgM and the maturation of the cell to the form of a small lymphocyte. Expression of surface IgD occurs slightly later. The mature but resting B-cell leaves the bone marrow and circulates via blood and lymph to the secondary lymphoid organs. The majority of circulating B-cells express both IgM and IgD on their surface. Maturation to this stage is independent of antigenic stimulation and of T-cells.

Surface immunoglobulin molecules act as receptors for antigen. Stimula-tion of these receptors leads to activation, proliferation, maturation to plasma cells, and finally to secretion of immunoglobulin. Activation involves the cell moving from G_0 to G_1 and then to S phase, which is accompanied by enlargement of the cell and decondensation of nuclear chromatin, before proceeding to mitosis. It is likely that different maturation pathways exist for different B-cell subtypes, but these are poorly worked out. For example, the production of centroblasts and centrocytes in the germinal centres of lymph node follicles is apparently quite separate from the generation of prolymphocytes and of lymphoplasmacytoid cells. The centrocytes found in the mucosal-associated lymphoid tissue also behave differently from those in lymph nodes and probably represent a different lineage.

Activation is frequently accompanied by class switching of immuno-globulin genes, so that the cell expresses surface IgG, IgA or IgE and the eventual plasma cell secretes the same class of immunoglobulin.

Activation of B-cells is under the control of growth factors, mainly produced by T-cells. The most important of these are interleukins-4, -5 and -6. The actions of these lymphokines are complex and most have effects on several different types of cell. In simple terms, interleukin-4 controls the activation and proliferation of resting B-cells, interleukin-4 and -5 acting together initiate immunoglobulin class switching, interleukin-5 controls proliferation and differentiation of activated B-cells, while interleukin-6 is concerned with the secretion of immunoglobulin.

Although immunoglobulin is the molecule most useful in defining B-cells, a whole range of cell markers which are present mainly or only on B-cells have been identified, principally by the use of monoclonal antibodies. These markers have been categorized by international workshops and given clusters of differentiation (CD) numbers.[3] The expression of some of them appears confined to certain stages of differentiation. The markers of most interest in B-cell differentiation are described in Table 5.1. The functions of most of these molecules are not yet determined but it is presumed that they form receptors concerned with cell activation and function.

Table 5.1 Classification of B-Cell Markers

Marker	Prototype antibody	Mol. wt. of Ag (kDa)	Distribution	Function
CD5	OKT1	67	Most T-cells B-CLL cells	CD5-pos. B-cells appear to represent a distinct lineage concerned with the basic idiotypic repertoire and autoimmunity
CD9	BA2	24	Early B-cells Platelets AML cells Myeloma cells	Unknown
CD10	J5	100	Early B-cells cALL Epithelial cells Some follicular lymphoma cells	Unknown
CD19	B4	95	All B-cells ? Dendritic cells	? Involved in B-cell stimulation by antigen and IL-4
CD20	B1	35	Most B-cells	Involved in B-cell activation
CD21	B2	140	Most B-cells Dendritic cells Some T-ALL cells	C3d receptor. EBV receptor
CD22	HD39	130	75% circulating B-cells Variably expressed on B-cell tumours	Involved in B-cell proliferation
CD23	MHM6	45	Late B-cells Dendritic cells	Fcε receptor. Receptor for B-cell growth factor
CD24	BA1	42	B-cells Granulocytes Monocytes Some T-ALL	Unknown
CD37	WR17	40	B-cells Granulocytes	Unknown

T-Lymphocytes

T-Cells arise from the same progenitors as B-cells, but differentiate in a discrete organ, the thymus, before seeding the secondary lympoid organs. T-Cells recognize antigen and major histocompatibility complex (MHC) molecules via a receptor (Ti) related in structure to immunoglobulin, but distinct from it. The Ti (T idiotype) receptor consists of two disulphide-linked dissimilar chains (α and β), each with a constant and variable region. The CD3 molecule is an essential part of the T-cell receptor and itself consists of three different non-covalently associated peptides (γ, δ and ε chains).

The genes which encode for Ti are similar to those of immunoglobulin, and idiotypic commitment is formulated in the same way by the selection of one V, D and J gene from the available repertoire of both α and β chains. It appears that the repertoire of V genes is considerably more restricted than that for immunoglobulin.[4] The Ti receptor is responsible for binding to antigen and the MHC molecule, but the role of the associated CD3 antigen is less clear. It is probably involved in signal transduction from Ti to cytoplasm.

Commitment of the T-cell takes place within the thymic cortex under the control of 'hormones' released from the thymic epithelial cells. At least four, thymosin, thymopoietin, thymulin, and thymic humoral factor, have been recognized, although the specific function of each is not clearly delineated.[5] Within the thymic medulla T-cells separate into two distinct sub-sets: helper/inducer cells which express the CD4 antigen, and suppressor/cytotoxic cells which express CD8. Early cortical T-cells express both CD4 and CD8. Both the CD4 and CD8 molecules are involved in specific interactions between cells in the immune response. CD4 is involved in the recognition by T-helper cells of MHC class II molecules on antigen-presenting cells, and CD8 is involved in the recognition by cytotoxic T-cells of MHC class I molecules on target cells.

Further heterogeneity of T-helper and -suppressor cells has recently been recognized and may be distinguished by antibodies of the CD45R group. In particular TH_1-cells, which mediate delayed hypersensitivity, proffer help to other T-cells, including T-suppressor cells, and secrete interleukin-2 (IL-2), are distinct from TH_2-cells which help B-cells and secrete IL-4 and IL-5.[6]

Mature TH- and TS-cells constantly recirculate via blood and lymph through the peripheral lymphoid system. Activation occurs on stimulation by antigen in association with MHC class II, and leads to the expression of the IL-2 receptor CD25. Lymphokine secretion occurs, but the range of different lymphokines is particular to specific sub-sets, IL-2 acting as an autocrine growth factor within such an immune response.

Other antigens are expressed during various stages of T-cell maturation (Table 5.2) but their function is at present obscure.

Null cells

Some lymphocytes express neither immunoglobulin nor the T idiotypic receptor. They are recognized as lymphocytes on morphological grounds but their designation as such is a semantic problem. One definition of a

Table 5.2 Classification of T-Cell Markers

Marker	Prototype Ab	Mol. wt. of Ag (kDa)	Distribution	Function
CD1	OKT6	45	Cortical thymocytes	Unknown
CD2	OKT11	50	Pan-T-cell	Sheep red cell receptor
CD3	OKT3	19	Pan-T-cell	Signal transduction
CD4	OKT4	55	T-helper/inducer cells	Recognition of MHC class II
CD5	OKT1	67	Pan-T-cell B-CLL	Unknown
CD6	OKT12	120	Medullary thymocytes and later T-cells	Unknown
CD7	3A1	47	Early T-cells	Unknown
CD8	OKT8	32	T-suppressor/cytotoxic cells	Recognition of MHC class I
CD25	Anti-TAC	55	Activated T-cells	IL-2 receptor

lymphocyte is of a cell capable of specifically recognizing and responding to antigen, and on these grounds null cells would be excluded.

Null cells are clearly heterogeneous. Among their number are haemopoietic progenitor cells, which contribute in particular to the bone marrow 'lymphocytes'.[7] (The morphological resemblance of these cells to lymphocytes led early authors to postulate that the small lymphocyte was the pluripotent stem cell.[8]) These cells are present in the peripheral blood and their numbers are increased during the recovery phase from marrow suppressive chemotherapy, a fact made use of by collecting the 'lymphocyte' fraction on a cell separator for the performance of stem cell autografts for bone marrow rescue after ablative chemotherapy.[9]

The majority of peripheral blood null cells are those responsible for natural killer (NK) activity, which when mature assume the appearance of large granular lymphocytes (LGLs).[10] Considerable confusion exists about this group of cells since not all LGLs are null cells, and not all cells exhibiting NK activity are either LGLs or null cells. Nevertheless, description is helped by assuming a reference population which has all three designations and then detailing exceptions. We will call this cell an N-cell.

N-Cells are of uncertain origin. One author refers to them as pre-thymic T-cells[11] but the fact that they behave as effector cells and carry some monocyte markers suggests a derivation from haemopoietic progenitors.[12]

The characteristic surface antigens possessed by N-cells are CD16 (the low-affinity Fcγ receptor) and Leu19 (also known as NKH-1). Although some N-cells exhibit CD2 (the sheep erythrocyte receptor) and CD8, they are CD3-negative. The monocyte marker OKM1 is also sometimes found.

The characteristic function displayed by N-cells is cellular cytotoxicity unrestricted by MHC class I recognition. In the laboratory this activity, known as NK activity, is demonstrated by the killing of a restricted group of tumour cell lines (e.g. K562). N-cells are capable of activation by IL-2, and following this their killing activity is much less restricted and may be demonstrated against lymphoblastoid cell lines (e.g. Daudi) and fresh tumour cells. This unrestricted cytotoxicity is known as lymphokine-activated killing (LAK).[13]

It seems that a small proportion of NK and LAK activity of human blood resides in a CD-3 positive, CD8-positive population.[12]

N-Cells are also capable of acting as effector cells in antibody-dependent cellular cytotoxicity (ADCC) through the CD16, Fcγ receptor. In the laboratory many other cells, including monocytes and granulocytes, are capable of acting as effectors in ADCC, but since high-affinity Fcγ receptors are easily inhibited by the monomeric IgG present in plasma, it is likely that N-cells are the major mediators of ADCC *in vivo*.[14] (This activity is also known as K-cell killing. Thus to add to the confusion it appears that operationally N-cells, K-cells and NK-cells are the same thing.)

Killing of target cells by N-cells involves the secretion of granule contents into the area between the closely opposed killer and target cell. A major component of the granules is perforin, which binds to the target cell membrane and polymerizes to form a transmembrane channel.[15] It is likely that other secreted products (possibly tumour necrosis factor) are also needed for cell killing.

In real life NK activity is thought to play a role in tumour surveillance, but N-cells are also important in defence against infectious agents, in the regulation of the immune response, in the control of haemopoietic stem cells, in transplantation rejection and graft-versus-host disease, and in autoimmunity.

The immune response

The prime purpose of lymphocytes is to respond to infections and eliminate the infecting organism. Although for the purposes of comprehension the immune response has been dissected into humoral and cell-mediated components, it must be realized that in life virtually all responses are mixed. Furthermore, all infective agents express several different antigens on their surfaces so that cell immune responses are polyclonal. B- and T-cells usually recognize different parts of the same antigen (epitopes). The response to each pathogen is distinct, and a study in its own right. Here, we will concentrate on common principles.

In order that most T-cells recognize the antigens of pathogenic organisms they must first be processed and then presented in association with MHC molecules. The antigen-presenting cells are mainly macrophages and lymphoid dentritic cells, and the process occurs mostly within secondary lymphoid organs. B-Cells do not require antigenic processing, but most require the antigen to be recognized by a T-helper cell before they can be activated. This cellular interaction is mediated by lymphokines and takes place within lymph nodes and spleen. The response to antigenic stimulation is activation, proliferation and differentiation.

Whether an infection is localized or systemic, the major changes in lymphoid tissue take place within the fixed lymphoid organ. Because both B- and T-cells continually recirculate, reflections of these processes are seen in the peripheral blood. Thus activated cells, which are larger and have nucleoli and basophilic cytoplasm, are frequently seen in infections, and the appearance of increased numbers of cytotoxic T-cells in the blood may reflect the proliferative response of these cells within the lymphoid organs.

Lymphocyte numbers

Absolute numbers of lymphocytes in the peripheral blood are given in Table 5.3. At birth high levels of circulating lymphocytes are found and these rise to a peak at 2 weeks. Thereafter a gradual decline occurs, reaching adult levels at about puberty. There is a diurnal variation, with a peak in the evening and a trough in the morning, reflecting changes in plasma cortisol levels. Levels do not vary significantly in pregnancy, nor between blacks and whites. Smoking does not affect the absolute numbers, nor does old age per se, although an interesting study from Baltimore demonstrated in men aged over 60 a persistent fall in lymphocyte count from 3 years before death, compared with that measured at 5 and 10 years before death.[17]

B-Cells comprise about 10% of peripheral blood lymphocytes (PBLs), a proportion that does not vary from birth. There are wide variations in T-cell numbers with age; a fall in numbers of T-cells accounting in the main for the fall in numbers from child to adult. Approximately 60% of PBLs are CD4 and 20% CD8 positive. Less than 10% bear the CD16 marker.

In bone marrow, absolute numbers are difficult to calculate because of contamination of aspirates by blood. The ratio of T-cells to B-cells is about 2.7 : 1 and the ratio of CD4-positive cells to CD8-positive cells is about 0.6 : 1.

LYMPHOCYTOSIS

The causes of lymphocytosis are given in Table 5.4. Lymphocytic proliferation is part of the normal immune response, but normally takes place within the secondary lymphoid organs. Thus most infections are associated with localized or generalized lymphadenopathy, and sometimes splenomegaly. Because of the lymphocytic recirculation through blood and lymph, proliferation is always liable to be represented in the peripheral blood, both by the appearance of activated cells and by a lymphocytosis. This is particularly marked in children, where even bacterial infections cause a reactive lymphocytosis.

Table 5.3 Normal Ranges for Lymphocyte Numbers in Peripheral Blood at Varying Ages

Age	Total lymphocytes (× 10⁹ per litre)	CD19+ B-cells	CD3+ T-cells	CD4+ TH	CD8+ TS	CD16+ N
Birth	2–11	0.2–1.1	0.68–6.6			
1 day	2–11.5					
7 days	2–17					
2 months	3–16					
6 months	4–13.5					
1 year	4–10.5					
2 years	3–9.5					
4 years	2–8					
8 years	1.5–7					
14 years	1.2–5.8					
Adult 20–60	1.2–3.5	0.08–0.28	0.8–2.2	0.5–1.7	0.3–0.9	0.05–0.3
60+	0.8–3.8					

After Ref. 16 and many others.

Table 5.4   Causes of Lymphocytosis

Infections
  Mononucleosis syndromes
    EBV
    CMV
    Toxoplasmosis
    Rubella
    Herpes simplex II
    HIV
    Adenovirus
  Acute infectious lymphocytosis
  Other viruses
    Measles
    Mumps
    Rubella
    Varicella (late)
    Influenza
    Infectious hepatitis
  Other infections
    Pertussis
    Brucellosis
    Syphilis (congenital and secondary)
    Tuberculosis (healing stage)

Malignant disorders
  Acute lymphoblastic leukaemia
  Chronic lymphocytic leukaemia
  Non-Hodgkin's lymphoma
  Prolymphocytic leukaemia
  Hairy cell leukaemia
  Waldenstrom's macroglobulinaemia
  LGL leukaemia
  Sezary syndrome
  Adult T-leukaemia lymphoma
  Plasma cell leukaemia
  Heavy-chain diseases

Miscellaneous
  Serum sickness
  Anti-epileptic drugs
  Thyrotoxicosis
  Addison's disease
  Post-splenectomy
  LGL lymphocytosis.

Infectious lymphocytosis

In certain infections characteristic types of lymphocytoses are seen.

Mononucleosis syndromes

Infectious mononucleosis is the name given to an acute self-limited infection by the Epstein–Barr virus (EBV). The characteristic clinical features: fever, pharyngitis, cervical lymphadenopathy and splenomegaly are well-known.

Peripheral blood lymphocytes are increased in number but are so atypical that for many years it was disputed whether they were lymphocytes or monocytes. The cells are large and irregular, with diffuse chromatin and prominent nucleoli, cytoplasmic basophilia and characteristically a scalloped margin where other cells are in contact. These are not the EBV-infected cells. The sequence of events is for the virus to gain entry via the epithelial cells of the oropharynx. B-Cells possess a specific receptor for EBV (CD22) and are preferentially infected. At the height of the infection one in 2000 of peripheral blood B-cells is infected. The lymphocytosis appears at the end of the first week of the infection and lasts for 2–3 weeks in most patients. The atypical cells are mainly CD8-positive T-cells which are specifically cytotoxic for lymphoid cells infected by EBV. Three months after the acute infection less than 5 in 10^9 peripheral blood B-cells are infected with EBV, although as with most herpes viruses this latent infection persists indefinitely.

EBV is a polyclonal mitogen and stimulates the production of the wide range of antibodies associated with infectious mononucleosis. The Paul–Bunnell test is sufficient to diagnose the great majority of patients, although a small number of false positives (mainly lymphomas) and a larger number of false negatives occur. For these patients measurement of EBV-specific IgM antibody is useful diagnostically.

Duncan's syndrome[18] is an X-linked recessive condition in which there is a specific inability to combat the EBV virus. The primary infection may be fatal or may be followed by agammaglobulinaemia, aplastic anaemia, agranulocytosis or B-cell lymphoma. The usual T-suppressor atypical lymphocytosis is absent but a B-cell lymphocytosis is seen.

Toxoplasmosis.   Acquired toxoplasmosis may mimic infectious mononucleosis although the lymphocyte count is seldom as high as in EBV infections. In most cases the infection does no harm and is not recognized, but lymphadenopathy, malaise, fever and sore throat may occur and be associated with a lymphocytosis. Symptoms often last for much longer than in EBV infections.

Toxoplasma gondii is a protozoan parasite which multiplies within nucleated cells. The definitive host is the cat, and it is spread to man by food contaminated with cat faeces or by eating undercooked meat from an infected animal. Diagnosis is confirmed by specific antibody tests. The parasite infects cells of the immune system, particularly antigen-presenting cells, and this leads to a degree of immunosuppression.

The nature of the lymphocytosis has not been described, but an increase in NK activity early in the infection has been recognized. Toxoplasma-secreted antigens have been shown to induce the proliferation of CD4-positive cells and other preparations enhance NK activity and proliferation of CD8-positive cells.[19]

In AIDS and other immunodeficiency syndromes, *Toxoplasma gondii* is an important pathogen.

Cytomegalovirus (CMV).   Although CMV infection is probably the commonest cause of Paul–Bunnell negative infectious mononucleosis, the majority of infections do not give rise to clinical symptoms. Lymphadenopathy is less marked than in EBV infections, but hepatitis and polyneuropathy commoner and more severe. Virus communication is by intimate contact or blood transfusion. The virus is one of several capable of infecting lymphocytes (Table 5.5). Using *in situ* hybridization, viral RNA has been found to be present in up to 2% of peripheral blood lymphocytes in seropositive individuals. CD4-positive cells were most frequently involved.

The nature of the lymphocytosis in CMV infections has not been dissected. However, since it is possible to generate CD8-positive cells capable of killing virally infected cells by incubating the virus with lymphocytes from a seropositive individual, it is likely that a similar sequence occurs as in EBV infections.[20]

In common with many of the viruses which infect lymphocytes, acute infection with CMV leads to a degree of immunosuppression, and it is itself a major pathogen in the immune deficient.

Table 5.5   Viruses that Infect Lymphocytes

Virus	Lymphocytes infected
Double-stranded DNA viruses	
Hepatitis B	T and B
Group C adenovirus	T, B and N
Herpes simplex	T
Epstein–Barr virus	B
Cytomegalovirus	TH
Positive-strand RNA viruses	
Polio	Lymphocytes
Rubella	T and B
Negative-strand RNA viruses	
Measles	T and B
Mumps	T and B
Respiratory syncytial virus	Lymphocytes
Influenza A	Lymphocytes
Parainfluenza	Lymphocytes
Retroviruses	
HTLV I & II	T, B and N
HIV	TH
HBLV	B

Acute infectious lymphocytosis

This syndrome was first reported in 1941[21] and subsequent epidemic outbreaks have been recognized in children and young adults. In most cases there have been either no symptoms or mild short-lived diarrhoea and fever. The striking abnormality in the blood is a lymphocytosis of between 20 and 30×10^9 per litre, although occasionally levels of greater than 100×10^9 per litre have been seen. The lymphocytes have the appearance of normal small lymphocytes and are mainly T-cells. The lymphocytosis is at its highest during the first week and falls gradually over the next 3 weeks. In some individuals a lymphocyte count of 10×10^9 per litre persists at 3 months. As the lymphocyte count falls, an eosinophilia of $2–3 \times 10^9$ per litre is often seen. No single virus has been found to cause acute infectious lymphocytosis, but most reports implicate one of the enteroviruses.[22]

Viral lymphocytosis

A moderate lymphocytosis is often seen in association with a range of viral infections as well as in some bacterial (e.g. brucellosis) and rickettsial infections. Activated lymphocytes and plasmacytoid cells are usually present and there may be an accompanying neutropenia.

Bordetella pertussis *infection*

Lymphocytosis is a characteristic finding in whooping cough. It appears at the end of the catarrhal stage and continues in the paroxysmal stage. It is most marked during the most severe coughing. Counts as high as 50×10^9 per litre occur although more usual levels are between 15 and 25×10^9 per litre. The lymphocytosis persists for about 3 weeks. Typical small lymphocytes are seen and a proportional increase in both T- and B-cells is usual. It has been postulated that the lymphocytosis results from a failure of recirculating lymphocytes to enter lymph nodes. A factor obtained from the supernatant of *B. pertussis* cultures is able to inhibit migration from blood to lymph nodes, leading to a gradual depletion of small lymphocytes in lymph nodes and an expansion of the recirculating pool.[23] In mice, this factor causes impaired delayed hypersensitivity and antibody responses.[24] However, other factors derived from pertussis cultures may act as adjuvants.

Malignant lymphocytosis

Acute lymphoblastic leukaemia

Acute lymphoblastic leukaemia (ALL), like cancers generally, becomes increasingly common in old age, but it is also characteristically common in childhood with a distinctive peak in incidence between the ages of 2 and 5. Patients usually present with the signs of marrow failure, but bone pain, lymphadenopathy and hepatosplenomegaly are all found reasonably commonly. At least a third of patients do not have a raised white count at diagnosis but almost all will have circulating lymphoblasts in the blood film. The diagnosis is dependent on the finding that at least 25% of bone marrow cells are lymphoblasts.

The French–American–British (FAB) study group has classified lympho-blastic leukaemia according to the morphological appearance of the lymphoblasts[25] (Table 5.6). L_1 is seen in 84% of childhood cases and carries the best prognosis. L_2 is seen in 14% of childhood ALL and has a rather worse prognosis. L_3 is present in only 2% of cases and has a dismal outlook. In adults, L_2 is roughly twice as common as L_1.

The cells of ALL are negative for the following cytochemical stains: peroxidase, Sudan Black, chloracetate esterase and usually α-naphthyl acetatesterase. Periodic Acid–Schiff is usually positive, but less than 20% show the characteristic coarse block positivity supposedly pathognomonic of ALL. In T-cell ALL acid phosphatase is strongly positive. Nuclear terminal deoxynucleotidyl transferase is usually detected by immunofluorescence and is positive in most cases of ALL (but not in L_3) as well as in less than 5% of acute myeloblastic leukaemia.

Other cell markers enable ALL to be classified according to B- and T-cell lineage and for the most part this classification is unrelated to the FAB classification. (The exception being B-cell ALL which is coincident with the L_3 sub-type). About 70% of ALLs can be demonstrated to be of B-cell lineage and most of the rest are of T-cell origin. No method of assigning lineage is absolutely reliable. Rearrangement of immunoglobulin heavy chain genes or T idiotype genes is the baseline standard, but in some cases both are

Table 5.6 FAB Classification of Lymphoblastic Leukaemia

	L_1	L_2	L_3
Size	Small cells	Large heterogeneous	Large homogeneous
Chromatin	Homogeneous	Variable	Finely stippled and homogeneous
Nuclear shape	Regular, occasional clefts	Irregular, clefts and indentations common	Regular, oval or round
Nucleoli	Small and inconspicuous	One or more large and obvious	One or more prominent
Cytoplasm	Scanty	Variable, often moderately abundant	Moderately abundant
Cytoplasmic basophilia	Slight or moderate	Variable, some-times intense	Very intense
Cytoplasmic vacuolation	Variable	Variable	Often prominent

After Ref. 25.

Table 5.7 Cell Markers in ALL

	Pre-B-ALL	B-ALL	Pre-T-ALL	T-ALL	Null ALL
TdT	+	−	+	+	+
MHC class II	+	+	−	−	−
CD1	−	−	−	+	−
CD2	−	−	−	+	−
CD3	−	−	−	+	−
CD5	−	−	−	+	−
CD7	−	−	+	+	−
CD9	+	+	−	−	−
CD10	+	+	−	−	−
CD19	+	+	−	−	−
CD20	+	+	−	−	−
CD24	+	+	−	−	−
Surface Ig	−	+	−	−	−
Cytoplasmic μ	+[a]	−	−	−	−

[a] In about 15% of cases

rearranged. Immunological markers are extremely helpful for assigning lineage, but a fairly large 'null' cell group remains, especially in adults. Cell marker patterns for pre-B-cell, B-cell, pre-T-cell, T-cell and null cell ALL are given in Table 5.7.

Chronic lymphatic leukaemias[26]

Chronic lymphatic leukaemia (CLL) is a name given with a varying degree of precision to a number of conditions in which there is a progressive accumulation of small, morphologically mature lymphocytes in the peripheral blood, bone marrow, lymph nodes and spleen. Careful study of the lymphocyte morphology and cell markers has enabled these diseases to be sub-classified (Table 5.8). By far the majority of such patients have classical B-cell CLL. Table 5.9 shows the incidence of CLL variants in two series: 1000 patients referred to the Hammersmith Hospital[27] and 303 patients arising in the Bournemouth area between 1972 and 1987.

B-Cell chronic lymphatic leukaemia (B-CLL).   Classical CLL is characterized by a persistent lymphocytosis in the blood and bone marrow. Various authors give lymphocyte counts of $>5 \times 10^9$ per litre,[28] $>10 \times 10^9$ per litre[27] and $>15 \times 10^9$ per litre[29] as criteria for diagnosis, but more important is evidence of monoclonality and the characteristic morphology. Monoclonality has been recognized by a single G6PD isotype, a single immunoglobulin idiotype, clonal chromosomal abnormalities and a single immunoglobulin gene rearrangement. More usually a single immunoglobulin light-chain isotype expressed on the cell surface is sufficient. Lymphocyte counts of up to 500×10^9 per litre are sometimes seen but in the vast majority of cases counts of less than 50×10^9 per litre are found.

Table 5.8 Cell Markers in CLL and Variants

	B-CLL	B-PLL	HCL	NHL cb/cc	NHL dcc	WM	T-CLL	T-PLL	ATLL	Sezary
CD2	−	−	−	−	−	−	+	+	+	+
CD3	−	−	−	−	−	−	+	+	+	+
CD4	−	−	−	−	−	−	−	+	+	+
CD5	+	±	−	−	+	−	−	+	+	+
CD8	−	−	−	−	−	−	+	−	−	−
CD10	−	−	−	+	−	−	−	−	−	−
CD19	+	+	+	+	+	+	−	−	−	−
CD20	+	+	+	+	+	+	−	−	−	−
CD21	+	±	−	−	−	−	−	−	−	−
CD22	+	+	+	+	+	+	−	−	−	−
CD24	+	+	+	+	+	+	−	−	−	−
CD37	+	+	+	+	+	+	−	−	−	−
SIg	+	+++	++	++	++	++	−	−	−	−
MRBC	+	±	±	−	−	−	−	−	−	−
FMC7	−	+	+	−	−	−	−	−	−	−
HNK-1	−	−	−	−	−	−	+	−	−	−
DR	+	+	+	+	+	+	−	−	±	−
PCA-1	−	−	+	−	−	+	−	−	−	−

Table 5.9 The Incidence of CLL Variants in Two Large Series

	Hammersmith series[a] (%)	Bournemouth series[b] (%)
B-cell tumours		
B-CLL	69	81.5
B-PLL	6.5	1.6
WM	1	1.3
NHL	13	8.2
HCL	6	3
T-cell tumours		
T-CLL	1	3
T-PLL	1.5	0.3
Sezary	1	0.3
ATLL	1	0

[a] 1000 patients referred to Hammersmith Hospital.[27]
[b] 303 patients seen in Bournemouth 1972–87.

The leukaemic lymphocytes are small, round monomorphic cells with a high nuclear/cytoplasmic ratio. The nucleus contains heavily clumped basophilic chromatin and sometimes an indistinct nucleolus may be seen. The cytoplasm is scanty and apparently fragile since 'smudge' cells are usually plentiful in blood films. Usually a small percentage of cells is large with a prominent nucleolus (prolymphocytes).

In most cases of B-CLL, IgM is found on the surface of cells either alone or in combination with IgD. IgG is sometimes seen on the surface of CLL cells but in most cases this is an artefact caused by cytophilic binding to Fcγ receptors. The quantity of Ig on the surface of CLL cells is usually very small and it may need extra sensitive methods to detect it. In most cases CLL cells have a receptor for mouse red blood cells and carry the CD5 antigen usually associated with T-cells. These two markers are helpful in distinguishing B-CLL from its variants.

The majority of cases of B-CLL are discovered by an incidental blood count, do not progress and require no treatment. Where progression occurs it is in many cases signalled by an increase in the number of prolymphocytes and although the presence of large numbers of prolymphocytes does not necessarily imply progression, survival is poorer in patients with greater than 15%. The cell markers of the prolymphocytes in B-CLL are usually the same as for the small lymphocytes, but in some cases the surface immunoglobulin is more dense and the FMC7 antigen is acquired.

B-Cell prolymphocytic leukaemia (B-PLL).   B-PLL occurs in the same aged population as B-CLL with a similar male preponderance. The characteristic clinical feature is splenomegaly in the absence of lymphadenopathy. The lymphocyte count is frequently greater than 100×10^9 per litre.

The prolymphocyte is larger than the characteristic CLL cells. The round nucleus has moderately condensed chromatin and a prominent central nucleolus. Cytoplasm is relatively abundant. Smudge cells are not usually seen. Cell markers characteristically show dense surface immunoglobulin, pan B-cell markers and FMC7 positivity, but mouse red blood cell receptors and the CD5 antigen are usually absent.

The disease is almost always progressive and is difficult to treat. Combination chemotherapy, splenic irradiation and leucapheresis have been recommended.

Hairy cell leukaemia (HCL).   This condition is also commoner in elderly males and is also characterized by splenomegaly without lymphadenopathy. Lymphocytosis is rare, being seen in less than 20% of cases. The majority have pancytopenia of varying degree but hairy cells are usually seen in the blood films. These are of moderate size and have an oval nucleus containing spongy cytoplasm and abundant pale blue cytoplasm with fine thread-like cytoplasmic projections. The cells are phagocytic for latex particles and show acid phosphatase activity which is resistant to treatment with tartrate. In most cases B-cell markers are found, including FMC7 positivity, but a rare T-cell type associated with the retrovirus HTLV II has been described.

Treatment is by splenectomy or with α-interferon or deoxycoformycin.

Waldenstrom's macroglobulinaemia (WM).   A peripheral lymphocytosis is seen in a minority of patients with WM. The lymphocytes may resemble those seen in B-CLL, but frequently lymphoplasmacytoid cells are also seen. IgM paraproteins may be seen in a number of other lymphoid malignancies including B-CLL and B-PLL. Distinction between these conditions may be difficult and require histological examination and marker studies.

Non-Hodgkin's lymphoma (NHL) spillover.   In low- and intermediate-grade NHL there is frequently a spillover of tumour cells into the peripheral blood, but a frank lymphocytosis is rare. The term 'lymphosarcoma cell leukaemia' was previously used for this phenomenon, but it is now archaic.

Among the lymphomas in which blood spillover occurs, two types predominate: follicular centroblastic/centrocytic (cb/cc) and diffuse centrocytic (dcc). The lymphoblastic lymphomas also spill over into the blood, but these diseases are essentially the same as the lymphoblastic leukaemias which have already been considered.

Cb/cc lymphoma is the commonest type of lymphoma in Europe and North America, and when a leukaemic phase is present there is usually widespread lymphadenopathy. Two types of cell are usually seen in the blood: the majority are small lymphocytes (centrocytes) which are larger than B-CLL cells, often with a notched or cleaved nucleus, chromatin that is less condensed than in B-CLL and a discernable nucleolus; the cytoplasm is normal. A proportion of larger cells have round nuclei with more open chromatin and one or more peripheral nucleoli and basophilic cytoplasm (centroblasts). Generally, cb/cc cells have denser surface Ig than B-CLL cells and frequently express the CD10 antigen.

Dcc lymphoma is not usually associated with widespread lymphadenopathy but involves spleen, blood and bone marrow and frequently extranodal tissues. Centrocytes predominate in the blood and centroblasts are generally not present. Dense surface immunoglobulin is the rule and the cells usually show the CD5 antigen but not the mouse red blood cell receptor.

T-Cell chronic lymphatic leukaemia (T-CLL).   The term T-cell CLL has been used to encompass a variety of conditions. Some of the early reports clearly referred to cases of B-CLL which expressed little surface immunoglobulin but formed anomalous sheep red cell rosettes. There is now common consent that T-CLL refers to a condition in which there is a proliferation of large granular lymphocytes, frequent splenomegaly and neutropenia. The characteristic cells have mature nuclei and abundant cytoplasm with azurophil granules. The lymphocytosis is moderate (5–20 × 10^9 per litre) and frequently non-progressive. In the majority of cases the cells are CD3-, CD8-, HNK-1-positive, CD5-negative and behave as cytotoxic/suppressor cells. Less commonly the cells are CD3-negative CD16-positive and behave as NK-cells. Rarely a T-helper phenotype has been found.

A number of patients give a history of rheumatoid arthritis and in these the condition needs to be distinguished from Felty's syndrome in which a polyclonal proliferation of large granular T-lymphocytes may be seen. The distinction is most easily made by looking for evidence of rearrangement of the T idiotype genes. In most patients T-CLL is a benign disease, but transformation to a high-grade T-cell lymphoma has been reported.

T-Cell prolymphocyte leukaemia (T-PLL).   In most respects T-PLL resembles T-CLL, but lymphadenopathy is rather more common and the leukaemic cells are more pleomorphic. The prognosis is poor, but responses to deoxycoformycin have been reported.

Sezary's syndrome.   Sezary's syndrome is the leukaemic variant of mycosis fungoides. Patients usually have exfoliative erythroderma with atypical lymphocytes in the peripheral blood. Often there are malignant plaques and tumours in the skin, and there may be involvement of lymph nodes, liver and spleen.

   The abnormal cells are moderate-sized lymphocytes with convoluted or cerebriform nuclei. In some patients the lymphocytes are small with scanty cytoplasm, and the nuclear convolutions may be hidden by the dark-staining chromatin. The cells are usually of T-helper phenotype.

Adult T-lymphoma/leukaemia.   This unusual syndrome is endemic in the Kyushu region of Japan and is also seen in Blacks of Caribbean origin. It is associated with infection by the HTLV I retrovirus. The disease primarily involves lymph nodes, skin and liver, and is present in blood and bone marrow in only one-third of cases. The atypical cells seen in the blood are of medium size and have a markedly irregular nuclear contour, often with multiple lobes. The cytoplasm is basophilic and may be vacuolated. Hypercalcaemia is a frequent finding in this condition and the prognosis is poor.

Miscellaneous causes of lymphocytosis

In serum sickness and other acute inflammatory conditions a lymphocytosis similar to that associated with the immune response to virus infections is often seen.

   In Addison's disease the absence of the corticosteroid suppression allows a lymphocytosis to occur as well as an eosinophilia. Lymphocytosis has been reported in thyrotoxicosis but the cause is obscure.

   Following splenectomy there is often a slight lymphocytosis with in particular increased numbers of large granular lymphocytes which have a T-suppressor phenotype.

   The pseudolymphomas associated with phenytoin are occasionally associated with a peripheral lymphocytosis.

LYMPHOCYTOPENIA

The causes of lymphocytopenia are given in Table 5.10.

Table 5.10 Causes of Lymphocytopenia

Congenital immunodeficiency syndromes (see Table 5.11)

Therapy
 Radiotherapy
 Cytotoxic drugs
 Corticosteroids
 Antilymphocyte globulin
 Thoracic duct drainage
 Lymphocytapheresis

Increased intestinal loss
 Intestinal lymphectasia
 Whipple's disease
 Severe right-sided heart failure
 Other causes of intestinal lymphatic obstruction

Miscellaneous causes
 Cushing's syndrome
 Aplastic anaemia
 Carcinomatosis
 Hodgkin's disease
 Sarcoidosis
 Systemic lupus erythematosus
 Renal failure
 Miliary tuberculosis
 AIDS

Immunodeficiency syndromes

Were we all completely immunocompetent we could walk through the sea of microorganisms that we are exposed to and never suffer an infection. As it is, the vast majority of these organisms hardly bother us and those that do are usually thrown off after a short battle and for the most part seldom bother us again. That this immunity is an active process must be obvious to any forensic pathologist who comes across a dead body left in a ditch for a week or two.

The immune sytem which allows us to live in harmony with our neighbours is complex and has many parts which can go wrong. Abnormalities in any of these parts are liable to render us susceptible to attack even by microorganisms which normally inhabit our bodies peacefully. For simplicity we usually divide the immune system into a humoral wing and a cell-mediated wing and recognize characteristic types of infection associated with a broken wing on either side. For classification purposes this is useful, but we must remember that while antibodies are made by B-cells, most require T-cell help, and that fundamental biochemical processes are common to most cells so that severe damage in one wing of the immune response may be mirrored by lesser impairment of the other. In simple terms, B-cell deficiencies lead to poor production of antibody which increases the risk of infection with bacteria such as *Haemophilus influenzae*,

Pneumococcus, Staphylococcus and *Campylobacter*; some viruses such as herpes zoster, polio and echo virus; and some protozoa such as *Giardia lamblia*. T-Cell deficiencies lead to poor cell-mediated immunity, and such patients are principally affected by fungal infections such as *Candida albicans, Aspergillus* and *Cryptococcus*; viruses such as herpes zoster and cytomegalovirus and protozoa such as *Pneumocystis carinii*. The immunodeficiency syndromes are summarized in Table 5.11. All of these diseases are excessively rare and only the least rare syndromes will be discussed. For an exhaustive description the reader is referred to *Diagnosis and Treatment of Immunodeficiency Diseases* by Asherson & Webster.[30]

Mainly B-cell defects

X-Linked agammaglobulinaemia.   Bruton's hypogammaglobulinaemia accounts for only a sixth of patients who are hypogammaglobulinaemic. As well as very low levels of serum immunoglobulin, these patients have virtually no B-cells in either blood or bone marrow. Pre-B-cells with small amounts of cytoplasmic μ chains are present in normal numbers in the bone marrow but their rate of division is reduced, suggesting that the defect is not in the structural gene for immunoglobulin but in a failure of maturation beyond the pre-B-cell stage. Ideas on why this might be include absence of a B-cell growth factor or its receptor or an inability to insert immunoglobulin into cell membranes. T-cells are normal in these patients and NK activity is intact. ADCC activity is very poor.

Common variable hypogammaglobulinaemia.   Late onset hypogammaglobulinaemia is a heterogeneous condition. A report for the World Health Organization (WHO)[31] recognized these separate causes for the hypogammaglobulinaemia: a B-cell defect is present in the largest group, a T-cell regulatory defect in the next, and a small group associated with auto-antibodies to either B-cells or T-cells or both. Four separate B-cell abnormalities have been recognized: a small group in which normal numbers of B-cells occur but only those bearing surface IgM and IgD together, and not other more mature sub-types; a larger group with very low B-cell numbers, and two different defects in the maturation of B-cells to plasma cells. T-cell immunoglobulin abnormalities may be caused either by decreased T-helper function or by increased T-cell suppression. In most patients K-cell and NK-cell activity is normal.

Thymoma-associated   hypogammaglobulinaemia.   Hypogammaglobulinaemia is part of a variable syndrome associated with thymomas. Other features include myasthenia gravis, red cell aplasia, neutropenia and thrombocytopenia. In most cases the thymoma is benign.

   In nearly every case B-cells are absent from blood and marrow and in some cases pre-B-cells are also missing. T-Cells are usually normal or increased in number. T-Cell function is usually objectively normal, but since some patients suffer from CMV infections or chronic mucocutaneous candidiasis, a subtle T-cell defect may be inferred.

Table 5.11 Immunodeficiency Syndromes

	B-cell numbers	T-cell numbers	Other abnormalities
Mainly B-cell defects			
X-linked hypogammaglobulinaemia	↓ or N	N	↓IgG ↓IgA ↓IgM
Hypogammaglobulinaemia with raised IgM	N	N	↓IgG ↓IgA ↑IgM
Selective IgA deficiency	N	N	↓IgA
Common variable hypogammaglobulinaemia			
With B-cell defect	↓ or N	N	↓IgG ↓IgA ↓IgM
With T-cell immunoregulatory defect	N	TH↓ or TS↑	↓IgG ↓IgA ↓IgM
Due to auto-antibodies	↓→	→	↓IgG ↓IgA ↓IgM
Thymoma-associated hypogammaglobulinaemia	↓→	TS↑	↓IgG ↓IgA ↓IgM
Mainly T-cell defects			
SCID			
Swiss type	↓→	→↓	↓IgG ↓IgA ↓IgM
ADA deficiency	N	N or →↓	↓IgG ↓IgA ↓IgM
Bare lymphocyte syndrome	N	→↓	DH↓ Ab responses ↓
Di George syndrome	N	→↓	
PNP deficiency	N	→↓	
Complex syndromes			
Ataxia telangiectasia	N	TH↓	↓IgA
Wiskott–Aldrich syndrome	N	N	↓IgM
Chediak–Higashi syndrome	N	N	NK↓

Mainly T-cell defects

Severe combined immunodeficiency (SCID).   SCID is a syndrome of variable aetiology presenting in the first 2 months of life and characterized by recurrent bacterial, viral and fungal infections, diarrhoea and failure to thrive due to severe loss of cell-mediated and humoral immunity. The serum immunoglobulins are low in the classical form but in Nezelof's syndrome one or more classes are normal or raised. Severe lymphocytopenia is the usual finding. T-Cells are very low and those that remain are poorly functional. The B-cell defect is less severe. Normal B-cell numbers are often found but in the absence of T-cell help the patients are rarely able to produce significant antibody.

The Swiss type of SCID represents only 10% of cases. There is an intrinsic defect of lymphoid stem cells leading to absence of both circulating B- and T-cells.

Adenosine deaminase (ADA) deficiency accounts for 50% of cases. ADA is an ubiquitous enzyme necessary in all cells to deaminate adenosine. Its absence leads to the accumulation of dATP which inhibits ribonucleotide reduction and of adenosine which inhibits the production of S-adenosylmethionine which is necessary for new DNA synthesis. T-Cells are more susceptible to these toxic effects than other tissues.

Bare lymphocyte syndrome.   Lymphocytes from affected infants lack MHC class II antigens, and most also lack class I antigens (including β_2-microglobulin). Selective deficiency of MHC class I antigen is compatible with normal health, but the full syndrome is associated with susceptibility to the kind of opportunistic infections characteristic of SCID. Most cases have arisen in North Africa, and the condition is inherited as an autosomal recessive character. Lymphocyte counts are normal but T-cell numbers are reduced in 50% of cases. PHA stimulation is normal but delayed hypersensitivity responses are absent. B-Cell numbers are variable but antibody responses to immunization are absent. Serum immunoglobulins are variable. K-Cell and NK activity are normal.

Di George syndrome.   This syndrome is acquired during foetal development, probably due to a teratogen. It is associated with abnormalities of the third and fourth branchial arches and characterized by absence of the thymus and parathyroid glands. Congenital cardiac abnormalities are common. There is selective loss of T-cell function. T-Cells are absent from the peripheral blood but B-cells are normal. Antibody responses and serum immunoglobulin levels are also normal. Patients have normal pre-T-cells in the bone marrow which mature *in vitro* on exposure to thymic hormones. The more severely affected infants often die of the associated cardiac abnormality. Otherwise they present with tetany and convulsions due to hypocalcaemia, and suffer from viral and fungal infections.

Purine nucleoside phosphorylase (PNP) deficiency.   Absence of PNP leads to raised plasma and urine levels of its substrates: inosine, deoxyinosine, guanosine and deoxyguanosine. The metabolite dGTP inhibits nucleotide reductase and is particularly toxic to T-cells so that the disease mimics thymic dysplasia. T-Cell numbers are reduced but B-cell numbers normal. After immunization the antibody is normal. About 25% of patients also have severe neurological disease with spasticity and poor muscular power.

Ataxia telangiectasia. This complex, inherited, autosomal recessive disorder presents in the second year of life when the child begins to walk. Progressive cerebellar ataxia is associated with telangiectasiae most notice-able in the conjunctivae from about the third year. The children have severe bronchopulmonary infections which lead to progressive bronchiectasis. The majority of patients have selective IgA deficiency, but a small proportion have panhypogammaglobulinaemia. T-Cell defects are present in roughly half, manifest as absent delayed hypersensitivity reactions and poor *in vitro* lymphocyte transformation to mitogens. T-Helper lymphocytes are reduced in number.

The underlying abnormality in ataxia telangiectasia seems to be a defect in DNA repair and this may explain the high incidence of lymphoid malignancies in this condition.

Wiskott–Aldrich syndrome. The triad of thrombocytopenia, eczema and immune deficiency describes this X-linked recessive condition. The main clinical problem is bleeding. Platelets are small, lack α granules and have a shortened half-life. The eczema has an allergic basis and is associated with raised IgE levels. Hypercatabolism of IgG, IgM and IgA occurs but the major immune defect is a poor antibody response to polysaccharide antigens with consequent low IgM levels. This is possibly related to the absence of Fc receptors on monocytes. A defect in delayed hypersensitivity reactions is associated with progressive loss of T-cell function as the patients grow older. All of these defects appear to be the result of an abnormality of membrane glycoproteins on T-cells, platelets and macrophages.

Even if they survive the problems of bleeding or infection patients frequently die in late childhood or adolescence from B-cell lymphomas. Early bone marrow transplantation is the treatment of choice.

Chediak–Higashi syndrome. This syndrome is a rare autosomal reces-sive disease in which partial occulocutaneous albinism, photophobia and nystagmus are associated with frequent pyogenic infections. The most striking laboratory abnormality is the presence of very large cytoplasmic granules which not only occur in lymphocytes, monocytes, granulocytes, neurones and melanocytes, but also in cells of renal tubules, gastric mucosa and pancreas. The underlying defect appears to be related to the control of microtubule assembly. The major cause of infections is the defect in granulocyte function, but there is an important NK-cell abnormality. These are unable to kill target cells, and this may account for the high incidence of chronic viral infections and lymphomas in this condition.

Therapeutic lymphocytopenia

Radiotherapy

Both the recirculating small lymphocytes and the organized lymphoid tissue are very radiosensitive. D_{37}-Values, the dose required to reduce the surviving population to 37% are around 0.7 Gy for lymphocytes compared to 1 Gy for other mammalian cells. B-Cells are more sensitive than T-cells. In contrast to most cells, lymphocytes are killed by ioinizing radiation without entering the mitotic cycle. Local radiotherapy can induce prolonged lymphocytopenia, with decreased numbers of both B- and T-cells. In addition, several functional tests are impaired, including mixed lymphocyte culture responses, ADCC and NK activity. In some cases there is a marked increase in suppressor activity and an increase in circulating null cells.[32]

Total nodal irradiation (TNI) is the treatment of choice of some types of lymphoma and a useful immunosuppressive regimen in autoimmune disease. The effect on the lymphocyte count is determined by the dose of irradiation used. Following TNI for Hodgkin's disease (44 Gy fractionated over 6 weeks) the total blood lymphocyte count falls to less than 0.5×10^9 per litre. Lymphocytes begin recovering shortly after completion of therapy but only reach pretreatment levels 2 years later. Even then, the level of T-cells is only half pretreatment values at 2 years and does not return to normal for 10 years. B-Cell numbers, on the other hand, begin to rise after 2 weeks and therafter overshoot pretreatment levels. B-Cell lymphocytosis remains until T-cell numbers are restored.[33]

In the treatment of intractable rheumatoid arthritis, doses of TNI of 20 Gy fractionated over 6 weeks are given. In a series of 11 patients so treated,[33] the mean lymphocyte count dropped precipitously to a nadir of 0.25×10^9 per litre. By 6 months a recovery to 0.6×10^9 per litre had occurred, but there was no further recovery up to 18 months. Studies of lymphocyte sub-sets suggested that although all types of lymphocytes were suppressed by TNI, recovery was reasonably rapid for all bar the CD4-positive sub-set. Even after 18 months CD4-positive cells were at 25% of pretreatment levels. Functional studies confirmed that the helper function of peripheral blood lymphocytes was suppressed, and the suppressor function enhanced. Experiments in animal models[33] suggest that in addition to enhanced T-suppressor activity there is an increase in non-specific suppression associated with the appearance of a bone-marrow-derived cell with null cell characteristics but without NK function.

Corticosteroids

Virtually all nucleated cells have a receptor for corticosteroids within their cytosol. The lipid soluble hormone passes freely through the cell membrane to gain access to the receptor, where it induces an allosteric change. The steroid–receptor complex moves to the nucleus where the net result is the synthesis of new mRNA which causes increased synthesis of certain proteins. Among these are an endonuclease in lymphocytes which causes DNA fragmentation, and an inhibitor of phosopholipase activity which interferes with the production of prostaglandins.[34]

Although mouse lymphocytes are lysed by corticosteroids, it is difficult to demonstrate that this occurs in man. The major steroid effect on lymphocytes appears to be its effect on cell traffic. After a bolus of corticosteroids the blood lymphocyte count falls rapidly, reaching a nadir approximately 4 h later. By 24 h the count returns to normal. The cause of this is the temporary redistribution of long-lived T-cells out of the blood and into the tissues, particularly the bone marrow. As steroid levels fall the reverse occurs. It is interesting to note that an opposite effect occurs on leukaemic B-cells in B-CLL when corticosteroids are administered.

The major 'immunosuppressive' effect of corticosteroids is really an anti-inflammatory one, involving the down-regulation of macrophage function. The diurnal variation of lymphocyte count, the lymphocytopenia of Cushing's syndrome and the 'stress' lymphocytopenia seen in burns patients are all related to changes in lymphocyte traffic.

Cytotoxic drugs

When given in large enough doses most cytotoxic drugs cause lymphocytopenia. With most, however, their myelosuppressive effect is more important than their immunosuppressive action, and these are seldom used as immunosuppressive agents.

Cyclophosphamide is one of the most widely used immunosuppressive agents and one of the most studied. Not widely appreciated in clinical circles is the degree of selectivity of cyclophosphamide for lymphocyte sub-sets. Single doeses of 100 mg/m^2 are capable of temporarily decreasing numbers of circulating B-cells; doses of 200 mg/m^2 significantly reduce CD8-positive T-cell numbers; but CD4-positive T-cells are not reduced until doses of 600 mg/m^2 are given.[35] The potential for enhancing immunity with low doses of cyclophosphamide has not been exploited clinically.

Continuous daily cyclophosphamide (100 mg/day) not only reduces T- and B-cell numbers but suppresses primary antibody and delayed hypersensitivity responses as well as K-cell and NK function.[36]

Azathioprine, the other commonly used immunosuppressive drug has been reported to have different effects on lymphocyte sub-sets in different conditions. When given to prevent renal transplant rejection it was preferentially toxic to CD4-positive cells, but in chronic active hepatitis and multiple sclerosis it was more toxic to CD8-positive cells.[37]

Interleukin-2 is currently undergoing trials as an anti-cancer agent. When high dose IL-2 is administered a profound lymphopenia ($<0.5 \times 10^9$ per litre) results. Two days after completing the infusion there is a rebound with overshoot, and a lymphocytosis of 20×10^9 per litre is common. The rebounding cells are of several phenotypes and include CD8-positive and CD16-positive cells.[38]

Anti-lymphocyte globulins

Polyclonal anti-lymphocyte globulins raised in horses, rabbits or goats still retain a role in the management of aplastic anaemia and transplant rejection despite the risk of serum sickness. Given by intravenous infusion on 5 successive days they cause profound lymphocytopenia (together with anaemia, thrombocytopenia and neutropenia as these cells are caught up as innocent bystanders). The main effect is on long-lived recirculating T-cells which are either lysed intravascularly or removed by the liver. Marked suppression of cell-mediated immunity is achieved.

More recently murine monoclonal anti-CD3 antibodies have been used to prevent transplant rejection. There is an initial lymphopenia which is reversed within 12 h. However, CD3-positive cells do not return until 24–48 h after the end of the infusion. The circulating cells carry other T-cell markers, and the reason for the discrepancy is antigenic modulation of the CD3 molecule. Since these monoclonal antibodies are effective immuno-suppressive agents it is clear that removal of the CD3 molecules renders the T-cells non-functional.[39]

Thoracic duct drainage and lymphocytapheresis

Thoracic duct drainage is an unnecessarily invasive and outmoded treatment for rheumatoid arthritis. Daily drainage of 5×10^{10} lymphocytes from the recirculating pool induced an improvement of rheumatoid synovitis that lasted for 3 months.[40] Lymphocytapheresis typically removes one-tenth as many lymphocytes per day. Nevertheless a study in rheumatoid arthritis demonstrated a fall in mean lymphocyte count from 2.9×10^9 to 0.67×10^9 per litre after nine treatments over 3 weeks. There was a proportional fall of all lymphocyte sub-sets.[41]

Increased intestinal loss

Dilatation of the lacteals within the villi of the small intestine may be a primary condition (lymphangectasia) in which there is congenital hypoplasia of the lymphatic vessels, or secondary to back pressure from right-sided heart failure caused by tricuspid incompetence, constrictive pericarditis or cardiomyopathy, or due to obstruction of the lymphatic vessels by infiltration, tumour or fibrosis. Whipple's disease is caused by a rod-shaped bacterium which leads to the deposition of PAS-positive material within the macrophages of the lamina propria of the small intestine leading to obstruction of the lymphatic drainage. Whatever the cause of the lymphatic obstruction, diarrhoea and steatorrhoea, caused by failure to transport lipid, are likely to occur together with loss of protein and lymphocytes into the gut lumen. Chylous ascites may also be present. Variable degrees of lympho-cytopenia occur.

Miscellaneous causes

Aplastic anaemia

Lymphocyte production is not considered to be impaired in aplastic anaemia. Nevertheless, levels of peripheral blood lymphocytes below 1.5 × 10^9 per litre are frequently found. The significance of this finding is not known since both delayed hypersensitivity reactions and immunoglobulin production are normal.

Carcinomatosis

In disseminated cancer lymphocytopenia is regularly seen. The reason for this is not clear but may be related to attraction of lymphocytes to the tumour or the production of factors by the tumour that affect lymphocyte traffic.

Hodgkin's disease

A defect in cell-mediated immunity is classically associated with Hodgkin's disease. Lymphocytopenia is particularly associated with older age, advanced stage and 'B' symptoms and as a poor prognostic factor independent of other variables. The major feature of the lymphocytopenia is a reduction in CD4-positive T-cells; the numbers of B-cells and CD8-positive T-cells are roughly normal unless the lymphocytopenia is very severe. Activated T-cells, recognized by MHC class II positivity, sometimes circulate. The cause of the fall in CD4-positive cells seems to be a redirection of lymphocyte traffic. Increased numbers of CD4-positive cells are seen in the spleen and unaffected lymph nodes but particularly in affected lymph nodes. The fall in T-helper cells in the blood does not fully explain the immune suppression seen in Hodgkin's disease. It is probable that suppressor factors derived from monocytes as well as T-cells play an active part. The overall picture is complicated by the effect of treatment and splenectomy.

Sarcoidosis

In active sarcoidosis there are impaired delayed hypersensitivity reactions to recall antigens and an inability to be sensitized to dinitrochlorbenzene. Circulating lymphocyte counts are low and both T- and B-cells are reduced. The remaining peripheral blood lymphocytes have increased suppressor activity. Cells obtained from the lung by bronchopulmonary lavage are rich in T-helper cells and it is presumed that the peripheral lymphocytopenia is mainly caused by sequestration of T-cells to the sites of active granulomas.

Systemic lupus erythematosus (SLE)

Patients with SLE are susceptible to viral and fungal pathogens even before treatment with immmunosuppressive drugs. Lymphocytopenia is common and is usually associated with the presence of anti-lymphocytotoxic antibodies. These antibodies are cytotoxic for T-suppressor cells which is the sub-class predominantly reduced in the circulation. Although the sequence lymphocyte antibody–reduced T-suppressor cells–uncontrolled B-cell proliferation, sounds too simplistic there appears no good reason to doubt that it plays a part in the pathogenesis of the disease.

Renal failure

There is suppression of delayed hypersensitivity in renal failure and prolonged allograft survival. The lymphocyte count is usually low and those present respond poorly in mixed lymphocyte cultures. Lymphocyte survival *in vivo* is shortened. Sub-set analysis may be confused by the cause of the renal failure, but in general it is the T-helper cells that are reduced. The cause is presumed to be a toxic factor removable by dialysis.

CHANGES IN LYMPHOCYTE SUB-SETS

Even when lymphocyte numbers are normal, variation in lymphocyte sub-sets has been observed in a number of diseases, and some have sought to gain insight into these diseases by looking at these variations. In particular the ratio of T-helper cells to T-suppressor cells in the blood has gained a certain notoriety.

The study of lymphocyte sub-types is deceptively difficult for the following reasons.

1. The marker chosen does not necessarily represent a functional sub-set. Early attempts to recognize T-cells and their sub-types relied on rosetting techniques; sheep red cell rosettes for T-cells, Fcγ rosettes for T-suppressor cells and Fcμ rosettes for T-helper cells. At a later stage, dot positivity with acid phosphatase, a non-specific esterase staining, was equated with the T-helper population, and more granular staining with the T-suppressor population. Nowadays, it is usual to separate helpers and suppressors with monoclonal antibodies of the CD4 (helper) and CD8 (suppressor) specificities. It is clear, however, using the various antibodies of the CD45R specificities that some T-helpers help B-cells and some help T-suppressors. Currently, no marker system correlates completely with functional studies.

2. *In vitro* functional studies may not reflect the *in vivo* situation. The demand for accessory cells in these assays is a source of error.

3. What is happening in the blood may reflect poorly what is happening in the tissues. An excess of a particular sub-type may reflect a whole body excess or a redirecting of the opposite sub-type from the blood to the site of infection or tumour.

4. Variation of lymphocyte sub-sets is time-dependent. Levels will rise and fall at different phases of an immune response so that single measurements are unlikely to be useful.

5. Measurements are frequently complicated by the effect of treatment.

Quite apart from the methodological hazards of measuring T and B sub-populations, there are very few clinical reasons for wanting to know the result. Apart from their value as a prognostic indicator in AIDS, and in separating different types of leukaemia, we know of no clinical situation where their determination affects clinical management. Claims have been made for their usefulness in detecting clinical relapse in multiple sclerosis, and it is certainly true that a fall in peripheral blood T-suppressor cells (however measured) together with a rise of CSF T-helper cells correlates well with relapse, but in practice the interval between change in lymphocyte sub-populations and the clinical evidence of relapse is so short that no real value attaches to the measurement.[42]

Table 5.12 gives a list of diseases in which changes in lymphocyte sub-populations occur.

Table 5.12 The Variation of Lymphocyte Sub-types in Disease

T-cells ↓
  AIDS
  Myelodyspasia
  Alcoholic cirrhosis
  Chronic active hepatitis
  Primary biliary cirrhosis
  Crohn's disease
  Ankylosing spondylitis
  Anterior uveitis
  Myasthenia gravis
  Multiple sclerosis
  Diabetes mellitus
  Autoimmune thyroid disease

B-cells ↑
  Post-splenectomy
  Chronic active hepatitis
  IgA nephropathy

Null cells ↑
  Post-splenectomy
  Rheumatoid arthritis
  Chronic active hepatitis
  Primary biliary cirrhosis

CD4-Cells ↓
  AIDS
  Hepatitis B
  Cutaneous leishmaniasis
  Myelodysplasia
  Aplastic anaemia
  Sepsis in the elderly
  Zinc deficiency
  Progressive systemic sclerosis

CD4-Cells ↑
  Angioimmunoblastic lymphadeno-
    pathy
  Immune thyroid disease
  Glomerulonephritis
  Diabetes mellitus

CD8-Cells ↓
  Multiple sclerosis
  SLE
  Juvenile rheumatoid arthritis
  Myasthenia gravis
  Diabetes mellitus
  Immune thyroid disease
  Chronic active hepatitis
  Proliferative polycythaemia

CD8-Cells ↑
  Post-splenectomy
  Hodgkin's disease in remission
  Minimal change glomerulonephritis
  Aplastic anaemia

SUMMARY

In the past 30 years the science of immunology has elbowed its way to the front of the haematologist's attention. The boring small lymphocytes have proved to be more than an uninteresting peasantry that populates the landscape. They are part of an infiltrating army complete with generals and foot soldiers. The haematologist must ask himself not only, 'Why is it there is such strength?' but when it is not there, 'Where has it gone to and why?' He must also be prepared to unmask the badges of rank on those individuals he captures, but he must still expect to be perplexed when he discovers a regiment consisting entirely of captains passing through.

ACKNOWLEDGEMENT

Our grateful thanks to Mrs K. Avery for typing this manuscript.

REFERENCES

1. Boyd, W.C. *Fundamentals of Immunology*, 3rd Edn. Interscience, New York, 1956.
2. Gowans, J.L. The effect of the continuous reinfusion of lymph and lymphocytes on the output of lymphocytes from the thoracic duct of unanaesthetized rats. *Br. J. Exp. Pathol.* **38**: 67–81, 1957.
3. Zola, H. The surface antigens of human B cell lymphocytes. *Immunol. Today* **8**: 308–15, 1987.
4. Barth, R.K., Kim, B.S., Lan, N.C., *et al.*. The immune T-cell receptor uses a limited repertoire of expressed Vβ gene segments. *Nature* **316**: 517–23, 1985.
5. Incefy, G.S. The role of thymic hormones on human lymphocytes. *Clin. Immunol. Allergy* **3**: 95–117, 1983.
6. Mossman, T.R. & Coffman, R.L. Two types of mouse helper T cell clone. *Immunol. Today* **8**: 223–7, 1987.
7. Goldschneider, I. Heterogeneity of bone marrow 'lymphocytes'. *Clin. Haemàtol.* **11**: 491–508, 1982.
8. Yoffey, J.M. *Bone Marrow Reactions.* Williams & Wilkins, Baltimore, 1966.
9. Bell, A.J., Hamblin, T.J. & Oscier, D.G. Peripheral blood stem cell autografting. *Haematol. Oncol.* **5**: 1–11, 1987.
10. Hersey, P. & Bolhuis, R. Nonspecific MHC-unrestricted killer cells and their receptors. *Immunol. Today* **8**: 233–46, 1987.
11. Kaplan, J. NK cell lineage and target cell specificity: a unifying concept. *Immunol. Today* **7**: 10–13, 1986.
12. Lanier, L.L. & Phillips, J.J. Evidence for three types of human cytotoxic lymphocytes. *Immunol. Today* **7**: 132–4, 1986.
13. Grimm, E.A., Ramsey, K.M., Mazumder, A., Wilson, D.J., Djeu, Y.T. & Rosenberg, S.A. Lymphokine-activated killer cell phenomenon. II. Precursor phenotype is serologically distinct from peripheral T lymphocytes, memory cytotoxic thymus-derived lymphocytes, and natural killer cells. *J. Exp. Med.* **157**: 884–97, 1983.
14. Dearman, R.J., Stevenson, F.K., Wrightman, M., Hamblin, T.J., Glennie, M.J. & Stevenson, G.T. Lymphokine activated killer cells from normal and lymphoma subjects are cytotoxic for cells coated with antibody derivatives displaying human Fcγ. *Blood* **72**: 1985–91, 1988.
15. Tschopp, J., Masson, D. & Stanley, K.K. Structural/functional similarity between

proteins involved in complement and cytotoxic T lymphocyte-mediated cytolysis. *Nature* **322**: 831–4, 1986.

16. Dittmer, D.S. Blood and other body fluids. *Fedn. Am. Soc. Exp. Biol.*, 125, 1961.
17. Bender, B.S., Nagel, J.E., Adler, W.H. & Andres, K. Absolute peripheral blood lymphocyte count and subsequent mortality of elderly men. *J. Am. Gerentol. Soc.* **34**: 649–54, 1986.
18. Purtilo, D.T. Pathogenesis and phenotypes of an X-linked recessive lympho-proliferative syndrome. *Lancet* **ii**: 882–3, 1976.
19. Britten, V. & Hughes, H.P.A. American trypanosomiasis, toxoplasmosis and leishmaniasis: intracellular infections with different immunological con-sequences. *Clin. Immunol. Allergy* **6**: 189–226, 1986.
20. McChesney, M.B. & Oldtone, M.B.A. Viruses perturb lymphocyte functions: selected principles characterising virus-induced immunosuppression. *Ann. Rev. Immunol.* **5**: 279–304, 1987.
21. Smith, C.H. Infectious lymphocytosis. *Am. J. Dis. Childh.* **62**: 231–61, 1941.
22. Nkrumah, F.K. & Addy, P.A.K. Acute infectious lymphocytosis. *Lancet* **i**: 1257–8, 1973.
23. Adler, A. & Morse, S.I. Interaction of lymphoid and nonlymphoid cells with lymphocytosis-promoting factor of *Bordetella pertussis*. *Infect. Immunol.* **7**: 461–7, 1973.
24. Ochiai, T., Okumura, K. & Tada, T. Effect of lymphocytosis-promoting-factor of *Bordetella pertussis* on the immune response. I. Suppression of cellular hypersensitivity reactions. *Int. Arch. Allergy Appl. Immunol.* **43**: 196–206, 1972.
25. Bennett, J.M., Catovsky, D., Daniel, M.-T. *et al.*. Proposals for the classification of the acute leukaemias. *Br. J. Haematol.* **33**: 451–8, 1976.
26. Hamblin, T.J. Chronic lymphocytic leukaemia. *Balliere's Clin. Haematol.* **1**: 449–91, 1987.
27. Catovsky, D. Chronic lymphocytic leukaemia, prolymphocytic and hairy cell leukaemias. In *Haematology*, Vol. 1, *Leukaemias* (eds J.M. Goldman & H.D. Preisler), pp. 266–98. Butterworths, London, 1986.
28. Sweet, D.L. Jr, Golomb, H.M. & Ultman, J.E. The clinical features of chronic lymphocytic leukaemia. *Clin. Haematol.* **6**: 185–202, 1977.
29. Rai, K.R., Sawitsky, A., Cronkite, E.P. *et al.* Clinical staging of chronic lymphocytic leukaemia. *Blood* **46**: 219–34, 1975.
30. Asherson, G.L. & Webster, A.D.B. *Diagnosis and Treatment of Immunodeficiency Diseases*. Blackwell, Oxford, 1980.
31. Rosen, F.S., Cooper, M.D & Wedgewood, R.J.P. The primary immuno-deficiencies (two parts). Medical Progress. *N. Engl. J. Med.* **311**: 235–42 and 300–10, 1984.
32. Eltringham, J.E. Effects of regional irradiation on immune responses. *Clin. Immunol. Allergy* **4**: 359–76, 1984.
33. Kotzin, B. & Strober, S. Total lymphoid irradiation. *Clin. Immunol. Allergy* **4**: 331–58, 1984.
34. Claman, H.N. Anti-inflammatory effects of corticosteroids. *Clin. Immunol. Allergy* **4**: 317–29, 1984.
35. Bast, R.C. Jr, Reinherz, E.L., Maver, C. *et al.* Contrasting effects of cyclophosphamide and prednisolone on the phenotype of human peripheral blood leukocytes. *Clin. Immunol. Immunopathol.* **28**: 101–14, 1983.
36. Tenberg, R.J.M., Van Walbeek, H.K. & Schellekens, P.T.A. Evaluation of the immunosuppressive effects of cyclophosphamide in patients with multiple sclerosis. *Clin. Exp. Immunol.* **50**: 495–502, 1982.
37. Spina, C.A. Azathioprine as an immune modulating drug: clinical applications. *Clin. Immunol. Allergy* **4**: 415–46, 1984.
38. Rosenberg, S.A. Immunotherapy of cancer using interleukin-2: current status and future prospects. *Immunol. Today* **9**: 58–62, 1988.

39. Chatenoud, L., Baudrihaye, M.F., Chkoff, N. *et al.* Immunologic followup of renal allograft recipients treated prophylactically by OKT3 alone. *Transplantation Proceedings* **15**: 643, 1983.
40. Panlus, H.E., Machleder, H.I., Levine, S., Yu, D.T.Y., MacDonald, N.S. Lymphocyte involvement in rheumatoid arthritis, studies during thoracic duct drainage. *Arthr. Rheum.* **20**: 1249–62, 1977.
41. Wallace, D.J., Goldfinger, D., Galli, R. *et al.* Plasmapheresis and lymphoplasmapheresis in the management of rheumatoid arthritis. *Arthr. Rheum.* **22**: 703–19, 1979.
42. Arnasen, B.G.W. Abnormalities of immunoregulating cells in demyelinating diseases. *Clin. Immunol. Allergy* **2**: 263–78, 1982.

6

Platelet abnormalities

H. Cohen
Clinical Lecturer in Haematology, University College and Middlesex School of Medicine, London, UK

S.J. Machin
Consultant Haematologist, University College and Middlesex School of Medicine, London, UK

INTRODUCTION

The normal haemostatic mechanism depends on several overlapping and sequential events including the vessel wall response to injury, platelet adhesion and aggregation, activation of the coagulation cascade leading to the formation of fibrin, which interdigitates with and reinforces the platelet plug, and finally activation of the fibrinolytic system to complete the repair process.[1] Platelets play a pivotal role in this mechanism and quantitative or qualitative pathological platelet defects have profound clinical effects leading to haemorrhagic and/or thrombotic episodes. Platelet abnormalities, both quantitative and/or qualitative, have been reported in a large number of acquired disorders of diverse aetiologies which are described in this chapter. An understanding of the physiology of platelet structure and activation enables the development of a structured approach to the investigation of platelet defects[2] and treatment of the various resultant disorders.

PHYSIOLOGY OF NORMAL PLATELET ACTIVATION

Platelets circulate as enucleate discs and structurally consist of a trilaminar phospholipoprotein membrane with sub-membrane circumferential contractile filaments, three types of secretory granules, an irregular internalized network from the outer membrane of canaliculi, whereby the granule contents can be released onto the platelet surface following activation, and the dense tubular system of smooth endoplasmic reticulum which has a high concentration of calcium ions.[3]

The granule types are: (1) dense granules which release ADP, ATP, serotonin and calcium ions; (2) α granules which release constituents including platelet-derived growth factor, platelet factor 4 which has heparin neutralizing activity, β-thromboglobulin, von Willebrand factor (vWF), Factor V, fibrinogen, fibronectin and thrombospondin; and (3) lysosomal granules which contain acid hydrolases.

The interactions with circulating platelets which follow vessel wall damage are summarized in Fig. 6.1. When the vessel wall is damaged, sub-endothelial structures including basement membrane collagen and micro-fibrils are exposed. Circulating platelets react with exposed collagen fibres and their adherence to the damaged surface is mediated by high molecular weight multimers of von Willebrand factor and probably fibronectin.[4] Von Willebrand factor is synthesized and stored in the Weibel Palade bodies of the vascular endothelial cells and in megakaryocytes (being stored in the α granules of platelets). When released into the circulation, von Willebrand factor forms an array of multimeric forms with molecular weights ranging up to 20 million Da.[5] Von Willebrand factor, particularly the higher molecular weight forms, interacts with two specific receptors on the platelet membrane, the glycoprotein Ib and glycoprotein IIb-IIIa complex, and also with insoluble components of the sub-endothelium at the site of vessel damage.[6] This enables a single layer of platelets to adhere to the damaged areas of the vessel wall.

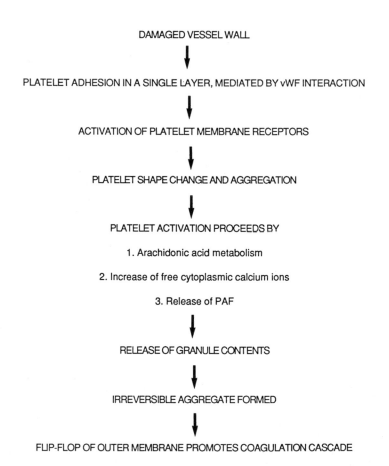

DAMAGED VESSEL WALL

PLATELET ADHESION IN A SINGLE LAYER, MEDIATED BY vWF INTERACTION

ACTIVATION OF PLATELET MEMBRANE RECEPTORS

PLATELET SHAPE CHANGE AND AGGREGATION

PLATELET ACTIVATION PROCEEDS BY

1. Arachidonic acid metabolism

2. Increase of free cytoplasmic calcium ions

3. Release of PAF

RELEASE OF GRANULE CONTENTS

IRREVERSIBLE AGGREGATE FORMED

FLIP-FLOP OF OUTER MEMBRANE PROMOTES COAGULATION CASCADE

Fig. 6.1. Platelet activation following vessel wall damage.

Following platelet adhesion, additional circulating platelets are activated. They immediately change shape, losing their discoid form and become tiny spheres with numerous projecting pseudopods. These activated platelets aggregate together and a primary platelet plug forms on the vessel wall. Certain physiological agonists react with specific platelet membrane surface receptors and initiate platelet aggregation and further activation.[7] These include exposed sub-endothelial collagen fibres, adenosine-5'-diphosphate (ADP) released from locally damaged and lysed red cells[8] and other activated platelets, adrenaline, serotonin, thrombin generated from the activated coagulation cascade and released platelet arachidonic acid metabolites, predominantly thromboxane A_2 (TXA$_2$) and prostaglandin H_2.

The mechanisms of platelet activation and aggregation proceed under the control of a balance of diverse physiological signals which may be either positive or negative.[9] The positive activating agonists listed above act as extracellular signals after binding to specific surface receptors. These signals pass information through the platelet membrane by means of so-called G-proteins which are guanine nucleotide-binding proteins. These activate amplifier enzymes on the inner surface of the platelet membrane, the most important of which is phospholipase C. Activated phospholipase C converts phosphatidylinositol biphosphate (PIP$_2$) into two separate but interrelated intracellular secondary messengers. Phosphatidylinositol biphosphate is thus converted into 1,2-diacylglycerol (DG) and inositol triphosphate (IP$_3$). 1,2-Diacylglycerol brings about the activation of protein kinase C which is responsible for the phosphorylation of the cytosolic protein P47, which helps to mediate the secondary response of the platelet granules. 1,2-Diacylglycerol also brings about the release of free arachidonic acid from the membrane-bound phospholipids by the action of diacylglycerol lipase. The other secondary messenger, inositol triphosphate, mobilizes free calcium ions from their storage site in the intracellular organelles, which is mainly the smooth endoplasmic reticulum or dense tubular system in the platelet. An increase of free cytosolic ionized calcium can also occur directly by influx of calcium ions across the platelet membrane from the extracellular medium. Free ionic calcium ions activate phospholipase A_2 which cleaves arachidonic acid from the carbon-2 position of the membrane phospholipids. Mobilized free calcium will also complex with the coenzyme calmodulin and bring about the platelet contractile response of the smooth muscle fibres after phosphorylation of the myosin chain which is known as P20. This activation signal transduction system in the platelet is shown diagrammatically in Fig. 6.2.

Approximately 50% of free arachidonic acid is converted by a lipoxygenase enzyme to a series of products including various leukotrienes which probably play a very small role in the control of haemostasis, being more important as chemoattractants of white cells. The remaining arachidonic acid is converted by the enzyme cyclo-oxygenase into the cyclic endoperoxides, prostaglandin G_2 (PGG$_2$) and prostaglandin H_2 (PGH$_2$), which are very labile.[10] Most of the endoperoxides are then rapidly converted by the thromboxane synthetase enzyme complex into TXA$_2$. TXA$_2$ has profound biological activity mediated by PGG$_2$/TXA$_2$ receptors causing platelet granule release, local vasoconstriction and also stimulating other platelets to aggregate locally. Release of the α and dense granule contents in relatively

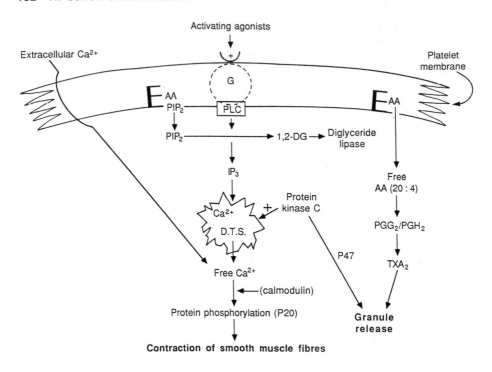

Fig. 6.2. Activation signal transduction system in the platelet. G: G-proteins; PLC: phospholipase C; AA: arachidonic acid; PIP$_2$: phosphatidylinositol biphosphate; 1,2-DG: 1,2-diacylglycerol; IP$_3$: inositol phosphate; DTS: dense tubular system; PGG$_2$, PGH$_2$: prostaglandins G$_2$ and H$_2$ respectively; TXA$_2$: thromboxane A$_2$.

high concentrations at the site of platelet aggregate formation further promotes the stabilization of the primary haemostatic plug. Adenine nucleotides, serotonin and calcium ions activate other platelets locally, von Willebrand factor stimulates platelet adhesion, fibrinogen and Factor V stimulate thrombin formation and platelet factor 4 and β-thromboglobulin bind to the vascular endothelial cell surface and inhibit heparin-like activity and prostacyclin release respectively.[11] TXA$_2$ is a very labile product with a half-life *in vivo* of approximately 45 s before being degraded to the inactive compounds thromboxane B$_2$ (TXB$_2$) and malondialdehyde. A small proportion of the cyclic endoperoxides are converted to the primary prostaglandins PGE$_2$, PGD$_2$ and PGF$_2$.

Another pathway of platelet activation involves the release of a lysolecithin compound called PAF (platelet activating factor) from the platelet membrane phospholipid which seems to be able to activate platelets independently of TXA$_2$ generation and calcium release.[12] The actual importance of PAF activation of human platelets has not been fully determined.

The aggregating platelets align together into initially a rather loose reversible aggregate but, following the release reaction of the platelet granule constituents, a larger interdigitating irreversible plug is formed. Changes in the platelet membrane configuration now occur which involves a 'flip-flop' rearrangement of the membrane surface so that the coagulant active negatively charged phospholipids; phosphatidylserine and phosphatidylinositol, which are concentrated in the resting platelet on the inner half of the phospholipid layer, become exposed on the outer surface of the activated platelet.[13]

INHIBITORY MECHANISMS OF PLATELET ACTIVATION

To prevent uncontrolled and inappropriate thrombus formation in the intact and undamaged vasculature, a large number of biological mechanisms exist.[11] The vascular endothelial cell is constantly being challenged and normally maintains an anticoagulant thrombo-resistant surface.[14] Platelets do not adhere to the intact vessel wall.

Endothelial cells synthesize prostacyclin from free arachidonic acid by the sequential action of cyclo-oxygenase and prostacyclin synthetase enzymes.[15] When released into the circulation, prostacyclin causes local vasodilation and is the most potent known inhibitor of platelet adhesion and aggregation. Prostacyclin probably does not circulate in biological quantities, but is released locally when the vessel wall is stressed or injured, thus controlling any excessive platelet activation. Prostacyclin is the most important negative or inhibitory extracellular signal to prevent excessive or inappropriate platelet activation. It binds to a specific platelet surface receptor which is linked to G-proteins that transmit inhibitory signals through the platelet membrane. This leads to stimulation of adenylate cyclase activity on the inner aspect of the platelet membrane which converts ATP (adenosine-5'-triphosphate) to cyclic-AMP (adenosine-3'5'-cyclic monophosphate). Increased levels of cyclic-AMP reverse or suppress any increase in cytosolic free calcium ions and decrease the formation of free arachidonic acid. This is controlled by cyclic-AMP decreasing the overall activity of phospholipase C. The platelet inhibitory actions of cyclic-AMP are ended when it is broken down to AMP by the action of the enzyme phosphodiesterase. Other physiological inhibitors of excessive platelet activation which also work by increasing cyclic-AMP activity include prostaglandin G_2, adenosine and adrenaline mediated via β-adrenoceptors on the platelet membrane surface.

INVESTIGATION OF A SUSPECTED PLATELET DISORDER

The causes of haemostatic failure are numerous and whenever a platelet defect is suspected, other abnormalities of the coagulation mechanism should always be excluded.[16] Excessive bleeding due to a deficiency in the circulating platelet mass or abnormal platelet function can usually be controlled by prolonged local pressure. Generally platelet bleeding starts immediately after the initiating event but once controlled it does not recur. Platelet disorders may be broadly classified into two main categories –

quantitative and qualitative. Platelet numbers may be reduced (thrombo-cytopenia) or increased (thrombocytosis). Platelet function defects have conventionally been regarded to imply impaired function predisposing to haemorrhage. This concept of platelet function defects should, however, be broadened to include enhanced platelet function which may play a role in the pathogenesis of thrombosis. In certain situations several platelet defects may coexist, for example, the thrombocytosis of myeloproliferative disorders may be associated with platelet dysfunction predisposing to both haemor-rhagic and thrombotic manifestations.

PLATELET DEFECTS IN SYSTEMIC DISORDERS

Thrombocytopenia

The peripheral platelet count and the bleeding time are the first-line basic laboratory tests of platelet involvement in the haemostatic process. If the results of these two tests are within normal limits, it is almost certain that a platelet defect is not responsible for excessive clinical bleeding. The normal range for the peripheral platelet count is $150–400 \times 10^9$ per litre. However, all very low values, below approximately 20×10^9 per litre should be checked manually and verified by inspection of a freshly stained blood film. Spurious thrombocytopenia may occur due to the presence of platelet agglutinins which may be EDTA-dependent. Although a platelet count of 150×10^9 per litre is the lower limit of the normal range, spontaneous bleeding due to thrombocytopenia alone is unlikely to occur until the count is below 50×10^9 per litre, and usually does not occur until it has fallen below 20×10^9 per litre. However, in the presence of a localized or generalized infection, serious platelet bleeding can occur when the count is at a higher level. Spontaneous platelet bleeding usually occurs initially from the mucous membranes, especially the mouth and gums, often being exacerbated by poor oral hygiene, or as in skin purpura, around areas of local pressure such as tight socks around the ankles or under the application site of a sphygmomanometer cuff.

Thrombocytopenia, a reduction in the number of platelets in the circulation, is often encountered in clinical medicine. The causes of thrombocytopenia can be classified as the result of decreased production of platelets, decreased survival of platelets due to increased destruction, utilization or loss from the circulation and abnormal distribution of platelets. Several causes may be operative in the same patient. A detailed history and clinical examination are essential in the evaluation of patients with thrombocytopenia. Information should be sought about the following factors which are of particular importance: (1) the family history may point to the possible presence of uncommon forms of thrombocytopenia associated with inherited disorders involving platelets; (2) the age of onset and duration and type of bleeding including the response to previous surgery or other trauma; (3) prior exposure to possible toxic substances including drugs, ethanol, chemicals and radiation – the occupational history may provide clues; (4) antecedent illnesses especially infections – enquiry regarding travel abroad may suggest particular infections; and (5) associated disorders such as neoplasms (carcinomas or lymphomas) or collagen vascular disorders. The physical examination should include determination of the type and location of haemorrhagic lesions, the presence or absence of lymphadenopathy or hepatosplenomegaly and other findings suggestive of associated disorders such as infection, malignancy, liver disease or severe pernicious anaemia. A bone marrow examination is mandatory in the investigation of thrombo-cytopenia unless the cause is very clear as in massive transfusion or disseminated intravascular coagulation. A trephine biopsy may provide additional information, for example when thrombocytopenia is secondary to bone marrow replacement with carcinoma or lymphoma, and should always be considered.

Thrombocytosis

Thrombocytosis, an increase in the number of circulating platelets, is a common clinical finding. It results from increased platelet production as platelet survival does not become prolonged beyond normal values. Thrombocytosis is either primary or reactive and the causes are listed in Table 6.1. Primary thrombocytosis, termed 'thrombocythaemia', occurs as a feature of primary diseases of the bone marrow such as the myeloproliferat-ive disorders. The most common causes of reactive thrombocytosis are haemorrhage, malignancy or diseases associated with tissue inflammation and/or necrosis. The clinical and laboratory approach is based on the differentiation of primary from reactive causes of thrombocytosis and identification of the cause of a reactive thrombocytosis. It has been said that a platelet count exceeding 1000×10^9 per litre suggests that the thrombocytosis is primary rather than reactive, but this belief may be misleading. In a large study of 372 patients, 11 patients with platelet counts above 1000×10^9 per litre had diagnoses other than myeloproliferative disease or malignancy.[17]

The history should include careful enquiry regarding haemorrhagic and/or thromboembolic manifestations as such symptoms are rare in patients with reactive thrombocytosis. A history of any concurrent disorders – such as malignancy, chronic inflammatory disease, acute or chronic infection, alcoholism or gastrointestinal haemorrhage, and a drug history – should be obtained. Pruritus, splenomegaly, microvascular thromboembolic manifesta-tions in the hands and feet, large ecchymoses or neurological signs may point to a myeloproliferative disorder. Particular attention should be given to signs of malignancy – breast and pelvic examination should be performed in women with thrombocytosis – and infection. In all cases, a peripheral blood count including a platelet count and blood film examination should be performed. Spurious thrombocytosis may result from aberrant automated counting of microspherocytes.[18] Platelet morphological abnormalities – platelet anisocytosis with giant platelets, decreased granulation and mega-karyocyte fragments – suggest a myeloproliferative disorder as do a polymorphonuclear neutrophil leucocytosis with basophilia and/or eosino-philia. A leucoerythroblastic film may indicate metastatic bone marrow infiltration. The presence of irregularly contracted red blood cells, target cells and Howell–Jolly bodies should be noted. These features indicate

Table 6.1   Causes of Thrombocytosis

Primary
  Myeloproliferative disorders
    Essential thrombocytosis (thrombocythaemia)
    Primary proliferative polycythaemia
    Myelofibrosis
    Chronic myeloid leukaemia
  Myelodysplastic syndromes
    Refractory anaemia with ring sideroblasts
    5q-syndrome

Reactive
  Haemorrhage and haemolytic anaemias
  Iron deficiency
  Infections – usually chronic rather than acute
  Inflammation
    Rheumatoid arthritis
    Ulcerative colitis, Crohn's disease
    Post-operative
  Malignancy
    Carcinoma, e.g. lung, ovary, breast, stomach
    Lymphoma – Hodgkin's disease
  Asplenia or hyposplenism
    Splenectomy
    Coeliac disease, dermatitis herpetiformis
    Sickle cell disease
  Drugs
    Vinca alkaloids
    Miconazole
  Redistribution
    Post-exercise
    Adrenaline
Rebound thrombocytosis (often after preceding thrombocytopenia)
    Withdrawal of cytotoxic drugs or alcohol
    Treatment of folate or vitamin B_{12} deficiency

---

splenectomy but asplenia or hyposplenism may result from repeated microinfarctions secondary to platelet thrombi in the splenic microcirculation in essential thrombocythaemia as well in other disorders such as coeliac disease. Hypochromic microcytic red cells may indicate iron deficiency anaemia secondary to primary polycythaemia, essential thrombocythaemia or bleeding from any source. Polycythaemia may be masked by bleeding resulting from a qualitative platelet defect associated with thrombocythaemia. Platelet function defects are found in the majority of patients with myeloproliferative disorders and therefore platelet function studies are useful in the discrimination of primary from reactive (secondary) thrombocytosis. Examination of the bone marrow and trephine biopsy appearances may also be useful. Although megakaryocytes are increased in thrombocytosis from any cause, in myeloproliferative disorders megakaryocytes are large, show increased ploidy and may be dyspoietic whereas in reactive thrombocytosis and chronic myeloid leukaemia, the mean volume of individual megakaryocytes is reduced to approximately two-thirds of normal.[19] In essential thrombocythaemia, there may be marrow fibrosis. Other useful investigations include cytogenetics, serum vitamin B_{12} and a chest radiograph.

Platelet function abnormalities

A prolonged bleeding time occurs when the platelet count falls below approximately 100×10^9 per litre and there is a progressive increase as the platelet count falls below this level.[20] If the platelet count is normal or raised, a prolonged bleeding time is suggestive of one of the many congenital or acquired qualitative disorders of platelet function. Other non-platelet haemostatic disorders which may prolong the bleeding time are vascular abnormalities, particularly if they involve skin collagen defects, von Willebrand's disease, afibrinogenaemia, dysproteinaemias, severe anaemia with a haematocrit of less than 0.20 and conditions in which the vessel wall may produce increased amounts of prostacyclin-like material such as in chronic renal failure.[21] There are several methods for performing a bleeding time test (Ivy, Duke and template methods), all of which rely on the time taken for a standard skin incision, breaking small subcutaneous vessels, to stop bleeding. However, the reproducibility is very variable and depends on several factors including operator experience, skin temperature, venous pressure, direction, length and depth of incision.[22] The template technique using a disposable, spring-loaded device (e.g Simplate II, General Diagnostics) standardizes at least the last three variables and should give reasonably comparable results for clinical use.

If such screening procedures suggest a platelet function defect or when there is a high degree of clinical suspicion despite a normal bleeding time, further platelet adhesion and aggregation tests should be planned in a systematic way.[23] Drugs and certain dietary practices are the commonest causes of platelet dysfunction[24] and patients must refrain from taking drugs with known anti-platelet effects for 10–14 days before blood sampling for more specific investigation. Clinically, the most important of these drugs and dietary foodstuffs and their proposed mechanisms of action are listed in Table 6.2.

Enhanced platelet function

There is good evidence that impaired platelet function can be detected by *in vitro* tests and that the abnormalities are associated with impaired haemostasis *in vivo*. However, despite the development of a number of tests to demonstrate enhanced activity of circulating platelets or to show that platelets have been activated *in vivo* by a thrombotic process, there is no conclusive evidence that enhanced platelet activity *in vitro* is important in the pathogenesis of thrombosis.

The interactions between platelets and the vascular endothelium are believed to be of fundamental importance in the development of thrombus formation and atherosclerosis.[25] In all vascular beds – arterial, venous and

Table 6.2   Agents Which Affect Platelet Function

Membrane stabilizing agents
  α-Antagonists
  β-Blockers
  Local anaesthetics (procaine)
  Antihistamines
  Tricyclic antidepressants
  Frusemide
Agents which affect prostanoid synthesis
  Aspirin and proprietary preparations containing aspirin
  Non-steroidal anti-inflammatory agents
  Corticosteroids
Antibiotics (usually only in high doses)
  Penicillins
  Cephalosporins
  β-Lactam derivatives
Agents which increase cyclic-AMP levels
  Dipyridamole
  Aminophylline
  Prostanoids[a]
Others
  Dextrans
  Phenothiazine
  Clofibrate
  Papaverine
  Heparin[a]
  Cyclosporin[a]
Dietary agents and toxins
  Garlic
  Ethanol[a]
  Cod liver oil (eicosapentaenoic acid)
  Saturated fatty acids[a]
  Cigarette smoke[a]

---

a These agents may lead to enhanced platelet function.

capillary – platelet adhesion to exposed sub-endothelium, in association with altered blood flow, hypercoagulability and/or increased platelet reactivity, precipitates thrombus formation. In the arterial vasculature, platelet interaction with perturbed vascular endothelium is thought to precipitate smooth muscle proliferation, an early event in the formation of atherosclerotic plaques. Platelets may play a role in a number of disorders associated with vaso-occlusive or vasospastic manifestations (Table 6.3) but the precise events leading to initiation of platelet activation and aggregation have not been defined.

    A number of *in vitro* measurements have been developed as indicators of hyperactive circulating platelets but their usefulness in clinical situations have by no means been established. The most generally employed measurements include detection of the presence of spontaneous platelet aggregation or enhanced platelet aggregation responses in platelet rich plasma or whole blood, the presence of circulating platelet aggregates,

Table 6.3 Conditions in which Enhanced Platelet Function May Play a Pathogenic Role in the Generation of Thrombosis

---

Atherosclerosis-related disorders
  Coronary heart disease
  Amaurosis fugax
  Cerebrovascular disease – transient ischaemic attacks and strokes
  Peripheral ischaemic vascular disease
  Cigarette smoking
  Hypercholesterolaemia
Diabetes mellitus
Vasospastic disorders
  Migraine
  Raynaud's phenomenon
Thromboembolism in alcoholics
Renal allograft rejection and cyclosporin nephrotoxicity
Microvascular thrombotic complications in myeloproliferative disorders
Thrombotic thrombocytopenic purpura and the haemolytic uraemic syndrome
Hypothermia

---

analysis of platelet release products such as β-thromboglobulin and platelet factor 4 and release of TXB_2 from maximally stimulated platelets. Spontaneous platelet aggregation in platelet-rich plasma occurs commonly in citrated platelet-rich plasma in patients with thrombocytosis associated with myeloproliferative disorders and has also been reported in patients with diabetes, cerebrovascular disease and post-renal transplantation in patients receiving cyclosporin immunosuppression. The mechanism of spontaneous platelet aggregation is uncertain. It may be indicative of increased sensitivity of the platelets to small amounts of ADP released from platelets when they are exposed to minor degrees of trauma or increased ability of the platelets to generate TXA_2 when stimulated by contact with a stir bar. The relationship of spontaneous platelet aggregation to thrombosis is uncertain but anecdotal reports suggest that patients with persistent thrombocytosis associated with myeloproliferative disorders who, not infrequently exhibit spontaneous platelet aggregation, have an increased risk of thrombosis.

Enhanced platelet aggregation *in vitro* has been described following thromboembolism or in disorders that predispose to thrombosis. A decreased threshold for aggregation to a variety of agonists such as ADP, adrenaline, thrombin and arachidonic acid may be indicative of increased sensitivity of the platelets as a result of continual low-grade platelet activation *in vivo*. Enhanced platelet aggregation *in vitro* has been reported in diabetics with vascular complications, angina pectoris and post-myocardial infarction, patients with hyperlipidaemia, particularly hypercholesterolaemia, chronic renal failure and post-renal transplantation. Decreased sensitivity to prostacyclin or its stable analogue has been observed in association with myocardial ischaemia, diabetes, Raynaud's phenomenon, haemolytic uraemic syndrome and in patients receiving cyclosporin immunosuppression post-renal transplantation. Prostacyclin is a very potent vasodilator and inhibitor of platelet aggregation and thus decreased sensitivity to its effects may lead to unchecked platelet aggregation and thrombus formation.

A method for the detection of circulating platelet aggregates was first described by Wu & Hoak in 1974.[26] Small aggregates of platelets may circulate in the blood of patients with thromboembolism and prothrombotic states. Measurements of these aggregates is based on the principle that platelet aggregates are fixed in blood collected in EDTA to which formalin has been added. The platelet aggregrates collected into this medium and platelets collected into EDTA alone are counted and the platelet aggregate ratio calculated. An increased platelet : aggregate ratio has been reported in patients with angina pectoris or post-myocardial infarction, transient cerebral ischaemia or strokes, recurrent venous thromboses and acute peripheral arterial insufficiency.

β-Thomboglubulin (β-TG) and platelet factor 4 (PF4) are released from the platelet α granules into plasma on activation or aggregration and can thus provide a means of monitoring platelet activation *in vivo* secondary to pathological processes. Both have been suggested to be indicators of prothrombotic states or thromboembolic events. Neither are present in plasma in significant amounts in normal individuals. PF4 is rapidly removed from plasma following its release presumably by binding to the vascular endothelium whereas β-TG remains in the circulation until filtered out by the kidneys. Measurement of both β-TG and PF4 enables differentiation of *in vivo* platelet activation from *in vitro* release during sample collection or handling – the ratio of β-TG to PF4 in normal plasma is 3 : 1. A raised plasma β-TG with a low PF4 suggests *in vivo* platelet activation but high levels of both suggests *in vitro* release. In renal impairment, β-TG may be raised due to decreased clearance. Increased levels of PF4 are found after heparin infusion due to displacement of PF4 from the vessel wall.

TXB_2, which can be measured by radioimmunoassay, is the stable inactive metabolite of TXA_2 formed by prostaglandin metabolism from membrane phospholipids via the cyclo-oxygenase pathway. TXA_2 has very potent vasoconstrictor and proaggregatory properties. Increased serum TXB_2 is probably indicative of increased ability of platelets to form TXB_2, and thus greater proaggregatory platelet activity, following a standardized maximal stimulation. Increased plasma TXB_2 may reflect platelet hyperaggregability within the circulation.

THROMBOCYTOSIS

The causes are listed in Table 6.1.

Primary thrombocytosis

Essential thrombocythaemia

Analysis of glucose-6-phosphate dehydrogenase (G6PD) isoenzyme types in selected black females with essential thrombocythaemia (ET) have demonstrated that ET, in which platelet production is autonomous, is a clonal disorder and circulating erythrocytes, granulocytes and platelets are the progeny of a single pluripotent haemopoietic stem cell.[27] The clonality of this disorder was established by application of the Lyon hypothesis which states that one X-chromosome in each female somatic cell is inactivated early in embryogenesis. Since the locus for G6PD is on the X-chromosome, a female heterozygous for the genes for the usual G6PD type B isoenzyme and the G6PD type A variant will have a population of cells synthesizing type B and a population of cells synthesizing type A. When females with ET were examined, circulating erythrocytes, granulocytes and platelets contained only one enzyme type, confirming the unicellular origin of the disease. Involvement of all three cell lines suggested that the cell of origin was an abnormal haemopoietic stem cell. Clonality has also been established in other myeloproliferative disorders, primary proliferative polycythaemia, myelofibrosis and chronic myeloid leukaemia.

In ET, platelet production appears to be autonomous and the platelet count is elevated because of an increased rate of platelet production, sometimes to as much as 15 times the normal rate. The peripheral platelet count may not fully reflect the increased rate of production because there may be some shortening of platelet survival and, if the spleen is enlarged, an increased proportion of the platelet mass will reside in it. The disease predominantly affects middle-aged patients and approximately 85% of patients are over 50 years of age. The ratio of male to females is 1.2 : 1. The spleen is palpably enlarged in 30% of patients but splenic atrophy is found in some patients, presumably secondary to repeated microinfarctions resulting from platelet thrombi in the microcirculation. Pruritus occurs in less than 10% of patients. Clinical manifestations from thrombocytosis per se result from haemorrhage or microvascular occlusions which may occur simultaneously, although some patients may be asymptomatic. Bleeding is often gastrointestinal, although epistaxis, mucous membrane bleeding and large ecchymoses may also occur. Many patients have evidence of microvascular occlusion of the extremities,[28] the central nervous system[29] or the coronary circulation.[30] The most common manifestation of microvascular occlusion is symptoms and signs of ischaemia in the fingers or toes, occasionally progressing to frank gangrene, with palpable peripheral pulses. Although there are anecdotal reports that patients with persistent thrombocytosis associated with myeloproliferative disorders have an increased risk of thromboembolic events it is questionable whether thrombocytosis increases the risk of large vessel occlusion and in one study, although retrospective, thrombotic episodes were no more frequent than those seen in an age-matched control group.[31]

ET is a diagnosis of exclusion and generally accepted diagnostic criteria have been devised by the Polycythaemia Vera Study Group.[32] Platelet counts frequently exceed 1000×10^9 per litre and there may be mild anaemia. The peripheral blood and bone marrow findings have been summarized above. Karyotype analysis of bone marrow showed aneuploidy in 21% of patients,[32] but a 21q-clonal abnormality has also been described.[33] Thrombocytosis may produce several spurious laboratory findings. Pseudo-hyperkalaemia, caused by *in vitro* release of potassium from platelets, may occur[34] and pseudohypoxaemia may result if arterial blood for measurement of oxygen tension is not chilled and analysed promptly.[35] Serum uric acid may be elevated. Platelet function tests are usually abnormal in ET. The bleeding time may or may not be prolonged. Spontaneous platelet aggregation and circulating platelet aggregates may occur in association with thrombocytosis and digital ischaemia.[36] Although the specificity of spontaneous platelet aggregation and its relationship to thromboembolism is uncertain, the abnormality in platelet aggregation and the clinical signs of ischaemia respond to aspirin administration. The most consistent platelet aggregation defect has been impaired platelet responsiveness to adrenaline, probably attributable to a reduction in the number of α-adrenergic receptors on the platelet membrane.[37] ADP-induced and collagen-induced aggregation may be impaired. PF3 availability has been reported to be impaired in patients with ET with clinical evidence of bleeding, whereas platelet coagulant hyperactivity has been reported in those with thrombotic complications.[38] Enzymatic and multiple platelet membrane defects have been described in ET which may account for the abnormal platelet function. Reported defects include abnormal arachidonic acid metabolism and, in some cases, lipoxygenase deficiency with increased platelet TXA_2 production presumably secondary to shunting of arachidonic acid through the cyclo-oxygenase pathway,[39] deficiencies in serotonin uptake and lipid peroxidation. Reported platelet membrane abnormalities include reduction in platelet membrane glycoproteins Ib and IIb with increased glycoprotein IV, decreased α-adrenergic receptors and prostaglandin D_2 receptors and inreased expression of Fc receptors. In addition, platelets of patients with ET may have a storage pool defect. Whether these defects arise from intrinsically abnormal platelet production by abnormal megakaryocytes or from platelet activation during intravascular platelet aggregation remains unclear.[40] Despite the occurrence of bleeding and thromboembolic complications in patients with ET with coexisting thrombocytosis and qualitative abnormalities, a study by Schafer[41] suggested that there is no correlation between bleeding or thromboembolic events and the level of the platelet count, the bleeding time or platelet aggregation studies in either ET or the thrombocytosis associated with other myeloproliferative disorders.

Thrombocytosis associated with other myeloproliferative disorders

Primary autonomous thrombocythaemia and qualitative platelet defects also occur in the other myeloproliferative disorders, primary proliferative polycythaemia, myelofibrosis and chronic myeloid leukaemia. In chronic myeloid leukaemia it is unusual to observe bleeding despite very high platelet counts. The clinical manifestations of thrombocytosis in patients with primary polycythaemia are similar to those with ET, but an uncontrolled increase in haematocrit and red cell mass may predispose to bleeding.[42] Indeed, haemorrhagic manifestations of thrombocytosis may be more frequent in patients with primary polycythaemia[31] who show a reduction in the incidence of bleeding following control of the red cell mass.

Myelodysplastic syndromes

Thrombocytosis is found in up to 30% of patients with refractory anaemia with ring sideroblasts[43] and in association with refractory macrocytic anaemia, low or normal white count and partial deletion of the long arm of chromosome number 5, the 5q-syndrome described by Mahmood *et al.*[44]

Reactive thrombocytosis

Thrombocytosis may occur in association with a number of pathological conditions. In a study of 372 patents with thrombocytosis, defined as a platelet count exceeding 500×10^9 per litre, 24% were related to infection, 19% to surgery, 17% to iron deficiency and bleeding, 9% to malignancy, 9% to splenectomy and 21% were miscellaneous.[17] Bleeding or thrombotic manifestations rarely occur in patients with reactive thrombocytosis, but two special situations, thrombocytosis seen post-splenectomy, and in association with iron deficiency, will be discussed.

Splenectomy

After splenectomy for non-haematological conditions, platelet counts rise twofold to sixfold within 1–2 weeks and usually return to normal over a period of weeks to months. Platelet survival remains normal in asplenic individuals. Since elimination of the splenic pool can account for platelet increases of no more than 50%, post-splenectomy thrombocytosis is most likely due to increased platelet production.[45] Studies involving large numbers of patients have found no differences in thrombotic tendency between splenectomized patients with thrombocytosis and other post-operative patients with normal platelet counts.[46] In contrast, Hirsh & Dacie[47] reported a 13% incidence of thrombotic complications following splenectomy in patients with haemolytic anaemias and haemoglobinopathies and Tso and co-workers[48] reported venous thrombosis and pulmonary embolism in two of nine patients with haemoglobin H disease post-splenectomy although thromboembolism is rare among the Chinese population. Splenectomy for haemolytic anaemia may result in persistent thrombocytosis if the haemolytic process is not corrected.[47] Several factors other than the thrombocytosis could contribute to post-splenectomy thromboembolism. Increased platelet adhesiveness has been reported post-splenectomy.[49] Red cells are known to contain clot-promoting activity.[50] Infusions of red cell haemolysates cause accelerated coagulation in experimental animals and the severity of the hypercoagulable state is increased after reticulo-endothelial cell blockade.[51] Reticulo-endothelial function is known to be depressed post-splenectomy.[52]

Iron deficiency

Patients with iron deficiency anaemia, usually secondary to bleeding but occasionally to nutritional deficiency, may develop marked thrombocytosis with platelet counts occasionally exceeding 2000×10^9 per litre. There are reports of thromboembolic complications in this setting.[53] The thrombocytosis responds dramatically to iron replacement, falling to normal levels within a week to 10 days of institution of iron therapy. Thrombopoiesis seems to be abruptly suppressed by iron replacement.

URAEMIA

Bleeding is a serious complication of renal failure and may sometimes be fatal. Clinical manifestations include purpura, epistaxis, gastrointestinal bleeding and occasionally haemorrhagic pericarditis and intracranial haemorrhage. The major haemostatic disturbance associated with uraemia is a defect in platelet function and the platelet–vessel wall interaction which is most readily assessed by the bleeding time.[54] Renal disease seldom results in deficiencies of coagulation factors unless complicated by uraemic enteritis (with concomitant malabsorption of vitamin K), liver disease or disseminated intravascular coagulation.

Many qualitative platelet defects have been recorded in renal failure but perhaps the single most important determinant of uraemic bleeding is the low haematocrit that accompanies long-standing renal failure.[21] The prolonged bleeding time seen in these patients largely corrects following blood transfusion[55] and has also done so after administration of recombinant erythropoietin for the treatment of anaemia.[56] In addition, platelets have been shown to have impaired aggregation to adrenaline, collagen and ADP but these *in vitro* defects do not seem to correlate well with bleeding in uraemic patients. Ristocetin-induced agglutination may aso be impaired and this would suggest an abnormal interaction between platelets and the von Willebrand factor. However, there is no convincing evidence in this setting of an abnormal von Willebrand factor, or, indeed, of the platelet membrane receptor for it, although some workers have been able to demonstrate proteolytic activity in uraemic blood which may enhance catabolism of von Willebrand factor.[57] Furthermore, the ristocetin-induced agglutination response of normal platelets suspended in uraemic plasma is reduced[58] and this, together with other data, is compatible with the hypothesis that uraemic plasma may contain an inhibitor of the von Willebrand factor–platelet interaction. Desmopressin (1-deamino-8-D-arginine vasopressin, DDAVP) has been shown to reduce the bleeding time in uraemia[59] and is known to cause direct release of the Factor VIII–von Willebrand factor complex from vascular endothelial cells; in this setting it may work by promoting a rise of plasma von Willebrand factor (especially the larger multimers), thereby overcoming any inhibitor to the von Willebrand factor–glycoprotein Ib interaction.[60]

Other qualitative abnormalities of platelets that have been documented include a storage pool defect with diminished serotonin and ADP content,[61] reduced arachidonic acid metabolism associated with a functional cyclooxygenase defect[62] and increased platelet calcium content correctable by vitamin D analogues.[63] The precise uraemic retention products that are responsible for these platelet functional defects have not been identified. So-called 'middle molecules' of molecular weight between 500 and 5000 Da have been shown to inhibit platelet function *in vitro*, although the levels of these compounds do not correlate with the risk of clinical bleeding,[64] as has parathormone, another possible uraemic toxin. It is interesting that while dialysis corrects the bleeding tendency of uraemic patients it does not always correct the platelet dysfunction.

Both peritoneal and haemodialysis will help reverse the haemostatic defect in uraemia, although they may not entirely correct it. Indeed, haemodialysis may occasionally be associated with increased bleeding as platelets may be activated by the artificial membrane and anticoagulation is required to maintain the patency of the extracorporeal circuit. For patients at high risk of bleeding, heparin may be administered in low doses or may even be substituted by citrate or prostacyclin infusions.[65] Treatment of the anaemia to bring the haematocrit up to 0.30 either by blood transfusion or erythropoietin therapy, will improve platelet function and shorten the bleeding time.[66] Short-term correction of the haemostatic defect has been achieved with infusions of cryoprecipitate,[67] but more recently with desmopressin, which has been used successfully. Thus, the bleeding time has been reduced for up to 4 h following an intravenous infusion of 0.3–0.4 µg/kg of desmopressin[59] and this may allow minor surgery and renal biopsies to be performed safely. Finally, there is evidence that conjugated oestrogens may restore the bleeding time for some days in uraemic patients[68] although their mechanism of action is uncertain and it is not yet clear whether they reduce clinical bleeding in renal failure.

RENAL TRANSPLANTATION

Microvascular thrombotic episodes are a well documented complication of allogeneic renal transplantation.

Renal allograft rejection may be accompanied by platelet consumption and there is some evidence that the rejection process is mediated by microvascular thrombosis. Platelet activation may occur as a result of circulating immune complexes[69] and platelet membrane antigens have been localized to the glomeruli in renal biopsy specimens obtained from rejecting grafts. These findings emphasize the potential role of platelets in the rejection process. Despite these observations, however, in a number of studies antiplatelet agents have not been successful in preserving graft functions although there is evidence that prostacyclin may be of benefit in this context.[70]

Following the first clinical trials in the late 1970s, cyclosporin A (cyclosporin; Sandoz Pharmaceuticals Ltd) has gradually superseded other forms of immunosuppression and is now used in virtually all renal allograft recipients to prevent allograft rejection, but nephrotoxicity is a major limiting side effect. Evidence from both clinical and animal studies has suggested that cyclosporin is associated with vascular endothelial damage, leading to microvascular thrombosis, and it has been proposed that this damage may play a role in cyclosporin induced nephrotoxicity. Human renal allograft recipients have been reported to develop platelet-fibrin thrombi in glomerular capillaries or afferent arterioles associated with high blood levels of cyclosporin,[71] and an arteriolopathy, which is usually irreversible and not seen in patients receiving immunosuppression with azathioprine.[72] Animal studies have shown that cyclosporin reduces plasma prostacyclin stimulating factor activity leading to a profound reduction in vascular release of prostacyclin.[73] Reduced prostacyclin, in conjunction with vascular endothelial cell damage, may result in unchecked platelet aggregation and microvascular thrombosis which would lead to infarction. However, in subsequent animal studies, toxic doses of cyclosporin did not induce increased platelet reactivity,[74] and chronic administration of cyclosporin did not affect the ability of circulating platelets to synthesize thromboxane A_2.[75] Human renal allograft recipients receiving cyclosporin show evidence of *in vivo* platelet activation, and *in vitro* hyperaggregability characterized by spontaneous aggregation, enhanced responsiveness to low doses of ADP and decreased sensitivity to the prostacyclin analogue Iloprost (Schering Chemical Co.), with changes persisting for at least one year post-transplantaton.[76] *In vivo* platelet activation and platelet hyperaggregability has also been documented in azathioprine-treated renal allograft recipients.[77] The increased platelet reactivity in these studies was not indicative of overt allograft rejection, but it is possible that platelet activation is secondary to immune-mediated vascular endothelial damage arising as a consequence of the hosts' response to foreign antigen. Activated platelets may in turn be contributary to vascular endothelial damage.

There have been occasional reports of the development of a frank haemolytic uraemic syndrome or thrombotic thrombocytopenic purpura following renal, bone marrow or liver transplantation and cyclosporin has been implicated, but this complication has also been reported in patients receiving immunosuppression with azathioprine and a causal role for cyclosporin has not been proven.

LIVER DISEASE

Patients with acute and chronic severe liver disease can exhibit significant haemostatic abnormalities which predispose to bleeding and may thus be contributory to morbidity and mortality. Platelet abnormalities, either thrombocytopenia or qualitative, are just one facet of the multiple haemostatic defects that complicate severe liver disease. Other haemostatic defects include decreased synthesis of all coagulation factors with the exception of Factor VIII. Plasma fibrinogen is normal or even increased in patients with stable chronic liver disease because although fibrinogen removal from the circulation is accelerated, the rate of synthesis is, in fact, normal or increased. However, hypofibrinogenaemia may be seen in advanced liver cirrhosis due to a combination of decreased synthesis, loss into the extracorporeal spaces (ascites, oedema) and consumption or increased catabolism of fibrinogen by plasmin. Dysfibrinogenaemia, characterized by abnormal fibrin polymerization, is common in liver disease and the functional defect may be related to excessive sialic acid in the fibrinogen molecules. The decreased functional levels of coagulation factors are balanced to a degree by decreased hepatic synthesis of antithrombin III, a naturally occurring inhibitor of coagulation. A hyperfibrinolytic state may occur secondary to decreased clearance of plasminogen activators and decreased levels of naturally occurring fibrinolytic inhibitors such as α_2-antiplasmin and histidine-rich glycoprotein. Superimposed on these abnormalities, a consumptive coagulopathy may lead to further derangement of haemostasis in patients with liver disease. Suggested triggering mechanisms include release of procoagulant substances into the blood from necrotic hepatocytes or liberation of clot-promoting intestine-derived endotoxins. In addition, impaired clearance of activated clotting factors and reduced levels of the naturally occurring anticoagulant, antithrombin III, may facilitate the development of disseminated intravascular coagulation.[78]

Thrombocytopenia, mild to moderate, is seen in approximately one-third of patients with liver cirrhosis and probably results from a combination of splenic pooling and shortened platelet survival. The number of mega-karyocytes in the bone marrow of such patients is normal or increased and the major mechanism of the thrombocytopenia is increased platelet pooling in the spleen. In normal individuals, the spleen contains one-third of the total platelet mass, whereas in patients with cirrhosis and congestive splenomegaly, 60–90% of the total platelet mass may be sequestered in the spleen. The mechanism of the shortened platelet survival is unclear – suggested mechanisms include thrombin-mediated platelet consumption and sequestration of platelets on incompletely endothelialized sinusoids of the regenerating liver.[79]

Prolonged bleeding times and various *in vitro* platelet abnormalities, including decreased platelet adhesiveness and platelet factor 3 (PF3) availability, impaired primary and secondary aggregation to ADP and impaired platelet aggregation to adrenaline, thrombin and ristocetin have been described in patients with chronic severe liver disease.[80–84] It has been suggested that the platelet functional abnormalities in chronic liver disease may be due to the inhibitory effect of increased plasma fibrin(ogen) degradation products (FDP) concentrations, but this seems unlikely in view of studies suggesting lack of correlation between platelet dysfunction and FDP levels in patients with liver disease[85] and that the FDP levels achieved in the circulation in fibrinolytic states are unlikely to cause significant impairment of platelet aggregation.[86] Furthermore, the platelet functional defect appears to be intrinsic as it is not inducible by incubation of normal platelets in plasma from cirrhotic patients.[83] Two double-blind placebo-controlled crossover studies have shown that DDAVP shortens the bleeding times of patients with liver cirrhosis.[87,88] Thus, DDAVP should be considered for cirrhotics with prolonged bleeding times who need invasive diagnostic procedures or when they suffer gastrointestinal bleeding.

The existence of platelet functional abnormalities in liver disease has been contested. Stein & Harker[79] failed to demonstrate any abnormality of the bleeding time, platelet retention to glass-bead columns and platelet aggregation to ADP, adrenaline and collagen in 60 patients with well-documented hepatic cirrhosis. Thus, the occurrence and biochemical basis of platelet dysfunction and its clinical importance in patients with liver disease remains to be established.

MICROANGIOPATHIC HAEMOLYTIC ANAEMIA AND THROMBOTIC THROMBOCYTOPENIC PURPURA

Thrombotic thrombocytopenic purpura (TTP) is a multi-system disease characterized by fever, fluctuating central neurological abnormalities, progressive renal failure, microangiopathic haemolytic anaemia and thrombocytopenia.[89] A microangiopathic haemolytic anaemia is present in virtually all cases with numerous bizarre fragmented red cells on the peripheral blood film. Peripheral thrombocytopenia is accompanied by marked marrow megakaryocytic hyperplasia and a shortened platelet survival. A coagulation screen and fibrinogen level usually show only minimal changes and so distinguish these cases from disseminated intravascular coagulation (DIC). However, some cases of severe TTP with extensive haemolysis or septicaemia may be further complicated with the added features of DIC. Several biochemical changes, including elevated bilirubin and lactic dehydrogenase (LDH) values, reflect intravascular haemolysis. Repeated monitoring of LDH levels provides a useful assessment in changes of the degree of haemolysis and disease progression. TTP is not a single disease entity but a clinical syndrome which has been associated with systemic lupus erythematosus, other connective tissue disorders, pregnancy, oral contraceptives and related to drug therapy with several compounds including cyclosporin and mitomycin and allogeneic transplantation. In addition, in certain rare instances, there seems to be a familial association and recurrent episodes of relapse have also been reported. However, in the majority of cases there is no known causal event or associated disease process. TTP is found in both sexes of all ages with a slight predominance in females and a peak incidence between 30 and 40 years of age.

Pathologically, there are intravascular thrombi consisting of platelet aggregates and fibrin in capillaries and pre-capillary arterioles predominantly involving the pancreas, adrenals, brain, heart and kidneys. The haemolytic uraemic syndrome (HUS) overlaps considerably with the clinical and pathological features of TTP but is often preceded by an acute infective illness which may be epidemic in nature and the intravascular thrombi are usually confined to the kidneys.[90] HUS is seen most frequently in children, varies considerably in its severity and has a much lower mortality rate than adult TTP. However, it is believed that the pathogenesis of both conditions is similar, only differing in the distribution of the thrombotic lesions. The pathogenesis of the diffuse microvascular thrombosis remains unknown. Presumably the initiating event is inappropriate platelet adhesion, aggregation and release on the microarterial surfaces.

Several workers have shown that plasma from patients with TTP and HUS lack a prostacyclin stimulatory factor and thus postulate that deficiency of such a factor was primarily responsible for reduced vascular prostacyclin synthesis and release and the initiation of platelet thrombi.[91] Subsequently in support of this hypothesis it has been reported that cultured endothelial cells show decreased prostacyclin production in the presence of TTP plasma compared with normal plasma. Prostacyclin is an unstable compound with a half-life *in vitro* of 2–4 min at a pH of 7.4, but when incubated in human plasma the half-life has been reported to be stabilized for up to 2 h. It has been suggested that plasma contains an active compound, other than albumin, which prolongs the activity of prostacyclin and that deficiency of this stabilizing factor will lead to reduced prostacyclin levels and thus favour platelet deposition and microvascular thrombosis.

It has also been demonstrated that the plasma from some patients with TTP induces aggregation of both normal and TTP platelets. Normal plasma contains an IgG which inhibits the platelet-aggregating factor of TTP plasma, whereas IgG purified from TTP plasma fails to inhibit this platelet-aggregating activity. It is therefore proposed that deficiency of an IgG which inhibits a platelet-aggregating factor present in normal plasma is responsible for inappropriate and excessive platelet activation in some cases of TTP.

Another related finding is the report of unusually large Factor VIII–von Willebrand factor multimers in plasma from patients with chronic relapsing TTP in remission but not in relapse. The multimer pattern reverts to normal following infusions of fresh frozen plasma or cryosupernatant of normal plasma, suggesting that these patients have a defect in the processing of these multimers which may bind to and agglutinate platelets *in vivo* and thus initiate intravascular agglutination and a clinical episode of TTP.[92] In seven cases of acute HUS, six of which were endemic, the same group reported a relative decrease in the higher molecular weight forms of von Willebrand factor and postulated that there was an alteration in von Willebrand factor metabolism, distribution or interaction with platelets.[93] These findings in HUS are at variance with the report of increased concentrations of high molecular weight von Willebrand factor multimers in patients with both sporadic and endemic HUS.[94]

Circulating cytotoxic anti-endothelial cell antibodies have been reported in TTP[95] and more recently in HUS.[96] These cytotoxic antibodies may play a role in the pathogenesis of vascular injury in TTP and HUS.

Therapy of TTP and HUS in the past has largely been empirical but with some basic understanding of the pathogenesis of this condition having recently emerged, a more reasoned approach can now be adopted. Because both are uncommon disorders and the use of multiple agents in severe cases are frequently employed, assessment of therapy is difficult to define accurately. Supportive therapy for acute renal failure and antibiotic prophylaxis should be instigated when appropriate.

Infusions of fresh frozen plasma should be started immediately after the diagnosis is confirmed.[97] The initial limitations to continual plasma infusions are the hazards of volume overload and the length of time required to infuse a large volume. It has been proposed that a plasma infusion would provide the so-called plasma factor which is presumably deficient. There is also evidence that cryoprecipitate infusions may be helpful in selected cases with factor VIII–von Willebrand factor complex abnormalities. Approximately 60–70% of patients respond to plasma infusions showing initially an improvement in neurological status followed by a spontaneous increase in the platelet count and a progressive decrease in the serum LDH levels. There seems to be very little correlation between disease severity and response rate. Those patients responding to plasma infusions exhibit a wide range in the volume infused and the duration the infusions require to be continued. Plasma exchange using a cell separator and replacement with fresh frozen plasma should be instituted in all patients not responding to plasma infusions alone after 48 h or earlier if the facilities are readily available or if the disease is becoming rapidly progressive. This allows 2–3 litres of plasma to be replaced daily with each exchange. Reported response rates are slightly improved ranging from 60 to 80% using an intensive plasma exchange and replacement regime. It is possible that the removal of a platelet-aggregating factor provides an additional benefit of exchange over simple plasma infusions. If replacement solutions other than plasma are used, such as artificial volume expanders or human albumin fractions, the results have been very disappointing. Although a significant number of patients will be severely thrombocytopenic with spontaneous bleeding and purpura, the use of platelet concentrates should be avoided. There are reports that platelet infusions may accelerate the disease process and are consistent with the view that the intravascular platelet aggregation is probably the initiating event.

The management of the small number of patients who do not respond to plasmapheresis and plasma replacement is extremely difficult. As local prostacyclin deficiency may be the primary defect at the vascular sites of platelet thrombi formation an intravenous infusion of prostacyclin may be helpful in refractory cases. There have also been several reports of the successful use of low-dose vincristine infusions in such circumstances.[98] The role of oral antiplatelet agents is difficult to assess. Used alone, they probably do not affect the underlying mechanisms causing the disorder.[99] However, they do appear to supplement plasma exchange in some reports and may be a useful form of maintenance therapy to prevent relapse. The ideal oral antiplatelet regime is also undetermined but low-dose aspirin and dipyridamole 400–600 mg daily in divided doses is the most widely used.

HAEMOSTATIC DEFECTS ASSOCIATED WITH MASSIVE TRANSFUSIONS

When a patient's blood volume is replaced by the administration of large quantities of stored banked blood in a short period of time, haemorrhagic manifestations are likely to follow.[100] Stored whole blood undergoes a progressive loss of mainly Factors V and VIII, with Factor VIII activity decreasing to 50% after 1 day, 30% after 5 days and 6% after 21 days and Factor V falling to 50% after 14 days.[101] There is no appreciable loss in the other coagulation factors after storage for 21 days. Platelet function, however, is quickly lost on storage and after 48 h there are practically no viable functioning platelets. If plasma-reduced red cells or red cells collected into an optimal additive solution are transfused, further dilution of coagulation factors will occur. Obviously, additional infusion of crystalloids, human albumin preparations or one of the artificial colloid substitutes will also cause further dilution of coagulation factors and platelets. The various red cell preparations may also precipitate disseminated intravascular coagulation owing to a combination of partial activation of clotting factors and breakdown of platelets, leucocytes and red cells releasing thromboplastin-like material during storage. There is also evidence that platelet function may be impaired in massively transfused patients.

Previously standardized schemes included the administration of platelet concentrates after the equivalent replacement of one blood volume (approximately 10 units in adults).[102] However, to prevent indiscriminate use of components, massively transfused patients should have routine haemostasis tests monitored early to define the precise abnormality.[103] Such patients primarily develop microvascular bleeding with oozing from mucosa, raw wounds and puncture sites due to thrombocytopenia with platelet counts $<50 \times 10^9$ per litre when approximately 1.5–2 times their blood volumes have been transfused. Thrombocytopenia can also be accentuated in these circumstances by accelerated platelet utilization. A standard dose of 6 units of platelet concentrates should be infused to control microvascular bleeding when this occurs. Generally, the haemostatic levels of the coagulation factors are well-maintained and fresh frozen plasma is not required prophylactically.[104] The use of fresh frozen plasma should be restricted to defined defects in the coagulation cascade with an increase in the international normalized ratio (INR) to 1.3 or more.

PLATELET DEFECTS ASSOCIATED WITH CARDIO-PULMONARY BYPASS SURGERY

A wide variety of haemostatic defects have been described in association with cardio-pulmonary bypass (CPB) surgery. These incude thrombocytopenia, acquired platelet functional defects, coagulation factor deficiencies, increased fibrinolysis and fibrinogenolysis, inadequate heparin neutralization and disseminated intravascular coagulation. In addition, haemodilution of viable platelets and coagulation factors by the fluid used to prime the extracorporeal circuit and the use of stored bank blood may further complicate the haemostatic picture. Despite all these *in vitro* disturbances, however, the coagulopathy of CPB is now seldom severe enough to result in excessive peri- or post-operative bleeding. In fact, most clinical bleeding problems arise in patients with added risk factors, such as prolonged surgery (for multiple valve replacements or repeat coronary artery grafting), pre-existing liver dysfunction (e.g. secondary to tricuspid incompetence) or a raised haematocrit of >0.55 (e.g. secondary to cyanotic heart disease).

Mild thrombocytopenia occurs in virtually all patients undergoing CBP surgery[105] but the platelet count seldom falls below 100×10^9 per litre unless the surgery is unduly prolonged. However, damage to the platelets as they pass through the pump and oxygenator system commonly causes a marked functional defect manifested by a prolonged bleeding time and associated with depletion of α granules and a reduced aggregation response to ADP.[106,107] The platelet defect usually corrects itself within 3 h following termination of bypass, but should the defect persist and be associated with excessive haemorrhage then the patient should receive platelet concentrates even when the platelet count is higher than 100×10^9 per litre.[105,106]

There have been several recent attempts to reduce blood loss associated with platelet dysfunction during cardiac surgery using pharmacological agents. Prostacyclin has been shown to increase platelet numbers at the end of bypass but does not seem to reduce transfusion requirements.[108] Most encouraging, however, has been the study by Salzman *et al.*[109] in which desmopressin was given as a short infusion at the end of bypass to 35 patients and found to reduce mean blood loss significantly from 2210 ml in control patients to 1317 ml in the study patients. The mechanism of action of desmopressin in this context is unclear, but there is recent evidence that desmopressin may cause von Willebrand factor to exceed a threshold concentration necessary for effective platelet–vessel interaction.[110]

PSEUDOTHROMBOCYTOPENIA

Pseudothrombocytopenia is the phenomenon of a falsely low platelet count due to non-specific agglutination *in vitro* in blood samples collected in a variety of anticoagulants. In most cases the agglutinating antibodies have been 'cold agglutinins', usually IgG or IgM and rarely IgA, reacting best at room temperature. However, some have reacted best at 37°C while others have not exhibited any temperature dependency. Agglutination appears to be complement-independent. The antibodies show no platelet group specificity and do not bind to platelets from patients with Glanzmann's thrombasthenia who lack the platelet membrane glycoprotein IIb/IIIa complex.[111] In one case an IgM agglutinating antibody has been shown to react specifically with platelet membrane glycoprotein IIb.[112] The agglutinating antibodies have been called 'EDTA-dependent' but pseudo-thrombocytopenia has also been observed in blood anticoagulated with citrate, oxalate or heparin. Although the *in vitro* agglutination occurs most readily with EDTA, the agglutination is abolished by excess EDTA (>40 mM). This inhibition has been attributed to concomitant lowering of the pH to below 6.0 which occurs with high concentrations of EDTA[113] but this cannot be the whole explanation as EDTA-induced inhibition persists when the pH is maintained at a higher level. It has been suggested that high concentrations of EDTA lead to solubilization of glycoprotein IIb resulting in loss of antigen-binding sites.[112]

The clinical significance of pseudothrombocytopenia is uncertain. Associated disorders include liver disease, cardiac disease, metastatic malignancy, Felty's syndrome and atherosclerotic cardio- or cerebrovascular disease.[114,115] However, these associations may be coincidental and in some cases, no associated disorder can be demonstrated. Pseudothrombo-cytopenia has been reported in patients receiving the drug mexiletene.[116] The agglutinins have not been implicated in platelet dysfunction and are not associated with clinical bleeding problems. Although pseudothrombo-cytopenia usually has no clinical manifestations, failure to recognize this entity may result in unnecessary treatment or unjustified withdrawal of drugs. Two situations in which the *in vitro* platelet agglutination could conceivably have important clinical consequences are during use of an extracorporeal circulation – for example in cardio-pulmonary bypass surgery, haemodialysis or plasmapheresis – and during heparin anticoagulation when anticoagulant-induced platelet agglutination may occur, resulting in profound loss of viable platelets.

ATHEROSCLEROSIS-RELATED CONDITIONS

The events involved in the progression of normal intima to atherosclerotic plaque are poorly understood but it has been suggested that the initiating event is endothelial cell denudation. Platelets adhere to the exposed sub-endothelium and release, from their α granules, platelet-derived growth factor, a mitogen which induces smooth muscle migration from the medial layer and subsequent proliferation resulting in intimal thickening.

The probable importance of platelets in the development of atherosclerosis as well as in acute vaso-occlusive events in patients with atheroscelerosis-related disorders such as coronary heart disease, hypertension, stroke, amaurosis fugax and peripheral ischaemia, has prompted many studies of platelet function in experimental models and in patients with such disorders, as well as clinical trials to determine whether platelet inhibitors reduce the incidence or severity of occlusive vascular disease.

Coronary and cerebrovascular disease

Patients with coronary heart disease who have unstable angina, exercise-induced ischaemia or acute myocardial infarction exhibit enhanced platelet function *in vitro* and evidence of *in vivo* platelet activation.[117–120] Reported changes include decreased platelet survival, increased plasma levels of β-TG and PF4, increased TXB_2 production, increased platelet sensitivity to ADP and arachidonic acid and decreased sensitivity to prostacyclin. These findings suggest that *in vivo* platelet activation and aggregation may be involved in the initiation and extension of myocardial infarction. Increased circulatory levels of TXA_2 in the local microarterial environment will also cause vasoconstriction and directly activate platelets, therefore facilitating the second phase of ADP-induced aggregation. The hypothesis that platelets are involved in the initiation of myocardial infarction has led to widespread interest in the use of antiplatelet drugs, particularly aspirin and dipyridamole in the primary prevention of myocardial infarction and in secondary prevention programmes.[121]

Several studies have recorded a marked circadian periodicity in the time of onset of myocardial infarction, sudden cardiac death and cerebral infarction with the peak onset in the occurrence in the morning.[122,123,124] These findings suggest that one or more diurnal alterations may be contributory and it is therefore of interest that platelet hyperaggregability has been demonstrated during the morning in normal human volunteers, specifically upon assuming an upright posture.[125,126] Associated with these aggregation changes, plasma adrenaline and noradrenaline levels showed a maximal diurnal increase. Although the levels of catecholamines are insufficient to directly stimulate platelet aggregation *in vitro*, they may have a synergistic effect on other platelet agonists including ADP.

A number of studies have shown encouraging results in the use of antiplatelet agents for secondary prevention in patients with a history of transient ischaemic attack, occlusive stroke, unstable angina and myocardial infarction. An overview of 25 randomized studies which included a total of 29,000 patients indicated, in both sexes analysed together, that antiplatelet treatment had no effect on non-vascular mortality but reduced vascular mortality by 15% and non-fatal vascular events (stroke, myocardial infarction) by 30%. There were no significant differences between the effects of the different types of antiplatelet treatment tested (300–325 mg aspirin daily, higher aspirin doses, sulphinpyrazone or high-dose aspirin with dipyridamole) nor between the effects in patients with histories of cerebral or cardiac disease.[127] Earlier results had suggested a benefit only in men with cerebrovascular disease but this may have been because men outnumbered women by 3 to 1 in most of those studies.[128,129] The balance of risk and benefit might be different for primary prevention among people at low absolute risk of occlusive disease if antiplatelet treatment produces even a small increase in the incidence of cerebral haemorrhage.[127]

Diabetes mellitus

Diabetics have a higher incidence of the clinical complications of atherosclerosis than non-diabetics.[130,131] Diabetics also develop a specific microangiopathy.[132] Considerable efforts have been directed at defining the role of platelets in the pathogenesis of the occlusive vascular complications in this disease. It is not clear whether the thromboembolic complications result from platelet hypersensitivity or from vessel wall changes that lead to platelet adhesion.[133] The majority of studies have reported abnormalities of platelet function in diabetics, particularly those with microvascular changes. Available evidence also suggests that the diabetic state is associated with vascular endothelial damage. Plasma von Willebrand factor is elevated in diabetics[132] which may be indicative of vascular endothelial cell damage or stimulation.[134] In addition, the ability of blood vessels to synthesize prostacyclin is reduced in rats with experimentally induced diabetes[135] and in the umbilical vessels of infants of diabetic mothers,[136] which may be a reflection of repeated endothelial injury or stimulation. The reported platelet abnormalities include increased platelet adhesiveness, circulating platelet aggregates, platelet hyperaggregability to ADP and collagen, increased serum TXB_2, increased plasma β-TG levels and decreased platelet life-span.[137-140] Platelets from diabetics also exhibit decreased sensitivity to prostacyclin *in vitro*.[141] Prostacyclin is a potent vasodilator and inhibitor of platelet aggregation and thus decreased sensitivity of platelets to its effects coupled with decreased vascular release of prostacyclin may lead to unchecked platelet aggregation and thrombus formation. There is some evidence suggesting that increased platelet reactivity, indicated by increased platelet sensitivity to arachidonic acid and increased platelet production of TXB_2, may contribute to the pathogenesis of diabetic neuropathy.[142]

Dietary lipids

In experimental animals, diets rich in saturated fatty acids are thrombogenic whereas those rich in polyunsaturated fatty acids are antithrombotic. The increased tendency to thrombosis may be due to increased platelet reactivity. Diets rich in saturated fatty acids have been shown to enhance platelet aggregation responses to thrombin in both rats and humans. Increased plasma cholesterol is associated with enhanced aggregation responses to platelet agonists. In contrast, platelets from human subjects fed diets rich in cod-liver oil (containing eicosapentaenoic acid) show decreased agonist-induced platelet aggregation responses.[143]

Smoking

A number of cytotoxic agents have been implicated in the perturbation of the vascular endothelial cell monolayer and subsequent formation of athero-sclerotic plaques. One such agent is cigarette smoke – many epidemiological studies have established the relationship between cigarette smoking and arterial disease and its complications[144] but the constituent of cigarette smoke that is responsible has not been identified. Exposure of vascular endothelium to cigarette smoke induces morphological changes including the formation of surface blebs, microvillus-like projections and increased numbers of plasmalemmal vesicles. These changes are associated with decreased release of prostacyclin and increased adhesion of platelets, suggesting that there is loss of the normal thrombo-resistance of the vascular endothelium.[145] It has been suggested that nicotine-mediated inhibition of vascular prostacyclin synthesis or release may contribute to cigarette smoke-induced vascular damage. However, exposure of vascular endothelial cells in culture to nicotine at concentrations comparable to those found in the plasma of cigarette smokers has no effect on either morphology or release of prostaglandins, suggesting that, although it may be contributory, nicotine is not the primary constituent of cigarette smoke responsible for inducing vascular damage.[146] A number of animal and human studies have suggested that smoking induces platelet hyperaggreability but Lazlo *et al.*[147] were unable to demonstrate any evidence of platelet activation after smoking. Pittilo *et al.*[148] found platelet aggregation response to ADP and collagen were unchanged by smoking in normally non-smoking human volunteers, and pointed out that studies demonstrating enhanced platelet aggregation responses following smoking in humans have been performed on regular smokers in whom the responses may well be different to those in non-smokers due to a cumulative effect of chronic smoking. Smoking leads to reduced platelet sensitivity to the inhibitory effects of prostacyclin, prostaglandins E_1 and D_2.[149]

VASOSPASTIC DISORDERS

Migraine

Migraine is an episodic disorder believed to be due to initial vasospasm leading to slowing of the cerebral circulation followed by vasodilatation and headache. The trigger is unknown but there is evidence for platelet activation with subsequent stimulation of the platelet release reaction indicated by increased plasma levels of β-TG and PF4. Platelet serotonin (5-hydroxytryptamine) increase during the prodrome and decreases during the headache phase presumably due to serotinin release from the dense granules. It may be that serotonin acts with bradykinin to produce the vascular pain. The role of platelets may explain the effectiveness in some patients of agents with antiplatelet activity such as aspirin or non-steroidal anti-inflammatory agents which inhibit platelet cyclo-oxygenase, pro-pranolol, a β-adrenergic blocker, or pizotifen, a serotonin-blocking agent.[150]

Raynaud's phenomenon

Raynaud's phenomenon is characterized by reduced blood flow in peripheral vessels precipitated by cooling and is sometimes complicated by local ischaemic lesions.[151] In this disorder, a functional imbalance may exist between prostacyclin, a potent vasodilator and inhibitor of platelet aggregation, synthesized and released from the vascular endothelium, and TXA_2, which is generated by platelets and has potent vascoconstrictor and proaggregatory effects. Platelets from patients with Raynaud's phenomenon show increased responsiveness to adrenaline, produce increased amounts of TXA_2 and are resistant to the prostaglandin inhibitors of platelet aggregation, prostacyclin and prostaglandin E_1. In addition, they have increased plasma levels of β-TG, circulating platelet aggregates and fibrinogen.[152] It has also been demonstrated that in patients with Raynaud's phenomenon as well as in normal individuals, platelets are more resistant to prostacyclin at temperatures below 37°C.[153,154] The enhanced platelet aggregation, decreased sensitivity to prostacyclin and decreased vascular synthesis of prostacyclin by the vascular endothelium at lower temperatures[155] may lead to a functional imbalance between prostacyclin and TXA_2 with unopposed action of the potent vasoconstrictor and proaggregatory effects of TXA_2. This hypothesis is supported by the observations of reversal of the platelet changes and clinical benefit in patients with Raynaud's phenomenon following the use of exogenous prostacyclin or other anti-aggregatory prostaglandins.[156] Serotonin, which is released from dense granules during platelet activation and causes platelet aggregation and vasoconstriction in peripheral and coronary vessels, has also been implicated in the pathogenesis of Raynaud's phenomenon. The vasoconstrictor response of blood vessels to serotonin is enhanced by cooling.[157] In a study of patients with Raynaud's phenomenon secondary to a connective tissue disorder, subjective and objective benefit was reported during treatment with ketanserin, a specific antagonist of S_2 serotoninergic receptors[158] which inhibits both platelet aggregation and vasoconstriction in response to serotonin.[159]

EFFECTS OF PHARMACOLOGICAL AGENTS AND TOXINS ON PLATELETS

Heparin and platelet interactions

Heparin-induced thrombocytopenia is an idiosyncratic reaction that has been reported to occur in between 0.5% and 20% of patients.[160] This complication is reported more frequently in the USA than in the UK and, in our experience, the actual incidence of heparin-induced thrombocytopenia is very low. It usually occurs after 6–8 days of treatment, but may develop earlier in patients who have been previously exposed to heparin. The mechanism of the thrombocytopenia is immune-mediated and raised levels of platelet-associated IgG are frequently found. However, some workers have also reported a heparin-dependent platelet-aggregating factor in the plasma of patients with heparin-induced thrombocytopenia.[161] The incidence of thrombocytopenia appears to be increased in patients receiving heparin extracted from bovine lungs, the principal source of heparin in the USA, than those receiving heparin from porcine intestinal mucosa, the chief source of heparin used in the UK. The molecular composition of heparin or contaminants from extracted tissues may account for this difference. Heparin-induced thrombocytopenia does not usually cause clinical problems, although occasionally it may be associated with a rebound arterial thrombosis which may be extensive. In addition, heparin has been reported to affect platelet function in a non-idiosyncratic fashion and *in vitro* has been shown to cause a variable degree of spontaneous platelet aggregation. Low molecular weight heparin fractions do not inhibit platelet function and there have been one or two case reports of patients with heparin-induced thrombocytopenia who have subsequently been treated with low molecular weight heparin and have maintained a normal platelet count.[162]

Antibiotics

Platelet dysfunction and a prolonged bleeding time have been reported after several days' therapy with a number of penicillins when administered at high doses. These include penicillin G,[163] carbenicillin,[164] ticarcillin[165] and piperacillin.[166] These effects are not due to inhibition of thromboxane synthesis[167] but may result from a global effect on platelet membrane receptors making them less responsive to physiological agonists. Shattil *et al.*[168] demonstrated that therapeutic clinically relevant concentrations of penicillin G and carbenicillin induced dose-dependent inhibition of ADP-induced aggregation by limiting the availability of the ADP receptor site of the platelet membrane. This deleterious effect may be due to the avid affinity of these drugs for cell membrane proteins and lipids.[169] The older carboxypenicillins (carbenicillin and ticarcillin) and moxalactam have consistently caused marked prolongation of the bleeding time. By comparison, the newer anti-pseudomonal acylureidopenicillins, mezlocillin, piperacillin and azlocillin, have caused less profound and less frequent prolongation of the bleeding time.[170] Of the cephalosporins, only moxalactam has consistently and severely affected platelet function *in vivo* and *in vitro*,[171,172] whereas cefotaxime, ceftizoxime, cefoperazone, cefotetan and cefriaxone have not affected platelets in clinical studies.[170,172–174] The monobactam, aztreonam, and the carbapenam, imipenem, have had minimal effects on platelet function *in vivo* and *in vitro*.[175,176]

In a retrospective analysis of 1493 patients using multiple logistic regression analysis, only moxalactam and cefoxitin were associated with a significantly increased risk of bleeding compared with other antibiotics.[177] Independent risk factors for bleeding were malnutrition, anti-ulcer therapy (indicating patients with a history of peptic ulceration or those in an intensive care unit) and renal dysfunction, which itself is associated with platelet dysfunction. In addition to inducing platelet dysfunction, cephalosporin antibiotics may cause a precipitous decrease in the hepatic cell synthesis of the biologically active γ-carboxylated forms of the vitamin-K-dependent coagulation factors[178] leading to hypoprothrombinaemia and clinical bleeding.

Alcohol

Alcohol has profound effects on haemostasis and the subject has been well reviewed by Cowan.[179] In alcoholic patients with cirrhosis both platelet and coagulation abnormalities may occur and the defects are similar to those found in patients with chronic liver disease from other causes. In alcoholic patients without cirrhosis the primary effect is on the blood platelet. The earliest observations linking alcohol to disorders of platelets were of thrombocytopenia in patients with alcoholic cirrhosis. The thrombocytopenia was attributed to splenomegaly and hypersplenism or dietary deficiency of folate. However, it became apparent that thrombocytopenia could occur in acutely ill alcoholics in the absence of these factors. This led to the recognition of the entity of alcohol-related thrombocytopenia. Subsequent research demonstrated inhibitory effects of alcohol on platelet production, survival, function, structure and metabolism.

Thrombocytopenia, with platelet counts below 100×10^9 per litre occurs in 3% of non-acutely ill patients with chronic alcoholism and in 26% of acutely ill alcoholics. Occasionally, the platelet counts fall as low as 10×10^9 per litre. Hepatomegaly and some degree of liver dysfunction is seen in 58% of these patients but there appears to be no relation between the presence or severity of abnormality of liver dysfunction and the presence or severity of thrombocytopenia. Splenomegaly is uncommon. Folate deficiency is seen in 50% of acutely ill alcoholics but although folate deficiency may cause thrombocytopenia, the development of thrombocytopenia does not seem to be dependent on low folate levels. The platelet counts in patients with alcohol-related thrombocytopenia return to normal after alcohol consumption has ceased. The platelet count begins to rise after 2–3 days and maximal counts may be seen 5–21 days after cessation of alcohol ingestion. This rise in platelet count also occurs in non-thrombocytopenic alcoholics and it is possible that rebound thrombocytosis may contribute to thromboembolic disease in some patients. The clinical importance of alcohol-related thrombocytopenia has been questioned as the range of platelet counts tends to be similar in those patients who bleed and those who do not. However, it seems reasonable to suppose that thrombocytopenia is one of several factors that predisposes the alcoholic patient to bleeding. Alcohol-related thrombocytopenia appears to be due to a combination of an increased rate of platelet destruction leading to decreased platelet survival and ineffective thrombopoiesis.

Platelet dysfunction in alcoholics may be related to underlying cirrhosis, folate deficiency or may arise as a direct consequence of the effects of alcohol. The template bleeding time in patients ingesting large amounts of alcohol increases twofold while platelet counts remain normal. The prolongation of the bleeding time is associated with abnormalities of platelet function in vitro which include abnormalities of platelet aggregation, the release reaction and platelet procoagulant activity. Patients in whom the blood alcohol level is >300 mg/dl for 7 days or more show decreased platelet aggregation responses to ADP, adrenaline, thrombin and collagen. The aggregation of normal platelets exposed to alcohol at doses above 240 mg/dl in vitro for 2 min or more is also significantly reduced. The aggregation defect observed in vitro primarily involves the secondary response. The storage pool concentrations of ADP and ATP are decreased and associated with decreased release of ADP following collagen stimulation. The acquired storage pool defect contributes to the defective secondary aggregation response seen with alcohol. At higher concentrations of alcohol, above 400 mg/dl, platelet factor 3 availability is impaired. Ingestion of alcohol is associated with changes in platelet metabolism but the precise relationships of metabolic alterations to the platelet functional abnormalities have not been established. During ingestion of alcohol, platelet cyclic-AMP concentrations decrease by 50% and this is associated with decreased platelet adenylate cyclase activity. Very high concentrations of alcohol lead to a dose-dependent inhibition of thromboxane synthesis in human platelets. Alcohol leads to an increase in serotonin influx as well as efflux from platelets. However, since the amount taken up is 25 times that which effluxes, serotonin metabolism by the platelet remains virtually unaffected.

Several hypotheses have been put forward to explain the mechanisms by which alcohol affects platelet function. Alcohol-related platelet dysfunction has been attributed to ethanol-induced hyperosmolality. Blood alcohol concentrations in excess of 300 mg/dl are associated with marked increases in plasma osmolality. It has been demonstrated that increasing plasma osmolality using a variety of solutes to levels observed in alcoholics impairs platelet function. The increased osmolality may inhibit the ability of the platelet membrane to interact with an agonist or may impair the transmission of a stimulus across the membrane. Alternatively, ethanol may impair the reactivity of the platelet membrane by acting as a local anaesthetic and 'stabilizing' the platelet membrane, thus leading to reduced platelet responsiveness. It is possible that some of the effects of ethanol may be related to its metabolites. Acetaldhyde or another metabolite may impair a membrane-bound protein and thus impair platelet membrane responses to agonists.

Although excess alcohol consumption is associated with thrombocytopenia and impaired platelet function which may predispose to bleeding, it is well-documented that excess alcohol consumption is also associated with an increased incidence of cerebrovascular stroke and thromboembolic disease. The incidence of these latter complications is probably greatest after cessation of alcohol ingestion. Alcohol-induced hypertension may be contributory, but there is evidence suggesting that platelets play a role in the pathogenesis of alcohol-related thromboembolic disorders. In addition to the 'rebound thrombocytosis' observed after cessation of drinking, alcohol withdrawal has been reported to be associated with platelet hyper-aggregability to ADP and adrenaline *in vitro* and evidence of *in vivo* platelet activation indicated by circulating platelet aggregates and increased plasma β-thromboglobulin concentrations. The cause of the enhanced platelet function is uncertain, but it has been suggested that it may be attributable to influx into the circulation of newly formed platelets with increased functional activity.[180]

Synthetic colloids

To maintain blood volume during the acute stages of hypovolaemic shock large volumes of synthetic colloids such as dextrans, gelatin solutions, hydroxyethyl starch or human albumin solutions are frequently infused.[181] In addition to their simple dilutional effect on all the coagulation factors and platelet count, they may further interfere with and inhibit haemostasis to variable degrees. Dextran has been shown to accelerate the action of thrombin on fibrinogen (thus shortening the thrombin time), to reduce plasma levels of factor VIII and von Willebrand's factor and induce an acquired von Willebrand's disease and, due to adsorption onto the platelet surface, to cause decreased platelet adhesiveness and aggregation by steric blockage of the surface membrane receptors.[182] These defects are additive and dose-dependent and may significantly prolong the bleeding time and activated partial thromboplastin time and predispose to clinical bleeding episodes. Similarly, hydroxyethyl starch, due to its macromolecular properties, will induce a slight shortening of the thrombin time and similar factor VIII defects *in vitro*,[183] but these effects are of negligible clinical significance with infused volumes of up to 1500 ml.[184] Human albumin solutions infused in large volumes have also been shown to further inhibit haemostasis, possibly by decreasing hepatic synthesis or by the presence of prekallikrein activator in the infused solution stimulating fibrinolysis.[195] The modified gelatins, although absorbed onto the platelet surface, do not induce any inhibitory haemostatic defect. However, gelatin solutions have been shown to significantly decrease plasma fibronectin levels and inhibit fibronectin function by gelatin–fibronectin interactions. This may potentially decrease the opsonization of noxious material and subsequent phagocytosis by the reticulo-endothelial system and delay early wound healing and cross-linkage of fibrin by Factor XIIIa.

REFERENCES

1. Machin, S.J. Haemostasis and blood clotting. In *Physiology in Surgical Practice* (eds M. Hobsley & F. Imms). Edward Arnold, London (in press).
2. Machin, S.J. & Preston, F.E. Guidelines on platelet function tests: prepared for BSH Haemostasis and Thrombosis Task Force. *J. Clin. Pathol.* **41**: 1322–30, 1988.
3. Mackie, I.J. & Neal, C.R. The platelet. In *Platelet–Vessel Wall Interactions* (eds R.M. Pittilo & S.J. Machin), pp. 1–32. Springer-Verlag, London, 1987.
4. Sixma, J.J., Sakariassen, K.S., Beeser-Visser, N.H., Ottenhof-Rovers, M. & Bolhuis, P.A. Adhesion of platelets to human artery subendothelium: effect of factor VIII–von Willebrand factor of various multimeric compositions. *Blood* **63**: 128–39, 1984.
5. Giddings, J.C. von Willebrand factor-physiology. In *Vascular Endothelium in Haemostasis and Thrombosis* (ed. M.A. Gimbrene), pp. 142–68. Churchill Livingstone, Edinburgh, 1986.
6. Ruggeri, Z.M. & Zimmermann, T.S. von Willebrand factor and von Willebrand disease. *Blood* **70**: 895–904, 1987.
7. Nurden, A.T. Platelet membrane glycoproteins and their clinical aspects. In *Thrombosis and Haemostasis* (eds M. Verstraete, J. Vermylen, R. Lijnen & J. Arnout). Leuven University Press, 1987.
8. Born, G.V., Bergquist, D. & Arfors, K.E. Evidence for inhibition of platelet

activation in blood by a drug effect on erythrocytes. *Nature* **259**: 233–5, 1976.

9. Haslam, R.J. Signal transduction in platelet activation. In *Thrombosis and Huemostasis* (eds M. Verstraete, J. Vermylen, R. Lijnen & J. Arnout), pp. 147–74. Leuven University Press, 1987.

10. Smith, J.B. Prostaglandins in platelet aggregation and haemostasis. In *Haemostasis and Thrombosis* (eds A.L. Bloom & D.P. Thomas), pp. 78–89. Churchill Livingstone, Edinburgh, 1987.

11. Bull, H.A. & Machin, S.J. The haemostatic function of the vascular endothelial cell. *Blut* **55**: 71–80, 1987.

12. Chignard, M., Le Couedic, J.P., Vargaftig, B.B. & Benveniste, J. Platelet activating factor (PAF-acether) secretion from platelets: effect of aggregating agents. *Br. J. Haematol.* **46**: 455–64, 1980.

13. Zwaal, R.F.A. & Hemker, H.C. Blood cell membranes and haemostasis. *Haemostasis* **11**: 12–39, 1982.

14. Nawroth, P.P, Handley, D.A. & Stern, D.M. The multiple levels of endothelial cell-coagulation factor interactions. *Clin. Haematol.* **15**: 293–322, 1986.

15. Moncada, S. & Higgs, E.A. Arachidonate metabolism in blood cells and the vessel wall. *Clin. Haematol.* **15**: 273–92, 1986.

16. Machin, S.J. & Mackie, I.J. Haemostasis. In *Laboratory Haematology* (ed. I. Chanarin). Churchill Livingstone, Edinburgh, 1989.

17. Robbins, G. & Barnard, D.L. Thrombocytosis and microthrombocytosis: A clinical evaluation of 372 cases. *Acta Haematol.* **70**: 175–82, 1983.

18. Gilmer, P.R., Williams, L.J. & Bessman, J.D. Spuriously elevated platelet count due to microspherocytes. *Am. J. Clin. Pathol.* **78**: 259, 1982.

19. Harker, L.A. & Finch, C.A. Thombokinetics in man. *J. Clin. Invest.* **48**: 963–74, 1969.

20. Harker, L.A. & Sclichter, S.J. The bleeding time as a screening test for the evaluation of platelet function. *N. Engl. J. Med.* **287**: 155–9, 1972.

21. Remuzzi, G. Bleeding in renal failure. *Lancet* **I**: 1205–8, 1988.

22. Poller, L., Thomsen, J.M. & Tomenson, J.A. The bleeding time: current practice in the UK. *J. Clin. Lab. Haematol.* **6**: 369–73, 1984.

23. Yardumian, D.A., Mackie, I.J. & Machin, S.J. Laboratory investigation of platelet function – a review of methodology. *J. Clin. Pathol.* **39**: 701–12, 1986.

24. Packham, M.A. & Mustard, J.F. Clinical pharmacology of platelets. *Blood* **50**: 555–67, 1977.

25. Ross, R. & Glomset, J.A. The pathogenenesis of atherosclerosis: I and II. *N. Engl. J. Med.* **295**: 420–5, 1976.

26. Wu, K.K. & Hoak, J.C. A new method for the quantitative detection of platelet aggregation in patients with arterial insufficiency. *Lancet* **II**: 924–6, 1974.

27. Fialkow, P.S., Fagnet, G.B., Jacobson, R.J., Vaidya, K. & Murphy, S. Evidence that essential thrombocythaemia is a colonal disorder with origin in a multipotent stem cell. *Blood* **58**: 916–19, 1981.

28. Singh, A.K. & Wetherley-Mein, G. Microvascular occlusive events in primary thrombocythaemia. *Br. J. Haematol.* **36**: 553–64, 1977.

29. Levine, J. & Swanson, P.D. Idiopathic thrombocytosis. *Neurology* **18**: 711–13, 1968.

30. Virmani, R., Popovsky, M. & Roberts, W.C. Thrombocytosis, coronary thrombosis and acute myocardial infarction. *Am. J. Med.* **67**: 498–506, 1979.

31. Kessler, C.M., Klein, H.G. & Harlik, R.J. Uncontrolled thrombocytosis in chronic myeloproliferative disorders. *Br. J. Haematol.* **50**: 157–62, 1982.

32. Murphy, S., Iland, H., Rosenthal, D. & Lazlo, J. Essential thrombocythaemia: an interim report from the Polycythaemia Vera Study Group. *Semin. Haematol.* **23**: 132–43, 1986.

33. Fuscaldo, K.E., Erlick, B.J., Fuscaldo, A.A. *et al.* Correlation of a specific chromosome marker. 21q-, and retroviral indicators in patients with thrombo-

cythaemia. *Cancer Lett.* **6**: 51–6, 1979.
34. Hartmann, R.C., Auditore, J.V. & Jackson, D.P. Studies on thrombocytosis. I. Hyperkalaemia due to release of potassium from platelets during coagulation. *J. Clin. Invest.* **37**: 699–707, 1958.
35. Hess, C.E., Nichols, A.B., Hunt, W.B. & Small, P.M. Pseudohypoxaemia secondary to leukaemia and thrombocytosis. *N. Engl. J. Med.* **301**: 361–3, 1979.
36. Wu, K.K. Platelet hyperaggregability and thrombosis in patients with thrombocythaemia. *Ann. Intern. Med.* **88**: 7–11, 1978.
37. Kaywin, P., McDonough, M., Insel, P.A. & Shattil, S.J. Platelet function in essential thrombocythaemia. Decreased epinephrine responsiveness associated with a deficiency of platelet alpha-adrenergic receptors. *N. Engl. J. Med.* **299**: 505–9, 1978.
38. Walsh, P.N., Murphy, S. & Barry, W.E. The role of platelets in the pathogenesis of thrombosis and haemorrhage in patients with thrombocytosis. *Thromb. Haemost.* **38**: 1085–96, 1977.
39. Schafer, A.I. Deficiency of platelet lipoxygenase in myeloproliferative disorders. *N. Engl. J. Med.* **306**: 381, 1982.
40. Boughton, B.J., Corbelt, W.E.N. & Ginsberg, A.D. Myeloproliferative disorders: a paradox of *in vivo* and *in vitro* platelet function. *J. Clin. Pathol.* **30**: 228, 1977.
41. Schafer, A.I. Bleeding and thrombosis in the myeloproliferative disorders. *Blood* **64**: 1–12, 1984.
42. Wassermann, L.R. & Gilbert, H.S. Surgery in polycythaemia vera. *N. Engl. J. Med.* **269**: 1226–30, 1963.
43. Kushner, J.P., Lee, G.R., Wintrobe, M.M & Cartwright, G.E. Idiopathic refractory sideroblastic anaemia. Clinical and laboratory investigation of 17 patients and review of the literature. *Medicine* **50**: 139–59, 1971.
44. Mahmood, T., Robinson, W.A., Hamstra, R.D. & Wallner, S.F. Macrocytic anaemia, thrombocytosis and nonlobulated megakaryocytes. The 5q-syndrome, a distinct entity. *Am. J. Med.* **66**: 946–50, 1979.
45. Shulman, N.R. & Jordan, J.V. Platelet kinetics. In *Haemostasis and Thrombosis* (eds R.W. Colman, J. Hirsh, V.B.J. Marder & E.W. Salzman). J.B. Lippincott Co, Philadelphia, 1987.
46. Boxer, M.A., Braun, J. & Ellman, L. Thromboembolic risk of postsplenectomy thrombocytosis. *Arch. Surg.* **113**: 808–9, 1978.
47. Hirsh, J. & Dacie, J.V. Persistent postsplenectomy thrombocytosis and thromboembolism: A consequence of continuing anaemia. *Br. J. Haematol.* **12**: 44, 1966.
48. Tso, S.C., Chan, T.K. & Todd, D. Venous thrombosis in haemoglobin H disease after splenectomy. *Aust. NZ J. Med.* **12**: 635–8, 1982.
49. Hirsh, J., McBride, J.A. & Dacie, J.V. Thromboembolism and increased platelet adhesiveness in post-splenectomy thrombocytosis. *Austral. Ann. Med. Sci.* **15**: 122–8, 1966.
50. Quick, A.J. Biochemistry of clotting factors in tissues and erythrocytes. *Proc. 4th Int. Congr. Biochem*, Vienna, 1958 (ed. E. Deutsch). Symposium X: Blood clotting factors, Pergamon Press, London, 1959.
51. Rabiner, S.F. & Rosenfield, S. Role of intravascular haemolysis and the reticuloendothelial system in the production of the hypercoagulable state. *J. Lab. Clin. Med.* **62**: 1005, 1963.
52. Kitchens, C.S. The syndrome of post-splenectomy fulminant sepsis. Case report and review of the literature. *Am. J. Med. Sci.* **270**: 523–4, 1975.
53. Knizley, H. & Noyes, W.D. Iron deficiency anaemia, papilloedema, thrombocytosis, and transient hemiparesis. *Arch. Intern. Med.* **129**: 483–6, 1972.
54. Steiner, R.W., Coggins, C. & Carvalho, A.C. Bleeding time in uraemia: a useful test to assess clinical bleeding. *Am. J. Haematol.* **7**: 107–17, 1979.
55. Livio, M., Gotti, E., Marchesi, D., Remuzzi, G., Mecca, G. & Gaetano, G.

Uraemic bleeding: role of anaemia and beneficial effects of red cell transfusions. *Lancet* ii: 1013–15, 1982.

56. Moia, M., Mannucci, P.M., Vizzatto, L., Casati, S., Cattaneo, M. & Ponticelli, C. Improvement in the haemostatic defect of uraemia after treatment with recombinant human erythropoietin. *Lancet* ii: 1227–9, 1987.

57. Lombardi, R., Mannucci, P.M., Seghatchian, M.J., Garcia, V.V. & Coppola, R. Alterations of factor VIII:von Willebrand factor in clinical conditions associated with an increase in its plasma concentration. *Br. J. Haematol.* **49**: 61–8, 1981.

58. Turney, J.H., Woods, H.F., Fewell, M.R. & Weston, M.J. Factor VIII complex in uraemia and effects of haemodialysis. *Br. Med. J.* **282**, 1663, 1981.

59. Mannucci, P.M., Remuzzi, G., Pusineri, F. *et al.* Deamino-8-D-arginine vasopressin shortens the bleeding time in uraemia. *N. Engl. J. Med.* **308**: 8–12, 1983.

60. Castaldi, P.A. & Gorman, D.J. Disordered platelet function in renal disease. In *Haemostasis and Thrombosis: Basic Principles and Clinical Practice* (eds R.W. Colman, J. Hirsh, V.J. Marder & E.W. Salzman), pp. 57–71. J.B. Lippincott, Philadelphia, 1987.

61. Eknoyan, G. & Brown, C.H. Biochemical abnormalities of platelets in renal failure: Evidence for decreased platelet serotonin, adenosine diphosphate, and Mg-dependent adenosine triphosphate. *Am. J. Nephrol.* **1**: 17–23, 1981.

62. Remuzzi, G., Benigni, A., Dodesini, A. *et al.* Reduced thromboxane formation in uraemia: evidence for a functional cyclo-oxygenase defect. *J. Clin. Invest.* **71**: 762–8, 1983.

63. Gura, V., Creter, D. & Levi, J. Elevated thrombocyte calcium content in uraemia and its correction by 1 alpha (OH) vitamin D treatment. *Nephron* **30**: 237–9, 1982.

64. Balilinski, N., Shaykh, M., Dunea, G., Mamdani, B., Patel, A., Czapek, E. & Ahmed, S. Inhibition of platelet function by uraemic middle molecules. *Nephron* **40**: 423–8, 1985.

65. Zusman, R.M., Rubin, R.H., Cato, A.E., Cocchetto, D.M., Crow, J.W. & Tolkoff-Rubin, N. Haemodialysis using prostacyclin instead of heparin as the sole antithrombotic agent. *N. Engl. J. Med.* **304**: 934–9, 1981.

66. Janson, P.A., Jubeliver, S.J., Weinstein, M.S. & Deykin, D. Treatment of bleeding tendency in uraemia with cryoprecipitate. *N. Engl. J. Med.* **303**; 1318, 1980.

67. Mannucci, P.M. Desmopressin: a nontransfusional form of treatment for congenital and acquired bleeding disorders. *Blood* **72**: 1449–55, 1988.

68. Livio, M., Mannucci, P.M., Vigano, G. *et al.* Conjugated oestrogens for the management of bleeding associated with renal failure. *N. Engl. J. Med.* **315**: 731–5, 1986.

69. Capitano, A., Mannucci, P.M., Ponticelli, C. & Pareti, F. Detection of circulating released platelets after renal transplantation. *Transplantation* **33**: 298–301, 1982.

70. Mundy, A.R., Bewick, M., Moncada, S. & Vane, J.R. Short term suppression of hyperacute renal allograft rejection in presensitized dogs with prostacyclin. *Prostaglandins* **19**: 595–603, 1980.

71. Neild, G.H., Reuben, R., Hartley, R.B. & Cameron, J.S. Glomerular thrombosis in renal allografts associated with cyclosporin therapy. *J. Clin. Pathol.* **38**: 253–8, 1985.

72. Mihatsch, M.J., Thiel, G., Spichtin, H.P. *et al.* Morphological changes in kidney transplants after treatment with cyclosporine. *Transplant Proc.* **15**: 2821–41, 1983.

73. Neild, G.H., Rocchi, G., Imberti, L. *et al.* Effect of cyclosporin A on prostacyclin synthesis by vascular tissue. *Thromb. Res.* **32**: 373–9, 1983.

74. Cohen, H. M.D. Thesis, Manchester University. pp. 168–188, 1989.

75. Perico, N., Benigni, A., Zoja, C., *et al.* Functional significance of exaggerated renal thromboxane A_2 synthesis induced by cyclosporin A. *Am. J. Physiol.* **251**:

F581–7, 1986.

76. Cohen, H., Neild, G.H., Patil, R. *et al.* Evidence for chronic platelet hyperaggregability and *in vivo* activation for cyclosporin-treated renal allograft recipients. *Thromb. Res.* **49**: 91–101, 1988.

77. Frampton, G., Parbatani, A., Marchesi, D. *et al. In vivo* platelet activation and *in vitro* hyperaggregability to arachidonic acid in renal allograft recipients. *Kidney International* **23**: 506–13, 1983.

78. Joist, J.H. Haemostatic abnormalities in liver disease. In *Haemostasis and Thrombosis* (eds R.W. Colman, J. Hirsh, V.J. Marder & E.W. Salzman). J.P. Lippincott, Philadelphia, 1987.

79. Stein, S.E. & Harker, L.A. Kinetic and functional studies of platelets, fibrinogen and plasminogen in patients with hepatic cirrhosis. *J. Lab. Clin. Med.* **99**: 217, 1982.

80. Mandel, E.F. & Lazerson, J. Thrombasthenia in liver disease. *N. Engl. J. Med.* **265**: 56, 1961.

81. Thomas, D.P., Ream, V.J. & Stuart, R.K. Platelet aggregation in patients with Laennec's cirrhosis of the liver. *N. Engl. J. Med.* **276**: 1342, 1967.

82. Castillo, R., Morragau, S., Rodes, J. *et al.* Increased factor VIII complex and defective ristocetin-induced platelet aggregation in liver disease. *Thromb. Res.* **11**: 899, 1977.

83. Owen, J.S., Hutton, R.A., Day, R.C. *et al.* Platelet lipid composition and platelet aggregation in human liver disease. *J. Lipid Res.* **22**: 423, 1981.

84. Langley, P.G., Hughes, R.D. & Williams, R. Platelet adhesiveness to glass beads in liver disease. *Acta Haematol.* **67**: 124, 1982.

85. Ballard, H.S. & Marcus, A.J. Platelet aggregation in portal cirrhosis. *Arch. Intern. Med.* **136**: 316, 1976.

86. Solum, N.O., Rigollot, C., Budzynski, A.Z. & Marder, V.J. A quantitative evaluation of the inhibition of platelet aggregation by low molecular weight degradation products of fibrinogen. *Br. J. Haematol.* **24**: 619, 1973.

87. Burroughs, A.K., Matthews, K., Wadiri, M., Thomas, N., Kernoff, P.B.A., Tuddenham, E.G.D. & MacIntyre, N. Desmopressin and bleeding time in patients with cirrhosis. *Br. Med. J.* **291**: 1377, 1985.

88. Mannucci, P.M., Vicente, V., Vianello, L., Cattaneo, M., Alberca, I., Coccato, M.P., Faioni, E. & Mari, D. Controlled trial of desmopressin (DDAVP) in liver cirrhosis and other conditions associated with a prolonged bleeding time. *Blood* **67**: 1148, 1986.

89. Machin, S.J. Thrombotic thrombocytopenic purpura. *Br. J. Haematol.* **56**: 191–7, 1984.

90. Levin, M. & Barratt, J.M. Haemolytic uraemic syndrome. *Arch. Dis. Childh.* **59**: 397–400, 1984.

91. Byrnes, J.J. & Moake, J.L. Thrombotic thrombocytopenic purpura and the haemolytic–uraemic syndrome: Evolving concepts in the pathogenesis and therapy. *Clin. Haematol.* **15**: 413–42, 1986.

92. Moake, J.L., Byrnes, J.J., Troll, J.H., Rudy, C.K., Hong, S.I., Weinstein, M.J. & Colannino, N.M. Effects of fresh-frozen plasma and its cryosupernatant fraction on von Willebrand factor multimeric forms in chronic relapsing thrombotic thrombocytopenic purpura. *Blood* **65**: 1232–6, 1985.

93. Moake, J.L., Byrnes, J.J, Troll, J.H., Rudy, C.K., Weinstein, M.J., Colannino, N.M. & Hong, S.L. Abnormal VIII: von Willebrand factor patterns in the plasma of patients with the haemolytic uraemic syndrome. *Blood* **64**: 592–8, 1984.

94. Rose, P.E., Enayat, S.M., Sunderland, R., Short, P.E., Williams, C.E. & Hill, F.G. Abnormalities of factor VIII related protein multimers in the haemolytic uraemic syndrome. *Arch. Dis. Childh.* **59**: 1135–40, 1984.

95. Burns, E.R. & Zucker-Franklin, D. Pathologic effects of plasma from patients

with thrombotic thrombocytopenic purpura on platelets and cultured vascular endothelial cells. *Blood* **60**: 1030–7, 1982.

96. Leung, D.Y.M., Moake, J.L., Havens, P.L., Kim, M. & Pober, J.S. Lytic anti-endothelial cell antibodies in haemolytic uraemic syndrome. *Lancet* **II**: 183–6, 1988.
97. Shepard, K.V. & Bokowski, R.M. The treatment of thrombotic thrombocytopenic purpura with exchange transfusions, plasma infusions and plasma exchange. *Semin. Haematol.* **24**: 178–93, 1987.
98. Gutterman, L.A. & Stevenson, T.D. Treatment of thrombotic thrombocytopenic purpura with vincristine. *J. Am. Med. Assoc.* **247**: 1433–6, 1982.
99. Rosove, M.H., Ho, W.G. & Goldfinger, D. Ineffectiveness of aspirin and dipyridamole in the treatment of thrombotic thrombocytopenic purpura. *Ann. Intern. Med.* **96**: 27–33, 1982.
100. Collins, J.A. Massive transfusion. *Clin. Haematol.* **5**: 201–27, 1976.
101. Counts, R.B., Haisch, C., Simon, T.L. *et al.* Haemostasis in massively transfused trauma patients. *Ann. Surg.* **190**: 91–9, 1979.
102. Gill, W., Champion, H.R., Lang, W.B., Austin, E.A. & Cowley, R.A. Volume resuscitation in critical major trauma. *J. R. Coll. Surg. Edinburgh* **20**: 166–73, 175, 1975.
103. Mannucci, P.M., Fedrici, A.B. & Sirchia, G. Haemostasis testing during massive blood replacement. *Vox Sanguinis* **42**; 113–23, 1982.
104. Jones, J. Abuse of fresh frozen plasma. *Br. Med. J.* **295**: 287, 1987.
105. Bick, R.L. Haemostasis defects associated with cardiac surgery, prosthetic devices, and other extracorporeal circuits. *Semin. Thromb. Haemost.* **11**: 249–80, 1985.
106. Harker, L.A., Malpass, T.W., Branson, H.E., Hessel, E.A. & Slichter, S.J. Mechanism of abnormal bleeding in patients undergoing cardiopulmonary bypass: acquired transient platelet dysfunction associated with selective alpha-granule release. *Blood* **56**: 824–34, 1980.
107. Mammen, E.F., Koets, M.H., Washington, B.D.C. *et al.* Haaemostasis changes during cardiopulmonary bypass surgery. *Semin. Thromb. Haemost.* **11**: 281–92, 1985.
108. Fish, K.J., Sarnquist, F.H., van Steennis, C. *et al.* A prospective, randomised study of the effects of prostacyclin on platelets and blood loss during coronary bypass operations. *J. Thor. Cardiovas. Surg.* **91**: 436–42, 1986.
109. Salzman, E.W., Weinstei, M.J., Weintraub, R.M. *et al.* Treatment with desmopresin acetate to reduce blood loss after cardiac surgery. A double blind randomised trial. *N. Engl. J. Med.* **314**: 1402–6, 1986.
110. Weinstein, M., Ware, J.A., Troll, J. & Salzman, E. Changes in von Willebrand factor during cardiac surgery: effect of desmopressin acetate. *Blood* **71**: 1648–55, 1988.
111. Pegels, J.G., Bruynes, E.C.E., Engelfriet, C.P. & van dem Borne, A.E.G. Kr. Pseudothrombocytopenia: An immunologic study on platelet antibodies dependent on ethylene diamine tetra-acetate. *Blood* **59**: 157–61, 1982.
112. van Vliet, H.H.D.M., Kappers-Klunne, M.C. & Abels, J. Pseudothrombocytopenia: a cold autoantibody against platelet membrane glycoprotein IIb. *Br. J. Haematol.* **62**: 501, 1986.
113. Berning, H. & Stilbo, I. Pseudothrombocytopenia and the haematology laboratory. *Lancet* **8813**: 1469–70, 1982.
114. Shreiner, D.P. & Bell, W.R. Pseudothrombocytopenia: manifestation of a new type of platelet agglutinin. *Blood* **42**: 541–9, 1973.
115. Watkins, S.P. Jr & Shulman, N.R. Platelet cold agglutinins. *Blood* **36**: 153–8, 1970.
116. Girman, G., Pees, H. & Scheurlen, P.G. Pseudothrombocytopenia and mexiletene. *Ann. Intern. Med.* **100**: 767, 1984.

117. Handin, R.I., McDonough, M. & Lesch, M. Evaluation of platelet factor four in acute myocardial infarction. *J. Lab. Clin. Med.* **91**: 340–7, 1978.
118. Salky, N. & Drydale, M. Platelet abnormalities in ischaemic heart disease. *Am. J. Cardiol.* **32**: 612–18, 1973.
119. Szczeklik, A., Serwanska, M., Lukusiewicz, W. *et al.* Arachidonate versus ADP-induced platelet abnormalities in acute myocardial infarction. *Thromb. Haemost.* **42**: 822–30, 1979.
120. Mehta, P. & Mehta, J. Platelet function studies in coronary heart disease: decreased platelet sensitivity to prostacyclin in patients with myocardial ischaemia. *Thromb. Res.* **18**: 273–7, 1980.
121. Gallus, A.S. The use of antithrombotic drugs in artery disease. *Clin. Haematol.* **15**: 509–59, 1985.
122. Muller, J.E., Stone, P.H., Ture, Z.G. *et al.* Circadian variation in the frequency of onset of acute myocardial infarction. *N. Engl. J. Med.* **313**: 1315–22, 1985.
123. Muller, J.E., Ludmer, P.L., Willich, S.N. *et al.* Circadian variation in the frequency of sudden cardiac death. *Circulation* **75**: 131–8, 1987.
124. Marshall, J. Diurnal variation in occurrence of strokes. *Stroke* **8**: 20–21, 1977.
125. Brezinski, D.A., Tofler, G.H., Muller, J.E. *et al.* Morning increase in platelet aggregability: association with assumption of the upright posture. *Circulation* **78**: 35–40, 1988.
126. Tofler, G.H., Brezinski, D.A., Schafer, Al. *et al.* Concurrent morning increase in platelet aggregability and the risk of myocardial infarction and sudden cardiac death. *N. Engl. J. Med.* **316**: 1514–18, 1987.
127. Antiplatelet trialists' collaboration: Secondary prevention of vascular disease by prolonged antiplatelet treatment. *Br. Med. J.* **296**: 320–31, 1988.
128. Fields, W.S., Lemak, N.A., Frankowski, R.F. & Hardy, R.J. Controlled trial of aspirin in cerebral ischaemia. *Stroke* **8**: 310–16, 1977.
129. Canadian Cooperative Study Group: A randomised trial of aspirin and sulfinpyrazone in threatened stroke. *N. Engl. J. Med.* **299**: 53–9, 1978.
130. Kannel, W.B. & McGee, D.C. Diabetes and cardiovascular disease: The Framingham study. *J. Am. Med. Assoc.* **241**: 2035–8, 1979.
131. Colwell, J.A., Wincour, P.D., Lopes-Virella, M. *et al.* New concepts about the pathogenesis of atherosclerosis in diabetes mellitus. *Am. J. Med.* **75**: 67–80, 1983.
132. Keen, H. & Jarrett, R.S. (eds) *Complications of Diabetes.* Edward Arnold, London, 1975.
133. Mustard, J.F. & Packham, M.A. Editorial retrospective: Platelets and diabetes mellitus. *N. Engl. J. Med.* **311**: 665–6, 1984.
134. Brinkhous, K.M., Sultzer, D.L. Reddick, R.L. *et al.* Elevated plasma von Willebrand factor (vWF) levels as an index of acute endothelial injury: Use of a hypotonic injury model in rats. *Fedn. Proc.* **39**: 630, 1980.
135. Gerrard, J.M., Stuart, M.J., Rao, G.H.R. *et al.* Alteration in the balance of prostaglandin and thromboxane synthesis in diabetic rats. *J. Lab. Clin. Med.* **95**: 950–8, 1980.
136. Stuart, M.J., Sunderji, S.G. & Allen, J.B. Decreased prostacyclin production in the infant of the diabetic mother. *J. Lab. Clin. Med.* **98**: 412–16, 1981.
137. Heaht, H., Brigden, W.D., Canever, J.V., Pollock, J., Hunter, P.R., Kelsey, J. & Bloom, A. Platelet adhesiveness and aggregation in relation to diabetic retinopathy. *Diabetilogica* **7**: 308–15, 1971.
138. Colwell, J.A., Halushka, P.V., Sarki, K.E. & Sagel, J. Platelet function and diabetes mellitus. *Med. Clin. North Am.* **62**: 753–66, 1978.
139. Preston, F.E., Ward, J.D., Mazzola, B., Porter, N.R., Timperley, W.R. & O'Malley, B.C. Elevated β-thromboglobulin levels and circulating aggregates in diabetic microangiopathy. *Lancet* **I**: 238–40, 1978.
140. Ferguson, J.C., Mackay, N., Philip, J.A.D. & Summer, D.J. Determination of platelet and fibrinogen half life with ^{75}Se selenomethionine studies in normal

and diabetic subjects. *Clin. Sci. Molec. Med.* **49**: 115–20, 1975.
141. Betteridge, D.J., El Tahir, K.E.H., Reckless, J.P.D. & Williams, K.I. Platelets from diabetic subjects show diminished sensitivity to prostacyclin. *Eur. J. Clin. Invest.* **12**: 395–8, 1982.
142. Ford, I., Newrick, P.G., Malik, R., Preston, F.E., Ward, J.D. & Greaves, M. Haemostatic parameters, endoneurial oxygen tension and sural nerve histology in diabetes mellitus. *Thromb. Haemost.* **58**: 308 (abstract), 1987.
143. Packham, M.A. & Mustard, J.F. The role of platelets in the development and complications of atherosclerosis. *Semin. Haematol.* **XXIII**: 8–26, 1986.
144. Doll, R. Smoking and death rates. *J. Am. Med. Assoc.* **251**: 2854–7, 1984.
145. Pittilo, R.M. Smoking and platelet–vessel wall interactions. In *Platelet–Vessel Wall Interactions* (eds R.M. Pittilo & S.J. Machin) pp. 87–98. Springer-Verlag, London, 1986.
146. Bull, H.A., Pittilo, R.M., Woolf, N. & Machin, S.J. The effect of nicotine on human endothelial cell release of prostaglandins and ultrastructure. *Br. J. Exp. Pathol.* **69**: 413–22, 1988.
147. Lazlo, E., Kaldi, N. & Kovacs, L. Alterations in plasma proteins and platelet function with ageing and cigarette smoking in healthy men. *Thromb. Haemost.* **49**: 150, 1983.
148. Pittilo, R.M., Clarke, J.M.F., Harris, D., Mackie, I.J., Rowles, P.M., Machin, S.J. & Woolf, N. Cigarette smoking and platelet adhesion. *Br. J. Haematol.* **58**: 627–32, 1984.
149. Sinzinger, H. & Kefalides, A. Passive smoking severely decreases platelet sensitivity to antiaggregating prostaglandins. *Lancet* **II**: 392–3, 1982.
150. Firkin, B.G. Involvement of platelets in non-haematological disorders and thrombosis. In *The Platelet and its Disorders*. Butler & Tanner, London, 1985.
151. Anonymous. Pathophysiology of Raynaud's phenomenon. *Br. Med. J.* **281**: 1027–8, 1980.
152. Hutton, R.A., Mikhailidis, D.P., Bernstein, R.M., Jeremy, J.Y., Hughes, G.V.R. & Dandona, P. Assessment of platelet function in patients with Raynaud's syndrome. *J. Clin. Pathol.* **37**: 182–7, 1984.
153. Mikhailidis, D.P., Hutton, R.A. & Dandona, P. Effect of cooling on prostaglandin mediated inhibition of platelet aggregation. *Clin. Sci.* **61**: 28P, 1981.
154. Mikhailidis, D.P., Hutton, R.A., Jeremy, J.Y. & Dandona, P. Cooling decreases the efficiency of prostaglandin inhibitors of platelet aggregation – a factor of possible relevance in cold induced pathology. *Microcirculation* **2**: 413–24, 1983.
155. Jeremy, J.Y., Mikhailidis, D.P., Hutton, R.A. & Dandona, P. Effect of cooling on prostacyclin-induced increase in intraplatelet cyclic AMP and on prostacyclin production. *Clin. Sci.* **62**: 42P, 1982.
156. Belch, J.J.F., Newman, P., Drury, J.K. *et al.* Intermittent epoprostenol (prostacyclin) infusion in patients with Raynaud's syndrome. *Lancet* **I**: 313–15, 1983.
157. Vanhoutte, P.M. & Shepherd, J.T. Effect of temperature on reactivity of isolated cutaneous veins of the dog. *Am. J. Physiol.* **218**: 187–90, 1970.
158. Van Neuten, J.M. Serotonergic amplification mechanisms in vascular tissues. In *5-Hydroxytryptamine in Peripheral Reactions* (eds F. De Clerck & P.M. Vanhoutte), pp. 77–82. Raven Press, New York, 1982.
159. Raold, O.K. & Seem, E. Treatment of Raynaud's phenomenon with ketanserin in patients with connective tissue disorders. *Br. Med. J.* **289**, 577–9, 1984.
160. Verstraete, M. & Machin, S.J. (eds) Clinical usage of heparin: present and future trends. *Scand. J. Haematol.* **25**: (Suppl. 36), 1980.
161. Green, D., Morris, K. & Reynolds, N. Heparin immune thrombocytopenia: evidence for a heparin platelet complex as the antigenic determinant. *J. Lab.*

Clin. Med. **91**: 167–72, 1978.
162. Mikhailidis, D.P., Barradas, M.A., Mikhailidis, A.M., Magnani, H. & Dandona, P. Comparison of the effect of a conventional heparin and a low molecular weight heparinoid on platelet function. *Br. J. Clin. Pharmacol.* **13**: 75–92, 1984.
163. Cazenove, J.P., Packham, M.A., Gucciane, M.A. & Mustard, J.F. Effects of penicillin G on platelet aggregation, release and adherence to collagen. *Proc. Soc. Exp. Biol. Med.* **142**: 159–66, 1973.
164. Ballard, J.O., Barnes, S.G. & Sattler, F.R. Comparison of the effects of the effects of mezlocillin, carbenicillin and placebo on normal haemostasis. *Antimicrob. Agents Chemother.* **25**: 153–6, 1984.
165. Gentry, L.O., Wood, B.A. & Natelson, E.A. Effects of sodium piperacillin on platelet function in normal volunteers. *Antimicrob. Agents Chemother.* **27**: 683–4, 1981.
166. Johnson, G.J., Rao, G.H.R. & White, J.G. Platelet dysfunction induced by parenteral carbenicillin and ticarcillin. *Am. J. Pathol.* **91**: 1440–2, 1978.
167. Johnson, G.J., Leis, L.A., Rao, H.R. & White, J.G. Prostaglandin synthesis remains intact in non-aggregating carbenicillin-treated platelets. *Circulation* **58**: 11, 1978.
168. Shattil, S., Sanford, J. & Bennet, J.S. Carbenicillin and penicillin G inhibit platelet function in vitro by impairing the interaction of agonists with the platelet surface. *J. Clin. Invest.* **65**: 329–37, 1980.
169. Padfield, J.M. & Kellaway, I.W. Rheological studies on mixed phospholipid sols and their interactions with penicillins: I. Continuous shear viscometry. *Chem. Phys. Lipids* **10**: 356–68, 1973.
170. Sattler, F.R., Weitekamp, M.R. & Ballard, J.O. Potential for bleeding with new beta-lactam antibiotics. *Ann. Intern. Med.* **105**: 924–31, 1986.
171. Bowcock, S., Mackie, I.J., Ho, D., Moulsdale, M., Billing, S.P. & Machin, S.J. Effects of various doses of latamoxef (moxalactam) on haemostasis. *J. Hosp. Infection* **8**: 193–9, 1986.
172. Weitkampe, M.R., Caputo, G.M., Al-Mondhiry, H.A.B. & Aber, R.C. The effects of latamoxef, cefotaxime, and cefaperazone on platelet function and coagulation in normal volunteers. *J. Antimicrob. Chemother.* **16**: 95–101, 1985.
173. Cohen, H., Mackie, I.J., Walshe, K. & Machin, S.J. The effects of cefotetan disodium on haemostasis. *J. Hosp. Infection* **10**: 51–7, 1987.
174. Weitekampe, M.R., Holmes, P. & Walker, P. A double-blinded study of the effects of cefoperazone (CPZ), ceftizoxime (CTZ), moxalactam (MOX), and placebo, (P) on platelet function and prothrombin time in normal volunteers (abstr 959). In *Program and Abstracts – 25th Interscience Conference on Antimicrobial Agents and Chemotherapy*, Minneapolis, Minnesota. Washington, D.C. American Society for Microbiology, 1985.
175. Tartaglione, T.A., Duma, R.J. & Quershi, G.D. *In vitro* and *in vivo* studies of the effect of aztreonam on platelet function and coagulation in normal volunteers. *Antimicrob. Agents Chemother.* **30**: 73–7, 1986.
176. Zieman, M., Shah, P.M., Bussman, H. & Breddin, H.K. Haemostasis during imipenam-cilastatin, therapy. *Infection* **14** (Suppl. 2): 139–42, 1986.
177. Brown, R.B., Klar, J., Lemeshow, S., Teres, D., Pastides, H. & Sands, M. Enhanced bleeding with cefoxitin or moxalactam: statistical analysis within a defined population of 1,493 patients. *Arch. Intern. Med.* **146**: 2159–64, 1986.
178. Mackie, I.J., Walshe, K., Cohen, H., McCarthy, P., Shearer, M., Scott, S., Karran, S.J. & Machin, S.J. The effects of an N-methyl-thiotetrazole cephalosporin on haemostasis in patients with reduced serum vitamin K_1 levels. *J. Clin. Pathol.* **39**: 1245–9, 1986.
179. Cowan, D.H. Effects of alcoholism on haemostasis. *Semin. Haematol.* **XVII**(2): 137–48, 1980.
180. Fink, R. & Hutton, R.A. Changes in the blood platelets of alcoholics during

alcohol withdrawal. *J. Clin. Pathol.* **36**: 337–40, 1983.

181. MacIntyre, E., Bullen, C. & Machin, S.J. Fluid replacement in hypovolaemia. *Intensive Care Med.* **11**: 231–3, 1985.

182. Mischlcr, J.M. Synthetic plasma volume expanders – their pharmacology, safety and clincial efficacy. *Clin. Haematol.* **13**: 75–92, 1984.

183. MacIntyre, E., Mackie, I.J., Ho, D., Tinker, J., Bullen, C. & Machin, S.J. The haemostatic effects of hydroxyethyl starch (HES) used as volume expander. *Intensive Care Med.* **11**: 301–4, 1985.

184. Lockwood, D.N.J., Bullen, C. & Machin, S.J. A severe coagulopathy following volume replacement with hydroxy ethyl starch in a Jehovah's Witness. *Anaesthesia* **43**; 391–3, 1988.

185. Lucas, C.E., Legerwood, A.M. & Mammen, E.P. Altered coagulation protein content after albumin resuscitation. *Ann. Surg.* **197**: 198–202, 1982.

7

Haemostatic defects

J.L. Hanslip
Lecturer in Ageing and Health, Ninewells Hospital and Medical School, Dundee, UK

C.D. Forbes
Professor and Hon. Consultant Physician, Ninewells Hospital and Medical School, Dundee, UK

CONTROL OF NORMAL HAEMOSTASIS

Haemostasis, the response of the body to vessel injury, results in the arrest of bleeding by the following mechanisms:

1. Local vascular constriction to decrease blood flow.
2. Platelet–vessel wall interaction with the formation of a haemostatic plug which will mechanically plug bleeding points in a vessel.
3. Local blood coagulation with the formation of a fibrin clot – the 'coagulation cascade'.
4. Appropriate fibrinolytic activity.

Normally, in undamaged vessels, these potential mechanisms are balanced in such a way that blood can flow freely through vessels until injury triggers the haemostatic system. The commonest and most important causes of bleeding are associated with defects in the formation of the haemostatic plug and fibrin clot. However, significant clinical bleeding can arise as a result of vascular abnormalities and abnormal fibrinolytic activity.

The vascular component and formation of a haemostatic plug

Following shearing injury to a vessel, there is rapid vasoconstriction which, initially, may completely prevent blood loss. The immediate vasoconstrictive response is mediated by local reflexes with little or no central control and is observed in denervated blood vessels. The artery wall may release vasconstrictor substances, e.g. angiotensin II, but serotonin and thromboxane A_2 liberated from platelets probably exert the main chemical vasoconstrictive effect.[1]

Tissue thromboplastin is the most important of the substances released from the vessel wall after injury. It is a lipoprotein which promotes haemostasis through combination with Factor VII, resulting in activation of the extrinsic coagulation pathway. Haemostasis at the vessel wall is likely to be affected by the von Willebrand factor and phospholipids which are released from the membranes of damaged cells. These phospholipids act as an extra source of phospholipid for reactions in the coagulation cascade.

The first cellular event in the haemostatic process is the adhesion of platelets to the collagen that has been exposed by endothelial damage. These platelets release adenine nucleotides and serotonin from specific storage granules. Accompanying this 'adhesion–release' mechanism is a change in the shape of the platelets with the development of surface membrane pseudopodial extensions resulting in 'sticky' platelets, platelet aggregation and platelet plug formation. These events are associated with metabolic changes which include the release of arachidonic acid from phospholipids in the cell membrane and subsequent induction of the prostaglandin pathways.

Prostaglandin I_2 (PGI$_2$, prostacyclin) is synthesized in the vessel wall, mainly by endothelial cells. Both platelet–surface adhesion and reactions between platelets can be inhibited by prostacyclin. Platelet prostaglandins, principally thromboxane A_2, promote platelet aggregation and it is possible that the balance between endothelial and platelet prostaglandin plays an important role in maintaining a fine balance between circulating platelets and the vessel wall. Local trauma alters this balance in favour of platelet adhesion, aggregation, and the formation of a haemostatic plug as described above. Platelets also contribute to coagulation in different ways.[1,2]

Local blood coagulation – the coagulation cascade

Modern understanding of blood coagulation is based on the 'cascade' or 'waterfall' hypothesis, in which each reaction, it was suggested, involved enzymatic conversion of an inactive precursor to an activated form which in turn acted as an enzyme in the activation of the succeeding factor. Although the skeleton of this hypothesis remains valid, it is evident that the system functions through a series of positive and negative feedback loops. The coagulation cascade (see Fig. 7.1) results in the generation of thrombin which produces fibrin from soluble fibrinogen. Appropriate fibrinolysis then takes place. The cascade can be considered in three parts which, *in vivo*, are closely interlinked. These are the intrinsic and extrinsic systems, and the final common pathway of thrombin formation. The plasma coagulation factors involved in the cascade are listed in Table 7.1.

Intrinsic system of coagulation

The intrinsic system is activated when blood comes into contact with non-endothelial surfaces. Normal contact activation requires the presence of Factors XI and XII, pre-kallikrein and high molecular weight (HMW) kininogen. Activated Factor XI, the product of contact activation, is a serine protease enzyme which splits Factor IX. A complex containing activated Factor IX, Factor VIII, calcium and phospholipid activates Factor X, the first molecule in the final common pathway. This reaction takes place on, or very close to the surface of platelets which act as a source of phospholipids in addition to providing a platform for assembly of molecules and an escape from the effect of plasma inhibitors.

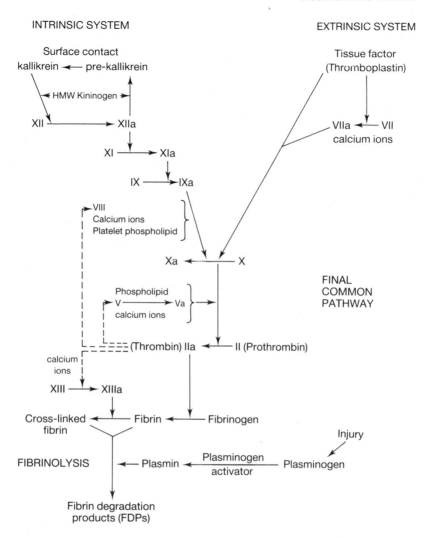

Fig. 7.1. Simplified diagram of the coagulation cascade and the interaction with fibrinolysis. 'a' denotes the active form of the coagulation factor; ----→ indicates known activation activities of thrombin.

Extrinsic system of coagulation

The extrinsic system provides a rapid response to injury. Generation of intrinsic activity in response to a stimulus can take seconds or even minutes, while generation of activated Factor X through the extrinsic system occurs almost immediately. The two unique components in the extrinsic system are tissue factor and Factor VII. Most human cells contain tissue factor. Factor X is activated by a complex containing tissue factor, activated Factor VII, calcium and phospholipid.

Table 7.1   The International Nomenclature of Clotting Factors

Factor	Common synonyms
I	Fibrinogen
II	Prothrombin
III	Thromboplastin (tissue factor)
IV	Calcium
V	Pro-accelerin
VI	No longer used
VII	Proconvertin
VIII	Anti-haemophilic factor (AHF)
	Anti-haemophilic globulin (AHG)
IX	Christmas factor
	Plasma thromboplastin component (PTC)
X	Stuart–Prower factor
XI	Plasma thromboplastin antecedent (PTA)
XII	Hageman factor, contact factor
XIII	Fibrin stabilizing factor
	Plasma transamidase

Final common pathway

The intrinsic and extrinsic systems converge on Factor X. Activated Factor X forms a complex with Factor V, calcium and phospholipid and thrombin is formed from prothrombin in a two-stage reaction. This reaction probably occurs on platelet plasma membranes and it is thought that platelet binding of activated Factor X results in increased thrombin generation. Factor V also appears to act as a surface binding agent, the binding of activated Factor X being reduced or absent in platelets from patients with congenital Factor V deficiency.

Coagulation inhibitors

Known inhibitory mechanisms regulating blood coagulation include neutralization of the serine protease enzymes – Factors IXa, Xa and thrombin – by the protease inhibitors antithrombin III and heparin cofactor II, and inhibition of the cofactors – Factors VIIIa and Va – by activated protein C.[6] Antithrombin III is the significant inhibitor of coagulation function in plasma and it has heparin-accelerated inhibitory activity against activated Factors XII, XI, IX, X and plasmin as well as thrombin. Congenital deficiency of antithrombin III resulting in a high risk of thromboembolism has been described in some families.

The above inhibitory mechanisms modulate the intermediate and late steps of blood coagulation. Little is yet known about inhibitory mechanisms that modulate the initiation of coagulation via the extrinsic pathway; however, a recent report described a mechanism inhibiting the initiation of the extrinsic coagulation pathway.[3]

Interactions between coagulation and other systems

Interactions exist between other physiological systems and blood clotting. Contact activation can cause generation of plasminogen activator, kinins, vascular permeability enhancing factor and chemotactic peptides. Activated Factor XII can initiate the formation of kallikrein from plasma pre-kallikrein and subsequently, kallikrein releases bradykinin from kininogens in plasma. Kinins produce effects on blood vessels, smooth muscles and vessel wall permeability.

Fibrin formation and fibrinolyis

Thrombin is essential for the conversion of fibrinogen to fibrin. Thrombin and fibrinogen in a pure system form a fragile unstable clot. Factor XIII stabilizes the fibrin clot. Once haemostasis is secured, there is concurrent activation of the fibrinolytic system to remove thrombus. Normally, plasminogen and fibrinogen are closely associated and as fibrin forms, both activator and plasminogen bind to it. Fibrinolysis evolves slowly and it only disturbs haemostasis when extensive tissue damage results in the production of large amounts of plasmin and the rapid dissolution of developing clots. This is discussed further later in the chapter.

TESTS OF HAEMOSTATIC FUNCTION

The screening tests commonly employed in the investigation of haemostatic disorders are the prothrombin time, partial thromboplastin time and the thrombin time. The prothrombin time, now usually reported as the international normalized ratio (INR) tests the extrinsic coagulation pathway and is prolonged by reduced levels of Factors VII, X, V, II and fibrinogen. The activated partial thromboplastin time (aPTT) and the kaolin cephalin clotting time (KCCT) test the intrinsic pathway and reflect changes in Factors VIII, IX, X, XI, XII and defects of the contact phase. To a lesser extent, the aPTT is prolonged by deficiencies in Factors II, V and fibrinogen.[4] Heparin also causes prolongation of the aPTT. The thrombin time detects abnormalities of the final common pathway and is prolonged by abnormalities in fibrinogen, raised fibrin degradation products (FDPs), and the presence of heparin.

If prolonged clotting times are found which can be corrected by the addition of normal plasma, a deficiency in coagulation factor(s) is present. No correction suggests the presence of an inhibitor as the immunoglobulin inactivates the clotting factor added. Once the above screening tests have helped to localize a haemostatic defect into one of the pathways, more specific tests, e.g. factor assays or inhibitor screens, will provide further information.[5]

GENERAL HAEMOSTATIC DEFECTS

Disorders of blood vessels

Simple easy bruising

This is a normal variant and is found usually in young women. Often single or multiple bruises appear spontaneously, usually on the upper arms, thighs and calves. The size of the bruise is usually less than 2 cm and it rapidly resolves. It is usually for cosmetic reasons that these patients present to their doctors. No changes in haemostatic factors are found and the patient (and relatives) can be reassured. It has sometimes been suggested that these patients bruise more readily after taking aspirin.

Senile purpura

Senile purpura is found commonly in the elderly, usually on areas exposed to recurrent trauma, i.e. backs of hands, wrists, forearms and face. The lesions may also be called 'age spots'. There are no abnormalities in tests of haemostasis but when the 'simplate' bleeding time is performed on the forearm the blood may seep subcutaneously to produce a typical lesion. These are usually dark purple to red and retain their colour for several weeks before turning brown.[7] With ageing it is now accepted that there is progressive loss of collagen and elastic fibres in the skin and this leads to lack of support for small blood vessels. Shearing forces lead to rupture and subcutaneous extravasation of blood. In some patients there has been shown to be defective cross-linking of collagen fibres[8] and in addition it has been suggested that there may be a reduction in phagocytic function of leucocytes which would normally rapidly reduce the red cells in the tissues to bilirubin. There is no specific treatment of value.

Congenital vascular disorders

This group includes hereditary haemorrhagic telangiectasia and giant cavernous haemangiomata. Both are rare but tend to be collected as curiosities in haematology clinics.

Hereditary haemorrhagic telangiectasia

This condition is transmitted as an autosomal dominant and the family of a diagnosed patient should be examined. The lesions are very typical telangiectasia and may be found in the mucous membranes of the nose, the whole alimentary tract (particularly on lips and mouth), skin (especially face and hands), in the urinary tract, vagina and lung. The lesions occur as individual venules or in small groups which are thin walled with no supporting muscular layer. They blanch easily on pressure with a glass slide and bleed easily when scratched. Because of absence of supporting structures they bleed for a prolonged period. With age the lesions tend to become more marked and new lesions appear. The liability to bleed also increases with advancing years. The commonest presentations are epistaxis and alimentary bleeding presenting as chronic iron deficiency anaemia.

In the majority of patients, no abnormality is present in tests of coagulation or platelet function. In a few patients there have been descriptions of associated Factor VIII deficiency or von Willebrand's disease. Diagnosis is based on the clinical history, family history and detection of the typical lesions. This may require endoscopy for gastric lesions or speculum examination for those on the nasal septum. There is no specific treatment of value. Recurrent iron deficiency may respond adequately to oral iron. Nasal bleeding requires local measures which include packing, balloon compression, topical agents (such as thrombin), local cautery and occasionally plastic surgery.[9] Use of oestrogens to convert columnar epithelium to stratified squamous epithelium may be of some value in individual patients[10] but others have failed to confirm this.[11] When the lesions are the source of blood loss from the upper alimentary tract they may be amenable to laser therapy via an endoscope. Bleeding from other sources such as kidney, vagina and lung may be recurrently troublesome and are usually treated conservatively. In the lung, arterio-venous malformations may result in profuse haemorrhage.[12]

The disease is also known eponomously as Rendu–Weber–Osler disease after its original descriptors.[13–15]

Giant cavernous haemangioma

These thin-walled venous abnormalities appear on the skin within a few months of birth and gradually enlarge up until puberty. They may also be found in internal organs especially the liver and spleen. They are not associated with any haemostatic defect in their own right, however they may very rarely be associated with disseminated intravascular coagulation (see later) with general effects on platelets and coagulation and prolongation of the bleeding time.[16] Spontaneous regression may occur in later life due to formation of microthrombi. Reduction of size of the lesions may be attempted with radiotherapy, laser therapy or with micro-embolization techniques.

Angio-keratoma corporis diffusum (Fabry's disease)

This is an extremely rare disorder of glycolipid metabolism and is due to deficiency of an enzyme found in skin fibroblasts (trihexosyl ceramide galactosyl hydrolase). The patient may present with renal involvement or to the dermatologists with multiple dark reddish-blue telangiectasia in the skin, especially of the trunk, thighs, scrotum and elbows. Other organs are also involved and lipid deposits may be found in the cerebral, cardiac and renal vessels which may become occluded.[17] There may also be vasomotor disturbances of the limbs. There are no generalized haemostatic defects. Diagnosis is made by estimation of enzyme levels in fibroblasts or by the finding of typical 'mulberry cells' in urine.

Hereditary connective tissue disorders

These are all rare conditions and are usually easily diagnosed from the clinical point of view. The resultant haemostatic disorders are usually mild to moderate.

Ehlers–Danlos syndrome[18,19]

This genetic condition is due to a range of defects in collagen and usually presents in families with hyperextensible skin, and hypermobile joints with recurrent episodes of bleeding into the skin and muscles due to poor support of blood vessels.[20] A variety of sub-types have been described, all with different clinical presentations; of interest is sub-type IV in which type III collagen is defective.[21] Recurrent stretching of the skin with subcutaneous haematoma formation leads to thin atrophic skin with paper-like scars over bony prominences. The haemosiderin deposited from the haematoma often colours the skin brown.

As blood vessels all over the body are affected, other sites of bleeding may be troublesome and these include the gut and lung. Major blood vessels also are liable to aneurysm formation and rupture. Bleeding may also occur after minor dental procedures and after surgery. A variety of defects of haemostasis may be found. These include a prolonged bleeding time, and abnormal tests of platelet function, indicating that there may also be structural platelet abnormalities[22] and abnormalities of collagen–platelet interaction. In addition, there have been described associations with Factor IX and XII deficiency.[23,24]

Pseudoxanthoma elasticum

This is a very rare disorder in which the elastic fibres are structurally and functionally abnormal. The skin and major blood vessels are usually affected and this results in the skin being lax with multiple telangiectasia.[25] There is recurrent skin bleeding as a result of the fragile blood vessels and bleeding may also occur from the alimentary tract. The bleeding time may be prolonged but there are no abnormalities of coagulation or platelet function.

Osteogenesis imperfecta

This is a rare disease in which there is an abnormality in type 1 collagen which results in defective bone matrix and resultant multiple fractures. Excess bleeding has been recorded into skin, from the nose, lungs and into the brain. Abnormal platelet function has been recorded but there is no abnormality in coagulation tests.[26]

Marfan's syndrome

The clinical features of this disease are well-documented, with long limbs, spider fingers, dislocation of the patellae and the lenses and aortic valve defects with aneurysm formation in large vessels. There is an abnormality in the cross-linking of collagen which reduces its strength and makes it more soluble.[27] There is a likelihood of excess bleeding after surgery and often lifelong easy bruising. This may be due to a defect in platelet function and an association with a defect in Factor VIII has been reported.[28]

Mechanical purpura

Alterations in capillary pressure are important in producing bleeding. These are difficult to measure but it is possible to measure the point at which capillaries rupture ('capillary fragility test') by application of a sphygmo-manometer cuff to obstruct the venous return (Hess test)[29,30] or alternatively by application of a suction cup to the skin surface and reducing the pressure.[31,32] None of these tests are particularly sensitive or specific for a particular disease. Large numbers of petechiae do appear in patients with thrombocytopenia or thrombasthenia; however, they may also be 'positive' in otherwise normal females and occasionally in diabetes mellitus. With advancing years and a reduction in capillary support the pressures required to cause capillaries to rupture is reduced and this may be an additional factor in the causation of senile purpura.

Increased venous pressure

Rapid rises in venous pressure may cause purpura. This can be seen diffusely after an epileptic seizure, violent coughing and vomiting or may be localized to the head and neck following strangling or obstruction to the superior vena cava. They are of little consequence and will rapidly disappear if the venous pressure returns to normal.

Skin trauma

Purpura and bruising may be produced by suction on the skin either by the persons themselves or by others. Use of suction toys may also produce characteristic lesions. Self-induced lesions are particularly difficult to diagnose in someone who is malingering. They are usually in areas of the body accessible to the mouth or to an instrument. They can be associated with other bleeding sites such as blood in the urine, vaginal bleeding and nasal bleeding, all of which may be induced in an attempt to deceive.

Abuse of a child may also produce multiple unexplained bruises and bleeding and result in referral for haemostatic testing. The characteristic feature of a traumatic bruise is breaking of the skin over the lesion and also marks of the instrument used. Admission to hospital results in regression of the lesions and often a marked cheerfulness of the victim – in contrast to any other normal child.

Metabolic causes of purpura

Scurvy

Scurvy is now a rare condition in clinical practice in the Western World and may now only be seen at the extremes of life. It is due to a deficient intake of vitamin C which is essential for the activation of the enzyme proline hydroxylase and this in turn results in a qualitative and quantitative decrease in collagen.[33] In addition, some workers have described decreased platelet adhesiveness in experimental situations and in human disease.[34,35] Clinically excess bleeding occurs from multiple sites especially the gums, joints, alimentary tract and brain. Perifollicular bleeding is also common and in young children subperiosteal haemorrhage occurs.[36]

The condition responds rapidly to taking a normal diet rich in vegetables and, of course, to supplements of vitamin C in the diet.

Diabetes mellitus

Purpura is an extremely rare abnormality in diabetes mellitus despite the commonly described abnormalities of retinal and renal vessels in which there can be shown to be abnormalities of capillary permeability. Tests of haemostasis are usually abnormal but favour thrombosis rather than haemorrhage.[37] The Hess test may be positive.

Amyloid

Purpura is a common feature in patients with amyloid, both primary and secondary. The lesions appear in the skin with minimal trauma and may be extensive enough to qualify as ecchymosis. Amyloid may be found around small blood vessels and this may partly explain the bleeding tendency. In addition, functional abnormalities of platelets and thrombocytopenia may be present. Deficiency of a range of clotting factors has also been described, especially Factor X which binds to amyloid.

Dysproteinaemias

In a variety of conditions in which there is massive elevation of immunoglobulin levels, purpura may occur. This is seen in benign hyperglobulinaemia, myeloma, cryoglobulinaemia and in a range of hyperviscosity syndromes. High levels of immunoglobulins interfere with platelet function as well as inhibiting normal fibrin polymerization.[38–41] Treatment is directed at the primary disease.

Drug-related purpura

Cushing's syndrome

Long-term administration of corticosteroids commonly results in purpura which is thought to be due to deficiency of collagen support for blood vessels in the skin which is also extremely thinned. There may also be defective white cell function. A similar type and distribution of purpura (arms and legs) is seen in Cushing's syndrome.[42]

Warfarin and protein C deficiency

Patients deficient in protein C have a tendency to venous and arterial thrombosis in the adult and disseminated intravascular coagulation in the newborn. Use of warfarin to treat the thrombotic event further depresses the levels of protein C, which is a vitamin K dependent factor, and purpuric skin necrosis may result.[43]

Allergic purpuras

Henoch–Schonlein purpura

This is probably the commonest form of vasculitic purpura and involves skin, joints, alimentary tract, kidneys, heart and central nervous system. There is often a history of preceding upper respiratory tract infection and often a B-haemolytic streptococcus has been implicated either by culture or a rising ASO titre. The condition may occur acutely in epidemics in children with a seasonal increase in the spring. It may start with fever followed by a purpuric rash which is often raised to the touch and affects the front of the legs, thighs and buttocks and may be more urticarial than purpuric. In addition, there may be acute arthritis, intestinal pain and bleeding, and nephritis with proteinuria. Rarely does it produce pleurisy, pericarditis or iritis. The skin lesions may continue to form in crops over several weeks. The most serious acute complications are central nervous system bleeding, acute intussusception or renal failure. In children the disease is often self-limiting but the symptoms often respond rapidly to corticosteroids and occasionally cytotoxic drugs have been claimed to be of value. Unfortunately because of the relative rarity of the syndrome no adequate controlled trials of therapy have been undertaken.

Tests of haemostasis show no consistent abnormality except for the demonstration that blood from a number of these patients lacks prostacyclin stimulating factor. This abnormality has also been found in close relatives.[44] Biopsy of skin and of the kidney may show massive deposits of IgA surrounding blood vessels in the affected site and also measurement of serum IgA shows an elevation in half the patients.[45,46]

Vasculitis

Inflammation and infiltration of the walls of blood vessels may be a reaction to a variety of agents including chemicals, toxins, infections and physical stimuli. Histological examination of the tissue (usually skin) shows a lymphocytic infiltrate. In addition, there may be evidence of antigen–antibody complex deposition and activation of the complement system.[47] The resultant endothelial damage facilitates platelet adhesion, aggregation and fibrin formation and the damaged vessel may leak red cells to produce purpura which is palpable to the finger. There may also be areas of skin which are necrotic and which ulcerate. Such lesions are the end-result of a large number of disease processes (Table 7.2).

Table 7.2   Causes of vasculitis

Infections	Streptococcal infections
	Subacute bacterial endocarditis
Drugs	Antibiotics
	Non-steroidal anti-inflammatory agents
	Hypnotics
	Anticoagulants
Cancers	Especially alimentary
	Haemopoietic
Collagen–vascular	SLE
	Systemic sclerosis
	Dermatomyositis

Psychogenic bleeding

This is a bizarre group of bleeding problems which have been attributed to psychological factors and include hysterical bleeding, auto-erythrocyte sensitization, factitial bleeding and religious stigmata. They have been well-reviewed by Ratnoff.[48]

Hysterical bleeding

This is a vague and difficult group of patients to classify and diagnose. There are often psychiatric overtones in the history and often the suspicion that the lesions are induced either by the patient or an associate. There may on occasion be religious overtones with bleeding or bruising occurring at sites corresponding to those in the crucifixion.

Auto-erythrocyte sensitization

This is again an ill-defined condition in which the patients, often middle-aged women with hysterical personalities and behavioural overtones, develop repeated episodes of bleeding and bruising which are usually painful and inflamed.[49] There is no history of direct immediate trauma but there is often a history of preceding physical insult in the prior months.[50] The lesions may be reproduced by the injection of the patient's red cell stroma or haemoglobin. Treatment consists of psychiatric counselling as all other conventional therapies have not proved of value. A similar condition has been described in which the lesions could be produced by injection of patient's own DNA.

Factitial bleeding and religious stigmata

These are a result of attempts to induce bleeding to try to mislead doctors or the public. Many of these patients have disturbed personalities and may only be found out after exhaustive testing for a bleeding defect. Bleeding may be induced by use of anticoagulant drugs or by direct trauma. Such individuals require psychiatric care.

DISSEMINATED INTRAVASCULAR COAGULATION

Disseminated intravascular coagulation (DIC) is a disruption of haemostasis in response to various 'trigger' mechanisms which can paradoxically produce simultaneous thrombosis and haemorrhage by concurrent activation of the coagulation and fibrinolytic systems. Many other terms have been used to describe this process including defibrination syndrome, consumption coagulopathy, and intravascular coagulation with fibrinolysis. The incidence of DIC has been reported to be 1:1000 of admissions to a busy general hospital.[51] At *post mortem*, 3% of hospital patients have histological evidence of DIC.[52]

This disordered haemostasis causes excessive bleeding and there may be ischaemic lesions, or even tissue necrosis due to thrombosis of small and large vessels by fibrin and platelet deposition. Kidneys, brain, heart and adrenals are most commonly affected. Venous thrombi also occur. Ultimately there may be organ failure. DIC is not a disease in itself. It occurs in a variety of clinical conditions and is associated with a wide spectrum of diseases. The presentation and subsequent course of DIC can be acute, subacute or chronic. Both the severity and chronicity of DIC depend on the haemostatic 'trigger'.

Pathogenesis of DIC (see Fig. 7.2)

At the initiation of DIC, there is activation of the coagulation sequence by various triggered mechanisms. This results in thrombin production and consumption of coagulation factors and platelets. Thrombin generated intravascularly at the start of DIC is regarded as an essential pathogenic factor in the continuation of the process. Intravascular coagulation can be directly induced by circulating thrombin. Many authors have presented DIC models in animals caused by intravenous injection of thrombin.[53–56] Animal

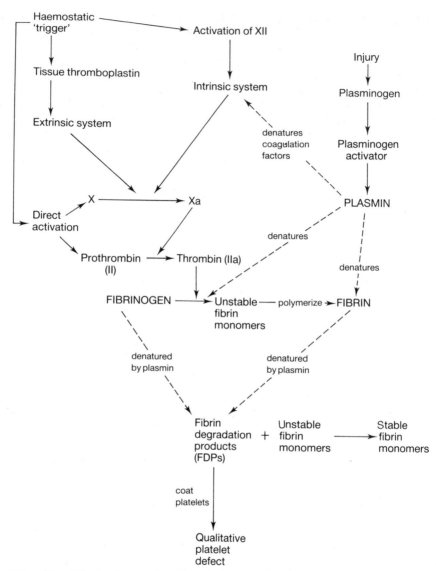

Fig. 7.2.   Simplified scheme showing the interaction between coagulation and fibrinolysis in the pathogenesis of DIC.

models have also been used to demonstrate that intravenous injection of homogenized thromboplastin-rich tissue resulted in a DIC state.[56-58] From these models, much information about thrombin and its haemostatic effects in DIC has been provided.

Role of thrombin

Thrombin is responsible for many haemostatic processes and these are seen in DIC. Fibrinogen, a fully soluble protein in plasma loses small terminal peptides (fibrinopeptides A and B) in the presence of thrombin, resulting in soluble fibrin monomers. In overt DIC, there is a definite increase in levels of fibrinopeptide A (FPA).[59] Polymerization of fibrin monomers results in an insoluble gel and this relatively unstable clot is stabilized by the action of a transamidase (Factor XIII) on the fibrin chains. Thrombin is responsible for the activation of Factor XIII in a calcium-dependent reaction. Total plasma fibrinogen is reduced as a result of the above reactions. There is a reduction in concentration of Factors VIII C[60] and V due to thrombin-mediated peptide release from each factor which results in factor activation and ultimately in a fall in factor concentration. Platelet aggregation occurs because of thrombin binding to platelets. The aggregated platelets can be cleared by the reticulo-endothelial system (RES) or are deposited in the microcirculation. Thrombin cleaves fibrinogen forming soluble fibrin which is either cleared by the RES or, as mentioned previously, precipitated and polymerized to an insoluble gel which can occlude blood vessels.

Thrombosis and bleeding in DIC

Mild forms of DIC can be seen in many conditions and can go unrecognized or are of little clinical importance. In these situations, small thrombi which form cause no apparent haemodynamic upset because of their size. In addition, the haemostatic balance is restored and vascular patency is maintained by the simultaneous triggering of the fibrinolytic system which removes such thrombi from the circulation as they form. Formation of localized occlusive thrombi can occur without fibrinolysis. In severe DIC haemostasis can be activated to such a degree that widespread thrombosis occurs in the microcirculation due to deposition of fibrin and platelets. This leads to organ ischaemia and microangiopathic haemolytic anaemia. Overwhelming activation of the coagulation system also causes consumption of coagulation factors and platelets resulting in a bleeding tendency which can be exacerbated by simultaneous and unbalanced fibrinolysis.

The role of fibrinolysis

Fibrinolysis in DIC has been shown in several animal models to be an important compensatory mechanism which prevents widespread organ damage due to vascular occlusion by fibrin. If fibrinolysis is inhibited by administration of antifibrinolytic agents, by pregnancy, or by injection of endotoxin widespread organ damage is observed.[61] Fibrinolysis can be a primary or secondary event and is usually the latter in DIC. Antifibrinolytic agents enhance DIC in man.[62]

Plasmin is the main enzyme involved in fibrin degradation. When intravascular and extravascular fibrin is laid down, plasminogen (an inactive precursor) is converted to plasmin (the active form) by tissue plasminogen activator (t-PA), resulting in plasminogen consumption, increased levels of t-PA, decreased levels of inhibitor (α_2-antiplasmin) and the presence of plasmin/antiplasmin complexes.

Plasmin cleaves fibrin into fibrin degradation products (FDPs). These FDPs form a complex with fibrin monomers before they can polymerize thus producing stable fibrin monomers which cannot polymerize.[63-65] FDPs can coat the surfaces of platelets causing platelet dysfunction.

Although dissolution of fibrin by plasmin has clearly beneficial effects, excessive plasmin (hyperplasminaemia) can cause adverse anticoagulant effects by (1) degrading Factors V, VIII, IX and XI which are already reduced in amount due to coagulation activation[66-68] and by (2) dissolving haemostatic thrombi as well as fibrin. The anticoagulant activity of circulating fibrin and FDPs exacerbates the bleeding tendency.

Plasmin also activates C1 and C3 complement sequence leading to red cell and platelet lysis, increased vascular permeability and shock. Release of kinins contributes to shock.[69,70] If, as in DIC, the fine balance between coagulation activation and effective compensatory fibrinolysis is disrupted, severe bleeding can be the catastrophic outcome.

Role of tissue plasminogen activator (t-PA)

t-PA in DIC is released from damaged endothelium, white cells or platelets or is generated through activation of Factor XII. An effective fibrinolytic response requires adequate endothelial synthesis and release of t-PA, and the expression of free t-PA activity at sites of fibrin formation. Free t-PA activity is regulated by one or more rapid specific plasma inhibitors.[71-73] It is possible to assay plasma t-PA antigen (the sum of free t-PA and inactive t-PA in complex with its inhibitors)[74,75] and t-PA activity (free t-PA).[76-78] Combined use of these assays in patients with thrombotic disorders has demonstrated that some patients with coronary artery disease[80] and venous thromboembolic disease[74,79] have either impaired t-PA release or increased levels of t-PA inhibitors, or both. If only activity assays are used, increased levels of the inhibitor may mask the true extent of endothelial t-PA release.[81]

Recently, a study of levels of t-PA antigen and activity in patients with DIC from various causes was carried out in an effort to clarify the mechanism of the fibrinolytic response in DIC.[82] Increased circulating levels of t-PA antigen were present in DIC regardless of the underlying cause. Elevated levels were also found in hospitalized subjects without DIC but these were lower than in the patients with DIC from similar illnesses, suggesting that increased levels of t-PA antigen in DIC represents more than a non-specific response to stress of an acute illness. The authors conclude that in DIC endothelium is strongly stimulated to release t-PA. In addition, detectable free t-PA activity was less frequently found in patients with DIC than in controls, DIC masking the increased endothelial secretion of t-PA.

As well as increased t-PA release from the endothelium in DIC, it has been postulated that there is a local factor involved at the sites of fibrin formation which encourages t-PA activity.[82] Activated protein C has been reported to inactivate t-PA inhibitor produced by cultured endothelial cells.[83] It is possible that in DIC activation of protein C by thrombin bound to thrombomodulin on the surface of endothelial cells prevents inhibition of endothelial t-PA aiding effective fibrinolysis. This theory is only applicable at a local endothelial level as, in the circulation at large, activated protein C is inhibited by its own circulating inhibitor[84,85] so that t-PA inhibitor would be unopposed and circulating t-PA would be rapidly inhibited.

Other haemostatic components in DIC

As a result of activation of the coagulation and fibrinolytic systems in DIC, the following haemostatic abnormalities can also be found. There are reduced plasma levels of vitamin K dependent coagulation factors. Fibronectin levels are low because fibronectin is used up in the formation of complexes with fibrin. These complexes are subsequently deposited in the microcirculation. Because of reduced fibronectin levels, soluble fibrin is inadequately cleared by macrophages.[86] Normally, antithrombin III, which is the main inhibitor of thrombin and Factor Xa, also inhibits other activated factors. However, in DIC, consumption of antithrombin III occurs and levels fall which accelerates the coagulation process.

In DIC, both quantitative and qualitative platelet defects occur. Platelets are activated, releasing platelet factor 3, factor 4, and β-thromboglobulin. Platelets are consumed in the process of thrombus formation, resulting in thrombocytopenia. Fibrin deposition in the microcirculation causes platelet trapping which contributes to thrombocytopenia.[87,88] Coating of platelets with circulating FDPs can cause defective platelet function.

The role of non-haemostatic factors in DIC

The following factors can be involved in modifying the course of DIC. The underlying cause of the DIC process will often determine the extent of the involvement of these other factors.

Reticulo-endothelial system

Normal haemostasis requires an intact reticulo-endothelial system (RES) which will remove activated clotting factors, soluble fibrin and triggers of DIC. Experimental blockade of the RES causes fulminant DIC as in the Schwartzman reaction.[89] In liver disease and pregnancy, blockade of the RES contributes to DIC.[90]

Catecholamines

Catecholamines have been shown experimentally[61] to be of importance in DIC. The production of microthrombi by different catecholamines during thrombin-induced DIC in rabbits was recently studied and the effects of the different catecholamines compared.[91] Only catecholamines stimulating α-adrenoreceptors trigger thrombosis during intravascular coagulation which supports previous findings. The α-adrenergic effects cause stasis of the microcirculation followed by deposition of fibrin.[92] It has been postulated that vasoactive agents and microcirculatory changes have an important role to play in the selection of target organs for microthrombi production in DIC.[91]

Lipids

Severe DIC has been induced in experimental animals by endotoxin injection combined with lipid infusion.[93]

Pregnancy

DIC occurs more frequently in pregnancy and is associated with several obstetric complications. In normal pregnancy, there are many changes in haemostasis which induce a hypercoagulable state. These changes include a progressive rise in coagulation factors, especially fibrinogen and Factor VIII, a decrease in fibrinolytic activity and decreased reticulo-endothelial clearance of activated coagulation factors.

Liver disease

DIC is especially common in liver disease because, in addition to a variety of metabolic problems, poor synthesis of coagulation factors and inadequate clearance mechanisms occur.

Initiation of DIC

DIC can be initiated by different mechanisms which occur in response to the underlying 'trigger' or cause of DIC. In a single case, more than one of the four main mechanisms now described may be involved.

Endothelial injury with activation of Factor XII (Hageman factor) and the intrinsic pathway

Endotoxins, extensive burns, acidosis, anoxia, viraemia, antigen/antibody complexes, vasculitis and hypotension can all cause severe endothelial damage which exposes the sub-endothelial collagen. This collagen can directly activate Factor XII which, in turn, can directly or indirectly activate the intrinsic coagulation system, complement cascade, kinin formation and fibrinolysis.

Tissue injury and activation of the extrinsic pathway

Release of tissue thromboplastin into the circulation directly activates the extrinsic coagulation pathway. Any tissue damage, e.g. septicaemia, surgical and obstetric trauma, breakdown of malignant cells and head injuries[94] can lead to tissue thromboplastin release. The brain is a rich source of thromboplastin. In granular promyelocytic leukaemia, damaged platelets, red cell stroma and blast cells can act as thromboplastins.[95]

Direct proteolytic cleavage

Life-threatening consumption coagulopathies can complicate severe snake venom poisonings. The venom of the snake *Echis carinatus* acts as a prothrombin activator causing rapid DIC *in vivo* due to direct activation of prothrombin and subsequent thrombin release.[60,96] Other venoms can directly cause proteolysis of fibrinogen resulting in thrombocytopenia and hypofibrinogenaemia, i.e. a 'DIC-like' syndrome.[97] DIC resulting from proteolytic cleavage of serine proteases of the coagulation cascade occurs in acute pancreatitis, when pancreatic enzymes enter the circulation, and in amniotic fluid embolism, when amniotic fluid enters the circulation.

Induction of platelet aggregation

Platelet aggregation and adherence to the endothelium rarely occurs in normal situations, i.e. free flowing blood and normal endothelium. The production of thromboxane A_2 (a potent platelet aggregating agent) by circulating platelets is constantly balanced by prostacyclin production from the vessel wall. Prostacyclin is a potent, naturally occurring, inhibitor of platelet aggregation.

This relationship between platelets and the vessel wall has been recently recognized as of probable importance in the initiation of DIC. Platelet aggregation can be induced by some known 'triggers' of DIC, including septicaemia (where bacterial endotoxin causes both endothelial damage and platelet defects), uraemia, immune complex disease and thrombin production (the result of coagulation activation). Irreversible platelet aggregation has been induced *in vitro* by bacterial isolates, particularly *Staphylococcus aureus* and *Pseudomonas aeruginosa*, both of which were associated with a high incidence of DIC in the individuals from whom they were isolated.[98]

Causes or 'triggers' of DIC

Many conditions can cause or 'trigger' the process of DIC (see Table 7.3). Sepsis, obstetric complications and malignant disease account for a large majority of cases. Some causes can be classified as to whether they produce acute, subacute or chronic DIC (see Table 7.4). Although activation of coagulation and subsequent consumption of coagulation factors and platelets usually occurs throughout the body in DIC, in certain conditions these processes can occur wholly at one site. This 'local consumption' still causes systemic effects but its treatment is different from that of other causes of DIC. 'Local consumption' is seen in patients with aortic aneurysms, giant haemangiomata, the dead foetus syndrome, and hyperacute renal allograft rejection.[99]

Sepsis

Approximately 70% of all cases of DIC are associated with infections.

Table 7.3   Causes or 'Triggers' of DIC

Sepsis
  Bacterial infection with these organisms
    Neisseria meningococcus
    Escherichia coli
    Pseudomonas aeruginosa
    Klebsiella
    Streptococcus pneumoniae
    Staphylococcus aureus
    Clostridium perfringens
    Chlamydia psittaci
    Mycoplasma pneumoniae
    Haemophilus influenzae
  Viral infection
    Varicella
    Hepatitis A and B
    Non-A non-B hepatitis
    Cytomegalovirus
    Haemorrhagic fevers, e.g. dengue
  Rickettsial infection, e.g. Rocky Mountain spotted fever
  Fungal infection
    Aspergillus
    Candida albicans
  Protozoan infection
    Malaria
    Schistosomiasis

Obstetric complications
  Abruptio placentae
  Amniotic fluid embolism
  Dead foetus syndrome ('local consumption')
  Retained placenta
  Abortion
  Pre-eclampsia/eclampsia

Malignancy
  Mucin-secreting adenocarcinomas
  Metastatic prostatic carcinoma
  Acute leukaemias (especially promyelocytic)

Hepatic disease
  Cirrhosis
  Acute liver failure

Trauma and surgery

Shock
  Septic
  Hypovolaemic
  Anaphylactic

Intravascular haemolysis
  Paroxysmal nocturnal haemoglobinuria
  Freshwater drowning
  Incompatible blood transfusion

cont'd over

Table 7.3 (cont.)   Causes or 'Triggers' of DIC

Vasculitis
  Collagen vascular diseases
  Haemolytic–uraemic syndrome
  Thrombotic thrombocytopenic purpura
  (Moschowitz' syndrome)

Snake venoms

Miscellaneous
  Burns
  Extracorporeal circulation
  Haemangiomatous lesions ('local consumption', e.g. Kasabach–Merritt
  syndrome and Klippel–Trelawney syndrome)
  Metabolic diseases, e.g. severe diabetes mellitus; hyperlipoproteinaemia
  Heat stroke
  Renal disease, e.g. glomerulonephritis
  Sarcoidosis
  Ingestion of acetic acid
  Aortic aneurysm ('local consumption')
  Hyperacute renal allograft rejection ('local consumption')
  Pulmonary embolism

Table 7.4   Some Causes of Acute, Subacute and Chronic DIC

Acute	*Subacute*	*Chronic*
Sepsis (e.g. meningococcal septicaemia)	Disseminated malignancy	Liver disease
Shock	Leukaemias	Malignant disease
Intravascular haemolysis	Eclampsia	Paroxysmal nocturnal
Extensive trauma or surgery	Sepsis (e.g. gram-negative infections)	haemoglobinuria
Heat stroke		Vasculitides
Burns		Renal disease
Obstetric causes (except eclampsia)		Sarcoidosis
SLE		Eclampsia

Meningococcal septicaemia was the first infection in which DIC was described.[100] A fulminant haemorrhagic picture is produced which is also seen in staphylococcal and streptococcal infections. Patients who have undergone splenectomy, or who are immunosuppressed, are particularly vulnerable to infection from *Streptococcus pneumoniae*. Such patients may develop a syndrome similar to the classical, potentially fatal, Waterhouse–Friderichsen syndrome of meningococcal septicaemia. Thus, routine prophylaxis with pneumococcal vaccine is advised in asplenic patients. Gram-negative infections can be responsible for a subacute form of DIC where haemorrhage is less severe. Endotoxin release from gram-negative organisms is responsible for activation of DIC as previously outlined. Many other bacterial infections are associated with DIC including 'sub-bacteria', e.g. *Mycoplasma pneumoniae.*[101]

In acute viral illnesses, e.g. varicella, hepatitis and CMV, the initiating mechanism of DIC is thought to involve antigen/antibody activation of Factor XII, platelet release and endothelial sloughing.[102,103] Fungal, rickettsial[87] and protozoan[63,88] infections are also recognized causes of DIC.

Obstetric complications

Pregnancy induces a hypercoagulable state with an increase in coagulation factors, depression of the fibrinolytic system and reduced reticulo-endothelial clearance of activated coagulation factors.[61,104,105]

Placental abruption is a relatively frequent complication of pregnancy and in a quarter of cases, hypofibrinogenaemia is seen within 8 h.[106,107] Delivery is usually carried out at an early stage in such cases to prevent the more serious haemorrhagic and thrombotic problems of acute DIC. Thromboplastin release into the maternal circulation is thought to be the likely mechanism behind DIC in placental abruption.[108]

In amniotic fluid embolism, uterine trauma or membrane tears allow amniotic fluid to enter the maternal circulation. The thromboplastic activity of amniotic fluid[109] is thought to be responsible for the coagulation abnormalities which occur. Severe DIC can develop as well as the cardiopulmonary collapse which is associated with embolism of amniotic fluid and fibrin thrombus in the pulmonary circulation. Another serious complication is uncontrollable uterine haemorrhage.[110] Patients with severe pre-eclampsia and eclampsia have changes in coagulation consistent with low-grade DIC[111] The main features present tend to be thrombocytopenia and decreased levels of clotting factors rather than raised levels of soluble fibrin and FDPs. The exact mechanism of coagulation activation is unknown.[112]

If a foetus dies in utero, DIC usually occurs within 3 weeks. Necrotic foetal tissues and enzymes are released and these act as thromboplastins which initiate DIC. Nowadays, septic abortions, previously a common cause of DIC, are rarer due to changes in abortion laws. Mild DIC can occur in abortions using hypertonic saline and urea. There have been occasional reports of DIC occurring in other methods of abortion.[113–115]

Malignancy

The severity of DIC in malignant disease is variable. It may not be clinically obvious, being diagnosed through laboratory investigations. The degree of metastatic disease often correlates with severity. Only 10–15% of patients with non-metastatic carcinoma may have clinical evidence of DIC compared with 40% of those with widespread metastatic disease. Thromboplastin synthesis and release from tumour cells, activation of coagulation by proteolytic enzymes and acceleration of fibrinolysis[116,117] are all thought to play a part in the initiation of DIC in malignancy. Carcinoma of lung, pancreas, prostate and ovary are particularly associated with DIC. Approximately 25% of cases of DIC have been attributed to prostatic carcinoma as the underlying pathophysiological defect.[118] Conversely approximately 13% of patients with prostatic carcinoma demonstrate some form of chronic DIC.[119]

The association between DIC and acute promyelocytic leukaemia (APL) is well-established. Procoagulant activity in leukaemia cells has been suspected to trigger the intravascular coagulation.[120] In APL and other acute non-lymphoid leukaemias (ANLL) in which DIC can also occur, the procoagulant activity in these leukaemia cells has been identified as tissue factor (TF).[121–123] Recently, it has been shown that DIC severity in ANLL may correlate mainly with the TF activity (TFA) of the leukaemia cells and that TFA is also affected by the bulk of leukaemia cells.[124] It has been suggested that TFA should be considered in the calculation of the heparin dosage to be used in the treatment of DIC in these leukaemias.[124]

DIC is rarely seen in lymphoid malignancies. There have been some reported cases in acute lymphoblastic leukaemia, and occasional reported cases in T-cell hairy cell leukaemia[125] and Burkitt's lymphoma/leukaemia.[126] In the latter case, cytogenetic investigations revealed a variant Burkitt's translocation t(8;22)(q24;q11) involving the λ light-chain gene region, and abnormalities of chromosomes 15 and 17 with breakpoints at q22 and q12, respectively, similar to those observed in t(15;17) in APL. It is suggested that there could be an association between a gene for coagulation factors and the above chromosome break sites. The authors also postulated that cytoplasmic crystalline inclusions seen on electron microscopy in the leukaemic blast cells may have had a role in precipitating DIC.

Hepatic disease

Hepatic disease affects coagulation in many ways as outlined later in this chapter. DIC is one haemostatic disorder that can arise.

Shock

DIC invariably accompanies severe shock.[127] Widespread vascular damage from endotoxins, immune complexes, hypoxia and acidosis is a major aetiological factor. Thrombocytopenia and raised fibrinogen levels are observed, leading to the postulate that platelet aggregation and micro-thrombus formation are 'triggering events'.[128]

Trauma and surgery

Any tissue damage can cause tissue thromboplastin release and DIC activation. Head injuries can cause severe DIC because the brain is a rich source of thromboplastin.

Intravascular haemolysis

The trigger for DIC in intravascular haemolysis is haemolysed red cells. Severe DIC can follow haemolytic reactions such as transfusion of incompatible blood and near drowning in fresh water.

Vasculitis

The association between chronic DIC and collagen vascular diseases has been widely accepted.[129] Recently, there have been case reports of acute DIC occurring as a complication of systemic lupus erythematosus (SLE)[130,131] and it may be that this is more prevalent than was previously thought. In SLE, circulating anticoagulants are associated with thrombotic events but they are not clearly associated with acute DIC. The exact mechanism by which coagulation is activated is unclear.[130] Haemolytic–uraemic syndrome and thrombotic thrombocytopenic purpura are other vasculitic processes associated with DIC.

Snake venoms

Disturbance of the haemostatic system is mainly an effect of the venom of snakes of the Viperidae family. Most of these venoms have strong procoagulant activity resulting in defibrination. Increased fibrinolysis and thrombocytopenia may occur due to vascular damage.[102]

Miscellaneous

There are many other reported causes of DIC as listed in Table 7.3. Heat stroke has been reported to cause DIC in humans.[132–135] It has been postulated that DIC is the mediator of adult respiratory distress syndrome (ARDS) in heat stroke patients[136] and that screening for DIC in heat stroke patients could serve as a predictor for the development of ARDS.

DIC has been described as an early complication of deliberate ingestion of acetic acid.[137]

The initiation of DIC in severe burns is thought to be due to thromboplastin release from damaged tissues and red cells. Other factors contributing to DIC in burns may be the development of septic or hypovolaemic shock and acute haemolysis.

Exposure of blood to a foreign surface as occurs in extracorporeal circulations causes protein adsorption, platelet adhesion and aggregation and coagulation activation resulting in DIC. The severity of the DIC process may be determined by the type of surface to which blood is exposed and the length of exposure time. Thus, in long procedures, e.g. cardio-pulmonary bypass, there is a greater chance of DIC than in short surgical procedures. Many other factors, e.g. the use of filters, the type of pump used to maintain the circulation, the need to oxygenate haemoglobin, the use of heparin and antiplatelet agents, plasma and blood transfusions will also determine the extent of DIC in extracorporeal circulations.

Haemangiomatous lesions can cause local platelet and coagulation factor consumption. Such 'local consumption' was originally described in an infant with a giant cavernous haemangioma who had thrombocytopenia and coagulation factor consumption, i.e. the Kasabach–Merritt syndrome. DIC has also been described in other vascular tumours and it is thought that sequestration and activation of platelets and coagulation factors in the abnormal vessels of these lesions are responsible.

Recently, it has been suggested that interleukin-I may act as a 'trigger' for DIC (unpublished).

Clinical features of DIC

DIC is not always clinically apparent and mild cases may only be detected because of minor abnormalities in clotting studies. At the other extreme, severe cases of DIC may have florid clinical features. The underlying cause of DIC usually determines whether the process is acute, subacute or chronic. Acute DIC is likely to have severe clinical consequences and subacute or chronic DIC is milder in its clinical manifestations (see Fig. 7.3). Acute DIC can progress from chronic DIC and less commonly the converse can occur.

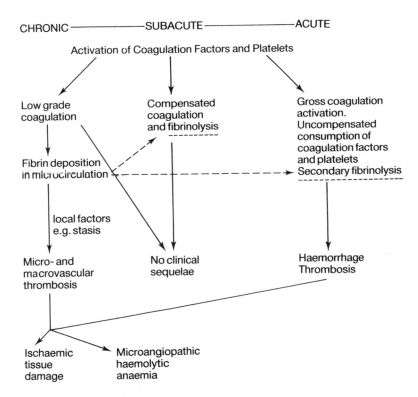

Fig. 7.3. Clinical manifestations of DIC.

In mild, usually subacute and chronic cases of DIC, the process is compensated, i.e. the increased consumption of coagulation factors and platelets is met by increased production. There is a reasonable balance between activation of coagulation and secondary (compensatory) fibrinolysis. Detectable levels of fibrin degradation products (FDPs) are present in the blood due to fibrin breakdown. Clotting studies may show mild abnormalities but often there is no clinical evidence of thrombosis or bleeding. Other factors, e.g. stasis or atheroma, may encourage thrombus formation.

In acute DIC, the balance between coagulation activation and adequate compensatory fibrinolysis is upset. The process of DIC now becomes uncompensated, resulting in a fall in levels of fibrinogen, platelets and coagulation factors. Clinically, the onset of DIC in such cases can be explosive with features of both haemorrhage and thrombosis. In general, patients with DIC can be severely ill showing signs of fever, hypotension, acidosis, hypoxia and proteinuria. Both the underlying cause of DIC and the DIC process itself can produce these signs and it is often difficult to clarify whether the clinical signs are due to the former or the latter. Haemorrhage is the commonest clinical manifestation in severe cases and is a presenting feature in up to 90% of some reported series. Petechiae, purpura, and ecchymoses are seen and are a reflection of skin bleeding. Spontaneous bleeding into muscles can occur. In addition, there can be haemorrhage from multiple sites, e.g. wounds, venepunctures, drain and catheter sites. Mucosal bleeding causes epistaxis, gum bleeding, vaginal haemorrhage, haematemesis and melaena. Intracerebral haemorrhage is another serious complication and bleeding into major organs, e.g. pulmonary haemorrhage, contributes to the organ dysfunction already caused by thrombosis and ischaemia.

Only 7% of patients have clinical signs of thrombosis at presentation of DIC[138] and thrombosis is apparent during the course of DIC in only about 25% of cases. Renal impairment, drowsiness, coma, confusion and cardiorespiratory failure can be caused by ischaemia resulting from micro- and macrovascular thromboses. Acral cyanosis, thrombophlebitis, digital and skin gangrene are also manifestations of thrombosis. Renal involvement in DIC is due to a combination of (1) ischaemic cortical necrosis due to thrombosis in the glomerular capillaries and arterioles and (2) acute tubular necrosis resulting from hypovolaemia or hypotension. Haematuria, oliguria or anuria can all occur. In one study, at necropsy of patients with DIC diagnosed before death, microthrombi were most often found in the lungs and kidney.[139] Microangiopathic haemolytic anaemia can arise because of fragmentation of red cells which are trapped in the fibrin network within the microvasculature. Finally, it is important to remember that the major organ dysfunction which can affect patients with DIC may be due to a combination of the underlying cause of DIC, associated circulatory failure, acidosis and disordered coagulation.

The laboratory diagnosis of DIC

When there is clinical suspicion of DIC, laboratory investigations are carried out which aim to detect evidence of platelet and coagulation activation and fibrinolysis. No single laboratory test, nor any particular combination of tests can be used to make a definite diagnosis of DIC.[140] Abnormalities of coagulation tests do, however, help to confirm a suspected diagnosis of DIC in patients who have conditions predisposing to DIC and/or whose clinical features suggest the development of DIC.

In acute DIC, it is important to confirm the diagnosis rapidly to enable the institution of prompt treatment. Thus, the tests which are most useful clinically are those which can quickly and accurately confirm the diagnosis, give information about the depletion of platelets and coagulation factors as well as giving an indication of the extent of the DIC process. The most useful initial screening investigations are shown in Table 7.5. It is important that samples for coagulation investigations are taken cleanly, by fresh venepuncture to prevent spurious results. Although the initial screening tests for diagnosing DIC are sensitive, most are non-specific and can be affected by the underlying conditions predisposing to DIC.

FDP determination is probably the most useful test, as many authorities require an elevation in its level before a diagnosis of DIC is entertained.[140,141] Assays of FDPs are semiquantitative and have limitations. Recently it has been suggested from a clinical evaluation of a prototype automated quantitative FDP assay that the quantitative assay has advantages over the semiquantitative assay, which include improved precision and ability to closely monitor changes in severity of the coagulopathy.[142]

DIC is a dynamic process and the results of the coagulation tests will be continually changing. It is important to interpret a single set of results cautiously. Sequential testing is of more value as it gives an indication of the pattern of change, i.e. any improvement or deterioration with time. Often, as indicated above, these initial investigations can give a clue as to whether the process is acute or chronic. In chronic DIC, coagulation changes may be minor. Additional tests (Table 7.6) can give more information. These tests are sometimes impractical or are not immediately necessary.

Many other detectable haemostatic abnormalities are reported in DIC. These are outlined in Table 7.7. These investigations can be time-consuming and they do not provide much extra information. Often, they are only performed in specialist centres.

Management of DIC

General principles

Often, there is uncertainty as to whether disrupted coagulation itself is responsible for pathological damage in DIC or whether the latter is mainly due to the underlying cause of the DIC process. As a result, there is some controversy about some aspects of the treatment of DIC. Many literature reports are based on small patient numbers or anecdotal observations. There are no reports of large controlled clinical trials concerning the treatment of DIC. However, it is generally agreed that the removal or treatment of the precipitating cause of the DIC process is an essential first step in management.[143] Normalization of coagulation usually follows soon after correction of the underlying cause or 'trigger'.

Table 7.5   Initial Investigations in the Laboratory Diagnosis of DIC

Investigation	Abnormality			Comment
	Acute	Subacute	Chronic	
Hb	↓	N or ↓	N or ↓	Usually reflects bleeding or haemolysis
Platelets	↓↓	↓ or ↑ or N	↓ or N or ↑	Platelet adherence and aggregation causes ↓ levels but local prostacyclin production can cause dispersal of platelet aggregates causing N or ↑ levels
Blood film	May be features of the underlying disease, e.g. target cells in liver disease. May show fragmentation of RBCs due to damage to RBCs from passage through fibrin in the microvasculature especially in intravascular haemolysis, renal disease and malignancy			
Prothrombin time	↑↑	↑	↓ or ↑ or N	Prolongation is due to factor consumption and presence of FDPs
Activated partial thromboplastin time	↑↑	↑	↓ or ↑ or N	
Thrombin time	↑↑	↑	↓ or ↑ or N	Measures conversion of fibrinogen → fibrin Prolonged by (1) lack of clottable fibrinogen, (2) presence of FDPs or (3) heparin[a]
Fibrinogen concentration	↓↓	↓ or N	N or ↓ or ↑	Can inspect clot in glass tube at bedside. In severe fibrinogen depletion, a small clot forms which is difficult to see
FDP concentration	↑↑	↑↑	N or ↑	Indicates activation of secondary fibrinolysis. Usually increased

[a] Heparin may contaminate sample, e.g. heparin in syringe or patient on heparin. Addition of protamine will reverse the heparin effect.

↑ = Increased or prolonged, ↑↑ = markedly increased, very prolonged; ↓ = decreased or shortened; ↓↓ = markedly decreased, very much shortened; N = normal.

Table 7.6 Additional Tests Used in the Diagnosis of DIC

Test	Result in DIC	Comment
Reptilase time	Prolonged	(1) Basis of test is that certain snake venoms act directly on fibrinogen to form fibrin (2) Unaffected by heparin – can distinguish between coagulation abnormalities due to heparin or DIC if the patient is on heparin (3) Can be unreliable if there are high levels of circulating FDPs
Ethanol gelatin test Protamine sulphate precipitation test	Positive	(1) Both tests are positive in the presence of fibrin monomer complexes in the blood (2) Both tests are non-specific. Fibrin monomer complexes can be found in trauma and infection

In septicaemia, appropriate intravenous antibiotics in high doses should be promptly started. In obstetric patients with abruption, dead foetus syndrome and pre-eclampsia, evacuation of the uterus should be carried out as soon as is feasible.[104,144,145] Usually, patients with acute DIC are critically ill because of both the underlying cause and the disordered coagulation in DIC. They often need to be managed in an intensive care unit. Haemorrhage and shock require rapid restoration of the circulating blood volume and transfusion of large volumes of fluid may be difficult if cardiac function is affected by ischaemia. Renal function should be closely monitored to detect evidence of renal failure. Haemorrhage can pose problems when inserting arterial or venous catheters which are required for monitoring the progress of the patient. Plasma expanders, e.g. dextrans and gelatin preparations can exacerbate haemorrhage and should not be used. Adequate arterial oxygenation is often difficult to achieve because oxygenation is impaired by the adult respiratory distress syndrome (ARDS). There is a close association between DIC and ARDS[136,146] but the cause–effect relationship between the two is unclear. Micro- and macrovascular thromboses can further impair tissue oxygenation. Correction of acidosis is important as there is an increased risk of thrombosis associated with acidosis.

Specific therapy

(1) Replacement therapy. (i) It is generally recommended that coagulation factor replacement should not be introduced solely on the basis of an abnormal coagulation screen. It should be instituted if there is uncontrolled bleeding or if the precipitating cause cannot be rapidly treated.[147] The necessary coagulation factors are provided by fresh frozen plasma (FFP) and cryoprecipitate. FFP contains all the non-cellular coagulation factors, including fibrinogen, at a concentration which is less than that of plasma.

Table 7.7   Other Detectable Haemostatic Abnormalities in DIC

1. Factors V, VIIIC, XIII	Decreased levels
2. Factor VIIIc, VIII:RAg	There is often a discrepancy between these values with FVIIIc being decreased. Measurement of the difference between the level of coagulant Factor VIII and the immunological level reflects thrombin generation
3. Factor XII, HMW kininogen, pre-kallikrein	May be decreased levels
4. Euglobulin lysis time	Indicates fibrinolytic activity Early DIC → short lysis times due to high activator levels (t-PA) Late DIC → long lysis times due to plasminogen depletion
5. BB 15–42 peptide levels (the result of digestion of fibrin monomer by plasmin)	Increased levels (indicates fibrinolytic activity)
6. Fibrinopeptides A and B	Increased levels Sensitive indicator of thrombin generation Levels elevated in inflammation and after injury
7. Platelet aggregation studies	Usually abnormal but no classical diagnostic abnormality specific for DIC
8. B-Thromboglobulin (BTG) Platelet factors 3 & 4 (Evidence of platelet activation and release of granules)	Increased levels in initial stages of DIC due to intravascular damage to platelets
9. Antithrombin III levels (AT III)	Decreased levels (which are also found in liver disease and congenital deficiency)
10. Plasminogen concentration	Reduced – indicates secondary fibrinolysis
11. α_2-Antiplasmin	Decreased levels due to fibrinolysis
12. Activator (t-PA)	May be increased levels due to fibrinolysis
13. Plasmin–antiplasmin complexes	Present

Large volumes of FFP are necessary to ensure the maintenance of adequate levels of coagulation factors which makes FFP less useful in practice than in theory. Cryoprecipitate contains both fibrinogen and Factor VIII. If there is profound depletion of fibrinogen, cryoprecipitate is especially useful. Its efficacy is monitored by transfusing approximately I0 U and rechecking the fibrinogen level shortly afterwards. The reluctance to use a concentrated source of coagulation factors to treat cases with abnormal coagulation tests and no overt bleeding stems from the theory that transfusion of coagulation factors may 'add fuel to the fire', i.e. rapid consumption of the coagulation factors occurs resulting in exacerbation of the thrombotic process in the microvasculature.[148,149]

(ii) In addition to coagulation factors, blood and platelet transfusions may be required in the presence of severe bleeding. Platelet transfusions are usually given if the platelet count is below 30×10^9 per litre. A platelet count checked 1 h after transfusion should show an increment. No increment suggests that there is rapid consumption of the transfused platelets, and that further platelet transfusions will be of little benefit. A high level of circulating FDPs causes platelet dysfunction which can affect transfused platelets.

(iii) Recently, there has been much interest in the use of antithrombin III concentrate (AT III). Prothrombin complex concentrates and fibrinogen concentrates are potentially thrombogenic and their use is inadvisable.

(2) Inhibition of activated coagulation.   Specific coagulation inhibitors such as heparin and AT III are sometimes used in the treatment of DIC in an attempt to stop the activated coagulation process which will, in turn, remove the drive to compensatory fibrinolysis. If coagulation inhibition can be achieved, this should theoretically resolve the DIC process.

(i) The use of heparin in DIC remains controversial because of the lack of controlled clinical trials,[150] variation of response to heparin and possible potentiation of the risk of bleeding. Heparin augments the role of AT III in inhibiting activated factors (mainly thrombin, X, IXa, and XIa) thus blocking the coagulation process which has been activated by thromboplastin release and thrombin formation in the circulation. Heparin therapy in DIC is not standard practice nowadays and some people advise its use when a satisfactory trial of replacement therapy has failed to improve clinically severe bleeding. Heparin may also be indicated when thrombosis is either responsible for organ damage or is potentially detrimental, e.g. pulmonary embolism or peripheral gangrene. Ultimately, the decision to institute heparin therapy in DIC depends upon the trigger to the DIC process and the clinical state of the patient and every case is considered individually.

Specific conditions where treatment with heparin should be considered at the first clinical suspicion of DIC include acute promyelocytic leukaemia (APL), other non-lymphoid leukaemias, amniotic fluid embolism, incompatible blood transfusion reactions, septic abortion, and heat stroke. Chronic DIC in malignancy may be helped by heparin.[151] DIC caused by 'local consumption' e.g. dead foetus syndrome, giant haemangiomata is a further indication for heparin therapy. The dose of heparin should be sufficient to be effective yet low enough to carry an acceptable risk of haemorrhage. The recommended dose of heparin is a bolus of 5000 U i.v.

and 1000 U/h as a continuous infusion.[149] Serial measurements of fibrinogen and platelet count should be performed to assess efficacy.

In a retrospective study of patients with acute non-lymphoid leukaemias and DIC successfully treated with heparin, an intimate correlation was noted between the dose of heparin administered and the tissue factor activity of the leukaemia cells. It was concluded that the dose of heparin administered should be proportional to tissue factor activity of leukaemia cells and that this dose could be calculated mathematically in an equation involving the logarithm of tissue factor activity.[124] During heparin therapy, replacement therapy with coagulation factors may also be necessary. For heparin to be effective in arresting intravascular coagulation, adequate plasma levels of the heparin co-factor AT III are required. Thus, where there are low levels of AT III, infusions of specific AT III concentrate (in addition to heparin) may be useful.[152] Oral anticoagulants have no place in the treatment of DIC.

(ii) AT III concentrate has been used with success as a single therapy in treating small groups of patients with DIC. AT III is known to be the most important inhibitor of serine protease in the coagulation system. In the treatment of DIC, it is important to neutralize the clotting activities of various serine proteases, especially Factor Xa and thrombin generated intravascularly – hence the use of AT III as a therapy in DIC. As AT III levels are usually low in DIC, it is thought that deceleration of the coagulation process will occur by increasing levels with infusions of specific AT III concentrate. The potential advantage of using AT III concentrate as a single therapy is that it sufficiently controls the symptoms of DIC without the risk of increased bleeding which is a problem in heparin therapy. In DIC due to obstetric causes, the presence of post-partum or post-operative wound bleeding makes heparin therapy more hazardous and AT III may be particularly useful in such cases.[153]

Conversely, in DIC due to APL, AT III levels do not decrease[154] and, in such cases heparin therapy alone suppresses coagulation sufficiently. Although more controlled clinical trials are required to justify widespread use of AT III in DIC, increased availability of supplies of AT III concentrate will probably lead to an increase in its use in the treatment of DIC.

(3) Inhibition of excessive fibrinolysis.   When laboratory tests indicate that fibrinolysis is a major factor in the DIC process, treatment with antifibrinolytic drugs such as ε-aminocaproic acid (EACA) or tranexamic acid (Cyklokapron) may be tried, particularly if haemorrhage is a problem. Fibrinolysis in DIC is usually secondary to increased intravascular coagulation. Primary fibrinolysis can be seen in situations where there is also DIC, e.g. neoplastic disease, carcinoma of prostate and pancreas, acute leukaemias, SLE and hepatic cirrhosis. In these cases, primary fibrinolysis can coexist but be independent of the coagulopathy of DIC as the stimulus to primary fibrinolysis is direct activation of plasminogen. To distinguish between primary and secondary fibrinolysis, assays of coagulation factors and tests of the fibrinolytic system are required. Although laboratory tests can be very similar in the two conditions, it is of clinical relevance to try to establish if primary fibrinolysis is a major cause of haemorrhage because treatment with antifibrinolytic agents may be more effective in controlling

the haemorrhage of primary fibrinolysis rather than secondary fibrinolysis in DIC.

EACA acts as both a competitive and non-competitive inhibitor of plasminogen, depending on the concentration used. It is usually given orally at a dose of 3 g 6-hourly. Tranexamic acid is given orally or intravenously. Antifibrinolytic agents in DIC can cause formation of unlysable thrombus which can appear in vessels or, if haematuria is present, can cause obstruction of the urinary tract. Simultaneous low-dose heparin is sometimes administered in an effort to prevent widespread thrombosis.

(4) Antiplatelet agents. There have been occasional reports of antiplatelet drugs, e.g. prostacyclin, being successful in the treatment of the haemolytic uraemic syndrome and thrombotic thrombocytopenic purpura. It is possible that in cases of DIC where platelet aggregation is thought to be an initiating mechanism, antiplatelet agents may be useful in treatment.

(5) DIC in prostatic carcinoma. There have been many case reports recently describing the successful use of ketoconazole in DIC associated with metastatic prostatic carcinoma.[155,156] Ketoconazole, an imidazole derivative, inhibits adrenal and testicular steroid synthesis and several studies show ketoconazole to have beneficial effects and prompt action in the treatment of prostatic carcinoma without DIC.[156] Ketoconazole seems to be an ideal method for hormonal manipulation of patients with life-threatening complications of prostatic carcinoma (including DIC) because of its prompt onset of action in decreasing circulating concentrations of androgens to castrate levels. In a patient with metastic prostatic carcinoma and spontaneous bleeding from DIC, treatment with 400 mg ketoconazole 8-hourly resulted in a cessation of bleeding within 48 h.[155] Other hormonal treatment is slower to act on prostatic carcinoma than ketoconazole and orchidectomy is contraindicated because of the bleeding diathesis associated with DIC.

Ketoconazole is probably effective in metastatic prostatic carcinoma because, by hormonal manipulation, it removes the 'trigger' to DIC via suppression of thromboplastin production or release by tumour cells as well as eradication of tumour cells. It is postulated that ketoconazole may have a direct effect on activators of fibrinolysis or intravascular coagulation; however, clinical trials are required to fully evaluate the role of ketoconazole in the treatment of DIC in prostatic carcinoma. There may be implications for its use in the management of DIC in other adenocarcinomas.[156]

(6) Synthetic thrombin inhibitors. Intravascular thrombin generation is considered to be an essential pathogenic factor in the initiation of the DIC process. With regard to this concept, the effects of synthetic thrombin inhibitors have been studied in animal models of DIC.[56,60] It is postulated that synthetic thrombin inhibitors may have a prophylactic and therapeutic use in the treatment of DIC. This theory still requires clinical evaluation.

(7) Removal of already formed thrombi. Both streptokinase and urokinase have been successful in animal experiments at removing fibrin from occluded vessels[157] but there is little evidence to support the use of

such agents in DIC in man. Recently, there has been much interest in the role of tissue plasminogen activator and coronary thrombolysis, and it may be that this activator will prove useful in the lysis of thrombi in the circulation in DIC.

Prognosis

The mortality of patients with DIC has been reported in one study of 346 patients to be 68%.[141] In most cases of DIC, this mortality is directly attributable to the underlying 'trigger' of the DIC process which emphasizes the importance of prompt treatment of this 'trigger' if a diagnosis of DIC is suspected.

Obstetric problems complicated by DIC carry a better prognosis, especially if treatment is instituted early.

LIVER DISEASE

Coagulation defects and their management

The important role of the liver in maintaining normal haemostasis is shown by the complex coagulation changes which can arise with liver disease. The liver is thought to be the main site of synthesis of fibrinogen, Factors II, VII, IX, X, V, XI, XII, XIII, plasminogen, antithrombin III, and inhibitors of fibrinolysis, e.g. α_2-antiplasmin. It is also responsible for clearing activated coagulation factors and plasminogen activator.[158] The 'vitamin K-dependent' factors (II, VII, IX and X) undergo post-synthetic modification of several glutamic acid residues in the microsomes of the hepatocytes under the influence of vitamin K. This modification is essential for calcium binding and subsequent factor activity.

The following mechanisms can result in haemostatic defects in liver disease. More than one mechanism can be present in a single case.

Failure of synthesis

Vitamin K-dependent coagulation factors.   Vitamin K is a fat-soluble vitamin whose absorption is reduced in obstructive liver disease due to lack of bile salts in the small intestine. Thus, as the vitamin K-dependent clotting factors (II, VII, IX and X) cannot be modified due to lack of vitamin K they are unable to participate in normal haemostasis but their initial synthesis is unaffected. However, in hepatocellular disease, production of the complete molecule is affected, resulting in low titres of the factors.

Factor V deficiency.   Low titres of Factor V can be found in a range of acute and chronic liver disorders but not in obstructive jaundice, primary biliary cirrhosis or metastatic liver disease. If fibrinolysis is present, plasmin production can cause a further fall in Factor V by degradation of the molecule.

Fibrinogen.   In severe liver disease, e.g. acute liver failure and the end stages of chronic liver disease, fibrinogen levels can be low. In other disorders, e.g. liver cirrhosis, hepatoma and chronic hepatitis, the levels can be normal or high. Abnormal fibrinogen with increased sialic acid content and abnormal fibrin polymerization has been reported.[159] Levels of fibrinogen can be affected by consumption if there is associated DIC, fibrinolysis, massive haemorrhage or transfusion.

Other factors.   The other coagulation factors synthesized in the liver may all be reduced in acute and chronic liver disease but such changes are probably of little clinical significance. Reduced levels of plasminogen, antithrombin, and α_1-antitrypsin have been described in cirrhosis and the mechanism is thought to be a combination of defective synthesis and increased consumption.[160]

Disseminated intravascular coagulation (DIC)

Acute DIC is associated with acute liver diseases and several mechanisms may contribute to its development including: (i) reduced hepatic or reticulo-endothelial clearance of activated coagulation factors;[161] (ii) reduced clearance of plasminogen activator;[162] and (iii) reduction in synthesis of α_2-antiplasmin and antithrombin III.[163]
    The trigger to DIC may be necrotic hepatocytes acting as thrombo-plastins[164] or endotoxins.[165] In addition to DIC, the other mechanisms in liver disease may contribute to haemostatic abnormalities (e.g. reduced synthesis of coagulation factors). This makes interpretation of laboratory tests for DIC more difficult as there may already be reduced titres of coagulation factors and thrombocytopenia.[161] In liver disease, a chronic DIC can exist which, in the presence of infection, trauma or bleeding, transforms into an acute process.

Fibrinolysis

Normally, plasminogen and antiplasmin are produced in the liver; while blood plasminogen activator, FDPs and other breakdown products that activate fibrinolysis are cleared by the liver. Liver disease can result in an increase or decrease in fibrinolysis depending upon which mechanism is affected, e.g. a reduction in antiplasmin will increase fibrinolysis whereas decreased fibrinolysis results from reduced plasminogen.[166] Liver cirrhosis is generally associated with increased fibrinolysis whereas obstructive jaundice and biliary cirrhosis have reduced fibrinolysis.

Role of vitamin K

As mentioned previously, vitamin K is required as a co-factor in a post-synthetic modification of Factors II, VII, IX and X. This modification involves γ-carboxylation of the factors to form γ-carboxyglutamic acid residue forms and is essential for normal activity of the factors. Deficiency of vitamin K causes defective function of these factors. Vitamin K is also required for the γ-carboxylation of protein C and protein S which both inhibit the active forms of Factors V and VIII. Vitamin K deficiency, e.g. in obstructive liver disease, causes a reduction in activity of these proteins which could lead to a potentially thrombotic state.

Lupus-like anticoagulants

These have been reported in association with hepatobiliary diseases, e.g. Budd–Chiari syndrome and sclerosing cholangitis.[167]

Platelet disorders

These are common in liver disease and are discussed earlier.

Clinical features of coagulation defects in liver disease

Patients with chronic liver disease may present with haematemesis and melaena due to bleeding from oesophageal varices, which are an indication of portal hypertension. In acute liver disease, despite prolongation of clotting times, bleeding may not be evident. If bleeding does occur, common sites are the nasopharynx, gastrointestinal tract, the retroperitoneal space, bronchial tree and the sites of venepunctures or catheters. DIC and massive blood transfusions can compound any bleeding problems. Despite the potential risk of thrombosis due to low AT III levels, thrombotic episodes are uncommon in liver disease.

Laboratory investigation of coagulation defects in liver disease (see Table 7.8)

The coagulation screen in liver disease may become abnormal before any other liver function test. Thus, in liver disease, coagulation tests have a role in the assessment of liver function as well as in the prediction of bleeding. The one-stage prothrombin time has a high prognostic value in acute liver disease, paracetamol poisoning (where it is used to detect early liver damage) and viral hepatitis.[168,169] Table 7.8 indicates the common abnormalities of coagulation tests in different liver diseases. The prothrombin time (PT) is the minimum investigation that should be done prior to liver biopsy. Bleeding problems are likely if the PT is more than 1.5 times the control value.

Table 7.8 Coagulation Tests in Liver Diseases

Investigation	Liver diseases					Comment
	Acute viral hepatitis	Acute liver failure/ paracetamol poisoning	Cirrhosis	Obstructive jaundice	Hepatoma/ liver metastases	
One-stage prothrombin time (PT)	N; ↑	↑↑	↑; N	↑↑	↑	Prolonged due to: ↓Factor synthesis. Defective utilization of Vitamin K. Consumption in DIC. Plasmin degradation
Activated partial thromboplastin time (aPTT)	N; ↑	↑↑	↑; ↓; N	↑; N	↑	
Thrombin time	N; ↑	↑↑	↑; N	↑; N	↑↑	Prolonged due to: Dysfibrinogenaemia. Hypofibrinogenaemia FDPs
Fibrinogen	N; ↑	↑	N; ↑; ↓	↑	↑; N; →	Low in advanced liver disease due to consumption
Platelet count	N	→	→	N	↑; N; →	Reduced due to splenic sequestration and decreased production

↑ = Prolonged, elevated; N = normal; → = shortened, reduced; ↑↑ = markedly prolonged, elevated.

The management of coagulation defects in liver disease

The majority of patients with liver disease may be asymptomatic requiring no treatment, but, if there is an element of biliary obstruction and prolongation of the PT due to vitamin K deficiency, oral or parenteral vitamin K may help. There are two main situations where treatment is indicated in the presence of a significant haemostatic defect.

(1) Prophylaxis to cover surgery or liver biopsy

For non-urgent procedures, vitamin K 10 mg orally for 5 days can be given and the PT checked before the procedure. If the ratio is <1.3, surgery or biopsy can proceed. If the PT is not improved or urgent surgery is required, fresh frozen plasma (FFP) can be given. Repeated transfusions of this may be necessary to secure haemostasis. Hypervolaemia can result and in such situations, prothrombin complex concentrates (PCC) may have to be considered. However, PCC are rarely used because of the risk of thrombotic complications and transmission of viruses, e.g. hepatitis B.[170] Prophylactic platelet transfusions may be required if severe thrombocytopenia is present. If a qualitative or quantitative fibrinogen defect is suggested by a prolonged thrombin time, cryoprecipitate transfusion may be of value.

(2) Severe bleeding

Bleeding usually occurs from the gastrointestinal tract – oesophageal varices, duodenal ulcer or gastric erosions. Correction of coagulation defects with FFP (sometimes PCC) and platelet transfusions are required. Parenteral vitamin K should be started. Hypovolaemia may require massive blood transfusions. Once bleeding is under control, further treatment should be aimed at the source of the bleeding, e.g. insertion of a Sengstaken tube or laser cautery for bleeding varices and surgery for peptic ulceration.

ACQUIRED INHIBITORS OF COAGULATION

In 1972, acquired inhibitors of coagulation were defined as 'pathologic substances which directly inhibit clotting factors or their reactions'.[171] The overall incidence of such inhibitors in the general population is unclear although it has been reported as 0.75% in a study based on the screening of 400 asymptomatic subjects.[172] If groups of patients with specific disorders are studied, the incidence will be much higher, e.g. 10% of those with SLE may have the 'lupus anticoagulant'.[173]

Acquired inhibitors are usually auto-antibodies which are directed against a single factor or enzymatic step. They may arise (a) as a result of treatment with factor concentrates in congenital factor deficiencies, (b) spontaneously in otherwise healthy (often elderly) individuals, (c) post-partum, or (d) in association with systemic diseases. The inhibitors which are commonest and the most important clinically are Factor VIIIc inhibitors. These and other acquired inhibitors will now be described.

Factor VIIIc inhibitors

In haemophilia A

About 6% of treated haemophilia A patients in the UK have inhibitors against the coagulant part of the Factor VIII molecule (FVIIIc). The inhibitor is usually an IgG antibody, although IgM has been implicated. The patients who acquire these inhibitors are usually severe haemophiliacs and in them the inhibitor usually persists. Haemophiliacs can develop inhibitors after transfusion of whole blood, plasma, cryoprecipitate or factor concentrates. An inhibitor to Factor VIIIc is diagnosed by demonstrating loss of FVIIIc activity in serial assays of a mixture of test plasma incubated with Factor VIII concentrate. The Bethesda method and units are those which are most commonly used and recognized in the demonstration and quantification of an inhibitor. Haemophiliacs with inhibitors can be classified as either high or low responders. In high responders (i.e. the majority of patients), the inhibitor level is high and treatment with Factor VIII is ineffective and may produce an anamnestic response. Although the high titre may fall if Factor VIII treatment is withheld, subsequent rechallenge causes a further rise in titre. Low responders have low inhibitor levels which do not rise after Factor VIII exposure. Thus, low responders can be successfully treated with high doses of Factor VIII when required, e.g. after injuries or operations. The plasma level of Factor VIIIc should be regularly checked to assess response. In high responders, short courses of Factor VIII concentrate can be tried but often even high doses of Factor VIII may be ineffective in producing adequate haemostasis. High purity porcine Factor VIII can be used but also causes antibody production. Other possible therapeutic options reported to be successful in individual cases include plasmapheresis, immunosuppression, activated Factor IX concentrates, and removal of the inhibitor by extracorporeal circulation through an immunoadsorbent.

In non-haemophiliacs

Acquired Factor VIIIc inhibitors in non-haemophiliac patients are rarely encountered in clinical practice. They have been described in the following conditions:[174–176]

1. 'auto-immune' disorders (e.g. SLE, rheumatoid arthritis, temporal arteritis, ulcerative colitis, pemphigus, multiple sclerosis);
2. post-partum women;
3. drug reactions (e.g. penicillin, phenytoin, ampicillin, chloramphenicol);
4. neoplastic disease (especially lymphoproliferative disorders, solid tumours, and paraproteinaemias);
5. normal individuals (often elderly females); and ·
6. respiratory disorders (e.g. asthma, lung abscess, sarcoidosis).

Usually, severe cases present with a haemorrhagic tendency. Spontaneous bleeding can occur, resulting in haemarthroses, intracranial haemorrhage, melaena, haematuria and haemoptysis. In one study of patients,[174] 22% of patients died either directly or indirectly as a consequence of having the inhibitor.

Laboratory diagnosis of Factor VIIIc inhibitors

The activated partial thromboplastin time (aPTT) is prolonged and the Factor VIIIc level will be low. When normal plasma is added to the plasma of a patient with Factor VIIIc inhibitor, these tests will not correct, whereas in a patient with a pure deficiency state they will correct. The titre of Factor VIIIc inhibitor can be assayed as in haemophiliacs. Most inhibitors are IgG antibodies.

Clinical course and treatment

The clinical course of these patients is variable. Post-partum, the inhibitor can diminish in titre over many months and spontaneously disappear. It may or may not reappear in subsequent pregnancies. Rarely, there can be transplacental transfer of an acquired Factor VIIIc inhibitor because they are usually of antibody class IgG.[177] In patients with autoimmune diseases, the inhibitor can persist and rise in titre.

The aim of treatment is to prevent haemorrhage. Acute bleeding can be treated with high doses of Factor VIII concentrates, porcine Factor VIII and activated Factor IX products (Feiba and Autoplex). It may be possible to reduce the inhibitor titre by plasmapheresis or immunosuppression, e.g. with azathioprine, cyclophosphamide, or steroids.[174] Suppression of the inhibitor after high-dose intravenous gammaglobulin has been reported in two patients.[178] An important aspect of the management of a patient with a known circulating inhibitor is to ensure that the patient is protected from any actions which could precipitate bleeding, e.g. avoidance of intramuscular injections, excessive venepunctures, and aspirin.

An important prognostic factor in the treatment of these patients is the initial titre of the inhibitor. Low titres indicate a better prognosis and a more likely response to immunosuppressive therapy.[179]

Finally, because the use of long-term cytotoxic immunosuppressive therapy is not without its own hazards, e.g. cytopenias, development of neoplasias, drug-induced haemorrhagic cystitis and gastroenteritis, short-term treatment is advised. Failure of response to such treatment after 6 weeks is considered an adequate trial and alternative therapy should be sought.[180]

Inhibitors against other factors (see also Table 7.9)

About 1–2% of patients with Factor IX deficiency (haemophilia B) have inhibitors to Factor IX. These inhibitors are exceptionally rare in non-deficient patients and are seen in clinical settings similar to those in which Factor VIII inhibitors arise, e.g. autoimmune disorders and post-partum women. Patients present with haemorrhagic problems similar to those seen with Factor VIII inhibitors. Treatment involves the use of immunosuppressive agents and activated Factor IX concentrates.

Inhibitors directed against von Willebrand factor (vWF) are rare and may be found in von Willebrand's disease, in previously healthy individuals, or

Table 7.9 Acquired Inhibitors of Coagulation – Types and Characteristic Features

Inhibitor	Coagulation and clinical abnormality		Associated conditions
VIIIC	↑ aPTT	Severe bleeding	Haemophilia A; elderly; post-partum; autoimmune diseases
VIII (vWF)	↑ Bleeding time ↑ aPTT Platelet dysfunction	Mucosal bleeding – can be severe	von Willebrand's disease treated with cryoprecipitate; rarely found in other conditions
IX	↑ aPTT	Severe bleeding	Haemophilia B (1–3%) Rarely found in non-haemophiliacs
V	↑ aPTT ↑ PT	Mild bleeding	Post-transfusion Infections Streptomycin therapy
XI; XII	↑ aPTT	Few bleeding problems	Autoimmune diseases Paraproteinaemias Chlorpromazine therapy
XIII	Unstable fibrin clot	Persistent severe bleeding	Isoniazid therapy
Directed against fibrin and fibrinogen	May have ↑ PT, ↑ aPTT, ↑ TCT	Mild bleeding tendency	Myeloma
Heparin-like anticoagulant	↑ TCT (reduced *in vitro* and *in vivo* by protamine sulphate)	Can be severe bleeding	Leukaemias Myeloma AIDS
Lupus & lupus-like anti-coagulants	↑ aPTT	No bleeding Recurrent thromboses	SLE & other autoimmune diseases Carcinomas Lymphomas Certain drugs, e.g. procainamide Apparently normal people

TCT = thrombin clotting time.
aPTT = activated partial thromboplastin time.
PT = prothrombin time.

in patients with disorders such as paraproteinaemias, lymphoma or SLE. The inhibitor may be an IgM or IgG antibody. Patients present with haemorrhagic problems including mucosal bleeding. Laboratory investigations reveal a prolonged bleeding time, platelet dysfunction, reduced levels of Factor VIIIc, vWF antigen, and the plasma factor necessary to support ristocetin-induced platelet aggregation. These inhibitors may disappear with treatment of the underlying pathology.

Inhibitors to Factor V have been described[171] and are extremely rare. They usually appear in patients with a genetic factor deficiency but have also occurred in patients with infections, post-transfusion, post-surgical patients or those treated with tetracyclines or streptomycin. The inhibitors can be IgG or IgM antibodies and the haemorrhagic tendency produced varies from minor bleeding to intractable, ultimately fatal haemorrhage. The natural history of the inhibitor is to gradually decline in titre. Steroids and immunosuppressive agents have been used in treatment. Transfusion with platelet concentrate has been successfully used to arrest haemorrhage.[184]

Inhibitors to Factors VII, X, XI, XII, XIII, prothrombin, fibrin, and fibrinogen have been described and are all exceptionally rare. Some cases are associated with drugs (e.g. chlorpromazine), autoimmune disorders, e.g. SLE, paraproteinaemias (especially Factor XI and XII inhibitors) or genetic deficiencies of the factors. Paraproteins arising in patients with myeloma may non-specifically block the aggregation of fibrin polymer.[181] Inhibitors against Factor XIII have occurred in patients after isoniazid therapy[182] and one case occurred in a lupus-like syndrome induced by practolol therapy.[183] Treatment of these rare inhibitors has usually been with steroids and immunosuppression.

Heparin-like anticoagulant

An acquired heparin-like anticoagulant has been found in patients with leukaemia,[185] systemic mastocytosis,[186] plasma cell myeloma[187] and the acquired immunodeficiency syndrome (AIDS).[188] This anticoagulant causes a prolonged thrombin time which is clearly reduced *in vivo* and *in vitro* by protamine sulphate. The reptilase time is usually normal and the patient's plasma can inhibit thrombin and activated Factor X (Xa). The anticoagulant is 'heparin-like' as it has been identified as a proteoglycan similar to heparan sulphate and heparin-like activity can be measured in patients. Patients may present with spontaneous, sometimes severe bleeding which can be rapidly corrected by protamine sulphate.[188]

Lupus-like anticoagulants (LLA)

Since the lupus circulating anticoagulant was first described in a patient with SLE in 1952,[189] similar substances often termed 'lupus-like' anticoagulants have been identified in conditions other than SLE such as carcinomas, lymphomas, eclampsia, autoimmune disorders, e.g. rheumatoid arthritis, in relation to drugs (chlorpromazine, Fansidar, procainamide, penicillin), in patients with opportunistic infections due to AIDS, and in many patients with no discernible underlying disease.[190-192] In addition, LLA have been observed and suggested to have a pathogenic role in recurrent spontaneous abortions, pulmonary hypertension, transverse myelitis and neurological disease associated with SLE and Bechet's disease.[193]

The lupus and lupus-like anticoagulants are IgG, IgM or combined IgG/IgM antibodies which are thought to be directed against the phospholipid portion of the prothrombin activator complex (Factor Xa, V, calcium and phospholipid) and occasionally against the phospholipids contained in the platelet membrane.[194,195] Their action at the junction of the extrinsic and intrinsic coagulation pathways causes inhibition of the interaction between prothrombin and the prothrombin activator complex.

The 'lupus' anticoagulant has been designated as an anticoagulant which prolongs the activated partial thromboplastin time (aPTT) and occasionally the prothrombin time (PT) of normal plasma but does not specifically inactivate any of the known clotting factors. A variety of tests can be used to diagnose LA and LLA and they have different sensitivities and specificities.[193] The PT and aPTT lack sensitivity for detecting the presence of LA. The most sensitive tests are those with a reduced phospholipid content, i.e. the kaolin clotting time and the prothrombin time performed with dilute thromboplastin.[198] The dilute Russell viper venom time has been described as a sensitive and relatively specific method for the detection of lupus anticoagulants.[199] Suspicion of a lupus or lupus-like anticoagulant is usually aroused by the finding of a prolonged aPTT that is not corrected by the addition of an equal volume of normal plasma. This can sometimes be a chance finding, e.g. on routine pre-operative clotting studies.

The clinical importance of these anticoagulants lies in their strong correlation with recurrent venous and arterial thromboses and foetal loss due to recurrent abortion.[196] Different hypotheses exist as to the exact mechanism responsible for the thrombotic tendency in these patients.[197,198] There is a strong correlation between the presence of the lupus anticoagulant and elevated titres of antibody to cardiolipin, and the presence of either or both is associated with a high incidence of thrombosis.[206] There is no evidence directly implicating anticardiolipin antibodies with anticoagulant activity in the pathogenesis of the thrombotic episodes. Despite the prolonged aPTT, few patients present with haemorrhagic problems even when undergoing major surgical procedures unless a second haemostatic defect, e.g. thrombocytopenia, hypoprothrombinaemia, or a second inhibitor, also exists.[190] Without therapy, the lupus anticoagulant usually persists, although spontaneous disappearance has been observed both with and without remission of the disease. Steroid therapy in the treatment of the primary disease may result in the reduction or disappearance of the anticoagulant activity if the disease remits.[190] Thrombotic events and recurrent abortions in pregnant patients may be treated by immunosuppressants and anticoagulants.[173,202,203] High-dose intravenous immunoglobulin infusions have been reported to transiently inhibit the lupus anticoagulant.[200] If there is evidence of platelet dysfunction and arterial insufficiency, inhibitors of platelet function, e.g. aspirin or dipyridamole, may be used.[201] In a case report of a lupus-type coagulation inhibitor appearing in hairy cell leukaemia, splenectomy resulted in disappearance of the inhibitor.[204]

In summary, patients who present with evidence of a haemorrhagic disorder, especially haematomas and haemarthroses, should be investigated for the presence of an antibody to a specific clotting factor. Acquired inhibitors should be particularly looked for in patients with persistent post-operative bleeding, despite the institution of normally adequate measures to control bleeding. A history of recurrent thromboses or repeated abortions in patients who have a prolonged aPTT and no bleeding suggests a lupus or lupus-like anticoagulant.

Table 7.9 outlines some of the characteristic features of the acquired inhibitors of coagulation.

REFERENCES

1. Davies, J.A. & McNicol, G.P. Haemostasis and thrombosis. In *Oxford Textbook of Medicine*, Vol. 2 (eds J.D. Weatherall, J.G.G. Ledingham & D.A. Warrell), pp. 19, 111–13. Oxford University Press, New York, 1983.
2. Bloom, A.L. Inherited disorders of blood coagulation. In *Haemostasis and Thrombosis* (eds A.L. Bloom & D.P. Thomas), pp. 394–6. Churchill Livingstone, Edinburgh, 1987.
3. Rao, L.V.M. & Rapaport, S.I. Studies of a mechanism inhibiting the initiation of the extrinsic pathway of coagulation. *Blood* **69**: 645–51, 1987.
4. Thomson, J.M. & Poller, L. The activated partial thromboplastin time. In *Blood Coagulation and Haemostasis. A Practical Guide*, 3rd Edn (ed. J.M. Thomson), pp. 301–39. Churchill Livingstone, Edinburgh. 1985.
5. Nilsson, I.-M. Assessment of blood coagulation and general haemostasis. In *Haemostasis and Thrombosis* (eds A.L. Bloom & D.P. Thomas), pp. 922–30. Churchill Livingstone, Edinburgh, 1987.
6. Clouse, L.J. & Comp, P.C. The regulation of hemostasis: the protein C system. *N. Engl. J. Med.* **314**: 1298–304, 1986.
7. Shuster, S. & Scarborough, H. Senile purpura. *Q. J. Med.* **30**: 33–40, 1961.
8. Shiozawa, S., Tanaka, T., Miyahara, T., Murai, A. & Kammeyamma, M. Age related change in the reducible cross-links of human skin and aorta collagens. *Gerontology* **25**: 247–54, 1979.
9. Saunders, W.H. Permanent control of nose bleeds in patients with hereditary haemorrhagic telangiectasia. *Ann. Intern. Med.* **53**: 147–52, 1960.
10. Blackburn, E.K. Long term treatment of epistaxis wth oestrogens. *Br. Med. J.* **2**: 159–60, 1963.
11. Harrison, D.F.N. Familial haemorrhagic telangiectasia: 20 cases treated with systemic oestrogen. *Q. J. Med.* **33**: NSI: 25–38, 1964.
12. Hodgson, C.H., Birchell, H.B., Good, C.A. & Clagett, O.T. Hereditary haemorrhagic telangiectasia and pulmonary arteriovenous fistula: Survey of a large family. *N. Eng. J. Med.* **261**: 625–36, 1959.
13. Rendu, M. Epistaxis répétées. Chez un sujet porteur de petits angiomes cutanés et muqueux. *Bull. Mem. Soc. Med. Paris* **13**: 731–3, 1896,
14. Weber, F.P. Multiple hereditary developmental angiomata (telangiectases) of skin and mucous membranes associated with recurring haemorrhages. *Lancet* **2**: 160–8, 1907.
15. Osler, W. On a family form of recurrent epistaxis associated with multiple telangiectases of the skin and mucous membranes. *Bull. Johns Hopkins Hosp.* **12**: 333, 1901.
16. Kasabach, H.H. & Merritt, K.K. Capillary haemangioma with extensive purpura. Report of a case. *Am. J. Dis. Childh.* **59**: 1063–70, 1940.

17. Wise, D., Wallace, H.J. & Jellinek, E.H. Angiokeratoma corporis diffusum. *Q. J. Med.* **31**: 177–206, 1962.
18. Ehlers, E. Cutis laxa, Neigung zu Haemorrhagien in der Haut, Lockerung mechrerer Artikulationum. *Dermatologische Zeitschrift* **8**: 173–4, 1901.
19. Danlos, M. Un cas de cutis laxa avec tumeurs par contusion chronique des coudes et des genoux. (xanthome juvenile pseudo diabetéque de MM. Hallopeau et Macé de Lépinay). *Bull. Soc. Francaise Dermatologie Syphiligraphie* **19**: 70–2, 1908.
20. Beighton, P. *The Ehlers–Danlos Syndrome*. Heinemann, London, 1970.
21. Pope, F.M., Martin, G.R. & Lichenstein, J.R. Patients with Ehlers–Danlos syndrome type IV lack type III collagen. *Proc. Natl. Acad. Sci. U.S.A* **72**: 1314–16, 1975.
22. Kashiwagi, H., Riddle, J.M., Abraham, J.P. & Frame, B. Functional and ultrastructural abnormalities of platelets in Ehlers–Danlos syndrome. *Ann. Intern. Med.* **63**: 249–54, 1965.
23. Lisker, R., Nogueron, A. & Sanchez-Medal, L. Plasma thromboplastin component deficiency in the Ehlers–Danlos syndrome. *Ann. Intern. Med.* **53**: 388–95, 1960.
24. Fantl, P., Morris, K.N. & Sawers, R.J. Repair of cardiac defect in patient with Ehlers–Danlos syndrome and deficiency of Hageman factor. *Br. Med. J.* **1**: 1202–4, 1961.
25. Goodman, R.M., Smith, E.W. & Paton, D. Pseudoxanthoma elasticum: A clinical and histopathological study. *Medicine* **42**: 297–334, 1963.
26. Siegel, B.M., Friedman, I.A. & Schwartz, S.O. Haemorrhagic disease in osteogenesis imperfecta: Studies of platelet function defect. *Am. J. Med.* **22**: 315–21, 1957.
27. Priest, R.E., Moinuddin, J.F. & Priest, J.H. Collagen of Marfan syndrome is abnormally soluble. *Nature* **245**: 264–6, 1973.
28. Erdohazi, M., Cowie, V. & Lo, S.S. A case of haemophilia with Marfan's syndrome. *Br. Med. J.* **1**: 102–3, 1964.
29. Leede, C. & Rumpel, D. Zur Beurteilung des Rumpel-Leedeschen Scharlach-phanomens. *Munchen Medizin Wochenschrift* **58**: 1673–4, 1911.
30. Hess, A.F. The involvement of the blood and blood vessels in infantile scurvy. *Proc. Soc. Exp. Biol. Med.* **11**: 130–2, 1914.
31. Gough, K.R. Capillary resistance to suction in hypertension. *Br. Med. J.* **1**: 21–4, 1962.
32. Kramar, J. The determination and evaluation of capillary resistance – a review of methodology. *Blood* **20**: 83–93, 1962.
33. Barnes, M.J., Constable, B.J. & Morton, L.F. Studies *in vivo* on the biosynthesis of collagen and elastin in ascorbic acid deficient guinea pigs. *Biochem. J.* **119**: 575–85, 1970.
34. Born, G.V.R. & Wright, H.P. Platelet adhesiveness in experimental scurvy. *Lancet* **1**: 477–8, 1967.
35. Wilson, P.A., McNicol, G.P. & Douglas, A.S. Platelet abnormality in human scurvy. *Lancet* **1**: 975–8, 1967.
36. Wallerstein, R.O. & Wallerstein, R.O., Jr. Scurvy. *Semin. Hematol.* **13**: 211–18, 1976.
37. Lowe, G.D.O., Lowe, J.M., Drummond, M.M., Reith, S., Belch, J.J.F., Kesson, C.M., Wyle, A., Foulds, W.S., Forbes, C.D., MacCuish, A.C. & Manderson, W. Blood viscosity in young male diabetics with and without retinopathy. *Diabetologia* **18**: 359–63, 1980.
38. Somer, T. Hyperviscosity syndrome in plasma cell dyscrasias. *Adv. Microcirculation* **6**: 1–55, 1975.
39. Preston, E., Cooke, K.B., Foster, M.F., Winfield, D.A. & Lee, D. Myelomatosis and the hyperviscosity syndrome. *Br. J. Haematol.* **38**: 517–30, 1978.

40. Lackner, H., Hunt, V., Zucker, M.B. & Pearson, J. Abnormal fibrin ultrastructure, polymerisation and clot retraction in multiple myeloma. *Br. J. Haematol.* **18**: 625–36, 1970.
41. Pachter, M.R., Johnson, S.A., Neblett, T.R. & Truant, J.P. Bleeding, platelets and macroglobulinaemia. *Am. J. Clin. Pathol.* **31**: 467–82, 1959.
42. Scarborough, H. & Shuster, S. Corticosteroid purpura. *Lancet* **1**: 93–4, 1960.
43. Broekmans, A.W., Bertina, R.M. & Loeliger, E.A. Protein C and the development of skin necrosis during anticoagulant therapy. *Thromb. Haemost.* **49**: 251–7, 1983.
44. Turi, S., Belch, J.J.F., Beattie, T.J. & Forbes, C.D. Abnormalities of vascular prostaglandins in Henoch–Schonlein purpura. *Arch. Dis. Child.* **61**: 173–7, 1986.
45. Trygstad, C.W. & Stiehm, E.R. Elevated serum IgA globulin in anaphylactoid purpura. *Pediatrics* **47**: 1023–8, 1971.
46. De La Faille-Kuyper, E.H., Kater, L., Kooker, C.J. *et al.* IgA deposits in cutaneous blood vessel walls and in Henoch–Schonlein syndrome. *Lancet* **1**: 892–3, 1973.
47. Fauci, A.S., Haynes, B.F. & Katz, P. The spectrum of vasculitis: clinical, pathologic, immunologic and therapeutic considerations. *Ann. Intern. Med.* **89**: 660–76, 1978.
48. Ratnoff, O.D. Psychogenic bleeding. In *Disorders of hemostasis* (eds O.D. Ratnoff & C.D. Forbes), pp. 549–53. Grune & Stratton, New York, 1984.
49. Gardiner, F.H. & Diamond, L.K. Autoerythrocyte sensitization. A form of purpura producing painful bruising following autosensitization to red blood cells in certain women. *Blood* **10**: 675–90, 1955.
50. Ratnoff, O.D. & Agle, D. Psychogenic purpura: A re-evaluation of the syndrome of autoerythrocyte sensitisation. *Medicine* **47**: 475–500, 1968.
51. Siegal, T., Seligsohn, U., Aghai, E. & Modan, M. Clinical and laboratory aspects of disseminated intravascular coagulation (DIC). A study of 118 cases. *Thromb. Haemost.* **39**: 122, 1978.
52. Kim, H.S., Suzuki, M., Lie, J.T. & Titus, J.L. Clinically unsuspected disseminated intravascular coagulation (DIC). An autopsy survey. *Am. J. Clin. Pathol.* **66**: 31, 1976.
53. Busch, C. & Saleen, T. Amount of fibrin in different organs after intravenous, intraportal and intraaortal injection of thrombin in rat. *Thromb. Diathes. Haemorrh.* **29**: 87–93, 1973.
54. Markwardt, F., Nowak, G., Meerbach, W. & Rudiger, K. Studies in experimental animals on D.I.C. *Thromb. Diathes, Haemorrh.* **34**: 513–21, 1975.
55. Markwardt, F., Nowak, G. & Hoffman, J. Comparative studies on thrombin inhibitors in experimental microthrombosis. *Thromb. Haemost.* **49**: 235–7, 1983.
56. Hara, H., Tamao, Y., Kikunoto, R. & Okamoto, S. Effect of a synthetic thrombin inhibitor MCI-9038 on experimental models of disseminated intravascular coagulation in rabbits. *Thromb. Haemost.* **57**: 165–70, 1987.
57. Slaastad, R. & Jeremic, M. The laboratory diagnosis of low-grade disseminated intravascular coagulation. *Scand. J. Haematol.* **11**: 50–8, 1973.
58. Pflug, J., Calnan, J. & Oslen, G.J. An experimental model for the study of thrombosis. *Br. J. Surg.* **25**: 63–9, 1968.
59. Cronlund, M., Hardin, J., Burton, H., Lee, L., Haber, E. & Block, K.J. Fibrinopeptide in plasma of normal subjects and patients with disseminated intravascular coagulation and systemic lupus erythematosus. *J. Clin. Invest.* **58**: 142–51, 1976.
60. Schaeffer, R.C., Briston, C., Chilton, S.-M. & Carlson, R.W. Disseminated intravascular coagulation following *Echis carinatus* venom in dogs: Effects of a synthetic thrombin inhibitor. *J. Lab. Clin. Med.* **107**: 488–97, 1986.
61. Muller-Berghaus, G. Pathophysiology of generalised intravascular coagulation. *Semin. Thromb. Hemost.* **3**: 209–46, 1977.

62. McKay, D.G. & Muller-Berghaus, G. Therapeutic implications of disseminated intravascular coagulation. *Am. J. Cardiol.* **20**: 392–410, 1967.
63. Bang, N.U. & Chang, M. Soluble fibrin complexes. *Semin. Thromb. Hemost.* **1**: 91, 1974.
64. Jakobsen, E., Ly, B. & Kieulf, P. Incorporation of fibrinogen with soluble fibrin complexes. *Thromb. Res.* **4**: 499, 1974.
65. Fletcher, A.P., Alkjaersig, N., Fisher, S. & Sherry, S. The proteolysis of fibrinogen by plasmin: the identification of thrombin-clottable fibrinogen derivatives which polymerise abnormally. *J. Lab. Clin. Med.* **68**: 780–802, 1966.
66. Sharp, A.A. Pathological fibrinolysis. *Br. Med. Bull.* **20**: 240, 1964.
67. Pechet, L. Fibrinolysis. *N. Engl. J. Med.* **273**: 966, 1965.
68. Donaldson, V. Effect of plasmin *in vitro* on clotting factors in plasma. *J. Lab. Clin. Med.* **56**: 644, 1960.
69. Schreiber, A.D. & Austen, K.F. Inter-relationships of the fibrinolytic, coagulation, kinin generation and complement systems. *Semin. Hematol.* **6**: 593, 1973.
70. Kaplan, A., Meier, H. & Mandle, R. The Hageman factor dependent coagulation pathways of coagulation, fibrinolysis and kinin generation. *Semin. Thromb. Hemost.* **3**: 6, 1976.
71. Verheijen, J.H., Chang, G.T.G. & Kluft, C. Evidence for the occurrence of a fast-acting inhibitor of plasminogen activator in human plasma. *Thromb. Haemost.* **51**: 392–5, 1984.
72. Kruithof, E.K.O., Tran-Thang, C., Ransijin, A. & Bachmann, F. Demonstration of a fast-acting inhibitor of plasminogen activators in human plasma. *Blood* **64**: 907–13, 1984.
73. Chmielewska, J., Ranby, M. & Wiman, B. Evidence for a rapid inhibitor to tissue plasminogen activator in plasma. *Thromb. Res.* **31**: 427–36, 1983.
74. Bergsdorf, N., Nilsson, T. & Wallen, P. An enzyme linked immunosorbent assay for determination of tissue plasminogen activator applied to patients with thromboembolic disease. *Thromb. Haemost.* **50**: 740–4, 1983.
75. Holvoet, P., Cleemput, H. & Collen, D. Assay of human tissue-type plasminogen activator (t-PA) with an enzyme-linked immunosorbent assay (ELISA) based on three murine monoclonal antibodies to t-PA. *Thromb. Haemost.* **54**: 684–7, 1985.
76. Mahmoud, M. & Gaffney, P.J. Bioimmunoassay (BIA) of tissue plasminogen activator (t-PA) and its specific inhibitor (t-PA/INH). *Thromb. Haemost.* **53**: 356–9, 1985.
77. Verheijen, J.H., Mullaart, F., Chang, G.T.G. *et al.* A simple sensitive spectrophotometric assay for extrinsic (tissue type) plasminogen activator applicable to measurements in plasma. *Thromb. Haemost.* **48**: 266–9, 1982.
78. Wiman, B., Mellbring, G. & Ranby, M. Plasminogen activator release during venous stasis and exercise as determined by a new specific assay. *Clin. Chim. Acta* **127**: 279–88, 1983.
79. Wiman, B., Ljunberg, B., Chmielewska, J. *et al.* The role of the fibrinolytic system in deep vein thrombosis. *J. Lab. Clin. Med.* **105**: 265–70, 1985.
80. Hamsten, A., Wiman, B., De Faire, U. & Blomback, M. Increased plasma levels of a rapid inhibitor of tissue plasminogen activator in young survivors of myocardial infarction. *N. Engl. J. Med.* **313**: 1557–63, 1985.
81. Brommer, E.J.P., Verheijen, J.H., Chang, G.T.G. & Rijken, D.C. Masking of fibrinolytic response to stimulation by an inhibitor of tissue-type plasminogen activator in plasma. *Thromb. Haemost.* **52**: 154–6, 1984.
82. Francis, R.B. Jr. & Seyfert, U. Tissue plasminogen activator antigen and activity in disseminated intravascular coagulation: Clinico-pathologic correlations. *J. Lab. Clin. Med.* **110**: 541–7, 1987.
83. Van Hinsbergh, V.W.M., Bertina, R.M., Van Wijingaarden, A. *et al.* Activated protein C decreases plasminogen activator-inhibitor activity in endothelial cell-

conditioned medium. *Blood* **65**: 444–51, 1985.

84. Francis, R.B. & Thomas, W. Behaviour of protein C inhibitor in intravascular coagulation and liver disease. *Thromb. Haemost.* **52**: 71–4, 1984.

85. Marlar, R.A., Endres-Brooks, J. & Miller, C. Serial studies of protein C and its plasma inhibitor in patients with disseminated intravascular coagulation. *Blood* **66**: 59–63, 1985.

86. Jilek, F. & Horman, H. Fibronectin (cold insoluble globulin) mediation of fibrin binding to macrophages. *Hoppe Seylers Z. Physiol. Chem.* **359**: 1603–5, 1978.

87. Lasdi, H.G., Henne, D.L., Huth, K. *et al.* Pathophysiology, clinical manifestations and therapy of consumption coagulopathy. *Am. J. Cardiol.* **20**: 381, 1967.

88. Owen, C.A., Bawie, E.J.W. & Cooper, H.A. Turnover of fibrinogen and platelets in dogs undergoing induced intravascular coagulation. *Thromb. Res.* **2**: 251, 1973.

89. Beller, F.K. The role of endotoxin in disseminated intravascular coagulation. *Thromb. Diathes. Haemorrh.* **36** (Suppl.): 125–50, 1969.

90. Evensen, S.A. & Hjort, P.F. Pathogenesis of disseminated intravascular clotting. Plenary sessions, scientific contributions. *XIII International Congress of Haematology*, Munich, pp. 109–120, 1970.

91. Latour, J.-G. & Léger-Gauthier, C. Vasoactive agents and production of thrombosis during intravascular coagulation. *Am. J. Pathol.* **126**: 569–80, 1987.

92. Latour, J.-G., Léger-Gauthier, C. & Solymoss, C.B. Vasoactive agents and production of thrombosis during intravascular coagulation: 2. Alpha-adrenergic stimulation: Effects and mechanisms. *Pathology* **17**: 429–36, 1985.

93. Huth, K., Schoenborn, W. & Knorpp, K. Experimentelle Verbranchskoagulopathie nach intravenoser Zufuhr von Fett und Endotoxin. *Thromb. Diathes. Haemorrh.* **16**: 228–42, 1967.

94. Goodnight, S.H., Kenoyer, G., Rappaport, S.I., Patel, M.J., Lee, J.A. & Kieze, T. Defibrination after brain-tissue destruction: A serious complication of head injury. *N. Engl. J. Med.* **290**: 1043, 1974.

95. Gralnick, H.R. & Abrell, E. Studies of the procoagulant and fibrinolytic activity of promyelocytes in acute promyelocytic leukaemia. *Br. J. Haematol.* **24**: 89–99, 1973.

96. Kornalik, F. & Blomback, B. Prothrombin activation induced by Ecarin – a prothrombin converting enzyme from *Echis carinatus* venom. *Thromb. Res.* **6**: 53–63, 1975.

97. Hasiba, U., Rosenback, L.M., Rockwell, D. & Lewis, J.H. DIC-like syndrome after envenomation by the snake, *Crotalus horridus*. *N. Engl. J. Med.* **292**: 505–7, 1975.

98. Kessler, C.M., Nussbaum, E. & Tuazon, C.U. *In vitro* correlation of platelet aggregation with occurrence of disseminated intravascular coagulation and subacute bacterial endocarditis. *J. Lab. Clin. Med.* **109**: 647–52, 1987.

99. Rodriguez-Erdman, F. & Gutmann, R.D. Coagulation in renal allograft rejection. *N. Engl. J. Med.* **281**: 1428, 1969.

100. McGehee, W.G., Rapaport, S.I. & Hjort, P.F. Intravascular coagulation in fulminant meningococcaemia. *Ann. Intern. Med.* **67**: 250, 1967.

101. Mulder, L.J.M.M. & Spierings, E.L.H. Stroke due to intravascular coagulation in mycoplasma pneumoniae infection. *Lancet* **2**: 1152–3, 1987.

102. Reid, A.H. Clinical haemostatic disorders caused by venoms. In *Disorders of Haemostasis* (eds O. Ratnoff & C.D. Forbes). Grune & Stratton, New York, 1984.

103. Wilmer, G.D., Nossel, H.D. & Le Roy, E.C. Activation of Hagemen Factor by collagen. *J. Clin. Invest.* **47**: 2608, 1968.

104. Kleiner, G.J. & Merskey, C. Defibrination in normal and abnormal parturition. *Br. J. Haematol.* **19**: 159, 1970.

105. Talbert, I.M. & Blatt, P.M. Disseminated intravascular coagulation in obstetrics. *Clin. Obstet. Gynecol.* **22**: 889, 1979.

106. Dieckmann, W.J. Blood chemistry and renal function in abruptio placentae. *Am. J. Obstet. Gynecol.* **31**: 734, 1936.
107. Pritchard, J.A. & Brekken, A.L. Clinical and laboratory studies on severe abruptio placentae. *Am. J. Obstet. Gynecol.* **97**: 681, 1967.
108. Schneider, C.L. "Fibrin embolism" (disseminated intravascular coagulation) with defibrination as one of the end results during placental abruption. *Surg. Gynaecol. Obstet.* **92**: 27, 1951.
109. Courtney, L.D. & Allington, M. Effect of amniotic fluid on blood coagulation. *Br. J. Haematol.* **22**: 353, 1972.
110. Wiener, A.E. & Reid, D.E. Pathogenesis of amniotic fluid embolism III. Coagulant activity of amniotic fluid. *N. Engl. J. Med.* **243**: 597, 1950.
111. Howie, P.W., Purdie, D.W., Begg, C.B. *et al.*. Use of coagulation tests to predict the clinical progress of pre-eclampsia. *Lancet* **2**: 323–5, 1976.
112. Howie, P.W., Prentice, C.R.M. & Forbes, C.D. Failure of heparin therapy to affect the clinical course of severe pre-eclampsia. *Br. J. Obstet. Gynaecol.* **82**: 711, 1975.
113. Grundy, M.F.B. & Graven, E.R. Consumption coagulopathy after intra-amniotic urea. *Br. Med. J.* **2**: 677, 1976.
114. Davis, G. & Liu, D.T. Mid-trimester abortion. Late dilatation and evacuation and DIC. *Lancet* **2**: 1026, 1972.
115. Savage, W. Abortion, Methods and sequelae. *Br. J. Hosp. Med.* **27**: 364, 1982.
116. Semeraro, N. & Donati, M.B. Pathways of blood clotting initiation by cancer cells. In *Malignancy and the Haemostatic System* (eds M.B. Donati, J.F. Davidson & S. Garattini). Raven Press, New York, 1981.
117. Pitney, W.R. Disseminated intravascular coagulation. *Semin. Hematol.* **8**: 65, 1971.
118. Straub, P.W. Chronic intravascular coagulation. Clinical spectrum and diagnostic criteria, with special emphasis on metabolism, distribution and localisation of I 131-fibrinogen. *Acta Med. Scand.* (Suppl.) **526**: 1, 1971.
119. Peck, S.D. & Reiquam, C.W. Disseminated intravascular coagulation in cancer patients: supportive evidence. *Cancer* **31**: 1114, 1973.
120. Jones, M.F. & Saleen, A. Acute promyelocytic leukaemia: a review of literature. *Am. J. Med.* **65**: 673–7, 1978.
121. Quingley, H.J. Peripheral leukocyte thromboplastin in promyelocytic leukaemias (Abstr) *Fed. Proc.* **26**: 648, 1967.
122. Gouault-Heilmann, M., Chardon, F., Sultan, C. & Josso, F. The procoagulant factor of leukaemic promyelocytes: Demonstration of immunologic cross reactivity with human brain tissue factor. *Br. J. Haematol.* **30**. 151–8, 1975.
123. Maekawa, T. & Gonmori, H. Tissue thromboplastin in leukocytes from various leukaemia and its localisation by immunoperoxidase staining method. (Abstr) *Thromb. Diathes. Haemorrh.* **38**: 151, 1977.
124. Andoh, K., Kubota, T., Takada, M., Tanaka, H., Kobayashi, N. & Maekawa, T. Tissue factor activity in leukaemia cells. *Cancer* **59**: 748–54, 1987.
125. Camba, L. & Joyner, M.V. T-cell hairy cell leukaemia presenting with disseminated intravascular coagulation: rapid response to alpha-interferon. *Br. J. Haematol.* **62**: 393–4, 1986.
126. Daly, P., Vasantha, B., Lawlor, E., Blaney, C., Parreira, A. & Catovsky, D. Varient translocation t(8;22) and abnormalities of chromosome 15(q22) and 17(q12–21) in a Burkitt's lymphoma/leukaemia with disseminated intravascular coagulation. *Br. J. Haematol.* **64**: 561–9, 1986.
127. Hardaway, R.M. The significance of coagulative and thrombotic changes after haemorrhage and injury. *J. Clin. Pathol.* **14** (suppl 33): 110–21, 1970.
128. Hardaway, R.M. Disseminated intravascular coagulation in experimental and clinical shock. *Am. J. Cardiol.* **20**: 161, 1967.
129. Owen, C.A. Jr. & Bowie, E.J. Chronic intravascular coagulation syndromes: A

summary. *Mayo Clin. Proc.* **49**: 673–9, 1974.

130. Kerr, L.D., Spiera, H. & Aledort, L. Acute disseminated intravascular coagulation as a complication of systemic lupus erythematosus. *N.Y. State J. Med.* **3**: 181–3, 1987.

131. Chellingsworth, M. & Scott, D.G. Case report: Acute systemic lupus erythematosus with fatal pneumonitis and disseminated intravascular coagulation. *Ann. Rheum. Dis.* **44**: 67–9, 1985.

132. Weber, M.B. & Blakely, J.A. The haemorrhagic diathesis of heat stroke: a consumption coagulopathy successfully treated with heparin. *Lancet* **1**: 1190–2, 1969.

133. Cornell, C.J., Fein, S.H., Reilly, B.I. & Cornwell, O.G. Heparin therapy for heat stroke (letter). *Ann. Int. Med.* **81**: 702–3, 1975.

134. Mustafa, M.K.Y., Khogali, M. & Gumaa, K. Disseminated intravascular coagulation among heat stroke cases. In *Heat Stroke and Temperature Regulation* (eds M.K. Khogali & J.R.S. Hales), pp. 109–17. Academic Press, Australia, 1983.

135. Choa, T.C., Sinniah, R. & Pakiam, J.E. Acute heat stroke deaths. *Pathology* **13**: 145–56, 1981.

136. El-Kassimi, F.A., Al-Mashhadani, S. & Akhtar, J. Adult respiratory distress syndrome and disseminated intravascular coagulation complicating heat stroke. *Chest* **90**: 571–4, 1986.

137. Grief, F. & Kaplan, O. Acid ingestion: Another cause of disseminated intravascular coagulation. *Crit. Care Med.* **14**: 990–1, 1986.

138. Hewitt, P.E. & Davies, S.C. The current state of DIC. *Intensive Care Med.* **9**: 249–52, 1983.

139. Wilde, J.T., Roberts, K.M., Greaves, M. & Preston, F.E. Association between necropsy evidence of disseminated intravascular coagulation and coagulation variables before death in patients in intensive care units. *J. Clin. Pathol.* **41**: 138–42, 1988.

140. Bick, R. Disseminated intravascular coagulation: A clinical/laboratory study of 48 patients. *Ann. N.Y. Acad. Sci.* **370**: 843–50, 1981.

141. Spero, J.A. Lewis, J.H. & Hasiba, U. Disseminated intravascular coagulation: Findings in 346 patients. *Thromb. Haemost.* **38**: 28–33, 1980.

142. Sigal, S.H., Cembrowski, G.S., Shattil, S.J., Brown, N.M., Schifreen, R.S. & Schwartz, M.W. Prototype quantitative assay for fibrinogen/fibrin degradation products – clinical evaluation. *Arch. Intern. Med.* **147**: 1790–3, 1987.

143. Hamilton, P.J., Stalker, A.L. & Douglas, A.S. Disseminated intravascular coagulation: A review. *J. Clin. Pathol.* **31**: 609, 1978.

144. Sharp, A.A. *et al.* Defibrination syndrome in pregnancy (value of various diagnostic tests). *Lancet* **2**: 1309, 1958.

145. Bailton, F.E. & Letsky, E.A. Obstetric haemorrhage: Causes and management. *Clin. Haematol.* **14**(3): 683, 1985.

146. Bone, R.C., Bailey, F.P. & Pierce, A. Intravascular coagulation associated with the adult respiratory distress syndrome. *Am. J. Med.* **61**: 585–9, 1976.

147. Bick, R.L., Schmelhost, W.R. & Fekete, L.F. Disseminated intravascular coagulation and blood component therapy. *Transfusion* **16**: 361, 1976.

148. Preston, F.E. Disseminated intravascular coagulation. *Br. J. Hosp. Med.* **28**: 129, 1982.

149. Prentice, C.R.M. Acquired haemostatic disorders. *Clin. Haematol.* Coagulation Disorders, 414, June 1985.

150. Prentice, C.R.M. Heparin and disseminated intravascular coagulation. In: *Heparin: Clinical Chemistry and Usage* (eds W. Kakkar & D.P. Thomas, p. 219. Academic Press, London, 1976.

151. Meishey, C. Defibrination syndrome. In *Human Blood Coagulation, Haemostasis and Thrombosis* (ed. R. Biggs), Blackwell Scientific Publications, Oxford, 1972.

152. Schipper, H.G., Kahle, L.H., Jenkins, C.S.P., Tencate, J.W., Veenhoff, C. &

Sinaasappel, M. Antithrombin III transfusions in disseminated intravascular coagulation. *Lancet* **1**: 209, 1978.

153. Maki, M. *et al.* Clinical evaluation of antithrombin III concentrate (BI 6.013) for disseminated intravascular coagulation in obstetrics. Well-controlled multicenter trial. *Gynecol. Obstet. Invest.* **23**: 230–40, 1987.

154. Drapkin, R.L., Gee, T.S., Monroe, D. *et al.* Prophylactic heparin therapy in acute promyelocytic leukaemia. *Cancer* **41**: 2484–90, 1978.

155. Lowe, F.C. & Somers, W.J. The use of ketoconazole in the emergency management of disseminated intravascular coagulation due to metastatic prostatic cancer. *J. Urol.* **137**: 1000–2, 1987.

156. Litt, M.R., Bell, W.R. & Lepor, H.A. Disseminated intravascular coagulation in prostatic carcinoma reversed by ketoconazole. *J. Am. Med. Assoc.* **258**: 1361–2, 1987.

157. Heene, D.L. Disseminated intravascular coagulation. Evaluation of therapeutic approaches. *Semin. Thromb. Hemost.* **3**: 291–317, 1977.

158. Prentice, C.R.M. Acquired coagulation disorders. *Clin. Haematol.* **14**: 413–42, 1985.

159. Francis, J.L. & Armstrong, D.J. Acquired dysfibrinogenaemia in liver disease. *J. Clin. Pathol.* **35**: 667–72, 1982.

160. Brozovic, M. Acquired disorders of coagulation. In *Haemostasis and Thrombosis* (eds A.L. Bloom & D.P. Thomas), pp. 519–20. Churchill Livingstone, Edinburgh, 1987.

161. Ratnoff, O. Haemostatic defects in liver and biliary tract disease and disorders of vitamin K metabolism. In *Disorders of Haemostasis* (eds O. Ratnoff & C.D. Forbes). Grune & Stratton, London, 1984.

162. Murray-Lyon, I.M., Clarke, H.G.M., McPherson, K. *et al.* Quantitative immunoelectrophoresis of serum proteins in cryptogenic cirrhosis, alcoholic cirrhosis and active chronic hepatitis. *Clin. Chim. Acta* **39**: 215, 1972.

163. Damus, P.S. & Wallace, G.A. Immunologic measurement of antithrombin III-heparin co-factor and α_2 macroglobulin in disseminated intravascular coagulation and hepatic failure coagulopathy. *Thromb. Res.* **6**: 27, 1975.

164. Verstraete, M., Vermylen, J. & Collen, D. Intravascular coagulation in liver disease. *Ann. Rev. Med.* **25**: 447–55, 1974.

165. Wardle, E.N. Fibrinogen in liver disease. *Arch. Surg.* **109**: 741, 1974.

166. Balkuv-Ulutin, S. Physiological response to enhanced fibrinolytic activity. In *Fibrinolysis. Current Fundamental and Clinical Concepts* (eds P.-J. Gaffney & S. Balkuv-Ulutin), pp. 27–36. Academic Press, London, 1978.

167. Kirby, D.F., Blei, A.T., Rosen, S.T., Vogelzang, R.L. & Neiman, H.L. Primary sclerosing cholangitis in the presence of a lupus anticoagulant. *Am. J. Med.* **81**: 1077–80, 1986.

168. Clark, R., Borirakchanyavat, V., Gazzard, B.G. *et al.* Disordered haemostasis in liver damage from paracetamol overdose. *Gastroenterology* **65**: 788–95, 1973.

169. Koller, F. Theory and experience behind the use of coagulation tests in diagnosis and prognosis of liver disease. *Scand. J. Gastroenterol.* (Suppl. 19) **8**: 51–61, 1973.

170. Chisholm, M. Haematological disorders in liver disease. In *Liver and Biliary Disease*, 2nd Edn (eds. R. Wright, G.H. Millward-Sadler, K.G.M.M. Albert & S. Karran), pp. 203–14. Baillière Tindall, London, 1985.

171. Feinstein, D.I. & Rapaport, S.I. Acquired inhibitors of blood coagulation. In *Progress in Hemostasis and Thrombosis*, Vol. 1 (ed. T.S. Spaet), p. 75. Grune & Stratton, New York, 1972.

172. Duran-Suarez, J.R. Incidence of circulating anticoagulants in a normal population. *Acta Haematol.* **67**: 217–19, 1982.

173. Shapiro, S.S. & Thiagarajan, P. Lupus anticoagulants. In *Progress in Haemostasis and Thrombosis*, Vol. 6 (ed. T.S. Spaet), pp. 263–85. Grune & Stratton, New

York, 1982.

174. Green, D. & Lechner, K. A survey of 215 non-hemophilic patients with inhibitors to factor VIII. *Thromb. Haemost.* **45**: 200–3, 1981.

175. Ganly, P.S., Isaacs, J.D., Laffan, M.A., Haslett, C. & Hows, J.M. Acquired factor VIII inhibitor associated with lung abscess. *Br. Med. J.* **295**: 811, 1987.

176. Hoyle, C. & Ludlam, C.A. Acquired factor VIII inhibitor associated with multiple sclerosis, successfully treated with porcine factor VIII. *Thromb. Haemost.* **57**: 233, 1987.

177. Broxson, E.H. & Hathaway, W.E. Transplacental transfer of acquired factor VIII: C inhibitor. *Thromb. Haemost.* **57**: 126, 1987.

178. Sultan, Y., Kazatchkine, M.D., Maisonneuve, P. & Nydegger, U.E. Anti-idiotypic suppression of autoantibodies to factor VIII (anti-haemophilic factor) by high dose intravenous gamma globulin. *Lancet* **2**: 765–8, 1984.

179. Green, D., Schuette, P.T. & Wallace, W.H. Factor VIII antibodies in rheumatoid arthritis: effect of cyclophosphamide. *Arch. Intern. Med.* **140**: 1232–5, 1980.

180. Green, D. Acquired inhibitors of blood coagulation. In *Haemostasis and Thrombosis* (eds A.L. Bloom & D.P. Thomas), p. 547. Churchill Livingstone, Edinburgh, 1987.

181. Coleman, N., Vigliano, E.N., Weksler, M.E., Nachman, R.L. Inhibition of fibrin monomer polymerisation by lambda myeloma globulins. *Blood* **39**: 210–23, 1972.

182. Lorand, L. Hemorrhagic disorders of fibrin-stabilisation. In *Haemostasis: Biochemistry, Physiology, Pathology* (eds D. Ogston & B. Bennet), pp. 405–23. Wiley, New York, 1977.

183. Milner, G.R., Holt, P.J.L., Bottomly, J. & MacIver, J.E. Practolol therapy associated with a systemic lupus erythematosus-like syndrome and an inhibitor to factor XIII. *J. Clin. Pathol.* **30**: 770–3, 1977.

184. Chediak, J., Ashenhurst, J.B., Garlick, I. & Desser, R.K. Successful management of bleeding in a patient with factor V inhibitor by platelet transfusions. *Blood* **56**: 835–41, 1980.

185. Bussel, J.B., Steinherz, P.G., Miller, D.R. & Hilgartner, M.W. A heparin-like anticoagulant in an 8-month-old boy with acute monoblastic leukaemia. *Am. J. Haematol.* **16**: 83–90, 1984.

186. Berrettini, M. & Nenci, G.G. Circulating heparin-like anticoagulants. *N. Engl. J. Med.* **311**: 1055, 1984.

187. Chapman, G.S., George, C.B. & Danley, D.L. Heparin-like anticoagulant associated with plasma cell myeloma. *Am. J. Clin. Pathol.* **83**: 764–6, 1985.

188. De Prost, D. Katlama, C., Pialoux, G., Karsenty-Mathonnet, F. & Wolff, M. Heparin-like anticoagulant associated with AIDS. *Thromb. Haemost.* **57**: 239, 1987.

189. Conley, L. & Hartmann, R. A haemorrhagic disorder caused by circulating anticoagulant in patients with disseminated lupus erythematosus. *J. Clin. Invest.* **31**: 621–2, 1952.

190. Schleider, M.A., Nachman, R.L., Jaffe, E.A. & Coleman, M. A clinical study of the lupus anticoagulant. *Blood* **48**: 499–509, 1976.

191. Cohen, A.J., Philips, T.M. & Kessler, C.M. Circulating coagulation inhibitors in the acquired immunodeficiency syndrome. *Ann. Intern. Med.* **104**: 175–80, 1986.

192. Jeffrey, R.F. Transient lupus anticoagulant and Fansidar therapy. *Postgrad. Med. J.* **62**: 893–4, 1986.

193. Green, D., Houghie, C., Kazmier, F.J., Lechner, K., Mannucci, P.M., Rizza, C.R. & Sultan, Y. Report of the working party on acquired inhibitors of coagulation: Studies of the "lupus" anticoagulant. *Thromb. Haemost.* **49**: 144–6, 1983.

194. Regan, M.G., Lackner, H. & Karpatkin, S. Platelet function and coagulation profile in lupus erythematosus: studies in 50 patients. *Ann. Intern. Med.* **81**: 462–8, 1974.

195. Bowie, E.J., Thompson, J.H., Pascuzzi, C.A. & Owen, C.A. Thrombosis in systemic lupus erythematosus despite circulating anticoagulants. *J. Lab. Clin. Med.* **62**: 416–30, 1963.
196. Feinstein, D.I. Lupus anticoagulant, thrombosis and fetal loss. *N. Engl. J. Med.* **313**: 1348–50, 1985.
197. Freyssinet, J.-M. & Cazenave, J.-P. Lupus-like anticoagulants, modulation of the protein C pathway and thrombosis. *Thromb. Haemost.* **58**: 679–81, 1987.
198. Carreras, L.O & Vermylen, J.G. "Lupus" anticoagulant and thrombosis – Possible role of inhibition of prostacyclin formation. *Thromb. Haemost.* **48**: 38–40, 1982.
199. Thiagarajan, P., Pengo, V. & Shapiro, S. The use of the dilute russell viper venom time for the diagnosis of lupus anticoagulants. *Blood* **68**: 869–74, 1986.
200. McVerry, B.A., Spearing, R. & Smith, A. SLE anticoagulant: Transient inhibition by high dose immunoglobulin infusions. *Br. J. Haematol.* **61**: 579–80, 1985.
201. Green, D. Acquired inhibitors of blood coagulation. In *Haemostasis and Thrombosis* (eds A.L. Bloom, & D.P. Thomas), p. 545. Churchill Livingstone, Edinburgh, 1987.
202. Carreras, L.O., Vermylen, J., Spitz, B. & Van Assche, A. 'Lupus' anticoagulant and inhibition of prostacyclin formation in patients with repeated abortion, intrauterine growth retardation and intra-uterine death. *Br. J. Obstet. Gynaecol.* **88**: 890–4, 1981.
203. Scott, J.S. Connective tissue disease antibodies and pregnancy. *Am. J. Reprod. Immunol. Microbiol.* **6**: 19, 1981.
204. Duncombe, A.S., Dalton, R.G. & Savidge, G.F. Lupus-type coagulation inhibitors in hairy cell leukaemia and resolution with splenectomy. *Br. J. Haematol.* **65**: 120–1, 1987.
205. Harris, E.N., Gharavi, A.E., Boey, M.L. *et al.* Anticardiolipin antibodies: detection by radioimmunoassay and association with thrombosis in systemic lupus erythematosus. *Lancet* **2**: 1211–14, 1983.

8

Connective tissue disorders

J.M. Hows
Senior Lecturer in Haematology, Royal Postgraduate Medical School,
Hammersmith Hospital, London, UK

INTRODUCTION

An approach to evaluating haematological abnormalities in connective tissue disorders

The connective tissue disorders (CTD) are an overlapping group of clinicopathological syndromes arising from widespread inflammatory damage to connective tissues and blood vessels. They are linked by the presence of disordered cellular immunity and a strong tendency to the formation of auto-antibodies. Although there is no evidence that CTD are induced by a single disease process, it is helpful to consider them as a group when discussing the associated haematological abnormalities.

The spectrum of haematological disorders seen in the CTD overlaps the different disease entities, for instance, autoimmune haemolytic anaemia, most commonly seen in systemic lupus erythematosus (SLE), is also present in some cases of rheumatoid arthritis (RA). Because of overlap, the pathogenesis, investigation and management of the main haematological disorders in the CTD will be discussed as haematological entities, with reference to the CTD in which they are most commonly found, rather than repetitious description of the haematological findings in each individual CTD. Finally, drug-associated cytopenias with platelet function abnormalities are common in the CTD. These are dealt with in detail in Chapter 10. For completeness they have been included in Tables 8.1 and 8.2 and in the summary flow chart (Fig. 8.2) at the end of this chapter. Drug-induced bone marrow failure as encountered in the CTD is covered in this chapter.

The spectrum of haematological abnormalities in CTD

Blood count abnormalities

The major haematological abnormalities seen in the CTD are listed in Table 8.1. The commonest findings are cytopenias, most frequently anaemia, although leucopenia and thrombocytopenia are also seen. Such cytopenias may occur singly, in pairs, or sequentially, in an individual patient. Occasionally, pancytopenia is seen. In contrast, cytophilias are unusual. Occasionally, reactive thrombocytosis is seen in active RA,[1] or

Table 8.1   Major Haematological Abnormalities Found in Connective Tissue Disorders

Haematological parameter	Pathogenesis	Main clinical association in CTD
Cytopenias		
Anaemia	Anaemia of chronic disease	All CTD
	Autoimmune haemolysis	Commonest in SLE
	Renal failure	Commonest in SLE
	Haematinic deficiency	Debilitated patients
	Blood loss	NSAID, aspirin, corticosteroids
	Sideroblastic	RA ?true association
Neutropenia	Felty's syndrome	RA
	Neutrophil-specific auto-antibody	Rare
	Immune complexes	SLE, RA
	Drug-induced	NSAID, penicillamine, gold
Lymphopenia	Active disease ⎫	All CTD
	Drug-induced ⎭	Corticosteroids
Thrombocytopenia	Platelet-specific auto-antibody	Most CTD
	Immune complexes	SLE, RA
	Drug-induced	NSAID, penicillamine, gold
Pancytopenia	Felty's syndrome	RA
	Aplastic anaemia	SLE (rare), gold, phenylbutazone
	Predictable marrow suppression	Azathioprine, alkylating agents
	Myelodysplasia	Alkylating agents
Cytophilia		
Eosinophilia	T-cell activation factors	Churg–Strauss
Thrombocytosis	Chronic inflammation	RA
	Blood loss	NSAID, corticosteroids, aspirin
Coagulation abnormalities		
Platelet function abnormality	Drugs	Aspirin, NSAID
Lupus anticoagulant	Antiphospholipid Inhibition of auto-antibody	SLE, lupus-like syndromes

secondary to gastrointestinal haemorrhage, caused by aspirin, cortico-steroids or non-steroidal anti-inflammatory drugs (NSAID). A rare cause of leucocytosis is the pulmonary variant of polyarteritis nodosa (PAN), the Churg–Strauss syndrome,[2] where eosinophilia accompanies intractable asthma and the appearance of recurrent pulmonary infiltrates.

Coagulation factors

In SLE and the lupus-like syndromes, a coagulation abnormality well-documented and characterized *in vitro* by prolongation of the partial thromboplastin time is found. This is due to formation of auto-antibodies specific for phospholipid molecules essential for activation of the intrinsic coagulation pathway. These auto-antibodies are known as 'lupus' anti-coagulants'[3] and surprisingly are associated with a thrombotic tendency *in vivo*, rather than a bleeding disorder.

Platelet function and the vessel wall

Spontaneous or excessive bleeding may be encountered in the CTD in the presence of a normal peripheral blood count and film. The commonest reason is platelet function abnormalities induced by aspirin or NSAID. In patients with a prolonged bleeding time, but normal platelet function studies, the possibility of vitamin C deficiency should be considered.

A classification of haematological abnormalities in CTD

It is useful to classify the haematological disorders seen in CTD into primary and secondary changes. (Table 8.2). The so-called primary abnormalities are a direct result of the disease process, e.g. red cell auto-antibodies leading to autoimmune haemolytic anaemia (AIHA). The secondary abnormalities are an indirect consequence of the disease, e.g. dietary iron and folate deficiency secondary to disability through arthritis. In some cases, the pathogenesis of the haematological abnormality detected will be multifactorial and have primary and secondary components. Even in these complex cases, it is useful to dissect out the primary and secondary components of the abnormality. For example, thrombocytopenia may be encountered in severely ill SLE patients with active disease receiving immunosuppressive therapy with azathioprine. Bone marrow examination usually reveals a hypoplastic picture with mildly or moderately decreased megakarocytes. Platelet antibodies and circulating immune complexes are frequently present. In this situation the primary cause of thrombocytopenia is immune platelet destruction by platelet-specific auto-antibodies and immune complexes, the thrombocytopenia being exacerbated by suppression of thrombopoiesis by the myelosuppressive drug azathioprine.

Assessment of CTD activity

An essential part of haematological evaluation in the CTD is a clinical and laboratory assessment of the activity of the CTD itself. This assessment is best carried out by a rheumatologist. In hospitals where a large number of CTD cases are treated, it is useful to have a combined Rheumatology/ Haematology Clinic, for assessment of CTD patients with significant haematological problems. It must be emphasized that it is impossible to interpret the haematological findings in CTD correctly without a clinical assessment of and laboratory tests for disease activity, as well as a detailed drug history.[4-6]

Non-haematological laboratory parameters of disease activity

Laboratory criteria for the diagnosis of the different CTD are relatively well-defined, however the parameters used to assess disease activity remain controversial and vary in the different CTD encountered. In RA available tests for disease activity are limited and most rheumatologists will follow the ESR and C reactive protein only, with careful assessment of the clinical disease status. In contrast, in SLE a plethora of tests for monitoring disease activity have been used, including assessment of serum complement levels, circulating immune complexes, levels of single- and double-stranded DNA auto-antibodies (DNA binding), levels of monoclonal anti-DNA idiotype antibody, and levels of IgM and IgG anticardiolipin antibody. Experience has shown that no single laboratory parameter can be used to monitor all cases of SLE for disease activity.[7-9] Certain tests are informative in well-defined disease sub-groups. For example, the levels of anticardiolipin IgM antibody reflect disease activity in SLE patients with spontaneous abortion/ thrombotic episodes, cerebral disease and the lupus anticoagulant.[10] In general, these non-haematological laboratory parameters reflect rather than predict disease activity.

Correlation of haematological abnormalities with disease activity

Primary haematological abnormalities correlate better with disease activity in the CTD than secondary abnormalities. (See Table 8.2). Unfortunately, there is no single haematological parameter which can be used to monitor disease activity. In a recent study of SLE by Isenberg et al., no patient with 'severe disease' had a lymphocyte count of above 1.9×10^9 per litre or haemoglobin above 11.7 g/dl.[4] It is important to note, however, that close correlations were seen between lymphopenia, monocytopenia, eosinopenia, and raised neutrophil peroxidase activity with steroid therapy, rather than with disease activity itself.

THE ANAEMIAS

Anaemia frequently accompanies the CTD, is usually mild to moderate (Hb 8.5–11.5 g/dl), and often multifactorial. The correct management depends on a clear understanding of the pathogenesis and the relative contributions of primary and secondary causes of the anaemia (see Table 8.2).

Anaemia of chronic disease

The main components in the pathogenesis are decreased haem synthesis due to failure of iron incorporation into the erythron, and marrow suppression due to active inflammatory disease. The anaemia is usually normochromic and normocytic, but can be hypochromic and/or microcytic. There is some correlation between the severity of the anaemia and overall disease activity, measured clinically and by elevations of the ESR and serum acute-phase proteins. More specific indicators of disease activity, e.g. DNA binding in SLE may also reflect the degree of anaemia. The plasma iron is decreased in the anaemia of chronic disease, and the total iron-binding capacity is either low or within normal limits. The bone marrow is usually normocellular, normoblastic, with dyserythropoietic features. Staining by Perl's method shows increased reticulo-endothelial iron stores. A block in iron incorporation into the erythron is seen with decreased erythroid siderotic granulation. It is important to differentiate the anaemia of chronic disease from cases of iron deficiency anaemia in the CTD. This distinction prevents the administration of unnecessary and potentially harmful iron therapy to patients with the anaemia of chronic disease.

The anaemia of chronic disease usually only improves when generalized disease activity can be brought under control. It is fortunate, therefore, that this type of anaemia is usually mild. A preliminary report by Means *et al.*.

Table 8.2 Classification of Main Haematological Abnormalities in CTD

Primary
  Immune
    Immune cytopenias
    Lupus anticoagulant
  Anaemia of chronic disease
  Anaemia of chronic renal failure
  Bone marrow suppression
  Felty's syndrome

Secondary
  Drug-associated blood loss anaemia
    Gastrointestinal erosion
    Platelet function abnormalities
  Drug-associated bone marrow failure
    Predictable marrow suppression
    Idiosyncratic aplastic anaemia
    Myelodysplasia
  Dietary deficiency anaemia
    Iron
    Folate
    Mixed

describes the successful treatment of the anaemia of chronic disease in two cases of RA with recombinant erythropoietin.[11] The rationale of this treatment is that in the anaemia of chronic disease, there may be a reduced sensitivity of erythroid precursors to the action of erythropoietin, which can be partially overcome by high concentrations of exogenous hormone.

Iron deficiency anaemia

This is frequent in patients with RA but may occur in the other CTD. It presents haematologically with the classical hypochromic microcytic anaemia, with tear-drop poikilocytes and pencil cells prominent on the peripheral blood film. The iron deficiency is usually due to a mixture of chronic gastrointestinal blood loss, associated with non-steroidal anti-inflammatory drugs (NSAID), aspirin or corticosteroids, and dietary deficiency. In older patients and those with abdominal symptoms, blood loss from localized benign and malignant lesions of the gut should be excluded. The serum iron and ferritin levels are always low, but, in the presence of active CTD, the total iron-binding capacity (TIBC) may not be elevated as in classical iron deficiency anemia. Demonstration of absent reticulo-endothelial iron stores by bone marrow aspiration is worthwhile to confirm the diagnosis of iron deficiency.

Treatment is to improve the patient's intake of dietary iron, to minimize gastrointestinal blood loss by withdrawing unnecessary drugs and introducing intensive antacid therapy and H2 receptor antagonists. A standard course of oral iron, e.g. ferrous sulphate 200 mg tds for 3–6 months should be given. In patients where the anaemia of chronic disease coexists, haematological response to oral iron will be suboptimal, the serum ferritin level should be used to monitor iron therapy.

Blood loss anaemia

Occasionally, a patient with RA or other CTD receiving treatment with aspirin, NSAID or corticosteroids, presents with a history of gastrointestinal bleeding and is found to be significantly anaemic. If the haemorrhage is of recent onset, the anaemia is usually normochromic and normocytic with obvious polychromasia and occasional nucleated red cells seen on the peripheral blood film. The platelet and white cell counts are often elevated. In cases of more chronic haemorrhage, evidence for iron deficiency anaemia is usually found, often associated with reactive thrombocytosis. Suspect drugs should be discontinued and the patient investigated to identify the source of blood loss. The commonest finding is of gastric erosions seen at gastroscopy. Carcinoma of stomach, colon or rectum, hiatus hernia, peptic ulceration, diverticular disease of the colon and haemorrhoids are the commoner lesions which require exclusion and, if found, appropriate treatment given. In cases where bleeding is attributed to drugs, anti-rheumatic treatment should be carefully re-evaluated.

Folate deficiency and mixed deficiency anaemia

Patients with advanced RA may eat poorly because of physical disability. The result is often a macrocytic, megaloblastic anaemia caused by folate deficiency. Dietary intake of iron may also be inadequate, or blood loss may be present, leading to a mixed iron and folate deficiency. In mixed deficiency, characteristic macrocytes and hypersegmented neutrophils are usually seen in addition to hypochromia on the peripheral blood film. The blood film may appear dimorphic with both microcytic and macrocytic red cells seen. Megaloblastic changes in the marrow may be partially masked by coexisting iron deficiency. Plasma iron levels, TIBC, serum folate and B_{12}, and red cell folate levels are required in addition to a peripheral blood film and marrow examination, to evaluate suspected mixed deficiency anaemia. Full dietary assessment is required and correction made, where possible. Most patients will require iron and folate supplements to prevent recurrence.

Autoimmune haemolytic anaemia (AIHA)

This is most frequently seen in patients with SLE, but may also occur in the other CTD, most often RA and mixed connective tissue disease. When a positive direct antiglobulin test (DAT) and/or clinical and laboratory evidence for haemolysis is identified, the approach to laboratory investigation and clinical management is the same, whatever the underlying CTD.[12]

Pathogenesis of AIHA in CTD

Extravascular haemolysis. Most cases of AIHA documented in the CTD are due to increased destruction of red cells by the macrophages of the reticulo-endothelial system, following coating of the red cells by immune complexes. Extravascular haemolysis is mediated through phagocytosis triggered by two separate macrophage receptor mechanisms. Firstly, the macrophage Fc receptor interacts with red cells coated with IgG1- and IgG3-containing immune complexes, but not IgG2, IgG4, IgM or IgA complexes. The spleen is the predominant site for clearance of red cells coated with IgG as the high haematocrit in the red cell pulp leads to reduced competition for the macrophage Fc receptor by free IgG molecules in the plasma.[12]

Secondly, red cells coated with complement-containing complexes are phagocytosed following interactions with the reticulo-endothelial macrophage complement (C3) receptors. This process takes place throughout the reticulo-endothelial system. Preferential destruction in the spleen does not occur as the native C3 molecules in the plasma are not ligands for the macrophage C3 receptors, hence competition between red-cell-bound C3 and plasma C3 does not occur. Two types of C3 receptor CR1 and CR3 have been identified on human macrophages. Immune adherence of C3-coated red cells to macrophages occurs primarily through the CR1 receptor, whereas the CR3 receptor triggers phagocytosis.[13]

Intravascular haemolysis.   This is unusual in patients with CTD and AIHA; however, an intravascular component may be present in those cases with the severest haemolysis. Intravascular haemolysis is complement-mediated, following deposition of immune complexes on the red cell membrane and activation of the classical complement pathway and the membrane attack sequence. Intravascular haemolysis may follow the deposition of either IgM- or IgG-containing immune complexes on the red cell membrane. IgM-containing complexes are most potent in precipitating intravascular haemolysis, although it may also occur as a result of IgG1- or IgG3-mediated complement activation.

Laboratory investigation of AIHA

Direct antiglobulin test (DAT).   The laboratory hallmark of AIHA is the positive DAT. In CTD testing with anti-C3 and IgG, specific antihuman globulin reagents reveal C3 and IgG on the red cell surface in about 70% of cases, reflecting the composition of the deposited immune complexes. In most of the remaining cases, C3 alone is detected. It is relatively difficult to detect IgM on the red cell by the DAT, so, many of the cases where C3 alone is detected are presumed to be associated with IgM-containing immune complexes.

Laboratory tests for haemolysis.   It is important to decide if patients with CTD and a positive DAT have active haemolysis, and if so, whether it is predominantly intravascular or extravascular. The subsequent need for full serological investigation of putative AIHA and treatment depends on haemolytic activity not on whether or not the patient has a positive DAT. All patients, therefore, should be tested for total bilirubin, reticulocyte count, serum haptoglobins, serum lactate dehydrogenase and urinary urobilinogen. The peripheral blood film may reveal autoagglutination, spherocytosis, polychromasia and the presence of nucleated red cells.

Bone marrow examination.   A bone marrow examination is useful in all patients with CTD and evidence for immune haemolysis. Findings such as megaloblastic erythropoiesis, dyserythropoiesis secondary to the anaemia of chronic disorder, or marrow hypoplasia secondary to myelosuppressive drug therapy, may be present and help explain why many patients with CTD have a suboptimal reticulocyte response to immune red cell destruction.

Serological investigation of AIHA in CTD.   Detailed investigations are indicated in patients who are actively haemolysing. Such investigations are best performed in immunohaematology laboratories with a special interest in AIHA or by the National Blood Transfusion Service Regional Centre Laboratory. In patients who have recently been transfused, it is critically important to exclude haemolysis due to allo-antibodies specific for circulating transfused red cells. Detection of clinically significant allo-antibodies may be hindered by auto-antibody present in patient's serum and in eluates prepared from the patient's red cells. A flow diagram for the laboratory investigations of patients with AIHA is shown in Fig. 8.1.

A

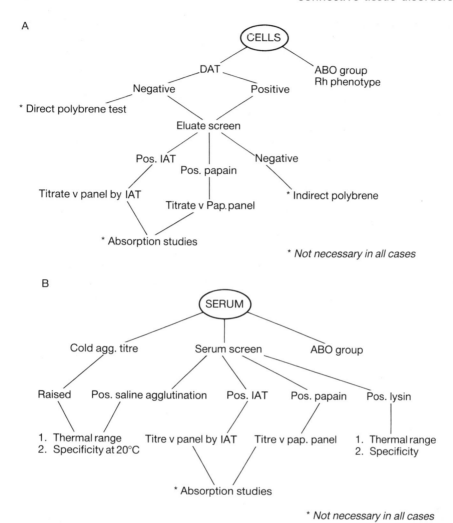

B

Fig. 8.1. A (cells) and B (serum) illustrate the flow of serological investigation of autoimmune haemolytic anaemia (AIHA). (A) Cells. *Positive DAT.* After performing the DAT and ascertaining patients ABO/Rh phenotype a red cell eluate is made and tested for antibody reactive by IAT or papainized pool O cells. Positive eluates are titrated by the appropriate technique to quantitate antibody present and determine specificity using routine panels of red cells. In recently transfused patients it is important to separate allo-antibodies from auto-antibodies in the eluate. This is done by differential absorption studies using allogeneic red cells. *Negative DAT.* If the DAT and/or the eluate is negative, but AIHA is strongly suspected on haematological and clinical grounds, the manual polybrene technique may give positive results. The direct polybrene method is used for testing intact red cells, the indirect polybrene method for the eluate. (B) Serum. Initially a serum screen at 20°C and 37°C, serum group and cold agglutinin titre are performed. If the cold agglutinin titre is raised, further investigations to establish thermal range and specificity are done. Antibody

Most patients with CTD have AIHA associated with warm reacting complement-fixing auto-antibodies. It is not always possible to be certain whether such antibodies detected in patient's serum are immune complex associated, or are specific for red cell membrane epitopes. Antibodies specific for serologically well-characterized red cell antigens, e.g. rhesus, are not often found in the AIHA associated with CTD, this means that most red cell auto-antibodies detected are 'non-specific' by routine serological testing.

Clinical features of AIHA

The diagnosis of AIHA may precede, coincide with or follow the diagnosis of the underlying CTD. About 25% of cases of AIHA associated with SLE present as idiopathic AIHA, the clinical and laboratory features of SLE only become apparent later in the disease. Most patients present with tiredness, pallor and mild jaundice. The activity of the underlying CTD is extremely variable, it may be clinically inactive. On examination, splenomegaly is a frequent but not invariable finding.

Management of AIHA in CTD

As noted above, the presence of a positive DAT in the absence of haemolysis is not an indication for treatment. Only cases with clinically significant haemolysis are treated specifically for AIHA.

Corticosteroids.   Initial treatment is the same as for idiopathic warm-type AIHA with oral prednisolone 1–2 mg/kg per day, and folic acid supplements. The dose is reduced after 7–10 days and tailed off over the subsequent 2–3 months, the exact regimen depending on the haematological response to treatment.

Transfusions.   All patients should be carefully monitored haematologically during the initial stages of corticosteroid therapy, as the haemoglobin may continue to fall. Urgent transfusions should be considered in those patients with a falling haemoglobin below 8 g/dl, especially in the elderly or if incipient heart failure develops. As mentioned earlier some patients with CTD may have an impaired erythropoietic response to peripheral red cell destruction; if so, transfusion is frequently required.

Splenectomy.   The place of splenectomy in the management of AIHA secondary to CTD is not so clear-cut as for idiopathic AIHA. In the CTD, the

---

detected in the serum screen is titred using the appropriate technique against a standard red cell panel to establish quantity of antibody present and specificity. In recently transfused patients differential absorption studies using allogeneic cells are necessary to exclude allo-antibodies. In patients who have been transfused in the past (more than 3 months previously) autologous red cells can be used for absorption studies.

spleen acts as a major site for clearance of circulating immune complexes. There is some evidence to suggest that after splenectomy the CTD and possibly haemolysis may be exacerbated by a build-up of immune complexes. In cases where the red cell is predominantly coated in IgG1 and IgG3, however, the spleen may be a major site of immune red cell destruction. This can be investigated *in vivo*, using ^{51}Cr radiolabelled autologous red cells and quantitative liver and spleen scanning. In cases where the spleen is the major site of red cell destruction and haemolysis is not controlled by steroids, splenectomy should be considered.

Azathioprine. Is the immunosuppressive drug of choice in patients not responding adequately to corticosteroids and/or splenectomy? The starting dose is 1–1.5 mg/kg per day orally. A trial of 3 months' treatment should be given, as response may not occur for 4–6 weeks. The patient's blood count should be carefully monitored for signs of myelosuppression evidenced by a falling white cell count.

Second-line immunosuppressive drugs. Cyclophosphamide either alone, or in resistant cases, combined with prednisolone and vincristine may be tried. The long-term complications of cyclophosphamide therapy, namely, haemorrhagic cystitis and myelodysplasia, should be taken into consideration. Cyclosporin may also be used as a second-line drug, although there is little clinical experience so far. A reasonable starting dose is 3 mg/kg twice daily by mouth. Cyclosporin is nephrotoxic and has a narrow therapeutic window. In all cases cyclosporin therapy should be carefully monitored by measuring serum or whole blood cyclosporin levels by radioimmunoassay.

High-dose immunoglobulin. High-dose immunoglobulin infusions are unlikely to be effective, as the main effect of such preparations is to block immune destruction of peripheral blood cells mediated by the Fc receptor mechanism. In the CTD the major mechanism for immune red cell destruction is C3 receptor interaction. Sometimes double dose intravenous immunoglobulin, e.g. Sandoglobulin 0.8 kg per day for 3–5 days may be effective when standard dose therapy fails. This is expensive.

Renal failure and anaemia

Renal failure in the CTD is most often seen in SLE when it is the consequence of immune complex-mediated glomerular injury, presenting as either the nephrotic syndrome, acute glomerular nephritis or asymptomatic proteinuria. In contrast, the kidney is not a primary target for the rheumatoid process. It may become involved, if amyloidosis develops, usually with the development of the nephrotic syndrome. Renal impairment may also result from drug nephropathy. Most frequent of the drug-associated nephropathies is the immune complex-induced glomerular nephritis secondary to gold and D-penicillamine therapy. If chronic renal failure develops, this may be accompanied by anaemia. The anaemia is moderate to severe, normochromic and normocytic. Characteristic schistocytes, target cells and burr cells are seen on the peripheral blood film. The platelet and white cell counts are usually normal, there is a reticulocytopenia. Serum erythropoietin levels are low. Iron deficiency, due to blood loss from impaired platelet function secondary to uraemia, and dietary deficiency of iron and folate coexist and contribute to the anaemia.

If effective treatment can be given for the renal failure, for example by withdrawal of toxic drugs, the anaemia will improve. Some increase in haemoglobin may be seen if iron and folate deficiency is treated appropriately. If the chronic renal failure becomes established and symptoms of anaemia are prominent, a transfusion programme may help. Alternatively, in carefully selected cases, the use of recombinant erythopoietin can be considered.[14]

Sideroblastic anaemia

The older textbooks quote rheumatoid arthritis as a cause of sideroblastic anaemia. Today, it is uncertain whether this is a real association or not. It is probable that most cases of sideroblastic anaemia arising in patients with RA and the other CTD are examples of myelodysplasia (primary acquired sideroblastic anaemia), either occurring by chance in the setting of a common pre-existing disorder, or secondary to treatment with alkylating agents. Myelodysplasia in CTD is covered later in this chapter under the heading of Bone marrow failure.

LEUCOPENIA

Lymphopenia

Lymphopenia is well-documented in RA, and it is often a feature of SLE. In general, lymphopenia is seen in those patients with CTD who have active disease more frequently than in those patients whose disease is quiescent. As Isenberg *et al.* have pointed out, it is not always possible to assess the relative importance of disease activity itself and that of corticosteroid therapy in the development of lymphopenia.[4] In active CTD, the lymphopenia may be in part induced by autoreactive lymphocytoxic antibodies. Corticosteroids are not only lympholytic in high concentrations, but also cause profound alterations in lymphocyte traffic and distribution *in vivo*.

Neutropenia

Neutropenia may be described under three headings: (1) Felty's syndrome, which is specifically seen in RA; (2) drug-associated neutropenia, also seen in other CTD disorders; and (3) immune neutropenia which, as an isolated cytopenia, is extremely rare.

Felty's syndrome

Clinical features.   Felty first described a syndrome consisting of classical RA, splenomegaly and neutropenia, in 1924.[15] The syndrome is uncommon, being seen in less than 1% of patients with RA. Ninety-eight per cent of cases of Felty's syndrome (FS) reported in the literature are seropositive for rheumatoid factors. In most cases, the rheumatic process is active and often severe.[16] The ESR and C-reactive protein are generally raised. There is a greater than expected incidence of extra-articular manifestations and constitutional symptoms such as weight loss. Prominent extra-articular abnormalities include rheumatoid nodules (76% of cases), Sjogren's syndrome (56%), lymphadenopathy (34%), leg ulcers (25%) and pleuritis (19%).[16]

Infections in Felty's syndrome.   Overall, significant infection has been documented in 60% of cases. Unfortunately, there are no controlled studies comparing the incidence of infections in FS with that in other cases of RA. Infection in RA can be due to disease-related factors other than neutropenia, e.g. corticosteroid administration, or to neutropenia due to other causes, such as drug toxicity. Most infections documented in FS are due to bacterial pathogens, including staphylococci, streptococci and gram-negative bacilli.[17,18]

Pathogenesis of splenomegaly in Felty's syndrome.   Abnormal liver function is documented in about 25% of patients with FS. A study from the King's College Hospital liver group showed that nodular regenerative hyperplasia of the liver is associated with FS. In contrast to cirrhosis, the nodules are not separated by collagen bundles and the portal vein radicles are not compressed. Despite this, the regenerative nodules are associated with mild portal vein fibrosis and some compression of the central veins. Hence pre-sinusoidal resistance, due to nodular regenerative hyperplasia, may lead to portal hypertension and splenomegaly.[16]

Pathogenesis of neutropenia in Felty's syndrome.   The pathogenesis of neutropenia in FS is multifactorial. Most investigators have defined neutropenia as less than 2.0×10^9 per litre circulating neutrophils, thus many cases described have been mildly neutropenic and not obviously associated with increased infections. The three main mechanisms which contribute to the neutropenia are:[19] (1) decreased neutrophil production due to cellular or humoral inhibitors of granulopoiesis; (2) immune complex-mediated peripheral destruction of neutrophils; and (3) sequestration of neutrophils within the enlarged spleen.

Marrow morphology usually shows active granulopoiesis with a relative decrease in myelocytes and metamyelocytes, suggesting that peripheral destruction is the major mechanism for the observed neutropenia. In the differential diagnosis of FS, it is important to exclude neutropenia associated with drug therapy.

Some experimental evidence for immune-mediated depression of myelo-poiesis in FS comes from *in vitro* studies of haemopoietic progenitor cells derived from blood or bone marrow. One study provided evidence for serum inhibitors, whereas in another study, in some cases the number of haemopoietic progenitor cells colonies increased after the removal of T-lymphocytes from the marrow. This suggested that cellular inhibition, mediated through suppressor or cytotoxic T-cells, may contribute to the neutropenia in some cases of FS.

Other haematological abnormalities in Felty's syndrome.   In some cases of FS, pancytopenia is apparent. The anaemia is multifactorial and can usually be attributed to splenic sequestration in addition to the anaemia of chronic disease. In about one-third of cases, thrombocytopenia due to splenic sequestration is also seen. This is rarely severe enough to cause clinically significant bleeding.

Treatment of Felty's syndrome.

(1) *Splenectomy.* The indications for splenectomy have not been standard-ized. The majority of patients with FS have an early rise in neutrophil count following splenectomy, reflecting the role of peripheral pooling/destruction of neutrophils in the spleen in the pathogenesis of the condition. In a proportion of patients the rise in neutrophils is temporary, as might be expected in cases where myelopoiesis is reduced. Furthermore, the reticulo-endothelial tissue elsewhere may take over from the spleen in removing neutrophils from the circulation. Most investigators agree that splenetomy is indicated in those patients who are experiencing life-threatening infections, have a granulocyte count of $<0.5 \times 10^9$ per litre and 'massive' spleno-megaly, i.e. >5–7 cm. Occasionally, patients with massive splenomegaly experience local pain and fullness, this, as well as the development of portal hypertension secondary to increased portal blood flow may occasionally be an indication for splenectomy.[16]

Not all patients cease to have infections after the correction of neutropenia by splenectomy. This is because other factors, e.g. corticosteroid adminis-tration, hypocomplementaemia may contribute to the increased risk of infection in FS as well as the neutropenia. It is essential that all splenectomized patients receive long-term prophylactic penicillin V 250 mg twice daily, to prevent overwhelming post-splenectomy infection with pneumococci or meningococci. Vaccination with Pneumovax is not sufficient protection for patients who may receive immunosuppressive or cytotoxic drugs post-splenectomy.

(2) *Corticosteroids.* Corticosteroids may be indicated to treat the primary rheumatoid process in patients with FS. The effect of these agents on the neutropenia is inconsistent. A proportion of patients may respond with improved counts and fewer infections. In others, infections may be exacerbated.

(3) *Lithium.* Lithium salts have been shown to raise the granulocyte count in FS. The mechanism of action is probably to increase the production of haemopoietic growth factors which stimulate granulopoiesis. The adverse effects of lithium therapy, namely, nephrotoxicity and hypothyroidism, and the need for careful pharmacological monitoring are relative contra-indications to the long-term use of this agent.

(4) *Levamisole.* Levamisole is an immunomodulatory agent which has been

shown to increase human granulopoietic activity *in vitro*. Studies of the use of this agent on FS have not been reported.

(5) *Haemopoietic growth factors.* Recombinant GM-CSF has been used to improve the granulocyte count in patients with AIDS and aplastic anaemia. There is some evidence that the use of this agent may decrease infection in neutropenic patients. Studies in FS have not yet been carried out.

Treatment of the rheumatoid process in Felty's syndrome.   Agents such as penicillamine and gold salts have been used to treat the underlying rheumatoid process in FS. There are reports of improved neutrophil counts and decreased rate of infection in FS using this approach, although controlled studies have not yet been performed.

The spleen may also enlarge in FS because of expansion of the white pulp, due to increased numbers of plasma cells and immunoblasts, as well as germinal centre hyperplasia. Increased splenic phagocyte function is not a consistent feature of FS. Enlargement of the spleen, through expansion of white pulp, may significantly increase portal blood flow and contribute to the development of portal hypertension.

THROMBOCYTOPENIA

Isolated thrombocytopenia in the CTD is usually immunologically mediated. Thrombocytopenia occurring with other cytopenias is usually secondary to drug-induced bone marrow suppression. Occasionally, the active CTD has a direct suppressive effect on bone marrow function. Bone marrow failure in the CTD is dealt with in the next section of this chapter.

Immune thrombocytopenia

Pathogenesis of immune thrombocytopenia in CTD

Immune thrombocytopenia (ITP) is most frequently seen in SLE and, as with AIHA in this disorder, may precede other symptoms and signs of the disease by several months or years. In SLE there is a clinical association of thrombocytopenia with recurrent abortions, a thrombotic tendency, pulmonary hypertension and the presence of the lupus anticoagulant and anticardiolipin antibodies.[20] The link between these clinical and laboratory features is the presence of antiphospholipid antibodies which have cross-reactivity with DNA.[8] The common epitope shared by DNA polynucleotides and phospholipid molecules present in many tissues are the phosphate groups in phosphodiester linkage separated by three carbon atoms of adjacent sugar molecules. In SLE, some cases of ITP may be due to auto-antibody specific for platelet membrane phospholipids. However, ITP in the CTD is most often associated with the binding of immune complexes to the platelet membrane. Premature destruction of immune complex-coated platelets occurs primarily by macrophage-mediated phagocytosis within the reticulo-endothelial system.

Laboratory investigation of immune thrombocytopenia

Haematology and coagulation screening tests.   Giant platelets indicative of increased platelet turnover are seen on the peripheral blood film. As in all putative cases of ITP, thrombotic thrombocytopenic purpura should be excluded by the absence of red cell fragmentation, and no laboratory signs of haemolysis or raised fibrin degradation products. In uncomplicated ITP coagulation screening should be normal. The exception to this is the prolonged partial thromboplastin time detected in patients with ITP associated with the lupus anticoagulant.

Bone marrow examination.   As in other cases of immune thrombocytopenia, increased numbers of megakaryocytes with prominent, morphologically normal, immature forms will be seen.

Platelet antibody studies.   Most methods of measurement of platelet antibodies will give positive results in thrombocytopenic patients with CTD. Simple platelet antibody tests include immunofluorescent antibody and enzyme-linked immunosorbent assay systems. Platelet antibody tests are usually positive in cases mediated by the immune complex mechanism and in cases where auto-antibodies specific for platelet membrane epitopes are present. Platelet antibodies should not be detected in cases where drug-induced bone marrow failure is the cause of the thrombocytopenia.

Clinical features of immune thrombocytopenia

As expected, patients may present with spontaneous haemorrhages of the skin and mucous membranes if the platelet count is below 20×10^9 per litre. Spontaneous haemorrhage is unusual when the platelet count is significantly above this level. Most patients with thrombocytopenia will have other clinical signs of active CTD. In SLE, the association of thrombocytopenia with recurrent abortion, a thrombotic tendency, pulmonary hypertension and the presence of anticardiolipin antibody and the lupus anticoagulant is often seen.

Treatment of immune thrombocytopenia

Corticosteroids.   As with idiopathic ITP, first-line treatment is with corticosteroids, for example, prednisolone 1–2 mg/kg per day for 10 days, then reducing over 2–3 months according to the clinical response.

Splenectomy.   The theoretical objection to splenectomy in CTD is that it may cause a build-up of pathogenic immune complexes normally cleared by the spleen macrophages. Despite this theoretical contraindication, splenectomy should be considered in those cases of immune thrombocytopenia where clinically significant bleeding persists despite an adequate trial of corticosteroid therapy.

Azathioprine.   In some corticosteroid-resistant cases of ITP, splenectomy may be avoided by a 3-month trial of azathioprine 1–1.5 mg/kg per day orally. This approach is indicated when the immune thrombocytopenia is associated with marked activity of the underlying CTD.

Alternative immunosuppressive drugs.   Cyclophosphamide 1–1.5 mg/kg per day orally may be tried in resistant cases. Cyclophosphamide has also been successful when combined with vincristine and prednisolone. Cyclosporin 3 mg/kg twice daily is another alternative, although successful therapy has only been documented in a few case reports. As in AIHA, cyclosporin therapy should be carefully monitored pharmacologically.

Vinca alkaloids.   The vinca alkaloids may be effective as single agents in the treatment of immune thrombocytopenia in the CTD. Their mechanism of action is prevention of phagocytosis by inhibition of the macrophage microtubular system. Vincristine 1.2 mg/m^2 (maximum dose 2 mg) given on days 0, 7, intravenously is a suitable regimen. In most patients especially those with chronic ITP only a temporary response lasting 1–4 weeks is observed.

High-dose intravenous immunoglobulin.   A 5-day course of intravenous human immunoglobulin, e.g. Sandoglobulin 0.4 g/kg per day may be used in resistant cases of chronic ITP associated with CTD. Cases caused by immune complex-mediated platelet destruction are unlikely to respond, as the C3 receptor mechanism predominates in the premature destruction of platelets. Immunoglobulin therapy primarily blocks immune destruction of platelets mediated by the Fc receptor mechanism. Most patients with chronic ITP only mount a temporary response of 1–6 weeks. Despite this high-dose immunoglobulin is a useful method of raising the platelet count perioperatively in patients with steroid-resistant chronic ITP. In addition it may be safely used during pregnancy.

BONE MARROW FAILURE IN THE CTD

Pathogenesis of bone marrow failure in the CTD

Bone marrow failure may be caused by two main mechanisms in the CTD. 'Primary' bone marrow failure may be the result of suppression of or cytotoxic damage to haemopoietic progenitor cells by the underlying autoimmune disease process. 'Secondary' bone marrow failure is due to the effects of drug therapy on bone marrow function and can be further divided into: (1) dose-dependent myelosuppression, (2) idiosyncratic aplastic anaemia, and (3) drug-associated myelodysplasia.

Primary bone marrow failure due to active CTD

Primary bone marrow failure has been well-documented in SLE.[21,22] Initial presentation is with pancytopenia and a hypocellular marrow on aspiration and trephine specimens, in the absence of splenomegaly. Most patients are acutely ill with gross signs of active SLE. Frequently, the interpretation of the blood and marrow findings is complicated by the recent use of azathioprine or other myelotoxic drugs, such as cyclophosphamide. The direct antiglobulin test and tests for platelet antibodies are classically negative. The initial approach to management is to support the patient with blood, platelets and antibiotics in combination with reverse barrier nursing in a single room, if the neutrophil count is $<0.5 \times 10^9$ per litre.

If possible, all myelosuppressive drugs should be stopped and an attempt made to control the patient's disease with high-dose corticosteroids. If the bone marrow failure does not improve *and* it is reasonably certain that prior use of myelosuppressive drugs is not contributing, high-dose cyclophosphamide given in an initial bolus dose of 600 mg/m^2 intravenously may be effective.[21,22] In one case of antibody-mediated bone marrow suppression, a response was seen after plasma exchange, although the disorder had been resistant to high-dose corticosteroid therapy.[23]

Bone marrow failure secondary to drug therapy in CTD

Dose-dependent drug-induced myelosuppression

This is the commonest form of bone marrow failure seen in the CTD. It is usually mild and recovery can be confidently predicted following dosage reduction or discontinuation of the responsible drug. The commonest drugs implicated are azathioprine and cyclophosphamide. The onset of more serious bone marrow failure can usually be prevented by close haematological monitoring of patients with CTD receiving myelotoxic drugs. In cases where the underlying CTD is active and/or there is clinical evidence of coexisting immune cytopenias, more detailed haematological studies, including ferrokinetic and red cell survival studies, may help elucidate the relative importance of bone marrow failure and peripheral destruction in producing the observed cytopenias.

Drug-associated idiosyncratic aplastic anaemia

The drugs used for treatment of the CTD most likely to cause idiosyncratic aplastic anaemia are gold salts, phenylbutazone and penicillamine. In this type of bone marrow failure, the onset is unpredictable and not dose-dependent. There is no guarantee that bone marrow function will improve when the drug is discontinued.

Diagnosis.   This is made by documenting peripheral pancytopenia and bone marrow hypoplasia, both by aspiration and trephine biopsy. Other causes of acquired aplastic anaemia should be excluded, such as non-A, non-B hepatitis, paroxysmal nocturnal haemoglobinuria, and in the case of SLE, activity of the disease itself. Occasionally, it is possible to demonstrate the toxic effects of the causative drug *in vitro*, using haemopoietic progenitor cell assay systems.

Prognosis. Prognosis is determined mainly by the severity of the bone marrow failure. Severe Aplastic Anaemia may be defined by the International Aplastic Anaemia Study Group criteria and is associated with two out of three of the following peripheral blood criteria neutrophils $<0.5 \times 10^9$ per litre, platelets $<20 \times 10^9$ per litre, reticulocytes (corrected for haematocrit) $<1\%$ in the presence of a severely hypocellular marrow containing $<30\%$ residual haemopoietic cells.

Treatment. Treatment of idiosyncratic drug-induced aplastic anaemia which does not improve on drug withdrawal is dependent on:[24] (1) disease severity, (2) age of patient, and (3) presence of a healthy HLA identical sibling. Non-severe cases not meeting the poor prognostic criteria detailed above and all patients over the age of 45 should be considered for treatment with anti-lymphocyte globulin. Patients under the age of 45 with severe disease, who have a suitable donor are candidates for early bone marrow transplantation.[25]

Drug-associated myelodysplasia

Treatment of the CTD with long-term alkylating agents, especially cyclo-phosphamide and chlorambucil, is associated with an increased risk of myelodysplasia and ultimately secondary acute myeloid leukaemia. Where possible, the use of these agents should be confined to short courses, especially in younger patients. Experience of long-term azathioprine therapy in renal allograft recipients suggests that the risk of myelodysplasia caused by this agent is much less than with the alkylating agents.

All patients with CTD receiving alkylating agents should be monitored haematologically. The peripheral blood film should be carefully examined with the peripheral blood count at each clinic visit to pick up early signs of myelodysplasia. In addition, the need for the continued use of these agents in the control of each patient's disease should be regularly reviewed.

LUPUS ANTICOAGULANTS

Pathogenesis of lupus anticoagulants (LA)

The so-called 'lupus anticoagulant' was first described as an acquired inhibitor of coagulation *in vitro* characterized by the finding of a prolonged partial thromboplastin time (PTT) in patients with SLE.[3] It is now known that the LA activity is due to auto-antibodies specific for phospholipid and which, by binding to phospholipid epitopes on the prothrombin complex, inhibit coagulation tests *in vitro* which are phospholipid-dependent.[26] Unlike other acquired inhibitors (e.g. to Factor VIII) the LA does not inhibit any specific coagulation factor assays.[9]

Clinical features associated with lupus anticoagulants

The LAs are most frequently documented in SLE, but as a result of increased pre-operative screening and coagulation tests carried out for other reasons, LA are now often detected in patients who do not have CTD. A recent review of 100 cases of LA indicates that in 53 cases, there was no evidence of autoimmune disease. Of the 47 with documented autoimmune features, 28 had SLE, 5 an SLE-like syndrome, 4 drug-associated SLE and 10 others CTD. In the non-autoimmune group, no particular pathology was predominant.[9]

In the CTD, the LA is associated with an *in vivo* thrombotic tendency involving both arteries and veins, with thrombocytopenia, recurrent abortions and pulmonary hypertension. The basis for this association is not fully understood, although these cases tend to have high levels of a spectrum of antiphospholipid antibodies, including anticardiolipins. The association between thrombosis and LA *in vivo* may be explained by inhibition of thrombomodulin activity by the LA leading to reduced protein C activation *in vivo*.

Laboratory diagnosis of lupus anticoagulant

The presence of an LA may be suspected on the basis of a prolonged partial thromboplastin time (PTT) not corrected by a 1:1 mixture of patient and normal plasma. Further confirmation is obtained by: (1) performing a diluted thromboplastin assay and demonstrating a prolongation of the patient's clotting time, not corrected by a 1:1 mixture of normal plasma; and (2) demonstrating that after incubating of patient plasma with normal plasma, specific factor assays are not inhibited.

Treatment of lupus anticoagulant

Patients who have a thrombotic tendency and/or primary hypertension should be considered for long-term anticoagulant therapy with a Coumarin derivative, and as arterial thrombosis may also occur, low-dose aspirin, e.g. 300 mg daily should also be considered. These measures are contraindicated in patients with severe thrombocytopenia or a platelet count $<20 \times 10^9$ per litre who, in contrast, usually have a haemorrhagic tendency. The management of pregnancy in patients with the LA is a specialized area and should be performed with close liaison between the rheumatologists, obstetrician and haematologist. The use of immunosuppressive therapy in patients with CTD and LA depends on the other clinical factors present and disease activity. Ideally, LA patients should be managed in a combined rheumatology/haematology clinic by physicians with a special interest.

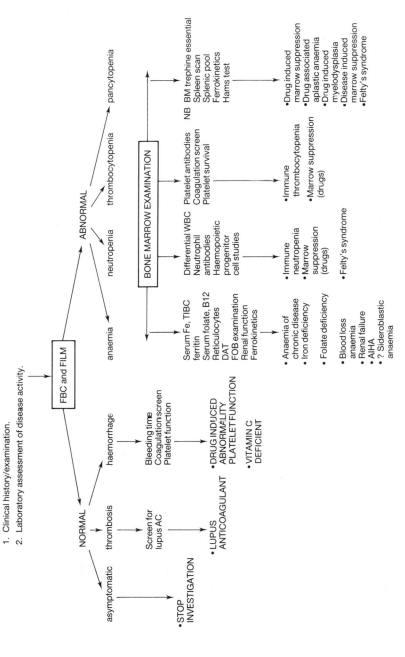

Fig. 8.2. Flowchart for investigating haematological abnormalities in Connective Tissue Disorders.

REFERENCES

1. Isenberg, D.A, Martin, P., Hajirouson, V., Todd-Pokropek, A., Goldstone, A.M. & Snaith, M.L. Haematological reassessment of rheumatoid arthritis. *Br. J. Rheumatol.* **25**: 152–7, 1986.
2. Churg, J. & Strauss, L. Allergic granulomatosis, allergic angiitis and polyarteritis nodosa. *Am. J. Pathol.* **27**: 277–301, 1951.
3. Feinstein, D.I. & Rapaport, S.I. Acquired inhibition of blood coagulation. *Prog. Hemost. Thromb.* **1**: 75–95, 1972.
4. Isenberg, D.A., Patterson, K.G., Todd-Pokropek, A., Snaith, M.L. & Goldstone, A.H. Haematological aspects of systemic lupus erythematosus: a re-appraisal using automated methods. *Acta Haematol.* **67**: 242–8, 1982.
5. Isenberg, D.A. & Shoenfeld, Y. The rheumatologic complications of haematologic disorders. *Semin. Arth. Rheumatol.* **12**: 348–58, 1983.
6. Morrow, W.J.W., Isenberg, D.A., Todd-Pokropek, A., Parry, H.F. & Snaith, M.L. Useful laboratory measurements in the management of systemic lupus erythematosus. *Q. J. Med.* **202**: 125–38, 1982.
7. Morrow, W.J.W., Isenberg, D.A., Parry, H.F. *et al.*. Studies on autoantibodies to polyadenosine diphosphate ribose in SLE and other autoimmune diseases. *Am. Rheumatol. Dis.* **41**: 396–402, 1982.
8. Isenberg, D.A., Colaco, C.B., Dudeney, C., Todd-Pokropek, A. & Snaith, M.L. A study of the relationship between anti-DNA antibody idiotypes and anticardiolipin antibodies with disease activity in systemic lupus erythematosus. *Medicine (Baltimore)* **63**: 450–8, 1986.
9. Ludvico, C.L., Ziverman, N., Myers, A.B., Herbert, J. & Green, P.A. Predictive value of anti-DNA antibody and selected laboratory studies in systemic lupus erythematosus. *J. Rheumatol.* **7**: 843–9, 1980.
10. Jude, B., Goudemand, J., Dolle, I. *et al.* Lupus anticoagulant: a clinical and laboratory study of 100 cases. *Clin. Lab. Haematol.* **10**: 41–51, 1988.
11. Means, R.T., Olsen, N.J., Krantz, S.B. *et al.* Treatment of the anaemia of rheumatoid arthritis with recombinant human erythropoietin: clinical and *in vitro* results. *Blood* **70**: Suppl. 1, abstract 413, 1987.
12. Hows, J.M. & Gordon-Smith, E.C. The acquired haemolytic anaemias. In *Postgraduate Haematology* 3rd Edn (eds A.V. Hoffbrand and S.M. Lewis), pp. 183–207, Heinemann Professional Publishing, 1989.
13 Ross, G.D. & Newman, S.L. Regulation of macrophage functions. In *The Reticuloendothelial System*, Vol. 6, *Immunology* (eds J.A. Bellanti & H.B. Herscowitz, pp. 173–99. Plenum Press, New York, 1984.
14. Winearls, C.G., Pippard, M.J., Downing, M.R. *et al.* Effect of human erythropoietin derived from recombinant DNA in the anaemia of patients maintained on chronic haemodialysis. *Lancet* **2**: 1175–8, 1986.
15. Felty, A.R. Chronic arthritis in the adult associated with splenomegaly and leukopenia. *Bull. Johns Hopkins Hosp.* **35**: 16–20, 1924.
16. Goldberg, J. & Pinals, R.S. Felty's syndrome. *Semin. Arth. Rheum.* **10**: 52–65, 1980.
17. Breedveld, F.C., Van den Barselaar, M.T., Leijh, P.C.J. *et al.* Phagocytosis and intracellular killing by polymorphonuclear cells from patients with rheumatoid arthritis and Felty's syndrome. *Arth. Rheum.* **28**: 395–404, 1985.
18. Breedveld, F.C. Factors influencing the incidence of infections in Felty's syndrome. *Arch. Intern. Med.* **147**: 915–20, 1987.
19. Vincent, P.C., Levi, J.A. & MacQueen, A. The mechanisms of neutropenia in Felty's syndrome. *Br. J. Haematol.* **27**: 463–75, 1974.
20. Miller, M.H., Urowitz, M.B. & Gladman, D.D. The significance of thrombocytopenia in systemic lupus erythematosus. *Arthritis Rheum.* **26**: 1181–1186, 1983.

21. Walport, M.J., Hubbard, W.N. & Hughes, G.R.V. Reversal of aplastic anaemia secondary to systemic lupus erythematosus by high-dose intravenous cyclophosphamide. *Br. Med. J.* **285**: 769–70, 1982.
22. Winkler, A., Jackson, R.W., Kay, D.S. *et al.* High-dose intravenous cyclophosphamide treatment of systemic lupus erythematosus associated aplastic anaemia. *Arthritis Rheum.* **31**: 693–4, 1988.
23. Fitchen, J.J., Cline, M.J., Saxon, A., *et al.* Serum inhibitors of hematopoiesis in a patient with aplastic anaemia and systemic lupus erythematosus: recovery after exchange plasmaphoresis. *Am. J. Med.* **66**: 537–42, 1979.
24. Marsh, J.C.W. & Gordon-Smith, E.C. The role of antilymphocyte globulin in the treatment of chronic acquired bone marrow failure. *Blood Rev.* **2**: 141–8, 1988.
25. Bacigalupo, A., Hows, J.M., Gluckman, E. *et al.* Bone Marrow Transplantation (BMT) versus immuno-suppression for the treatment of severe aplastic anaemia (SAA); a report of the EBMT SAA Working Party. *Br. J. Haematol.* **70**: 177–82, 1988.
26. Koffler, D., Biesecker, G. & Katz, S.M. Immunopathogenesis of systemic lupus erythematosus. *Arthritis Rheum.* **25**: 858–61, 1982.

9

Paraproteinaemia

Robert A. Kyle

Chairman, Division of Haematology and Internal Medicine, Mayo Clinic and Mayo Foundation, William H. Donner Professor of Medicine and Laboratory Medicine, Mayo Medical School, Rochester, Minnesota, USA

Each paraprotein (monoclonal protein, M-protein) consists of two heavy-chain polypeptides of the same class and sub-class and two light-chain polypeptides of the same type. The different monoclonal proteins are designated by capital letters that correspond to the class of their heavy chains, which are designated by Greek letters, γ in IgG, α in IgA, μ in IgM, δ in IgD, and ε in IgE. Their sub-classes are IgG1, IgG2, IgG3 and IgG4 or IgA1 and IgA2 and their light-chain types are kappa ($\varkappa$) and lambda (λ).

A paraprotein (having a single heavy-chain class and single light-chain type) appears as a narrow peak (like a church spire) on the densitometer tracing or as a dense, discrete band on the cellulose acetate membrane in the γ, β or α_2 globulin regions (Fig. 9.1A). The differential diagnosis of paraproteins is shown in Table 9.1.

In contrast to a paraprotein, a polyclonal increase in immunoglobulins consists of one or more heavy-chain classes and both light-chain types. On electrophoresis, a polyclonal increase is characterized by a broad peak or band usually of γ mobility (Fig. 9.1B). A polyclonal increase in immunoglobulins is associated with connective tissue (autoimmune) diseases, chronic liver disease, chronic infections, and lymphoproliferative diseases, although it is seen in some apparently normal persons.

Paraproteins should be differentiated from polyclonal increases in immunoglobulins because the former are associated with a neoplastic or potentially malignant process, whereas the latter are associated with an inflammatory or reactive process.

Although paraproteins had been considered to be abnormal proteins, they are now considered to be only excessive quantities of normal immunoglobulins. Paraproteins are individual antibodies and are products of a single or closely related clone of plasma cells. Some monoclonal proteins represent known antibodies but others do not. The one-cell, one-immunoglobulin concept is supported by the fact that nearly all plasma cells contain either $\varkappa$ or λ light chains but not both.

RECOGNITION OF PARAPROTEINS

Analysis of the serum and urine for paraproteins requires a sensitive, rapid, dependable screening method and a specific technique to identify the heavy-

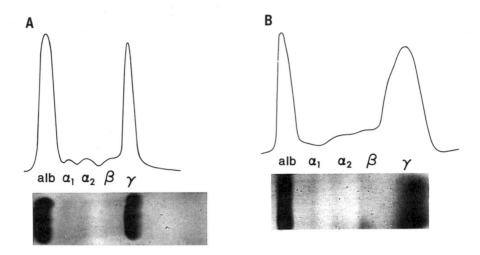

Fig. 9.1. (A) Top: Pattern of serum paraprotein from densitometer tracing after electrophoresis of serum on cellulose acetate (anode on left): tall, narrowbased peak of γ mobility; bottom: pattern from electrophoresis of serum on cellulose acetate (anode on left): dense, localized band representing paraprotein in γ area. (B) Top: Polyclonal pattern of serum protein from densitometer tracing after electrophoresis on cellulose acetate (anode on left): Broad-based peak of γ mobility; bottom: polyclonal pattern from electrophoresis of serum on cellulose acetate (anode on left): γ band is broad. (From Ref. 75 by permission of Mayo Foundation.)

chain class and light-chain type.

Electrophoresis on cellulose acetate membrane is satisfactory for screening but may not detect small monoclonal proteins. High-resolution agarose gel electrophoresis is more sensitive than cellulose acetate membranes.[1] Either immunoelectrophoresis or immunofixation[2] or both should be used to confirm the presence of a paraprotein and to identify the heavy-chain class and light-chain type.

Serum protein electrophoresis should be done in all cases in which multiple myeloma, macroglobulinaemia, amyloidosis or a related disorder is suspected. In addition, the test is indicated in any patient with unexplained weakness or fatigue, anaemia, elevation of the erythrocyte sedimentation rate, back pain, osteoporosis, osteolytic lesions or fractures, immunoglobulin deficiency, hypercalcaemia, Bence Jones proteinuria, renal insufficiency or recurrent infections. Because a localized band or spike is strongly suggestive of primary amyloidosis, serum protein electrophoresis should also be performed in cases of peripheral neuropathy, carpal tunnel syndrome, refractory congestive heart failure, nephrotic syndrome, orthostatic hypotension or malabsorption. Electrophoresis is an excellent screening test because it can be done easily, rapidly and economically.

A paraprotein may be present even when the total serum protein concentration, β and γ globulin levels, and quantitative immunoglobulins

Table 9.1 Differential Diagnosis of Paraproteins

I. Paraproteins of undetermined significance
  A. Benign (IgG, IgA, IgD, IgM, and, rarely, free light chains)
  B. Associated with neoplasms of cell types not known to produce monoclonal proteins
  C. Biclonal paraproteins

II. Malignant paraproteins
  A. Multiple myeloma (IgG, IgA, IgD, IgE, and free light chains)
    1. Overt multiple myeloma
    2. Smouldering multiple myeloma
    3. Plasma cell leukaemia
    4. Non-secretory myeloma
    5. IgD myeloma
    6. Osteosclerotic myeloma
  B. Plasmacytoma
    1. Solitary plasmacytoma of bone
    2. Extramedullary plasmacytoma
  C. Malignant lymphoproliferative diseases
    1. Waldenström's (primary) macroglobulinaemia
    2. Malignant lymphoma
  D. Heavy-chain diseases (HCD)
    1. γ HCD
    2. α HCD
    3. μ HCD
  E. Amyloidosis (AL)
    1. Primary
    2. With myeloma
      (secondary, localized, and familial amyloidosis have no paraprotein)

Modified from Ref. 76.

are all normal. The cellulose strip must be examined visually because the densitometer tracing may not detect a small paraprotein. A small paraprotein also may be concealed among the β and γ components. Bence Jones proteinaemia (monoclonal light chain) is rarely seen in the cellulose acetate tracing. A localized band is occasionally seen in μ heavy-chain disease but is never observed in α heavy-chain disease. In γ heavy-chain disease, a broad band rather than a sharp localized band is often seen on electrophoresis. A paraprotein may be seen as a rather broad band or spike and may be mistaken for a polyclonal increase in immunoglobulins. Hence, immunoelectrophoresis or immunofixation is necessary to identify a paraprotein.

Immunoelectrophoresis

Immunoelectrophoresis is a useful technique for the identification of a paraprotein and should be performed in all cases in which a sharp peak or localized band is found on electrophoresis or in which multiple myeloma, macroglobulinaemia, amyloidosis or a related disorder is suspected. The immunoelectrophoretic pattern of an IgG $\varkappa$ monoclonal protein is shown in Fig. 9.2. All sera should be screened using Ouchterlony immunodiffusion for IgD and IgE paraproteins. Screening is essential when there is bowing of the $\varkappa$ or λ arcs but no accompanying abnormality of the IgG, IgA, or IgM arcs.

Immunofixation

This is useful when results of immunoelectrophoresis are equivocal. The technique is often helpful when a paraprotein is suspected and bowing of only a single heavy chain or a single light chain is found on immunoelectrophoresis (Fig. 9.3). Immunofixation is also useful in detecting a small paraprotein in the presence of a polyclonal increase in immunoglobulins. It is particularly advantageous in (1) treated myeloma or macroglobulinaemia when the localized band has disappeared on electrophoresis; (2) suspected amyloidosis when an attempt is made to detect a small paraprotein; (3) apparent solitary plasmacytoma or extramedullary plasmacytoma after treatment with radiation and subsequent follow-up; and (4) recognition of the second component of a biclonal gammopathy.

Despite the advantages of immunofixation, immunoelectrophoresis is recommended as the initial procedure because it is technically easier and more economical and the results generally are satisfactory. In addition,

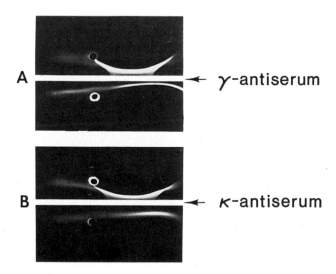

Fig. 9.2. Immunoelectrophoretic pattern of serum. (A) Top: Antiserum to IgG (γ) shows a thickened arc; bottom: antiserum to IgG (γ) show a normal arc. (B) top: Antisera to $\varkappa$ chains shows a thickened arc similar to the IgG arc; bottom: antiserum to $\varkappa$ shows a normal arc. The patient's serum contains an IgG $\varkappa$ paraprotein. (From Ref. 75 by permission of Mayo Foundation.)

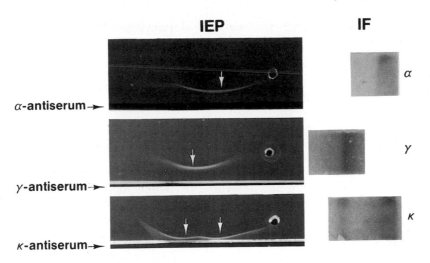

Fig. 9.3. Immunoelectrophoresis and immunofixation of serum. Left: Serum immunoelectrophoresis (IEP; anode to left) shows bowing of IgA and IgG arcs corresponding to double bowing of ϰ. Right: Serum immunofixation (IF) shows a localized IgA (α) band in the top position corresponding to a ϰ band in the lower position. The localized IgG (γ) band in the middle position corresponds to a similar ϰ band in the lower position. This patient has a biclonal gammopathy (IgA ϰ and IgG ϰ). (From Ref. 76 by permission of the publisher.)

interpretation of immunofixation may be misleading and can result in overdiagnosis or underdiagnosis of paraproteins because the dilution of the serum or urine specimen is crucial.

A rate nephelometer using monospecific anti-ϰ and anti-λ antisera to identify the light-chain component is satisfactory when large paraproteins are present. However, small paraproteins will have a normal or almost normal ϰ:λ ratio and consequently may not be recognized with this technique.

Quantitation of immunoglobulins

Use of a rate nephelometer is a practical method for quantitation of immunoglobulins. In this system, the degree of turbidity produced by antigen–antibody interaction is measured by nephelometry in the near ultraviolet region. Because the method is not affected by the molecular size of the antigen, as is radial immunodiffusion, the nephelometric technique measures 7S IgM, polymers of IgA or aggregates of IgG accurately. We have seen many instances in which the quantitative immunoglobulin level, as determined by rate nephelometry, is more than 2000 mg/dl greater than that determined by densitometry. The use of a densitometer tracing of the cellulose acetate electrophoresis is preferred for the follow-up of a paraprotein because of this discrepancy and the ease, reproducibility, and economy of the cellulose acetate tracing. In any event, follow-up must involve evaluating either the size of a paraprotein by serum protein electrophoresis or the quantitation of the immunoglobulins, but the method used must remain the same.

ANALYSIS OF URINE FOR PARAPROTEINS

The use of sulphosalicylic acid or of Exton's reagent is best for the detection of a paraprotein. In many laboratories, dipstick tests are used to screen for protein. However, these tests are often insensitive to Bence Jones protein and should not be used when the possibility of Bence Jones proteinuria exists. The heat test for the detection of Bence Jones proteinuria is not satisfactory because both false-positive and false-negative results occur. The recognition of Bence Jones proteinuria depends on the demonstration of a monoclonal light chain by immunoelectrophoresis or immunofixation.

Electrophoresis

This should be performed in all cases of multiple myeloma, macro-globulinaemia, amyloidosis, monoclonal gammopathy of undetermined significance (MGUS), heavy-chain diseases (HCD) or suspicion of these entities.

A 24-h collection of urine must be made for determination of the total amount of protein excreted each day. This determination is important when the level of a urinary paraprotein is used for following the course of a patient, because the amount of paraprotein correlates directly with the size of the plasma cell burden.

A urinary paraprotein is seen as a dense, localized band on the cellulose strip or as a tall, narrow, homogeneous peak on the densitometer tracing (Fig. 9.4). Occasionally, two discrete globulin bands may be seen in the cellulose acetate tracing. These bands may represent a paraprotein plus an immunoglobulin fragment from the serum, or they may be monomers and dimers of the monoclonal urinary paraprotein (Fig. 9.5). Therefore, immunoelectrophoresis or immunofixation of the appropriate heavy- and light-chain antisera is necessary. It is not unusual for the protein reaction to be negative and for immunoelectrophoresis or immunofixation of a concentrated urine specimen to reveal a paraprotein. Sometimes, electrophoresis of urine shows a large amount of albumin and insignificant amounts of globulin (nephrotic pattern) and the urine contains a paraprotein. This is seen most often in patients with primary systemic amyloidosis (AL). Consequently, immunoelectrophoresis or immunofixation should be done in all older patients in whom the nephrotic syndrome develops and the cause is unknown. Immunofixation is more sensitive than immunoelectrophoresis but is technically more difficult. Particular care must be taken to obtain the appropriate dilution because either overdiagnosis or underdiagnosis of a paraprotein is possible with this technique.

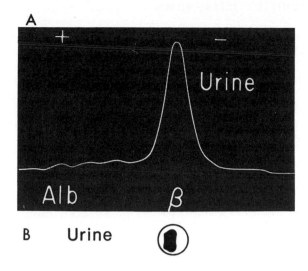

Fig. 9.4. Urine paraprotein. Top: Densitometer tracing showing a tall, narrow-based peak of β mobility; bottom: cellulose acetate electrophoretic pattern showing a dense band of β mobility. This is consistent with a urinary paraprotein (Bence Jones protein). (From Ref. 75 by permission of Mayo Foundation.)

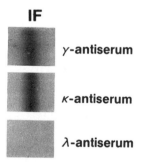

Fig. 9.5. Urine immunofixation. The localized IgG (γ) band in the top position corresponds to the localized ϰ band in the middle position. This patient has an IgG (ϰ) paraprotein fragment in the urine. (From Ref. 76 by permission of the publisher.)

CLINICAL PARAPROTEINAEMIAS

Paraproteins may be classified according to Table 9.1. Paraproteins without evidence of myeloma, macroglobulinaemia, amyloidosis or related diseases have been found in approximately 3% of persons more than 70 years old in Sweden[3] and in the United States.[4] In Sweden, among 6995 normal persons more than 25 years old, the overall prevalence of paraproteins was 1%;[3] among 1200 patients 50 years old or older who were residents of a small Minnesota community, 1.25% had a paraprotein.[4] In a survey of 17,968 adults 50 years old or older in Finistère, France, 303 (1.7%) had a paraprotein.[5]

More sensitive techniques will detect a higher incidence of paraproteins. For example, Papadopoulos et al.,[6] using agarose electrophoresis, detected paraproteins in the serum of 30 (5%) of 600 healthy adults who were 22–65 years of age. Immuno-isoelectric focusing, an even more sensitive technique, identified a paraprotein in the sera of 11% of patients more than 45 years of age who had been hospitalized for surgery of a non-malignant condition. Agarose electrophoresis revealed that only 2% had a paraprotein.[7]

Paraproteins are being recognized in clinical practice much more commonly than in the past. At present, approximately 50,000 serum protein electrophoretic strips are screened each year at the Mayo Clinic. During 1986, 888 new cases of serum paraproteins were identified. The clinical diagnoses included benign paraproteinaemia (monoclonal gammopathy of undetermined significance, MGUS, benign monoclonal gammopathy, BMG), 68%; multiple myeloma (MM), 11%; primary systemic amyloidosis (AL), 8%; lymphoproliferative disease, 6%; chronic lymphocytic leukaemia, 2%; solitary or extramedullary plasmacytoma, 2%; macroglubulinaemia, 1%; and other diagnoses, 2%. Thus, the prevalence of benign paraproteinaemia (MGUS) is considerable, and it is important to both the patient and the physician to determine whether the paraprotein will remain benign or progress to multiple myeloma, macroglobulinaemia, lymphoma or amyloidosis.

We are continuing to gather follow-up data on 241 patients who had a serum paraprotein recognized at the Mayo Clinic before 1 January 1971.[8] Patients with multiple myeloma, macroglobulinaemia, amyloidosis, lymphoma or a related disease were excluded. The patients were classified as follows: group 1, patients without an increase in serum paraprotein during follow-up (benign); group 2, patients with more than a 50% increase of serum paraprotein or the development of urine paraprotein but no diagnosis of myeloma or related disease; group 3, patients who died from unrelated causes; and group 4, patients in whom multiple myeloma, macroglobulinaemia, amyloidosis, or a related disease developed.

Group 1 (stable)

At the end of 10 or more years (median, 13 years), the number of patients whose paraprotein had remained stable and could be classified as 'benign' paraproteinaemia had decreased to 88 (37%). Indeed, 22 patients (25%) had been followed up for 15–26 years and had not developed multiple myeloma, macroglobulinaemia, amyloidosis or lymphoproliferative disease. In one patient, the paraprotein disappeared from the serum. There were no significant differences between the stable or benign disease and the total group, in size of the serum paraprotein peak, type of serum heavy and light chains, reduction of uninvolved immunoglobulins, sub-class of IgG heavy chain and the number of plasma cells in the bone marrow.

Group 2 (increase of paraprotein only)

In all 13 patients of this group the serum paraprotein level increased by 50% or more (median increase, 1.1 g/dl; range, 0.7–1.5 g/dl), but multiple myeloma, macroglobulinaemia or amyloidosis did not develop. The median interval from the finding of the paraprotein to an increase of 50% or more was 10.5 years (range 5–15 years).

Group 3 (died without developing multiple myeloma or related disease)

The 94 patients in this group died without having evidence of a plasma cell proliferative process. The median duration from diagnosis of the paraprotein to death was 67 months (range, 0–221 months). Eighteen patients survived more than 10 years after diagnosis of the paraprotein. Cardiac disease was the most frequent cause of death (38%) followed by cerebrovascular disease (14%). Seven patients died of a malignancy not associated with a plasma cell proliferative process.

Group 4 (developed multiple myeloma, macroglobulinaemia, amyloidosis, or related diseases)

Multiple myeloma, macroglobulinaemia, amyloidosis, or a malignant lymphoplasma proliferative process developed in 46 patients (19%). The actuarial rate at 10 years was 16.2%. Among this group, 32 (70%) had multiple myeloma. The interval from the recognition of the paraprotein to the diagnosis of multiple myeloma ranged from 2 to 21 years (median, 8.2 years). The median survival after the diagnosis of multiple myeloma was 35 months.

Macroglobulinaemia of Waldenström developed in six patients 4–20 years after recognition of the paraprotein. In an additional six patients, systemic amyloidosis was recognized 6–14 years after a serum paraprotein was found. Two other patients developed a malignant lymphoproliferative process – chronic lymphocytic leukaemia in one and an aggressive undifferentiated non-Hodgkin's lymphoma in the other.

DIFFERENTIATION OF BENIGN PARAPROTEINAEMIA FROM MULTIPLE MYELOMA AND MACROGLOBULINAEMIA

Patients with benign paraproteinaemia (MGUS) have <3 g/dl of paraprotein in the serum and no or small amounts of Bence Jones proteinuria; fewer than 5% plasma cells in the bone marrow aspirate; and no anaemia, hypercalcaemia, renal insufficiency or osteolytic lesions unless caused by other diseases. The only basis for deciding that the patient has benign paraproteinaemia is the absence of an increase of the paraprotein level or the development of a plasma cell–lymphoproliferative process during long-term follow-up.

In contrast to the patient with benign paraproteinaemia, the patient with smouldering multiple myeloma (SMM) has a paraprotein level >3 g/dl in the serum, >10% atypical plasma cells in the bone marrow, and a very low plasma cell labelling index (LI). In addition, the patient with SMM frequently has a small amount of Bence Jones protein in the urine and a reduction of uninvolved immunoglobulins in the serum. However, anaemia, renal insufficiency and skeletal lesions do not develop and the patient's condition remains stable. These patients should not be treated unless laboratory study shows progression of disease or symptoms of myeloma develop.[9]

Differentiation of the patient with benign paraproteinaemia from the patient in whom myeloma or macroglobulinaemia eventually develops is very difficult at the time that the paraprotein is recognized. The size of the serum M-protein is of some help – higher levels are associated with a greater likelihood of malignancy.[10] The presence of >3 g/dl of paraprotein usually indicates overt multiple myeloma or macroglobulinaemia, but some exceptions such as SMM do exist. Levels of immunoglobulin class not associated with the paraprotein (normal polyclonal background immunoglobulins) may aid in differentiating benign from malignant conditions. In most patients with multiple myeloma, the levels of polyclonal immunoglobulins are reduced, although a similar reduction in levels in patients with benign paraproteinaemia also may occur. Thus, such a reduction is not a satisfactory differentiating feature. The association of Bence Jones proteinuria with a serum paraprotein usually indicates a neoplastic process, although there are many patients with a small amount of Bence Jones proteinuria and a paraprotein in the serum whose conditions have remained stable for years. The presence of >10% plasma cells in the bone marrow is suggestive of multiple myeloma, but the conditions of some patients with a greater degree of plasmacytosis have remained stable for long periods. Plasma cells in multiple myeloma are usually atypical, but these features also may be seen in benign paraproteinaemia. The presence of osteolytic lesions is suggestive of multiple myeloma, but metastatic carcinoma may produce lytic lesions and plasmacytosis and be associated with an unrelated serum paraprotein.

Levels of β_2-microglobulin are not helpful in differentiating benign paraproteinaemia from low-grade multiple myeloma because there is too much overlap. The presence of J-chains in malignant plasma cells or the acid phosphatase levels in plasma cells are also unreliable for differentiation. Reduced numbers of OKT4+ T-cells, increased numbers of idiotype-bearing peripheral blood lymphocytes, and increased numbers of immunoglobulin-secreting cells in the peripheral blood are characteristic of multiple myeloma, but there is an overlap with benign paraproteinaemia.

The plasma cell labelling index (LI) using tritiated thymidine is helpful in differentiating benign paraproteinaemia or SMM from multiple myeloma.[11] Patients whose plasma cells are not synthesizing DNA (LI = 0%) most likely have a stable condition and should be followed up closely without treatment. Recently, a more practical LI procedure has been developed. A monoclonal antibody (BU-1) reactive with 5-bromo-2-deoxyuridine (BrdUrd) was raised in mice.[12] This monoclonal antibody can be used in a slide-based immunofluorescent assay. Fluorescein-conjugated immunoglobulin antisera ($\varkappa$ and λ) identifies monoclonal plasma cells and plasmacytoid lymphocytes. The immunofluorescent LI can be done in 4–5 h and is superior to the use of tritiated thymidine.[13]

In summary, there is no single dependable technique for differentiating a patient with benign paraproteinaemia from one who subsequently will develop multiple myeloma or other related disorders. The most reliable means of differentiating benign from a malignant course is the serial measurement of the paraprotein level and periodic evaluation of the patient to determine whether the features of multiple myeloma, systemic amyloidosis, macroglobulinaemia or another malignant lymphoproliferative process develop.

PARAPROTEINS IN OTHER DISEASES

Although benign paraproteinaemia frequently exists without any other abnormalities, certain diseases are associated with it, as would be expected in an older population. The association of two diseases in a person depends on the frequency with which each disease occurs independently. For example, association of benign paraproteinaemia and hyperparathyroidism has been noted in several instances. In an effort to clarify the relationship, we reviewed the records of patients with surgically proven parathyroid adenoma in whom serum protein electrophoresis had been done within 6 months preceding parathyroidectomy. Among 911 patients who met these criteria and who were more than 50 years of age, immunoelectrophoresis revealed a paraprotein in 9 (1%).[14] This prevalence of paraprotein is similar to that found in previous studies of normal populations. Thus, the association of hyperparathyroidism and benign paraproteinaemia seems to be due to chance alone. This demonstrates the need for comparison with an adequate control population before an assumption is made that an association exists between benign paraproteinaemia and any disease.

Lymphoproliferative disorders

For 30 years, paraproteins have been recognized in lymphoma. Alexanian[15] reported an IgM protein in 29 (4.5%) of 640 patients with diffuse lymphoproliferative disease and in none of 292 patients with a nodular lymphoma. The incidence of an IgM protein was approximately 100 times greater than that found in a normal population.

Leukaemia

Paraproteins have been found in the sera of some patients with acute leukaemia. Noel & Kyle[16] described 100 patients with chronic lymphocytic leukaemia (CLL) and a paraprotein in the serum or urine. The protein was IgG in 51% and IgM in 38%. There was no important difference in patients with CLL whether they had an IgG or an IgM paraprotein.

Other haematologic diseases

Paraproteins have been found in a wide variety of haematologic diseases, including pernicious anaemia, acquired von Willebrand's disease, Gaucher's disease, pure red cell aplasia, polycythaemia vera, myelofibrosis, chronic myelocytic leukaemia, primary thrombocythaemia and myelodysplasia.

Connective tissue diseases

Rheumatoid arthritis, lupus erythematosus, polymyalgia rheumatica, poly-myositis and discoid lupus erythematosus have been associated with a paraprotein.

Neurologic disorders

In a series of 279 patients with clinically recognized sensorimotor peripheral neuropathy of unknown cause, Kelly et al.[17] found 16 with benign paraproteinaemia. A monograph on neurologic disorders associated with paraproteins has recently been published.[18]

Latov et al.[19] demonstrated that a small IgM λ paraprotein in a patient with peripheral neuropathy was directed against peripheral nerve myelin. This protein was subsequently identified as a specific glycoprotein component of myelin and referred to as myelin-associated glycoprotein (MAG). In approximately half the patients with peripheral neuropathy and an IgM paraprotein, the paraprotein binds to MAG.[20] These patients usually present with paraesthesias and numbness of the feet, which progresses proximally in a stocking-glove distribution. Motor involvement is less prominent than sensory. Cranial nerves and autonomic functions are usually intact.

Patients with IgG paraprotein and peripheral neuropathy have been reported, but the relationship of the paraprotein to the peripheral neuropathy has not been well-documented.

Motor neurone diseases (including amyotrophic lateral sclerosis and spinal muscular atrophy) associated with paraproteins have been reported.[21] Myasthenia gravis, ataxia telangiectasia and multiple sclerosis have been found with paraproteins, but the association may be only fortuitous.

Dermatologic diseases

Lichen myxoedematosus (papular mucinosis, scleromyxoedema) is a rare dermatologic condition frequently associated with an IgG λ paraprotein that has cathodal mobility.[22] Pyoderma gangraenosum has been associated with paraproteins usually of the IgA class.[23] An IgG paraprotein is frequently found with necrobiotic xanthogranuloma.[24] Paraproteins have been associated with subcutaneous T-cell lymphomas such as Sézary syndrome and mycosis fungoides.

Miscellaneous

Gelfand *et al.*[25] described a patient with angioedema and acquired deficiency of C1-esterase inhibitor and reviewed the records of 14 others reported in the literature. Five patients had a 7S IgM paraprotein. Of nine patients with the periodic systemic capillary leak syndrome (increased capillary permeability), eight had a paraprotein in the serum.[26] Paraproteins have been associated with liver disease and acquired immune deficiency syndrome (AIDS), as well as renal, bone marrow and liver transplantations.

Henoch–Schönlein purpura, bacterial endocarditis, Hashimoto's thyroiditis, septic arthritis, purpura fulminans, idiopathic pulmonary fibrosis, pulmonary alveolar proteinosis, thymoma, hereditary spherocytosis, Doyne's macular heredodystrophy, subcorneal pustular dermatosis, corneal crystalline deposits and proliferative glomerulonephritis have all been associated with paraproteins, but the relationship is not clear and the association may be fortuitous in many of these entities.

Paraproteins with antibody activity

In some cases of benign paraproteinaemia, myeloma or macroglobulinaemia, the paraprotein has shown unusual specificities – for example, to dextran, antistreptolysin O, von Willebrand factor, thyroglobulin, insulin, double-stranded DNA, apolipoprotein B, thyroxin and antibiotics as well as showing antinuclear activity. Transient paraproteins with antibody activity have been recognized after infections. Paraproteins with antibody activity have been reviewed by Merlini *et al.*[27]

Binding of calcium by a paraprotein may produce hypercalcaemia without symptomatic or pathologic consequences. This situation should be recognized in order to avoid treating the patient for hypercalcaemia.[28] A copper-binding paraprotein has been found in multiple myeloma, as well as in benign paraproteinaemia.

Biclonal paraproteinaemia

Biclonal paraproteinaemia of undetermined significance (biclonal gammopathy of undetermined significance, BGUS) has been reported in one group of 37 patients with the clinical findings similar to those in MGUS.[29] In one patient, symptomatic multiple myeloma developed after 2 years. In another, the biclonal paraprotein disappeared for no apparent reason. Riddell et al.[30] reported that in 2.5% of 1135 patients who had paraprotein, the paraprotein was biclonal. The authors postulated that the paraprotein arises from two separate plasma cell clones in some patients while in others the paraprotein behaves in a concordant manner that is consistent with incomplete class switching in a single plasma cell clone.

Triclonal paraproteinaemia

This type has been found in a patient with plasma cell dyscrasia in whom AIDS subsequently developed and in a patient with non-Hodgkin's lymphoma. We have also seen some patients with triclonal paraproteinaemia.

IDIOPATHIC BENCE JONES PROTEINURIA

The possibility of a benign paraproteinaemia of the light-chain type must be considered even though Bence Jones proteinuria is a recognized feature of multiple myeloma, macroglobulinaemia, primary amyloidosis, and occasionally lymphoma. We have described seven patients who at presentation had Bence Jones proteinuria (>1 g/24 h) but no paraprotein in the serum and no evidence of multiple myeloma or related diseases. Multiple myeloma developed in one patient after 20 years and after 8.8 years in another. In a third patient, severe renal insufficiency developed after two episodes of acute renal failure. A fourth patient had a slowly evolving multiple myeloma during a 9 year period but died of an unrelated cause. A fifth patient developed systemic amyloidosis, while a sixth patient died of an extensive squamous cell carcinoma. The seventh patient has continued to excrete 1–1.8 g of $\varkappa$ light chain daily for 12 years without developing evidence of multiple myeloma or related disease. Although idiopathic Bence Jones proteinuria may remain stable for years, multiple myeloma or amyloidosis often develops. Consequently, these patients must be observed indefinitely.[31]

MULTIPLE MYELOMA

Multiple myeloma (myelomatosis or Kahler's disease) is characterized by a neoplastic proliferation of a clone of plasma cells engaged in the production of a paraprotein.

Incidence and diagnosis

Multiple myeloma accounts for about 1% of all types of malignant disease and slightly more than 10% of haematologic malignancies. The annual incidence is approximately 3 per 100,000. The cause of multiple myeloma is unknown, but radiation, exposure to industrial or agricultural toxins or a genetic predisposition may have a role in some cases.

Multiple myeloma has a peak incidence in the seventh decade of life. Only 2% of patients are <40 years of age.[32] Bone pain, particularly in the back or chest, is present in more than two-thirds of patients at diagnosis. The pain is usually aggravated by movement. Weakness and fatigue are common and often are associated with anaemia. Pallor is the most frequent physical finding. The liver is palpable in about 20% of patients and the spleen in 5%.

A normocytic, normochromic anaemia eventually occurs in almost every patient with multiple myeloma. Increased plasma volume from the osmotic effect of a large amount of paraprotein may produce a spurious decrease in haemoglobin and haematocrit values. The serum protein electrophoretic pattern has a peak or localized band in 80% of patients, hypogammaglobulinaemia in almost 10%, and no apparent abnormality in 10%. Almost all patients with hypogammaglobulinaemia have a paraprotein in the urine. Experience indicates that 50% of the paraproteins are IgG, 22% are IgA, 17% are light chain only (Bence Jones proteinaemia), 2% are IgD, and 1% are biclonal; and in 8%, there is no paraprotein. Immunoelectrophoresis or immunofixation of the urine reveals a paraprotein in approximately 80%. Almost all (99%) of patients with multiple myeloma have a paraprotein in the serum or urine at the time of diagnosis. At diagnosis, the serum creatinine level is 176 μmol/litre (≥2 mg/dl) in about one-fourth of patients, while hypercalcaemia is present in 30%. Conventional roentgenograms reveal lytic lesions, osteoporosis or fractures in about 80% of patients. In myeloma, technetium-99m bone scans are inferior to conventional roentgenograms in the detection of lesions. Computed tomography (CT) is helpful for the detection of lytic lesions in patients with myeloma who have skeletal pain but no abnormality on the roentgenograms.[33]

The normal plasma cell is a B-lymphocyte that has undergone differentiation and transformation. It has the capacity to synthesize and secrete immunoglobulin and, in the process of differentiation, loses certain surface markers, such as surface immunoglobulin, Ia antigen and receptors for the Fc portion of IgG, C3b and C3d. The myeloma plasma cell may retain SIg and may possess earlier differentiation markers, such as CALLA or R1-3. Among the peripheral blood T-lymphocytes, OKT4+ helper cells are reduced and OKT8+ suppressor cells are increased in patients with myeloma. Lymphocytes or plasma cells in the peripheral blood share idiotypic characteristics with myeloma cells in the bone marrow. The demonstration of the paraprotein idiotype and the production of the patient's paraprotein by peripheral blood lymphocytes indicate that these cells are part of the malignant clone. Hybridoma technology has been used to raise specific reagents to identify cell-surface differentiation antigens in myeloma. Monoclonal antibodies identifying antigens on human plasma cells have been described.[34,35] Patients with plasmablastic myeloma cells or with a high tumour burden and an elevated plasma cell labelling index are more likely to have increased numbers of circulating cells expressing the plasma cell antigens R1-3 and OKT10.[36]

The criteria for the diagnosis of multiple myeloma include the presence of at least 10% abnormal, immature plasma cells in the bone marrow or histologic proof of an extramedullary plasmacytoma, the usual clinical features of multiple myeloma, and at least one of the following abnormalities: a paraprotein in the serum (usually >3 g/dl), paraprotein in the urine, or osteolytic lesions. Connective tissue diseases, chronic infections, metastatic carcinoma, lymphoma and leukaemia may simulate some of the characteristics of myeloma and should be included in the differential diagnosis.

Treatment

Not all patients who fulfil the minimal criteria for the diagnosis of multiple myeloma should be treated. Patients with smouldering multiple myeloma (SMM) should not be given therapy. The plasma cell LI is helpful in differentiating a patient with benign paraproteinaemia or SMM from one with multiple myeloma. Patients should not be treated unless progression occurs. The most dependable means of differentiating a benign from a malignant plasma cell proliferative process is the serial measurement of the paraprotein. Because multiple myeloma is not curable and therapy entails cost and morbidity, treatment should be delayed until evidence of progression develops, the patients becomes symptomatic or complications become imminent.[37]

Chemotherapy is the preferred initial treatment for overt, symptomatic multiple myeloma. Palliative radiation should be limited to patients who have disabling pain from a well-defined focal process that has not responded to chemotherapy. The major controversy, still not resolved, is whether melphalan and prednisone or a combination of alkylating agents should be used. The oral administration of melphalan (Alkeran) (0.15 mg/kg daily for 7 days) and prednisone (20 mg three times daily for the same 7 days) every 6 weeks is a satisfactory regimen and produces objective response in 50–60% of patients. Leucocyte and platelet counts must be determined at 3 week intervals and the dose of melphalan altered in order to achieve modest cytopenia at mid-cycle because absorption of melphalan is variable. Many combinations of chemotherapeutic agents have been used because of the obvious shortcomings of melphalan and prednisone. The best-known combination, the M-2 Protocol, includes melphalan, cyclophosphamide, carmustine (BCNU), vincristine and prednisone. This regimen produced objective response in almost 80% of patients and a median survival of 38 months.[38] In a randomized trial comparing VBMCP with a combination of melphalan and prednisone, objective response was noted in 72% of patients receiving the combination and in 51% of those receiving melphalan and prednisone. The median survival times of 31 and 30 months, respectively, were not significantly different. There was greater toxicity associated with the combination chemotherapy.[39]

The ideal duration of chemotherapy is unknown. Cessation of treatment after 1–2 years usually results in relapse, and response to resumed therapy may be both of lesser degree and frequency than that after initial chemotherapy. However, chemotherapy may lead to a myelodysplastic syndrome or acute leukaemia. Cuzick et al.[40] reported a 5-year actuarial prevalance of 3% and an 8-year prevalence of myelodysplastic syndrome or acute leukaemia of 10% in patients treated with melphalan or cyclophosphamide (or both). In most patients, abnormal karyotypes usually involving chromosome 5 and 7 have been observed.[41]

Treatment for refractory myeloma

Almost all patients with multiple myeloma who have a response to chemotherapy will eventually suffer a relapse if they do not die of another disease. In addition, approximately one-third of patients treated initially will not experience an objective response with chemotherapy. The highest response rates reported for patients with multiple myeloma that is resistant to alkylating agents have been with vincristine, doxorubicin (Adriamycin) and dexamethasone (VAD). Vincristine and Adriamycin in a 4 day continuous infusion with dexamethasone (40 mg daily) produced a response in 14 (70%) of 20 patients with resistant multiple myeloma.[42] VBAP – a combination of vincristine (2 mg), carmustine (BCNU) (30 mg/m^2), doxorubicin (Adriamycin) (30 mg/m^2) and prednisone (60 mg daily × 5) – has produced some benefit in approximately 40% of patients. Interferon has had considerable notice in both the lay and medical press, but the number of patients with objective benefit has been disappointing.[43]

New considerations for therapy include large intravenous doses of melphalan. Selby *et al.*[44] reported that 11 of 41 (27%) patients with previously untreated myeloma who were ≤63 years of age achieved a complete remission after a single intravenous dose of melphalan (140 mg/m^2). The median duration of the remission was 19 months. Further follow-up is necessary.

Bone marrow transplantation from an identical twin has resulted in long-term survival in one of five patients.[45] Gahrton *et al.*[46] reported that 10 of 14 patients with multiple myeloma who received an allogeneic bone marrow graft from an HLA-compatible sibling survived for a median of 12 months. Five patients had no signs of active myeloma, while four others had minimal persistent disease. Barlogie *et al.*[47] have used melphalan (140 mg/m^2) and total body radiation (850 rad or 8.5 Gy) followed by autologous or allogeneic bone marrow transplantation in six patients with multiple myeloma refractory to chemotherapy. All patients survived for longer than 2–14 months.

Autologous bone marrow transplantation is potentially applicable to far more patients than is allogeneic transplantation because the problems of graft-versus-host disease and graft rejection are circumvented. Two major problems exist. First, multiple myeloma is difficult to eradicate from the bone marrow, even with large doses of chemotherapy and radiation. The second major problem is the difficulty in removing the myeloma cells and their precursors from the autologous bone marrow before reinfusion. A panel of monoclonal antibodies directed against myeloma cells and their precursors or chemotherapy (or both) may be helpful.

The therapeutic use of monoclonal antibodies to plasma cell antigens conjugated to immunotoxins or radionucleotides are of interest, but many hurdles must be overcome.[48]

Course and prognosis

Multiple myeloma runs a progressive course with a median survival of 2–3 years. A clinical staging system based on a combination of laboratory findings that correlates with the myeloma cell mass has been frequently utilized. The median survival was 61 months for patients with stage IA and 14.7 months for those with stage IIIB.[49] Survival is shorter for patients with plasmablastic myeloma than for patients with more mature morphology.[50] The immunofluorescence plasma cell labelling index utilizing a monoclonal antibody (BU-1) to 5-bromo-2-deoxyuridine (BrdUrd) is a useful prognostic tool.[13]

The serum β_2-microglobulin (β_2-M) level is an important prognostic factor in multiple myeloma. Cuzick et al.[51] reported that the β_2-M level, uncorrected for serum creatinine level, was the single most powerful prognostic factor in a study of 476 patients with multiple myeloma. In a study of 100 patients with newly diagnosed multiple myeloma who were followed up for at least 3.5 years, the independent prognostic value of β_2-M as well as of the bone marrow plasma cell labelling index was demonstrated. Patients with a β_2-M value <4 µg/ml and a LI <0.4% had a median survival of 48 months, while patients with a β_2-M value ≥4 µg/ml had a median survival of 12 months.[52] Smith et al.[53] reported that 9 of 10 patients with hypodiploid DNA levels and low RNA content had no response to chemotherapy and had shortened survival. For patients with untreated multiple myeloma, survival is shorter for those with chromosomal abnormalities than for those with normal chromosomes.[54] Response to treatment is a very important factor in prognosis. The prognosis seems to be poorer for patients who show a rapid response to therapy.

VARIANT FORMS OF MYELOMA

Smouldering multiple myeloma

(See page 308.)

Plasma cell leukaemia

Patients with plasma cell leukaemia have >20% plasma cells in the peripheral blood and an absolute plasma cell content of at least 2000/µl. Plasma cell leukaemia may be classified as primary when it is diagnosed in the leukaemic phase or as secondary when there is leukaemic transformation of a previously recognized multiple myeloma. Approximately 60% of patients have the primary form. Patients with primary plasma cell leukaemia are younger, have a greater incidence of hepatosplenomegaly and lymphadenopathy, a higher platelet count, fewer lytic lesions, a smaller serum paraprotein and a longer survival than do patients with secondary plasma cell leukaemia. Treatment of plasma cell leukaemia is unsatisfactory, the median survival being 7–9 months. Patients with secondary plasma cell leukaemia rarely respond, the median survival being approximately 1 month.[55]

Non-secretory myeloma

Patients with non-secretory myeloma have no paraprotein in either the serum or the urine. Experience indicates that about 1% of patients with multiple myeloma have the non-secretory form. For certainty of diagnosis, a paraprotein must be identified in the plasma cells by immunoperoxidase or immunofluorescence. In some cases, no evidence of a paraprotein can be found within the cells, suggesting that no such protein is synthesized. More than a dozen such patients have been described.[56] Treatment for non-secretory myeloma is the same as for multiple myeloma. Survival is longer than in typical myeloma.

IgD myeloma

IgD myeloma differs enough from IgG and IgA myeloma to warrant discussion as a separate entity. More than 130 cases[57] have been reported since the discovery of an IgD immunoglobulin in 1965. Monoclonal λ paraproteins have been reported in 90% of cases, but our experience has shown that only 55% had a monoclonal λ protein. Bence Jones proteinuria is common. Plasma cell leukaemia, amyloidosis and extramedullary plasma-cytomas are more common with IgD myeloma than with other types. Survival is probably less than with other types, although IgD myeloma often is not diagnosed until later in its course. We have seen several patients with IgD myeloma who have survived >5 years.

Osteosclerotic myeloma

The major clinical feature in osteosclerotic myeloma is a chronic inflammatory–demyelinating polyneuropathy with predominantly motor disability. Single or multiple osteosclerotic lesions are characteristic. Takatsuki & Sanada[58] described the diverse features of the syndrome and emphasized its frequency in Japanese males. Bardwick *et al.*[59] suggested the acronym POEMS (polyneuropathy, organomegaly, endocrinopathy, M-proteins, and skin changes). Sensory symptoms consisting of tingling and paraesthesias precede motor involvement. The symptoms begin in the feet and spread proximally. The autonomic nervous system and cranial nerves are not involved, except for papilloedema. Hyperpigmentation and hypertrichosis may be striking. Gynaecomastia and atrophic testes may be seen. The haemoglobin level is usually normal, and thrombocytosis occurs in more than half the patients.[60] Renal insufficiency and hypercalcaemia are rarely found. The bone marrow aspirate usually contains few plasma cells and the serum paraprotein is usually small. Almost all patients have a λ light chain. If the patients have a single or multiple osteosclerotic lesions in a limited area, they should be treated with radiation. More than half the patients will improve. If the patient has widespread osteosclerotic lesions, chemotherapy is necessary.

Solitary plasmacytoma (solitary myeloma) of bone

The diagnosis is based on histologic evidence that the tumour consists of plasma cells identical to those seen in multiple myeloma. In addition, complete skeletal roentgenograms must show no other lesions of myeloma; the bone marrow aspirate must contain no evidence of multiple myeloma; and immunoelectrophoresis or immunofixation of the serum and concentrated urine should show no paraprotein. Some exceptions occur but therapy for the solitary lesion should result in the disappearance of the paraprotein. In a review of 96 published cases of solitary plasmacytoma and 18 personal cases, Bataille & Sany[61] found that at the end of 10 years, the plasmacytoma remained solitary without local recurrence in only 15%. Knowling *et al.*[62] reported that 12 of 25 patients with a solitary plasmacytoma developed multiple myeloma at a median time of 6.5 years and only 4 were free of progression at 10 years. Treatment for solitary plasmacytoma consists of radiation in the range of 4000–5000 rad (40–50 Gy).

Extramedullary plasmacytoma

This plasma cell tumour arises outside the bone marrow. The upper respiratory tract, including the nasal cavity and sinuses, nasopharynx and larynx, is the most frequent location of the lesions.[63] Extramedullary plasmacytoma infrequently develops into overt multiple myeloma, in contrast to solitary plasmacytoma of bone. Meis *et al.*[64] reported that only 3 of 13 patients (23%) with an extramedullary plasmacytoma developed multiple myeloma 8–52 months after the extramedullary plasmacytoma was diagnosed. Solitary extramedullary plasmacytoma may occur in virtually any organ. The diagnosis is made on the basis of a plasma cell tumour in an extramedullary site and the absence of multiple myeloma on the basis of bone marrow, roentgenography, and appropriate studies of blood and urine.

WALDENSTRÖM'S MACROGLOBULINAEMIA

This malignant lymphoplasma cell proliferative disorder produces a large IgM paraprotein. It has a predilection for older men. Weakness, fatigue and oronasal bleeding are common presenting symptoms. Patients may have symptoms of hyperviscosity. Pallor, hepatosplenomegaly and peripheral lymphadenopathy are common.

Almost all patients have normocytic, normochromic anaemia. The bone marrow aspirate is often hypocellular, but fixed sections or biopsy specimens show hypercellularity and extensive infiltration with lymphoid and plasma cells.

The liver is palpable in 25% of patients and the spleen in 20%. Lymphadenopathy is present in 17%. In one study[65] 80% of patients had Bence Jones proteinuria.

A combination of typical symptoms, physical findings, an IgM paraprotein in the serum and lymphoplasma cell proliferation of the bone marrow provides the diagnosis of Waldenström's macroglobulinaemia. The median survival is approximately 5 years and is no different whether the paraprotein is greater than or less than 3 g/dl.

Chlorambucil, in an initial daily dose of 6–8 mg, is an effective agent. The dosage must be reduced, depending on the leucocyte and platelet counts. Cyclophosphamide may also be beneficial.

HEAVY-CHAIN DISEASES (HCD)

Gamma heavy-chain disease (γ-HCD)

This lymphoplasma cell proliferative syndrome produces a monoclonal γ heavy chain in the serum or urine or both. Patients usually present with a lymphoma-like illness, but the clinical findings are diverse and range from an aggressive lymphoproliferative process to an asymptomatic state. Weakness, fatigue and fever are common, but other features including extranodal non-Hodgkin's lymphoma, autoimmune haemolytic anaemia, thrombocytopenic purpura, neutropenia and an atypical lymphoproliferative process have all been noted. Hepatosplenomegaly and lymphadenopathy occur in about 60% of patients. Anaemia is found in about 80%.[66] Treatment is not indicated for the asymptomatic patient. Many different agents have been used, but a trial of cyclophosphamide, vincristine and prednisone is recommended for patients with symptomatic γ-HCD.

Alpha heavy-chain disease (α-HCD)

Most patients with α-HCD are from the Mediterranean region and have involvement of the digestive tract with severe malabsorption, loss of weight, diarrhoea and steatorrhoea.[67] Patients in their second or third decade of life are affected most frequently; 60% are men. The serum protein electrophoretic pattern is normal in half of the cases; in the remainder, an unimpressive broad band may appear in the α_2 or the β regions. Bence Jones proteinuria does not occur. The diagnosis depends on the recognition of a monoclonal α heavy chain not associated with a light chain.

Most often, α-HCD is progressive and fatal, yet remissions using melphalan or cyclophosphamide or prednisone – and, unexpectedly, antibiotics – have been recorded. Spontaneous remission has occurred in a few cases.

Mu heavy-chain disease (μ-HCD)

In this condition, chronic lymphocytic leukaemia or a lymphoma-like pattern is most common. A stable, asymptomatic state also has been noted. The clinical spectrum of μ-HCD should broaden, as it has in γ-HCD. Serum electrophoresis usually reveals hypogammaglobulinaemia; a localized peak or band is uncommon. Bence Jones proteinuria has been found in two-thirds of patients,[68] but μ-chain fragments in the urine are rare. The presence of vacuolated plasma cells in the bone marrow aids in the diagnosis. The demonstration of a monoclonal μ heavy chain in the serum is necessary for diagnosis. Treatment with alkylating agents and corticosteroids has produced benefit.

AMYLOIDOSIS

A workable classification of amyloidosis is provided in Table 9.2. The diagnosis requires the demonstration of amyloid deposits in tissue. Congo red staining of the deposits produces an apple-green birefringence under polarized light and is the most widely accepted stain. In some instances, electron microscopy is necessary for recognizing the typical amyloid fibrils. The unlabelled immunoperoxidase technique utilizing antisera to $\varkappa$, λ, AA

Table 9.2 Classification of Amyloidosis

Amyloid type[a]	Classification	Major protein component
AL	Primary: no evidence of preceding or coexisting disease, except multiple myeloma	Ig-V_L[b]
AA	Secondary: coexistence with other conditions such as rheumatoid arthritis or chronic infections	Protein A
AL	Localized: involvement of a single organ without evidence of generalized involvement (that is, urinary bladder, ureter, urethra, tracheo-bronchial, and so forth)	Ig-V_L
AF	Familial	
	AF$_p$ Portuguese	Prealbumin (transthyretin)
	AF$_j$ Japanese	Prealbumin
	AF$_s$ Swedish	Prealbumin
	Familial amyloidotic cardiomyopathy (Danish)	Prealbumin
	Hereditary cerebral haemorrhage with amyloidosis (HCHWA)	Gamma trace
AA	Familial Mediterranean fever	Protein A
AS$_{c1}$	Senile systemic amyloidosis	Prealbumin
HA	Carpal tunnel syndrome in chronic haemodialysis patients	β$_2$-Microglobulin

[a] AL, amyloid light chains, may be $\varkappa$ or λ; AA, amyloid, protein A.
[b] IgV$_L$, variable portion of light chain.
Modified from Ref. 69.

and pre-albumin would be helpful in classifying the different types of amyloid but satisfactory antisera are not readily available.

PRIMARY AMYLOIDOSIS (AL)

Clinical findings

The possibility of primary amyloidosis (AL) must be considered in any patient who has a paraprotein in serum or urine and refractory congestive heart failure, nephrotic syndrome, sensorimotor peripheral neuropathy, carpal tunnel syndrome, orthostatic hypotension or steatorrhoea. Primary amyloidosis is found more often in men (65%) than women. The median age at diagnosis is 65 years, and 99% are 40 years old or older.[69]

Weakness and fatigue are the most frequent symptoms. Loss of weight may be striking, and many patients lose more than 20 kg. Dyspnoea, pedal oedema, paraesthesias, light-headedness, syncope, purpura, claudication and changes in the voice may occur. Hepatomegaly is found in one-third of patients, but splenomegaly occurs in <5%. Macroglossia is present in one-fifth of patients. Purpura is common and often involves the neck and face, particularly the upper eyelids. Ankle oedema usually results from congestive heart failure or the nephrotic syndrome.

At diagnosis, one-third of patients have a nephrotic syndrome, one-fourth have a carpal tunnel syndrome, one-fourth have congestive heart failure and about 15% each have peripheral neuropathy or orthostatic hypotension.

Laboratory findings

Anaemia is uncommon and when present is usually due to renal insufficiency, multiple myeloma or gastrointestinal bleeding. Thrombocytosis is present in 5–10% of patients. Results of liver function tests are frequently normal, even in the presence of hepatomegaly. The serum protein electrophoretic pattern shows a localized band or spike in only 40% of cases, while hypogammaglobulinaemia is seen in approximately one-fourth. Immunoelectrophoresis or immunofixation (or both) reveals a paraprotein in two-thirds of cases. Bence Jones proteinuria is found in 65% of cases. Light chains of the λ type (65%) are more common than ϰ. The serum or urine of approximately 85% of patients with primary amyloidosis contains a paraprotein. Modest plasmacytosis of the bone marrow is common.

Cardiac and circulatory involvement

Congestive heart failure occurs in more than one-third of patients with primary amyloidosis. Amyloid may infiltrate the conduction system and produce the sick sinus syndrome or an atrioventricular block. Constrictive pericarditis may be difficult to differentiate from the restrictive cardio-myopathy of cardiac amyloidosis. The electrocardiogram frequently has a pattern indicative of an anteroseptal myocardial infarction. Echocardiography is very helpful in recognizing cardiac involvement and for estimating survival.[70]

Other organ involvement

Proteinuria is present initially in more than 80% of patients, while renal insufficiency is found in more than half. The kidneys are usually normal in size. Gross haematuria is rare. Although microscopic evidence of respiratory tract involvement is common, primary amyloidosis rarely produces pulmonary symptoms.[71] Pseudo-obstruction or diarrhoea may result from extensive infiltration by amyloid or, more frequently, from involvement of the autonomic nervous system. Peripheral neuropathy occurs in about 15% of patients. Dysaesthetic numbness is distal, symmetric and progressive. The lower extremities are more frequently involved than the upper. Petechiae, ecchymoses, papules, plaques, nodules, tumours, bullous lesions, alopecia and thickening of the skin may occur from amyloidosis. Bleeding may be a major manifestation. In addition to the well-known deficiency of factor X, decreased vitamin K-dependent clotting factors, increased antithrombin activity, increased fibrinolysis and intravascular coagulation may all contribute to bleeding.

Diagnosis

The diagnosis depends on the demonstration of amyloid in tissues. Biopsy of subcutaneous abdominal fat is positive in approximately 80% of cases, but both false-positive and false-negative results can occur.[72] Aspiration and biopsy specimens of the bone marrow are positive for amyloid in only 30% of patients but provide an estimate of the degree of plasmacytosis and should be taken. If the bone marrow and subcutaneous fat contain no amyloid, rectal biopsy, which is positive in 70% of patients, should be done. The biopsy specimen must contain submucosa. If these tissues do not contain amyloid, then biopsy specimens should be taken of the kidney, liver, carpal tunnel tissue, small intestine, sural nerve or endomyocardium, depending on the organ involved.

Prognosis

The median survival of patients with primary amyloidosis is 2 years. The median survival ranges from 5 months for patients presenting with congestive heart failure to more than 4 years for those presenting with peripheral neuropathy. The presence of congestive heart failure, paraprotein in the urine, hepatomegaly, and multiple myeloma are major factors adversely affecting survival during the first year after diagnosis. Elevated serum creatinine level and the presence of multiple myeloma, orthostatic hypotension and serum paraprotein are the most important variables adversely affecting survival for patients surviving after 1 year.[73]

Therapy

The treatment of primary amyloidosis is not satisfactory. In a prospective randomized study, the median survival was 25 months for patients receiving melphalan and prednisone and 18 months for those receiving colchicine. The difference was not statistically significant. When the survival of patients who received only one regimen was analysed or when survival was analysed from study entry until death or progression of disease, a significant survival difference favouring melphalan and prednisone was evident. This study suggests that melphalan–prednisone is superior to colchicine in the treatment of primary amyloidosis.[74]

Secondary, localized and familial amyloidoses have no paraprotein and are not included in this discussion.

ACKNOWLEDGEMENT

Supported in part by Research Grants CA-16835 and CA-15083 from the National Institutes of Health, Public Health Service.

REFERENCES

1. Howerton, D.A., Check, I.J. & Hunter, R.L. Densitometric quantitation of high resolution agarose gel protein electrophoresis. *Am. J. Clin. Pathol.* **85**: 213–18, 1986.
2. Roberts, R.T. Usefulness of immunofixation electrophoresis in the clinical laboratory. *Clin. Lab. Med.* **6**: 601–5, 1986.
3. Axelsson, U., Bachmann, R. & Hällén, J. Frequency of pathological proteins (M-components) in 6,995 sera from an adult population. *Acta Med. Scand.* **179**: 235–47, 1966.
4. Kyle, R.A., Finkelstein, S., Elveback, L.R. *et al.* Incidence of monoclonal proteins in a Minnesota community with a cluster of multiple myeloma. *Blood* **40**: 719–24, 1972.
5. Saleun, J.P., Vicariot, M., Deroff, P. *et al.* Monoclonal gammopathies in the adult population of Finistère, France. *J. Clin. Pathol.* **35**: 63–8, 1982.
6. Papadopoulos, N.M., Elin, R.J. & Wilson, D.M. Incidence of γ-globulin banding in a healthy population by high-resolution electrophoresis. *Clin. Chem.* **28**: 707–8, 1982.
7. Sinclair, D., Sheehan, T., Parrott, D.M.V. *et al.* The incidence of monoclonal gammopathy in a population over 45 years old determined by isoelectric focusing. *Br. J. Haematol.* **64**: 745–50, 1986.

8. Kyle, R.A. 'Benign' monoclonal gammopathy. A misnomer? *J. Am. Med. Assoc.* **251**: 1849–54, 1984.
9. Kyle, R.A. & Greipp, P.R. Smoldering multiple myeloma. *N. Engl. J. Med.* **302**: 1347–9, 1980.
10. Møller-Petersen, J. & Schmidt, E.B. Diagnostic value of the concentration of M-component in initial classification of monoclonal gammopathy. *Scand. J. Haematol.* **36**: 295–301, 1986.
11. Greipp, P.R. & Kyle, R.A. Clinical, morphological, and cell kinetic differences among multiple myeloma, monoclonal gammopathy of undetermined significance, and smoldering multiple myeloma. *Blood* **62**: 166–71, 1983.
12. Gonchoroff, N.J., Greipp, P.R., Kyle, R.A. *et al.* A monoclonal antibody reactive with 5-bromo-2-deoxyuridine that does not require DNA denaturation. *Cytometry* **6**: 506–12, 1985.
13. Greipp, P.R., Witzig, T.E., Gonchoroff, N.J. *et al.* Immunofluorescence labeling indices in myeloma and related monoclonal gammopathies. *Mayo Clin. Proc.* **62**: 969–77, 1987.
14. Mundis, R.J., Kyle, R.A. Primary hyperparathyroidism and monoclonal gammopathy of undetermined significance. *Am. J. Clin. Pathol.* **77**: 619–21, 1982.
15. Alexanian, R. Monoclonal gammopathy in lymphoma. *Arch. Intern. Med.* **135**: 62–6, 1975.
16. Noel, P. & Kyle, R.A. Monoclonal proteins in chronic lymphocytic leukemia. *Am. J. Clin. Pathol.* **87**: 385–8, 1987.
17. Kelly, J.J. Jr, Kyle, R.A., O'Brien, P.C. *et al.* Prevalence of monoclonal protein in peripheral neuropathy. *Neurology* **31**: 1480–3, 1981.
18. Kelly, J.J. Jr, Kyle, R.A. & Latov, N. *Polyneuropathies Associated with Plasma Cell Dyscrasias.* Martinus Nijhoff, Boston, 1987.
19. Latov, N., Sherman, W.H., Nemni, R. *et al.* Plasma-cell dyscrasia and peripheral neuropathy with a monoclonal antibody to peripheral-nerve myelin. *N. Engl. J. Med.* **303**: 618–21, 1980.
20. Hafler, D.A., Johnson, D., Kelly, J.J. *et al.* Monoclonal gammopathy and neuropathy: Myelin-associated glycoprotein reactivity and clinical characteristics. *Neurology* **36**: 75–8, 1986.
21. Shy, M.E., Rowland, L.P., Smith, T. *et al.* Motor neuron disease and plasma cell dyscrasia. *Neurology* **36**: 1429–36, 1986.
22. James, K., Fudenberg, H., Epstein, W.L. *et al.* Studies on a unique diagnostic serum globulin in papular mucinosis (lichen myxedematosus). *Clin. Exp. Immunol.* **2**: 153–66, 1967.
23. Powell, F.C., Schroeter, A.L., Su, W.P.D. *et al.* Pyoderma gangrenosum and monoclonal gammopathy. *Arch. Dermatol.* **119**: 468–72, 1983.
24. Finan, M.C. & Winkelmann, R.K. Necrobiotic xanthogranuloma with paraproteinemia. A review of 22 cases. *Medicine (Baltimore)* **65**: 376–88, 1986.
25. Gelfand, J.A., Boss, G.R., Conley C.L. *et al.* Acquired C1 esterase inhibitor deficiency and angioedema: A review. *Medicine (Baltimore)* **58**: 321–8, 1979.
26. Löfdahl, C.-G., Sölvell, L., Laurell, A.-B. *et al.* Systemic capillary leak syndrome with monoclonal IgG and complement alterations. A case report on an episodic syndrome. *Acta Med. Scand.* **206**: 405–12, 1979.
27. Merlini, G., Farhangi, M., Osserman, E.F. Monoclonal immunoglobulins with antibody activity in myeloma, macroglobulinemia and related plasma cell dyscrasias. *Semin. Oncol.* **13**: 350–65, 1986.
28. Annesley, T.M., Burritt, M.F. & Kyle, R.A. Artifactual hypercalcemia in multiple myeloma. *Mayo Clin. Proc.* **57**: 572–5, 1982.
29. Kyle, R.A., Robinson, R.A. & Katzmann, J.A. The clinical aspects biclonal gammopathies. Review of 57 cases. *Am. J. Med.* **71**: 999–1008, 1981.
30. Riddell, S., Traczyk, Z., Paraskevas, F. *et al.* The double gammopathies. Clinical

and immunological studies. *Medicine (Baltimore)* **65**: 135–42, 1986.
31. Kyle, R.A. & Greipp, P.R. 'Idiopathic' Bence Jones proteinuria: Long-term follow-up in seven patients. *N. Engl. J. Med.* **306**: 564–67, 1982.
32. Kyle, R.A. Multiple myeloma: Review of 869 cases. *Mayo Clin. Proc.* **50**: 29–40, 1975.
33. Kyle, R.A., Schreiman, J.S., McLeod, R.A. *et al.* Computed tomography in diagnosis and management of multiple myeloma and its variants. *Arch. Intern. Med.* **145**: 1451–2, 1985.
34. Anderson, K.C., Park, E.K., Bales, M.P. *et al.* Antigens on human plasma cells identified by monoclonal antibodies. *J. Immunol.* **130**: 1132–8, 1983.
35. Gonchoroff, N.J., Katzmann, J.A., Garton, J.P. *et al.* A monoclonal antibody reactive with a subset of human plasma cells. *Br. J. Haematol.* **62**: 619–30, 1986.
36. Ruiz-Argüelles, G.J., Katzmann, J.A., Greipp, P.R. *et al.* Multiple myeloma: Circulating lymphocytes that express plasma cell antigens. *Blood* **64**: 352–6, 1984.
37. Kyle, R.A. Is there a correct time to begin treatment of multiple myeloma? (Editorial) *Haematologica* **72**: 107–110, 1987.
38. Lee, B.J., Lake-Lewin, D. & Myers, J.E. Intensive treatment of multiple myeloma. In *Controversies in Oncology* (ed. P.H. Wiernik), pp. 61–79. John Wiley & Sons, New York, 1982.
39. Oken, M.M., Tsiatis, A., Abramson, N. *et al.* Evaluation of intensive (VBMCP) vs. standard (MP) therapy for multiple myeloma. (Abstract). *Proc. Am. Soc. Clin. Oncol.* **6**: 203, 1987.
40. Cuzick, J., Erskine, S., Edelman, D. *et al.* A comparison of the incidence of the myelodysplastic syndrome and acute myeloid leukaemia following melphalan and cyclophosphamide treatment for myelomatosis. A report to the Medical Research Council's working party on leukaemia in adults. *Br. J. Cancer* **55**: 523–9, 1987.
41. Pedersen-Bjergaard, J. & Philip, P. Cytogenetic characteristics of therapy-related acute nonlymphocytic leukaemia, preleukaemia and acute myeloproliferative syndrome: Correlation with clinical data for 61 consecutive cases. *Br. J. Haematol.* **66**: 199–207, 1987.
42. Barlogie, B., Smith, L. & Alexanian, R. Effective treatment of advanced multiple myeloma refractory to alkylating agents. *N. Engl. J. Med.* **310**: 1353–6, 1984.
43. Costanzi, J.J. & Pollard, R.B. The use of interferon in the treatment of multiple myeloma. *Semin. Oncol.* **14** (Suppl. 2): 24–8, 1987.
44. Selby, P.J., McElwain, T.J., Nandi, A.C. *et al.* Multiple myeloma treated with high dose intravenous melphalan. *Br. J. Haematol.* **66**: 55–62, 1987.
45. Fefer, A., Cheever, M.A. & Greenberg, P.D. Identical-twin (syngeneic) marrow transplantation for hematologic cancers. *J. Natl. Cancer Inst.* **76**: 1269–73, 1986.
46. Gahrton, G., Tura, S., Flesch, M. *et al.* Bone marrow transplantation in multiple myeloma: Report from the European Cooperative Group for bone marrow transplantation. *Blood* **69**: 1262–4, 1987.
47. Barlogie, B., Alexanian, R., Dicke, K.A. *et al.* High dose melphalan (HDM) and total body irradiation (TBI) for refractory multiple myeloma. (Abstract). *Proc. Am. Soc. Clin. Oncol.* **6**: 192, 1987.
48. Embleton, M.J. Drug-targeting by monoclonal antibodies. *Br. J. Cancer* **55**: 227–31, 1987.
49. Durie, B.G.M., Salmon, S.E. & Moon, T.E. Pretreatment tumor mass, cell kinetics, and prognosis in multiple myeloma. *Blood* **55**: 364–72, 1980.
50. Bartl, R., Frisch, B., Fateh-Moghadam, A. *et al.* Histologic classification and staging of multiple myeloma. A retrospective and prospective study of 674 cases. *Am. J. Clin. Pathol.* **87**: 342–55, 1987.
51. Cuzick, J., Cooper, E.H. & MacLennan, I.C.M. The prognostic value of serum β2 microglobulin compared with other presentation features in myelomatosis. *Br. J.*

Cancer **52**: 1–6, 1985.
52. Greipp, P.R., Katzmann, J.A., O'Fallon, W.M. *et al.* Value of β2-microglobulin level and plasma cell labeling indices as prognostic factors in patients with newly diagnosed myeloma. *Blood* **72**: 219–23, 1988.
53. Smith, L., Barlogie, B. & Alexanian, R. Biclonal and hypodiploid multiple myeloma. *Am. J. Med.* **80**: 841–3, 1986.
54. Dewald, G.W., Kyle, R.A., Hicks, G.A. *et al.* The clinical significance of cytogenetic studies in 100 patients with multiple myeloma, plasma cell leukemia, or amyloidosis. *Blood* **66**: 380–90, 1985.
55. Noel, P. & Kyle, R.A. Plasma cell leukemia: An evaluation of response to therapy. *Am. J. Med.* **83**: 1062–8, 1987.
56. Franchi, F., Seminara, P., Teodori, L. *et al.* The non-producer plasma cell myeloma. Report of a case and review of the literature. *Blut* **52**: 281–7, 1986.
57. Jancelewicz, Z., Takatsuki, K., Sugai, S. *et al.* IgD multiple myeloma. Review of 133 cases. *Arch. Intern. Med.* **135**: 87–93, 1975.
58. Takatsuki, K. & Sanada, I. Plasma cell dyscrasia with polyneuropathy and endocrine disorder: Clinical and laboratory features of 109 reported cases. *Jpn. J. Clin. Oncol.* **13**: 543–55, 1983.
59. Bardwick, P.A., Zvaifler, N.J., Gill, G.N. *et al.* Plasma cell dyscrasia with polyneuropathy, organomegaly, endocrinopathy, M protein, and skin changes: The POEMS syndrome. Report on two cases and a review of the literature. *Medicine (Baltimore)* **59**: 311–22, 1980.
60. Kelly, J.J. Jr, Kyle, R.A., Miles, J.M. *et al.* Osteosclerotic myeloma and peripheral neuropathy. *Neurology* **33**: 202–10, 1983.
61. Bataille, R. & Sany, J. Solitary myeloma: Clinical and prognostic features of a review of 114 cases. *Cancer* **48**: 845–51, 1981.
62. Knowling, M.A., Harwood, A.R. & Bergsagel, D.E. Comparison of extramedullary plasmacytomas with solitary and multiple plasma cell tumors of bone. *J. Clin. Oncol.* **1**: 255–62, 1983.
63. Wiltshaw, E. The natural history of extramedullary plasmacytoma and its relation to solitary myeloma of bone and myelomatosis. *Medicine (Baltimore)* **55**: 217–38, 1976.
64. Meis, J.M., Butler, J.J., Osborne, B.M. *et al.* Solitary plasmacytomas of bone and extramedullary plasmacytomas. A clinicopathologic and immunohistochemical study. *Cancer* **59**: 1475–85, 1987.
65. Kyle, R.A. & Garton, J.P. The spectrum of IgM monoclonal gammopathy in 430 cases. *Mayo Clin. Proc.* **62**: 719–31, 1987.
66. Kyle, R.A., Greipp, P.R. & Banks, P.M. The diverse picture of gamma heavy-chain disease: Report of seven cases and review of the literature. *Mayo Clin. Proc.* **56**: 439–51, 1981.
67. Haghighi, P., Kharazmi, A., Gerami, C. *et al.* Primary upper small-intestinal lymphoma and alpha-chain disease. Report of 10 cases emphasizing pathological aspects. *Am. J. Surg. Pathol.* **2**: 147–57, 1978.
68. Brouet, J.-C., Seligmann, M., Danon,F. *et al.* μ-Chain disease. Report of two new cases. *Arch. Intern. Med.* **139**: 672–4, 1979.
69. Kyle, R.A. & Greipp, P.R. Amyloidosis (AL). Clinical and laboratory features of 229 cases. *Mayo Clin. Proc.* **58**: 665–93, 1983.
70. Cueto-Garcia, L., Reeder, G.S., Kyle, R.A. *et al.* Echocardiographic findings in systemic amyloidosis: Spectrum of cardiac involvement and relation to survival. *J. Am. Coll. Cardiol.* **6**: 737–43, 1985.
71. Grégoire, J.M., Close, P., Dourov, N. *et al.* Pulmonary alveoloseptal amyloidosis. *Acta Clin. Belg.* **41**: 388–94, 1986.
72. Gertz, M.A., Li, C.-Y., Shirahama, T. *et al.* Utility of subcutaneous fat aspiration for the diagnosis of systemic amyloidosis (immunoglobulin light chain). *Arch. Intern. Med.* **148**: 929–33, 1988.

73. Kyle, R.A., Greipp, P.R. & O'Fallon, W.M. Primary systemic amyloidosis: multivariate analysis for prognostic factors in 168 cases. *Blood* **68**: 220–4, 1986.
74. Kyle, R.A., Greipp, P.R., Garton, J.P. *et al.* Primary systemic amyloidosis. Comparison of melphalon/prednisone versus colchicine. *Am. J. Med.* **79**: 708–16, 1985.
75. Kyle, R.A. & Greipp, P.R. The laboratory investigation of monoclonal gammopathies. *Mayo Clin. Proc.* **53**: 719–39, 1978.
76. Kyle, R.A. Classification and diagnosis of monoclonal gammopathies. In *Manual of Clinical Laboratory Immunology*, 3rd Edn (eds N.R. Rose, H. Friedman & J.L. Fahey), pp. 152–67. American Society for Microbiology, Washington, D.C., 1986.

10

Drug-induced cytopenias

E.C. Gordon-Smith
Professor of Haematology, St George's Hospital, London, UK

Drugs may cause a reduction in circulating blood cells either as a direct consequence of their therapeutic action or as an idiosyncratic reaction seen only in a proportion of people exposed to the drug. The former group consist mainly of the cytotoxic agents used in chemotherapy for malignant disease and their effects on the blood will not be considered in this chapter. Within the latter group, two main sub-groups may be considered: (1) those drugs where cytopenias are dose-related and inevitable in all people exposed to them, but some people, for individual reasons of genetics or environment, will develop cytopenias at a much lower dose than the majority; and (2) those drugs where the cytopenia is unpredictable and truly idiosyncratic. The dose-dependent cytopenias are mainly the consequences of interference in metabolic processes, the idiosyncratic reactions are immune or unknown. In both instances it may be the prescribed drug which produces the cytopenia or one or more of its metabolites. The major mechanisms of drug-induced cytopenias are outlined in Table 10.1.

Drug-induced cytopenias caused by interference in metabolic pathways are more common than the immune cytopenias and will be considered first, but mostly the effects are less serious than the truly idiosyncratic cytopenias which may produce devastating results. In part this distinction arises because the drugs which affect metabolic pathways mostly produce

Table 10.1 Mechanisms of Drug-induced Cytopenias

Mechanism	Pathway	Most common cytopenias
1. Metabolic	Oxidative stress	Haemolytic anaemia Methaemoglobinaemia
	Interference with DNA replication	Megaloblastic anaemia Pancytopenias
	Mitochondrial damage	Reticulocytopenia Sideroblastic change
2. Immune	Immune complex formation Drug-related allo-antibodies Autoimmune	Acute cytopenia Subacute cytopenia Variable; usually haemolytic anaemia
3. Unknown	Unknown	Aplastic anaemia

anaemias, which are readily correctable, whereas the immune processes are as likely to affect granulocytes or platelets. Also the onset of cytopenia is relatively slow in the former group, with the exception of some cases of oxidative haemolysis.

CYTOPENIAS INDUCED BY INTERFERENCE WITH METABOLIC PATHWAYS

The major causes of haematological disorders produced by drugs acting chemically are oxidative haemolytic anaemia and megaloblastic anaemia. Drugs which interfere with mitochrondrial metabolism mostly produce interesting changes in the marrow without causing significant anaemia.

Oxidative haemolytic anaemia

Oxidative substances produce a number of changes in red blood cells, the observed effects depending upon the strength of the oxidative potential, the competence of the reducing system of the red cells and the site at which most of the oxidative stress is delivered. Oxidative drugs may attack the red cell membrane, the haemoglobin or interfere with the reduction of methaemoglobin. The haematological syndromes produced depend upon the interplay between these effects. The main syndromes are (1) acute intravascular haemolysis, usually without renal failure; (2) chronic intra-vascular haemolysis with Heinz body formation; (3) methaemoglobinaemia with or without some degree of intravascular haemolysis.

Reducing mechanisms of the red cell

It is not the intention to review here in detail the metabolism of the red cell. Many good reviews are to be found in standard textbooks or special issues.[1,2] The relationship between the inherited characteristics of the various reducing pathways, drug metabolic pathways and exposure to oxidative substances provides a good example of the importance of genetic factors in the response to disease producing agents. Susceptibility to oxidative stress may be increased in a number of ways in any individual. The important pathways in the provision of reducing power for the red cell are the pentose phosphate pathway which produces reduced nicotinamide adenine dinucleotide phosphate (NADPH), the glutathione cycle which links the NADPH produced to the production of reduced glutathione (GSH), the major reducing substance for the red cell membrane, and the methaemoglobin reducing pathways, particularly through the activity of NADH-methaemoglobin reductase.

The pentose phosphate pathway (hexose monophosphate shunt)

In the normal red cell about 10% of glucose metabolized is cycled through the pentose phosphate pathway. In this system glucose-6-phosphate, produced from glucose by the action of hexokinase, is oxidized to 6-phosphogluconate a reaction catalysed by glucose-6-phosphate dehydrogenase (G6PD). The oxidation is provided by NADP which is converted to NADPH. The second step is a second oxidation and decarboxylation to ribose-5-phosphate catalysed by 6-phosphogluconate dehydrogenase, again with the production of one molecule of NADPH for each molecule of 6-phosphogluconate passed along the pathway. The rate-limiting mechanism for this pathway in normal red blood cells is the supply of NADP which is dependent on the rate of oxidation of NADPH through the glutathione cycle. In the presence of increased oxidative stress the proportion of glucose metabolized by this pathway, and hence the reducing capacity of the red cell, is increased, leading in effect to a reserve of reducing power.

Glucose-6-phosphate dehydrogenase deficiency

Inherited deficiency of G6PD is amongst the most common genetic disorders worldwide.[3-5] The gene which codes for G6PD is located on the X-chromosome so the disorder is sex-linked. Female heterozygotes are protected from falciparum malaria to some extent, which would explain the presence of a balanced polymorphism of G6PD-deficient genes and normal genes in many parts of the world and the presence of many (over 100) variants of the gene with deficient enzyme activity. The survival of red blood cells in most individuals with G6PD deficiency is normal under unstressed conditions, though there are rare variants with particularly low activity who have a congenital non-spherocytic haemolytic anaemia.[5] In the presence of increased oxidative stress, however, acute intravascular haemolysis will occur. Which substances produce haemolysis in any individual depends upon the type of enzyme inherited and its residual activity. The two main types of variant are those with severe deficiency (less then 1%), which causes favism, and those variants which have some residual activity (up to 10% of normal) where haemolysis only occurs when oxidative drugs are ingested. Favism, which is classically found in the Mediterranean variant, is defined clinically by the tendency of those patients to experience haemolysis if they eat broad beans (fava beans). They will also haemolyse if exposed to the oxidative drugs which cause haemolysis in the other, less severe, variants, for example, the A− variant found in Africa.

In susceptible individuals oxidative stress produces acute intravascular haemolysis with haemoglobinaemia, haemoglobinuria and a rapid fall in haemoglobin. In the Mediterranean-type deficiency there may be systemic symptoms with fever and abdominal pain, though renal failure is rare unless there are additional factors such as hypotension or dehydration associated with the oxidative stress.

Mostly the acute haemolytic episodes associated with G6PD deficiency bring the patient to the attention of the haematologist but the general physician may be perplexed by the knowledge that a patient has G6PD deficiency (or is likely to have) and has to make a decision about which drugs may be used to manage a serious condition. Most confusion arises in the treatment or prophylaxis of malaria but worries may also arise when faced with other serious diseases. Lists of drugs which may cause haemolysis in these patients tend to be long, all-embracing and unhelpful.

Clearly a patient with falciparum malaria has to be treated even if there is a risk of haemolysis, the haemolysis anticipated and its potential nephrotoxicity minimized by giving a high fluid intake. Even so it is possible to choose regimens which are less likely to produce significant haemolysis than others. In general the 8-aminoquinolines are more oxidative than the 4-aminoquinolines. The former include primaquine and pamaquine, used for the treatment of *P. vivax* infections. Choroquine, amodiaquine and hydroxychloroquine are 4-aminoquinolines. They do not produce haemolysis in black patients who have A− deficiency and do not normally produce significant haemolyis in patients with favism when administered at the usual prophylactic doses. Some degree of haemolysis may occur in Mediterranean G6PD deficiency if there is infection present at the same time, which increases the oxidative load through the release of hydrogen peroxide and free oxygen radicals from macrophages and neutrophils.

Primaquine in standard doses of 15 mg per day for 14 days combined with 1.5 g of chloroquine base for 3 days for cure of *P. vivax* will not produce significant haemolysis in black patients but will cause haemolysis in Mediterranean G6PD deficiency. At 20 mg per day or higher primaquine will induce haemolysis in the A− variant but it will be self-limiting as the reticulocyte count rises with a higher content of G6PD enzyme.[6] At higher doses, 60 mg per day or more, primaquine will produce methaemoglobinaemia even in subjects with normal G6PD activity. If it is necessary to use potentially haemolytic drugs in G6PD-deficient patients, careful monitoring of the blood and urine for evidence of intravascular haemolysis is required. High fluid intake to maintain a good urine flow is important.

Other antimalarials, pyrimethamine and proguanil, are not oxidative, though pyrimethamine may produce megaloblastic anaemia (see below). Dapsone, a powerful oxidative drug, has been combined with pyrimethamine as Malaporim for chemoprophylaxis of malaria in areas where chloroquine resistance is common. Dapsone will cause haemolysis in G6PD-deficient subjects and Heinz body haemolytic anaemia in normal individuals if taken in sufficient doses.[6] It should be avoided in G6PD-deficient subjects.

Some confusion also exists about whether it is safe to use chloramphenicol in G6PD-deficient subjects. The propensity of chloramphenicol to cause aplastic anaemia is discussed later but it may be stated that, alone, chloramphenicol does not produce significant haemolysis in G6PD-deficient patients who do not have a severe infection. However, chloramphenicol is usually given to patients who do have bacterial infections and the combined oxidative stress of the infections and the drug may be enough to produce haemolysis.[7]

Drugs which will produce oxidative haemolysis in different groups are listed in Table 10.2. It should be remembered that any drug which causes oxidative haemolysis in all G6PD-deficient patients will produce the haemolysis at lower doses in the severely affected individuals. More detailed accounts of the dose dependency of haemolysis have been published.[6,8]

The glutathione cycle

Reduced glutathione (GSH) is the main proton donor in the red cell to counteract oxidative stress to the red cell membrane and to reduce

Table 10.2 Drugs which Cause Oxidative Haemolysis at Therapeutic Doses

Indications	Drugs[a]		
	All patients	All G6PD-deficient patients	Severe G6PD deficiency
Antimalarials	Dapsone	Primaquine Pamaquine	Chloroquine[b]
Antibiotics	Salazopyrine	Sulphapyridine Sulphamethoxypyridazine Nalidixic acid Nitrofurantoin	Chloramphenicol[b]
Analgesics/ antipyretics		Phenacetin	Antipyrine (phenazone)
Cytotoxic drugs		Adriamycin BCNU	
Miscellaneous		Nitidazole Nitrofurazone Phenazopyridine Diazoxide Dimercaprol Menadiol (vit K analogue)	

[a] All drugs listed cause haemolysis in severe G6PD deficiency.
[b] Cause haemolysis in infected patients only.

inappropriate disulphide bonding. NADPH is linked to the pentose phosphate pathway via glutathione reductase which catalyses the reduction of oxidized glutathione (GSSG) to GSH. Glutathione peroxidase is the enzyme that catalyses the reduction of hydrogen peroxide with the formation of GSSG from GSH. Deficiency of glutathione reductase[9] and glutathione peroxidase[10] have been reported in association with drug-induced haemolytic anaemia but they are very rare. However, in neonates, particularly premature babies, the activity of these enzymes is reduced, which accounts for the increased sensitivity of infants to oxidative drugs.[6,11]

NADH-methaemoglobin reductase

There are two NADH-methaemoglobin reductase enzymes, type I which accounts for 90% of methaemoglobin reduction and type II. Deficiency of type I leads to methaemoglobinaemia. As with other enzyme deficiencies there are several genetic variants which lead to deficient activity in the gene product.[12] Deficiency leading to congenital methaemoglobinaemia is rare but there may be variants in the normal population which have reduced activity and lead to methaemoglobinaemia manifest as cyanosis in response to oxidative stress. The use of Maloprim (pyrimethamine and dapsone) as malarial prophylaxis leads to significant methaemoglobinaemia in some people who have normal G6PD activity but reduced NADH-methaemoglobin activity. Neonates have transiently reduced levels of NADH-methaemoglobin reductase leading to increased susceptibility to oxidizing compounds such as nitrates which cause cyanosis.

Drugs which cause oxidative haemolytic anaemia in normal subjects

Dapsone[13] and sulphasalazine (salazopyrin)[14] are two drugs which may cause chronic intravascular haemolysis with some degree of methaemoglobinaemia and Heinz body formation in normal subjects when given at acceptable doses. There is some individual variation even amongst patients with normal reducing systems depending upon the efficiency of the acetylation process of drug detoxification on the liver.[15] Slow acetylators are more likely to develop significant haemolysis than fast ones.

Dapsone given at a dose of 300 mg per day will produce a shortening of the red cell survival in all patients. If the anaemia becomes significant the dose should be reduced but the intravascular haemolysis alone is not a reason for stopping the drug if it is indicated. Dapsone is used in the treatment of dermatitis herpetiformis which may be associated with functional hyposplenism. In this case Heinz bodies may be seen in the peripheral blood.

Salzopyrin is used mainly in the treatment of ulcerative colitis. It is metabolized in the gastrointestinal tract to sulphapyridine which is absorbed and aminosalicylate which appears in the stool. The sulphapyridine is the oxidative compound.[14] Some shortening of the red cell survival is seen in most patients taking 8 g or more per day. A more serious toxicity is aplastic anaemia or agranulocytosis (see below).

Drugs which affect DNA biosynthesis

Drugs which interfere with DNA biosynthesis, either directly or indirectly will produce megaloblastic change and may lead to megaloblastic anaemia.[16] In some instances the interference may be so marked that neutropenia and thrombocytopenia occur. In most cases the drugs concerned are used because of their action on DNA synthesis, they are cytotoxic agents and so will not be considered in detail here. Scott & Weir[16] divided the ways in which drugs interfere with DNA synthesis into six groups (Table 10.3). As will be seen from the table, in the majority of cases megaloblastic change is rare if the drug is given on its own but clinically significant anaemia may arise if combinations of drugs having megaloblastic potential are given at the same time or if the patient is potentially folate deficient. Certain drugs or combinations require special mention.

Pyrimethamine and trimethoprim

These two drugs are 2,3-diaminopyrimidines in wide use worldwide, pyrimethamine as an antimalarial agent, particularly where chloroquine resistance is common, trimethoprim as an antibiotic. Each drug may be combined with a sulphonamide which enhances their activity but also increases the toxicity. The rationale of adding the sulphonamide is that the two compounds inhibit sequential steps in the microbial utilization of folate. The sulphonamide inhibits the formation of folate from para-aminobenzoic acid in microbes, which cannot accumulate preformed folate; the 2,4-aminopyrimidine inhibits dihydrofolate (DHF) reductase, the microbial DHF reductase at much lower concentrations than eukaryotic. For example, 50% inhibition of mammalian DHF reductase occurs at concentrations of trimethoprim about 60 μM, whereas bacterial DHF reductase is inhibited at 5 nM.[17] The addition of the sulphonamide does not increase the tendency to cause megaloblastic anaemia but does lead to an increase in idiosyncratic cytopenias, particularly agranulocytosis and aplastic anaemia (see later sections).

Pyrimethamine, used as malarial prophylaxis, is usually given as 25 mg once a week, perhaps with an initial dose of 50 mg. At this dose schedule megaloblastic anaemia is rare but the prophylaxis may be continued for a long time and other events may overtake the subject, sometimes requiring the use of other drugs which interfere with folate metabolism, including trimethoprim (often in combination with sulphamethoxazole (Septrin, Bactrim). The two 2,4-aminopyrimidines taken together are a potent cause of megaloblastic anaemia, often with a rapid fall in haemoglobin and a degree of pancytopenia. The not uncommon addition of oral contraceptives to the pharmacological exposure increases the risk of developing anaemia. Oral contraceptives enhance the effects of folate deficiency but do not cause changes in folate replete women. However, folate deficiency is more likely in areas where pyrimethamine is required than in malaria-free areas.

Trimethoprim, with or without sulphamethoxazole, is unlikely to produce megaloblastic anaemia when taken in conventional doses for a bacterial infection. Megaloblastic anaemia is usual however in the high-dose Septrin

Table 10.3 Drugs which Cause Megaloblastic Change

Nature of inhibition	Drug examples	Incidence of megaloblastosis	Mechanism of action
1. DNA assembly	Cytosine arabinoside	Frequent	Inhibits polymerase
	Cyclophosphamide	Infrequent	Cross-links DNA
2. Ribonucleotide reduction	Hydroxyurea	Frequent	Inhibits ribonucleotide reductase
3. Thymidylate biosynthesis			
(i) Thymidylate synthetase	5-Fluorouracil	Frequent	Inhibits synthesis
(ii) DHF reductase	Methotrexate	Frequent	Decrease folate availability
	Pyrimethamine	See text	
	Triamterene	Infrequent	
	Trimethoprim	See text	
(iii) Inadequate or inactive folate	Phenytoin	Frequent	
	Primidone	Frequent	
	Phenobarbitone	Frequent	
	Oral contraceptives	Infrequent	
	Alcohol (chronic)	Frequent	
	Sulphasalazine	Infrequent	
(iv) Inadequate or inactive vitamin B_{12}	Nitrous oxide	Infrequent	Inhibits folate at B_{12} dependent step
	Neomycin	Infrequent	
	Metformin	Infrequent	
4. Pyrimidine precursor biosynthesis	Azauridine	Infrequent	Inhibits orotidylate synthetase
5. Purine precursor biosynthesis	Azathioprine	Infrequent	Inhibits several sites of purine synthesis
	6-Mercaptopurine	Infrequent	
6. Unknown	Tetracycline	Infrequent	Unknown
	Nitrofurantoin	Infrequent	
	Azidothymidine (AZT)	Frequent	Possibly inhibits DNA synthesis

regimens used for the treatment of *Pneumocystis carinii*. Patients receiving high-dose Septrin should receive folinic acid supplements to prevent the occurrence of megaloblastic anaemia. Folinic acid should be used to correct the megaloblastic anaemia of the combination described above and folate supplements should be given to people on long-term pyrimethamine prophylaxis.

Anticonvulsants

Long-term administration of anticonvulsants to patients with epilepsy is usual. Phenytoin, primidone and phenobarbitone all interfere with folate uptake and possibly increase folate catabolism though the precise mechanisms are not known.[19] Patients with epilepsy tend to have low folate anyway, particularly if the epilepsy is severe, because of poor nutrition. Folate supplements should always be given when these anticonvulsants are administered over a prolonged period of time.

Alcohol

The haematological effects of chronic or excessive alcohol have been reviewed on a number of occasions[20] and it is not the purpose of this chapter to review them in detail. Alcohol and alcoholism may lead to folate deficiency and therefore potentiate the megaloblastic effects of drugs which do not usually produce anaemia. Thus triamterene-induced megaloblastic anaemia has been described in patients with alcoholic cirrhosis.[21]

Azidothymidine (AZT)

AZT (3'-azido-3'deoxythimidine) has been introduced for the treatment of patients infected with human immunodeficiency virus (HIV). It appears to have useful therapeutic effects in the short term when given to patients with acquired immunodeficiency syndrome (AIDS), but these benefits are not sustained.[22] Its antiviral activity appears to rest on inhibition of viral reverse transcriptase.[23] Its clinical use is limited to some extent by bone marrow toxicity.[24] Macrocytosis is present in nearly all patients (associated with anaemia). Transfusions may be required. Neutropenia is also common, with sometimes severe thrombocytopenia. The precise mechanism of action in producing these haematological effects is unclear but AZT may inhibit DNA synthesis.[24,25]

Interference with mitochondrial metabolism

Mitochondria are essential for haem synthesis.[26] The first step takes place within the mitochondrion with formation of 5-aminolaevulinic acid from succinyl-CoA (derived from the tricarboxylic acid cycle) and glycine. The reaction, catalysed by ALA synthetase, requires pyridoxal-5-phosphate as a coenzyme, the phosphate being produced from pyridoxine (vitamin B_6) by pyridoxal-kinase. The formation of haem is also intramitochondrial, the incorporation of iron into the protoporphyrin IX ring taking place through the action of ferrochetalase.

Drugs which interfere with mitochondrial protein synthesis or decrease the availability of pyridoxal-5-phosphate cause the formation of ringed sideroblasts with deposition of iron in the mitochondria and may occasionally lead to sideroblastic anaemia.

Chloramphenicol

Chloramphenicol exerts its antibacterial action by binding to the bacterial 50S ribosomal subunit and preventing the binding of the aminoacyl tRNA to the ribosomes, hence inhibiting protein synthesis.[27,28] It will also bind to eukaryotic mitochondrial ribosomal subunits but not to cytoplasmic ribosomes.[29] Mitochondrial protein synthesis is thus inhibited and the mitochondria of erythroid precursors seem to be particularly sensitive, probably because of specific effect of chloramphenicol on ferrochetalase. In a dose-dependent fashion chloramphenicol will reduce iron clearance and iron utilization, cause vacuolation and maturation arrest in erythroid and, less commonly, myeloid precursors, produce reticulocytopenia and occasionally anaemia with ringed sideroblasts in the marrow. These effects are all reversible.[30] Whether these predictable effects are related to the development of aplastic anaemia in a proportion of patients exposed to chloramphenicol is unknown. Mehta and colleagues demonstrated the presence of a substitution in the mitochondrial DNA which encodes for the ribosomal subunit in a patient with chloramphenicol-induced aplastic anaemia who recovered.[31] The substitution was close to the region where substitutions in yeasts and bacteria promote chloramphenicol resistance.[32] However, other patients with chloramphenicol-induced aplasia did not show changes in mitochondrial DNA and its significance is still uncertain.

Antituberculous drugs

Isoniazid, pyrazinamide and cycloserine may each produce sideroblastic change, with or without anaemia.[26] These drugs interfere with the availability of pyridoxal-5-phosphate. Isoniazid is the most extensively studied. It forms a hydrazone with pyridoxal phosphate which not only reduces the availability of pyridoxal-5-phosphate but also inhibits pyridoxal kinase strongly. In patients with good supplies of pyridoxine and normal or high pyridoxal phosphate levels in the blood, sideroblastic anaemia is rare but in vitamin B_6 deficient patients the anaemia may be significant unless supplements are given. Such patients are found more commonly amongst the elderly and the black population,[33] though the reason for the lower levels of pyridoxal-5-phosphate in the black population is not known.

IMMUNE CYTOPENIAS PRODUCED BY DRUGS

Agranulocytosis, neutropenia, thrombocytopenia and haemolytic anaemia may each be produced through the action of antibodies induced by drugs or their metabolites. Amongst these immune-mediated cytopenias are some of the most devastating adverse effects of drugs which have led to a number of them being withdrawn from the market. Although in most cases the risk of inducing immune cytopenia is small, the effects are so marked that it is essential for the haematologist and physician to be alert to the possibility and to report all suspected cases to the appropriate drug monitoring body.

There are three major ways in which drugs may induce an immune cytopenia which may be classified as the immune complex mechanism, the drug absorption mechanism and the induction of auto-antibodies.[34,35] Each of these mechanisms may apply in the reduction of one of the cell lines, granulocytes, platelets or red cells, though why one particular cell line is targeted in any particular case or why particular drugs affect predominantly one particular cell line is not clear. The mechanisms have been studied most extensively in relation to haemolytic anaemia, mainly because the techniques for establishing the mechanisms are more readily available than with white cells or platelets, but the same mechanisms apply equally to these cytopenias.

Cytopenias produced by the immune complex mechanism

This mechanism produces the most acute type of drug-induced cytopenia. The supposition is that the drug or metabolite acting as a hapten, binds to a plasma constituent to produce a full antigen which generates an antibody reaction.[36,37] The antibodies were originally thought to be IgM but IgG class antibodies are probably equally important.[38] The antigen–antibody complex is absorbed on to the surface of the involved cell and there binds and activates complement. The activated complement lyses the cell, producing an acute cytopenia. The binding of the drug–antibody complex to the affected cell is probably not random but may depend on specific binding sites[35,39,40] which bind the complex by the Fab portion.[41]

The characteristic features of cytopenias produced by this mechanism are (i) an acute fall in the cell count, in the case of haemolytic anaemia by acute intravascular haemolysis, (ii) development of the cytopenia following exposure to a small amount of the offending drug, particularly if the patient has been exposed to the drug before, (iii) detection of complement only on the surface of the cell (these studies mainly in immune complex haemolytic anaemia), (iv) the frequent occurrence of systemic symptoms and signs, derived from the activation of complement and/or release of cell contents. These effects are described in more detail in the sections relating to specific cytopenias.

Drug absorption mechanism

Certain drugs are bound to cell membranes as an inevitable consequence of their structure. If the presence of the drug leads to the formation of antibodies these antibodies will be bound by the Fab end to the drug on the cell surface. If sufficient antibody is bound to the cell surface the cell will be removed by phagocytosis following binding of the Fc portion of the antibody to the Fc receptors of macrophages, particularly in the liver and spleen. The characteristic features of this mechanism are (i) a high concentration of the drug is required on the cell surface, the cytopenia is dose-dependent, (ii) antibody can be detected in the cell surface, (iii) the removal of cells is extravascular and subacute when compared to the immune complex mechanism, and (iv) systemic features do not occur.

Autoimmune cytopenias

In these cases antibodies are produced during the time that the drug is being taken which have specificity for constituents of the patient's cells. The first example described was the production of antibodies which had specificity for the rhesus complex of red cells in patients taking methyl DOPA.[42,43] Autoimmune cytopenias involving platelets or granulocytes have been less readily demonstrated but probably occur. In haemolytic anaemias caused by drug-induced anto-antibodies, the antibody characteristically develops after relatively long exposure to the drug and remains for several weeks or months after the drug is withdrawn. The clinical features are discussed in greater detail in the section on drug-induced autoimmune haemolytic anaemia.

The mechanisms of drug-induced cytopenias have been introduced in this way as a convenient classification but it should be realized that in many cases it is not possible to identify the precise mechanism of cell destruction and the same drug may produce cytopenias by different pathways both in different individuals and in the same individual at different times.[44]

Drug-induced immune haemolytic anaemias

The clinical and haematological features of the haemolytic anaemia produced by each of the three mechanisms outlines above are shown in Table 10.4.

Drugs which cause immune complex haemolytic anaemia

A large number of drugs have been reported as causing acute intravascular haemolysis, though the number of reported instances for each drug tends to be small, suggesting marked idiosyncrasy. The haemolysis is acute, often leading to gross haemoglobinuria and not infrequently acute renal failure with oliguria. The haemolysis may develop suddenly in a patient receiving a prolonged course of the drug, which may delay recognition of the association, or may appear immediately after re-exposure to a previously innocuous drug. Some patients may have received the drug several times before the haemolysis occurs.

A list of drugs which have been reported as causing acute intravascular

Table 10.4 Drug-induced Immune Haemolytic Anaemias

Mechanism	Example	Clinical features	Antibody characteristics
1. Immune complex	Quinidine Many others (see text)	Acute intravascular haemolysis, systemic features and renal failure Small dose of drug May be fatal	DAT: complement only Serum reacts with rbc in presence of drug Eluate does not react
2. Drug absorption	Benzyl penicillin	Extravascular haemolysis Large doses of drug	DAT: IgG ± complement Serum reacts with drug-treated cells Eluate reacts with drug-treated cells
3. Auto-antibody production	Methyl DOPA	Typically gradual onset with mild or no anaemia (but see text)	DAT: IgG only. Strong Antibody in serum and eluate May have Rh specificity (may not react with Rh null cells)

haemolysis appears in Table 10.5 but some drugs require special mention. The list is not comprehensive and care must be taken when new drugs are introduced to the market that all possible haemolytic episodes are reported promptly. The experience with nomefensine, reported below, is salutory. Many of the drugs listed in Table 10.5 may also cause thrombocytopenia or agranulocytosis but it is uncommon to find more than one cell line affected in the same patient. Cross-reactivity of the antibody with drugs closely related to the sensitizing drug may occur but is uncommon. The patient reported by Worlledge[45] who developed recurrent haemolytic episodes when exposed to phenacetin, also haemolysed following two tablets of paracetamol. However, the latter is a metabolite of phenacetin and the antibodies may have been directed against this metabolite.

Drugs producing haemolytic anaemia by the absorption mechanism

Benzylpenicillin, given intravenously, usually for bacterial endocarditis, in large doses is now well-recognized as a cause of haemolytic anaemia.[46,47] Administration of the drug has usually been for a week or more before the haemolysis becomes apparent. A fatal case has been reported[48] but this type of haemolysis is not usually life-threatening unless the penicillin is continued in high dose. It should also be remembered that penicillin may also cause acute haemolysis by the immune complex mechanism.[49,50] Once the drug is withdrawn the haemolysis begins to diminish promptly but the

Table 10.5   Drugs Causing Acute Intravascular Haemolysis by Immune Mechanisms

Drug	Ref.	Drug	Ref.
Antilymphocyte globulin	199	5-Fluorouracil	222
Anti-inflammatory drugs	120, 200	Glibenclamide	223
Antihistamines	40, 201	Hydrochlorothiazide	224–226
Azapropazone (apazone)	202	Ibuprofen	227–229
Captopril	203	Ketoconazole	230
Carbamazepine	204	Methotrexate	231
Carbimazole	205	Naproxen	232
Cefamandole	206	Probenecid	203, 204
Cefoxitin	207	Procainamide	235
Chlorpropamide	208–210	Rifampicin	236
Cimetidine	211, 212	Sulphsalazine	237
Cyclofenil	213, 214	Sulphonylurea	238
Diclofenac	215	Sulindac	235, 240
Dimethylsulphoxide	216	Tenopiside	241, 242
Dipyrone	217	Tetracycline	243, 244
Erythromycin	218	Thiopental	245
Fenbufen	219	Ticarcillin	246
Fenoprofen	220	Tolmellin	247
Feprazone	221	Triamterine	248

direct antiglobulin test will remain positive until all drug-coated cells are removed or until the drug or responsible metabolite is completely eliminated from the plasma.

Cephalosporins may also produce a positive direct antiglobulin test by a similar mechanism but are much less likely to produce a haemolytic anaemia.[53,54] There may be cross-reactivity with antipenicillin antibodies.[55] Other penicillins may have a similar effect[51,52] but the semisynthetic compounds seem much more likely to produce an immune neutropenia (see below).

Autoimmune haemolytic anaemia caused by drugs

In 1966 Carstairs and colleagues reported the occurrence of a positive direct antiglobulin test and antinuclear factor in hypertensive patients receiving methyl DOPA.[42] Further extensive investigations on a large number of patients showed that about 25% of the patients receiving the drug developed a positive direct antiglobulin,[56] but less than 1% of patients showed evidence of haemolysis.[45] Patients who received higher doses of the drug were more likely to develop a positive test but even at high dosage no more than 40% of patients became positive. The direct antiglobulin test became positive some 3–6 months after the onset of treatment, usually remained positive whilst the drug was continued and became negative only some months or even years after withdrawal.[57]

The antibody is IgG in type and reacts with all cells except Rh null cells. In all cases tested, absorption with Rh null cells leaves antibody which will react with cells having the rhesus stem.[58,59] Re-exposure of the patient to methyl DOPA leads to a similar pattern of slow emergence of a positive direct antiglobulin test.

Other drugs have been reported to have a similar effect in producing a positive direct antiglobulin test with or without haemolytic anaemia.

L-DOPA, chemically closely related to methyl DOPA but used in the treatment of Parkinson's disease, has also been reported to cause a positive direct antiglobulin test but significant haemolysis seems to be rarer than with methyl DOPA.[60,61]

Mefenamic acid (Ponstan), a non-steroidal anti-inflammatory agent, was first described as producing an autoimmune haemolytic anaemic in 1968.[63] The authors reported three patients with rheumatoid arthritis who were on long-term treatment with mefenamic acid, who developed haemolysis, but as autoimmune haemolytic anaemia may arise spontaneously in patients with rheumatoid arthritis the association of the drug with the haemolysis was not initially accepted.[44] However, several other cases have been reported and the causal relationship seems undoubted.[34] Most patients have significant haemolysis.

Procainamide, an anti-arrhythmic drug, produces a number of auto-immune phenomena including drug-induced lupus erythematosus, the development of antinuclear antibodies and lymphocytotoxic antibodies. It may also induce red cell antibodies. Kleinman and colleagues[63] studied the incidence of a positive direct antiglobulin test in 100 patients taking the drug compared with 100 age- and disease-matched controls. Twenty-one per cent of the procainamide-treated group developed a positive DAT, of whom the majority had IgG on the surface of the red cells, with or without complement. This compared with 10% in the control group, 7 of these 10 patients having complement only on the red cell surface. As with methyl DOPA the test became positive after 2–3 months therapy and the DAT remained positive for many months after withdrawal of the drug. Three of the 21 patients with positive DAT developed haemolytic anaemia which resolved promptly when the drug was stopped. Two other cases of haemolytic anaemia have been reported.[64]

Nomefensine, an antidepressant, was of particular interest in its production of immune haemolytic anaemia. In 1979 Bounerias & Habibi reported immune haemolytic anaemia with renal failure in a patient re-exposed to the drug.[65] The mechanism appeared to be the immune complex, complement activation pathway. Several other reports appeared sub-sequently, mostly with a similar pattern, acute intravascular haemolysis, usually with renal failure and systemic symptoms. Some patients died. The drug was withdrawn voluntarily from the market by the manufacturers as this side-effect became alarmingly common. Mueller-Eckhardt and col-leagues demonstrated conclusively that the patients had an antibody directed, in most cases, against metabolites of the drug.[38,44] However, amongst the reports there were some which suggested that an auto-antibody-producing autoimmune haemolytic anaemia was present.[44] These instances were in patients who took the drug continuously, just like the methyl DOPA patients, and the haemolysis was relatively mild. In one remarkable case a patient on continuous nomefensine developed auto-immune haemolytic anaemia. She stopped the drug for a period. The direct antiglobulin test became negative. Re-exposure to the drug produced a prompt, catastrophic intravascular haemolysis with renal failure. The nomefensine story is interesting because it highlights the need for careful reporting and investigation. Although the case of autoimmune antibody production remains obscure, it is intriguing that nomefensine interferes with dopamine metabolism which perhaps provides a link with methyl DOPA.

Other drugs which have been reported to cause autoimmune haemolytic anaemia but where the information is not complete to be certain are ibuprofen,[66,67] cimetidine,[68] fenfluramine,[70] methysergide,[69] chlor-promazine[45] and chlorpropramide.[71] In each of these there are features of the haemolytic anaemia which might be explained in other ways than incriminating the drug. If the observed features of methyl DOPA, L-DOPA, nomefensine and mefenamic acid induced autoimmune haemolytic anaemia apply in other cases one would expect a prolonged course of treatment to precede the onset of positive direct antiglobulin test, for the antibody to be IgG in type and to react with all cells in the absence of the drug except for cells lacking rhesus specificity as outlined above.

Microangiopathic haemolytic anaemia

Microangiopathic haemolytic anaemia is characterized by intravascular haemolysis, fragmentation of red cells and pathology of small blood vessels, the last feature often being assumed in the absence of biopsy material. One mechanism of microangiopathy is the deposition of fibrin within the vessels of the kidney with or without evidence of diffuse coagulopathy. Although complement and/or immune globulin may be found on the glomerular basement membrane it is not clear what role immune mechanisms play in the pathogenesis of this syndrome and it is included here more for convenience than strict classification. Two drugs, mitomycin C and cyclosporin, are well-known to produce renal toxicity and may be associated with a microangiopathic haemolytic anaemia, accompanied in many cases by thrombocytopenia and renal impairment consistent with a haemolytic uraemic syndrome.

Mitomycin C is used in the treatment of a variety of cancers including gastrointestinal tract, bladder, breast and prostate. It causes a dose-related depression of the bone marrow, occasional pulmonary toxicity and renal function impairment. In a proportion of patients with renal impairment microangiopathic haemolytic anaemia may occur.[72,73] Thrombocytopenia frequently accompanies the haemolytic anaemia but may also be due to bone marrow depression. Nephrotoxicity occurs in 2–10% of patients receiving mitomycin C, about half of them showing evidence of microangiopathic haemolytic anaemia.[74,75,76] The clinical picture may resemble thrombotic thrombocytopenic purpura with neurological changes as well as haemolytic anaemia and thrombocytopenia. Histology of the kidney shows glomerular sclerosis and fibrin deposition in glomerular capillaries. Plasma exchange may halt and reverse the haematological abnormalities but does not affect the renal function.[77]

Cyclosporin is an immunosuppressive agent used extensively to prevent rejection in solid organ transplants and to modify graft-versus-host disease after bone marrow transplantation. It has a dose-dependent nephrotoxicity which is mostly reversible when the dose is reduced or the drug withdrawn. Occasionally a haemolytic uraemia-like syndrome may arise with marked fragmentation of red cells in the peripheral blood, microangiopathic haemolytic anaemia, hypertension and renal failure.[78,79] The haemolytic anaemia responds to withdrawal of the drug or reduction in the dosage, the renal failure, which is associated with fibrin deposition in the glomerulae, may recover slowly.

Other drugs which have been associated with a microangiopathic haemolytic anaemia include cisplatin[80] and metronidazole,[81] though it must be remembered that microangiopathic haemolytic anaemia may be a complication of malignant disease per se.

Drug-induced pure red cell aplasia

A number of drugs have been recorded as causing an isolated arrest of erythroid development with an anaemia accompanied by reticulocytopenia. This particular association is very rare and the mechanism poorly understood; in only a few instances has it been possible to identify a drug-dependent inhibitor in the serum of affected patients. Direct toxicity on the marrow seems to be a possibility. The drugs implicated are shown in Table 10.6.

DRUG-INDUCED NEUTROPENIA

Adverse reactions to drugs are the most common cause of isolated neutropenia if haematological disease, collagen disorders and exposure to cytotoxic drugs are excluded.[100] Although a rare event, drug-induced neutropenia is important because it carries a high risk of mortality. Vigilance is also required because some drugs which cause neutropenia may be available as non-prescription preparations; detailed questioning may be needed to discover that the patient took such self-medication. Dipyrone is one such drug.

Mechanisms of drug-induced neutropenia

There are two clinical syndromes which accompany drug-induced neutropenia.

Drug-induced agranulocytosis

In the first, and more dangerous, there is a rapid fall in neutrophil count following ingestion of a small amount of the drug – often a single dose – usually within 12–24 h of exposure in a patient who has taken the drug before. Systemic symptoms are common with fever, oral or pharyngeal ulceration, abdominal pain and prostration,[101,102] though these features can be mild or absent. The neutrophil count often falls to zero. This type of adverse drug reaction will be referred to as drug-induced agranulocytosis. There is good evidence that there is antibody present which is directed

Table 10.6 Drugs Associated with Pure Red Cell Aplasia

Drugs	References
Azathioprine	82, 83
Carbamazepine	84
Cephalothin	85
Chloramphenicol	86
Chlorpropamide	87
Co-trimoxazole	88, 89
Diphenylhydantoin	90, 91
Fenbufen	92
Fenoprofen	93, 94
Gold	95
Indomethacin	120
Isoniazid	96, 97
L-Methyl DOPA	98
D-Penicillamine	99
Phenylbutazone	120

against the drug or metabolite and that immune complexes play an important part in the destruction of the granulocytes, though the cells are probably not complete 'innocent by-standers' but have specific receptors for the immune complexes in the individuals affected. The bone marrow is most commonly cellular in these patients but shows an absence of granulocyte precursors beyond the myelocyte or promyelocyte stage – an appearance which has been termed, rather misleadingly, 'maturation arrest'. Occasional reports describe a bone marrow in which granulocyte precursors are completely absent and *in vitro* culture may show inhibition of CFU-C by drug and patient's serum together.[103,104] Recovery of peripheral granulocyte counts usually begins 7–14 days after withdrawal of the drug depending upon the rate of clearance of the drug or its metabolites from the plasma. The antibody may persist for many months so that re-exposure to the drug will produce another swift episode of agranulocytosis.

Drug-induced neutropenia

This term is reserved here for those drug-induced episodes where the onset of the neutropenia is slower than above and follows prolonged exposure to the drug, often in high doses. There are two main mechanisms by which this type of neutropenia may develop.[105] The first, and more common, is akin to the drug absorption mechanisms described at the beginning of this chapter.[106] Neutropenia usually begins to develop at about 10 days after the drug has been started and although the fall in neutrophils is not so abrupt as in the drug-induced agranulocytosis, the final neutrophil count may be equally low if the complication is not identified and the drug stopped. Recovery is usually rapid following withdrawal, granulocytes appearing within 2–3 days of stopping the drug. Exceptions occur when the drug or its metabolite remain present in high concentration following withdrawal.[107] The most commonly implicated drugs in this group are the semi-synthetic penicillins and cephalosporins (see below).

In the second group with this slower onset of neutropenia are drugs which seem to have a direct effect upon the bone marrow, whether by an immune mechanism or by direct toxicity is not always clear. Gold salts and metiamide are two drugs where such a mechanism may operate, the latter having been replaced by newer H-2 antagonists because of this side-effect. β-Lactam antibiotic-induced neutropenia may also sometimes occur through this mechanism.[108] Recovery of the neutrophil count may be slower in this type of drug-induced neutropenia.

Specific groups of drugs causing neutropenia

Very many drugs have been reported to cause neutropenia by one or other mechanism and a representative list appears in Table 10.7. Other lists may be found in previous reviews.[101,102] It is, however, possible to detect groups of drugs which have a higher risk of inducing neutropenia than others, an increased risk which is linked in some way to their structure. Cross-reactivity may occur within the groups.[109] Some patients seem particularly

Table 10.7   Drugs Associated with Idiosyncratic Agranulocytosis and
Neutropenia

Group	Examples	Representative references
Analgesics, antipyretics, NSAIDs		100, 113, 120, 249, 250
	Amidopyrine	102, 110–112, 251
	Dipyrone	100, 116–118, 252, 253
	Diflunisal	254
	Fenbufen	120
	Fenoprofen	255, 256
	Gold salts	257, 258
	Ibuprofen	123
	Indomethacin	113, 120
	Naproxen	259
	Penicillamine	260
	Pentazocine	261–263
	Phenylbutazone Oxyphenbutazone	113, 120
	Sulindac	121, 122, 264
	Tolmetin	265
Antiarrythmics		266
	Aprindine	267, 268
	Flecanide	269
	Procainamide	132–135
	Quinidine	130
	Tocainide	136, 137
Antithyroid drugs		124–127
	Carbimazole	126, 127
	Methimazole	271–273
	Propylthiouracil	124–127, 274, 275
Antihypertensive drugs		142
	Captopril	142, 147, 148
	Analopril	147
	Nifedipine	297
Psychotropic drugs		160
	Amitriptyline	162
	Carbamazepine	298, 299
	Chlorpromazine	160, 161, 300
	Desimipramine	301
	Dothiepin	302
	Mianserin	164–168
	Phenothiazines	303, 304
	Chlorpheniramine	305
	Clozapine	306, 307
	Meprobamate	308
	Metachlopramide	309

Table 10.7 continued

Group	Examples	Representative references
Antibiotics		105
	Cephalosporins	150, 276–278
	Cefotaxime	179
	Ceftriaxone	280
	Cephradine	281
	Fusidic acid	282, 283
	Norfloxacin	284
	Penicillins	105–108, 276, 277
	Ampicillin	278, 285
	Augmentin	286
	Benzyl penicillin	287, 288
	Cloxacillin	289
	Methicillin	290
	Mezlocillin	291
	Piperacillin	291
	Ticarcillin	292, 293
	Sulphonamides	
	Sulphadiazine	294
	Sulphamethoxazol	141
	Sulphasalazine	138–140
	Vancomycin	151, 152
Antimalarial agents		
	Amodiaquine	153–157
	Chloroquine	295
	Fansidar	296
	Maloprim	158, 159
Drugs which inhibit gastric acid secretion		
	Cimetidine	310–312
	Metiamide	312
	Ranitidine	313, 314
	Pirenzapine	315
Miscellaneous		
	Chlorpropamide	316, 317
	Laetrile	318
	Pentamidine	319
	Phenytoin	320
	Sodium valproate	321
	Spironolactone	322

susceptible to drug-induced complications, which observation raises intriguing questions about the tendency of certain immune systems to mount inappropriate responses.

The pyrazolones

This group of drugs deserves pride of place in any discussion of drug-induced agranulocytosis because two of the archetypal drugs in this group, amidopyrine (aminophenzone) and dipyrone (noramidopyrine methanesulphonate) are notorious for provoking agranulocytosis and yet there has been great resistance to removing them completely from the market. Other drugs in this group include phenylbutazone and oxyphenbutazone, apazone and the closely related compounds chloramphenicol and thiamphenicol. It will be appreciated from this list that some drugs are more likely to cause agranulocytosis, others aplastic anaemia, but the tendency to produce blood dyscrasias does seem to be related to the presence of the pyrazolone ring, though phenazone (antipyrine) itself has not been directly implicated.

Many cases of amidopyrine-induced agranulocytosis have been described, many of them fatal. An earlier literature review has been presented and clinical features described by Hartl.[102] The drug had a chequered history since its discovery in 1896. It was widely prescribed in continental Europe, Africa and Asia as an antipyretic. It was less popular in the USA and UK and its dangers were appreciated. In 1939 it was made a prescription-only drug in the USA but in much of the rest of the world it was marketed as a non-prescription compound with catastrophic results for a few. Fatal agranulocytosis in babies born to mothers taking amidopyrine has been reported,[110] and in one intriguing case only one of dizygotic twins was affected. Typically the agranulocytosis followed the taking of a single dose of amidopyrine by a patient who had taken the drug before. Often there is fever and malaise which confuses the issue by suggesting septicaemia which is rarely present, at least at presentation. The bone marrow is cellular with maturation arrest at the myelocyte stage. It has been estimated that about 8 in 1000 patients who had taken amidopyrine for 14 days or more developed agranulocytosis[111,112] and about half of them died though it should be noted that this is a statistical analysis and agranulocytosis is most likely to occur as described above, not in someone who takes the drug for 14 days.

Phenylbutazone and oxyphenbutazone are more likely to cause aplastic anaemia than agranulocytosis,[113] though many cases of the latter have been described with each drug. They are powerful non-steroidal anti-inflammatory agents and are still appropriately used though their propensity to cause blood dyscrasias is widely publicized.[114-116] The International Agranulocytosis and Aplastic Anaemia Study (IAAAS) found an excess risk of agranulocytosis with phenylbutazone of about 3.8 compared with 8.7 for aplastic anaemia and about 24 for agranulocytosis caused by dipyrone,[113] though the method for calculating excess risk has been questioned.[114] Phenylbutazone is extensively used in horse racing to prevent joint inflammation in race horses but cases of agranulocytosis or aplastic anaemia have not been recorded in horses. Similar controversy surrounds the related compound dipyrone[116] which, for obscure reasons, still continues to be sold.

Dipyrone-induced agranulocytosis is well-described and it used to be amongst the most common causes of drug-induced agranulocytosis in Sweden until it was banned.[100] Its marketing in Asia causes considerable concern.[118]

Chloramphenicol toxicity will be considered under aplastic anaemia. It is interesting that its potential haematological toxicity was predicted on the basis of the similarity of its structure to amidopyrine before the first case of aplastic anaemia was reported.[119]

Other non-steroidal anti-inflammatory drugs (NSAID)[120]

Indomethacin is a widely prescribed NSAID which has appreciable haematological toxocity.[113] The IAAAS found an increased risk of both agranulocytosis and aplastic anaemia with indomethacin and individual reports of agranulocytosis have appeared. Sulindac, a closely related compound, was more recently introduced to avoid toxicity but reports of agranulocytosis have already appeared.[121,122] A case of ibuprofen-induced agranulocytosis with drug-dependent antibodies which inhibited granulocyte colony formation *in vitro* has been described.[123] Ibuprofen is a propionic acid derivate, a class of compound which has been used for their anti-inflammatory action. The tendency to produce blood dyscrasias is lower than with the pyrazolones but is not negligible.

Benoxaprofen (Opren) was withdrawn from the market because of its effects on the liver and skin in the elderly, but it also produced blood dyscrasias including agranulocytosis and aplastic anaemia.

Antithyroid drugs

Methimazole, carbimazole and propylthiourea have been used for several decades in the control of thyrotoxicosis and serious, but rare side-effects are well recognized.[124] The nature of their use means that they are often prescribed for a prolonged period of time. Methimazole and carbimazole often produce a mild neutropenia when used in this way with a neutrophil count around 1.0×10^9 per litre.[125] This neutropenia is not clinically significant and reverses with removal of the drug. A much more marked fall in the granulocyte count occurs more rarely[126] with an incidence of about 1 in 500, but is potentially fatal. The IAAAS recorded 45 cases of agranulocytosis in patients taking antithyroid drugs, compared with only 3 in the control group, the largest single group in the population studied.[126] The pattern of exposure to methimazole and carbimazole in one study suggested that older patients (over 40) who had taken the drug for 2 months or less were most likely to develop agranulocytosis.[127] The mechanism of the agranulocytosis has been more extensively studied with propylthiourea. Both drug-dependent and auto-antibodies have been described.[128] Recovery of neutrophil counts may be much slower than in the acute agranulocytosis described above, sometimes taking several weeks, suggesting that a different mechanism from the immune complex one operates, though the precise mechanism is not known.

Anti-arrhythmic drugs

Quinidine is best known for its tendency to produce thrombocytopenia (see below) but it may also induce agranulocytosis,[129,130] either alone or with thrombocytopenia. In one carefully studied case the antibodies directed against the platelets were different from those directed against the granulocytes, the leucocyte antibodies being drug-dependent.[131]

Procainamide has already been mentioned in the section on drug-induced autoimmune haemolytic anaemia. Cases of severe neutropenia have been reported.[132,133] Procainamide also produces a drug-induced lupus syndrome and the blood dyscrasias may accompany the syndrome or be separate[134] and more than one cytopenia may occur in the same patient. Mostly the agranulocytosis occurs within 24 h of taking the drug, but occasionally prolonged usage ends with agranulocytosis, perhaps indicating that both drug-dependent and auto-antibodies may occur. Meyers and colleagues studied the incidence of neutropenia in patients taking procainamide in a well-defined hospital patient population in the USA. In a 4 year period they found 17 cases, an incidence of 5.7 per 1000 people taking the drug.[135] There was no difference in risk between people taking procainamide hydrochloride and those taking a slow release preparation. The bone marrow in these patients showed maturation arrest.

Tocainide, an analogue of lidocaine, is used to treat ventricular arrhythmias. Agranulocytosis with a hypocellular bone marrow has been recorded.[136] The neutropenia may be part of a lupus-like syndrome.[137]

Sulphonamides

Blood dyscrasias, including agranulocytosis, have long been associated with sulphonamide treatment. Sulphasalazine (salicylazosulphapyridine, salazo-pyrine) may produce agranulocytosis[138–140] in addition to its tendency to produce oxidative damage and haemolytic anaemia (see above). Sulpha-methoxazole is combined with trimethoprim in Septrin (Bactrim) and has a low, but significant tendency to produce immune agranulocytosis.[141] This is in addition to the megaloblastic pancytopenia which may be produced by high dosage. Other sulphonamides associated with agranulocytosis are listed in Table 10.7.

Sulphydryl compounds

Penicillamine, captopril and enalopril are widely used sulphydryl com-pounds. Less used are 5-thiopyridoxine, pyrithioxine and α-glycine. The first three are well-recognized as mercapto propionyl agents causing blood dyscrasias.[142]

Penicillamine is an important drug in the management of rheumatoid arthritis. Early toxicity includes agranulocytosis,[142–144] pure red cell aplasia[99] and aplastic anaemia,[145,146] allergic reactions and nephrotoxicity. Toxicity after prolonged usage includes a lupus-like syndrome. Penicillamine may cross-react with penicillin sensitivity. The agranulocytosis produced by penicillamine is uncommon and reversible; the aplastic anaemia even rarer but not readily reversible.

Captopril, an angiotensin-converting enzyme inhibitor used to treat hypertension, has been associated with severe and even fatal agranulocytosis in a number of reports. Patients with renal failure and collagen disease are particularly at risk; patients without these features rarely, if ever, have been reported to have developed neutropenia.[147,148] It has been suggested that the toxic effect might be related to using too high a dose in patients with renal function impairment.[149] Special care should thus be taken to monitor blood counts of patients with renal failure who receive the drug. Enalopril is a newer analogue of captopril with a longer plasma half-life than captopril which is used once daily but may also produce agranulocytosis. The incidence of this complication appears to be lower than with captopril,[147] but since the drug is newer and has been less widely prescribed it is not possible to be certain.

Penicillins and cephalosporins

The β-lactam antibiotics as a group induce neutropenia through the drug absorption mechanism[106] or through direct inhibition of granulopoiesis.[108] Typically the antibiotic has been given in high dose for a period of 7 or more days. The neutropenia develops over a period of a few days though it may be severe, with fatal consequences, if not identified in time. Leuco-agglutinins may be detected in the peripheral blood and the bone marrow usually shows maturation arrest. Recovery occurs within 5–10 days of stopping the drug and, if essential for therapy, the drug may be re-introduced at a lower dose. The semi-synthetic penicillins are the most commonly reported group causing neutropenia, though cephalosporins have been implicated.[150] Cross-reactivity may occur. A more detailed list appears in Table 10.7. A particular difficulty arises when β-lactam antibiotics are used for a prolonged period of time for the treatment of fever in patients with neutropenia.[105] There is some evidence that the use of ceftazidime, for example, may prolong neutropenia, though the same is likely to be the case with the penicillins also. Whilst initial treatment with such antibiotics may be advisable, a switch to an appropriate antibiotic which does not produce neutropenia so regularly would be advisable after 10 days if the antibiotics cannot be stopped altogether.

Other antibiotics

It is important in certain clinical situations to have some idea of the likelihood of one of several antibiotics administered at the same time being responsible for a neutropenia. The aminoglycosides, for example, seem to have a very low propensity for producing blood dyscrasias, though agranulocytosis has been described.

Vancomycin, on the other hand, may produce severe neutropenia, particularly in patients with renal failure, where the drug has a very prolonged plasma half-life,[151] measured in weeks.[152] It is not dialysable. The bone marrow often shows granulocytic aplasia.

Antimalarial agents

Quinine, and compounds derived from it, produce a number of blood dyscrasias. Oxidative haemolysis has already been mentioned. Quinine itself is most likely to produce thrombocytopenia (see below), but agranulocytosis following quinine therapy is described.

Amodiaquine is a 4-aminoquinoline which has been introduced in the battle against chloroquine-resistant falciparum malaria. Its tendency to cause blood dyscrasia, particularly agranulocytosis,[153–155] has led to the recommendation that it should not be used for malaria prophylaxis, though agranulocytosis has been reported both when it is used for prophylaxis and therapy. Recovery may take up to 3 weeks. The bone marrow usually shows granulocytic hypoplasia,[154] though some cases show maturation arrest.[155] Circulating IgG antibodies dependent on the drug or its metabolite, mono-desethyl amodiaquine, have been detected which act against mature neutrophils but not against CFU-C.[153] However, in another instance antibodies which inhibited colony growth have been detected.[156]

This serious side-effect has resulted in the preparation being withdrawn for malaraia prophylaxis except for chloroquine-resistant areas with appropriate warnings given.[157]

Maloprim, a mixture of pyrimethamine (12.5 mg) and dapsone (100 mg) has a low incidence of agranulocytosis when used once a week, a higher rate when taken twice weekly.[158,159]

Drugs used in the treatment of psychoses

The management of psychiatric illnesses has been greatly improved by the introduction of effective drug therapy, beginning with the clinical trials of phenothiazines for psychotic illnesses and the structurally related tricyclic antidepressant drugs in the 1950s. Millions of people have been treated with these compounds and it is not surprising that some cases of agranulocytosis, clearly related to the drugs, have been reported for most of them. The benzodiazepines appear to have a very low incidence of blood dyscrasias, the tricyclic antidepressants an almost equally low tendency and the phenothiazines a higher, but nevertheless low, incidence. Mianserin, a tetracyclic antidepressant seems to have a more substantial tendency to produce agranulocytosis (see below). In most instances the blood dyscrasia develops 4–12 weeks after starting the drug and special care should be taken during this period to warn patients to report infections such as sore throats, face or mouth ulcers at once and where possible to monitor the blood count at monthly intervals.

Chlorpromazine therapy, particularly at high dosage, may be associated with a leucopenia which is mild, stable and not clinically important. More serious cases of agranulocytosis occur rarely, an estimated incidence of 1 in 10,000 exposures being suggested,[160] usually appearing within 12 weeks of starting treatment. Although agranulocytosis is most commonly seen in elderly patients, children may be affected.[161] The bone marrow may show maturation arrest or complete absence of granulocyte precursors. Recovery usually occurs within 2 weeks of stopping the drug, though more prolonged courses have been described. It is not clear whether immune mechanisms or direct effects on the bone marrow are responsible but the time course makes the former a little more likely.

Amitryptyline is the most widely prescribed tricyclic antidepressant and the incidence of agranulocytosis seems to be very low. Clink,[162] in a comparison of amitryptiline with mianserin mentions 83 cases of agranulocytosis with the former, reported over 17 years from 1964 to 1981. The denominator in this collection was not recorded but must have been over a million prescriptions.

Mianserin was introduced into clinical practice because it has a low incidence of serious toxicity in overdose, clearly an advantage for a drug used to treat depression. Cases of blood dyscrasia, particularly agranulocytosis with or without other cytopenias, accumulated slowly at first but have now reached the stage where major controversy, both medical and legal, surrounds the drug's use.[163] Two cases were reported in 1979, one where mianserin was the only drug being taken at the time[164] the other in conjunction with thyroxine.[165] These were thought to be the first cases reported. By 1983 there were some 26 reports, 3 of them fatal, of which 19 appeared to be definitely associated with the drug.[162] In most cases the agranulocytosis appeared 4–6 weeks after starting the drug. By 1986 the manufacturers had received notification of 279 cases of white cell disorders, 14 pancytopenia, 129 cases of leucopenia with granulocytopenia and 136 cases of agranulocytosis, 22 of them fatal. The company put out a position document[166] reporting these figures which occurred on the background of 11 million prescriptions. In 162 of the cases other drugs were prescribed at the same time and as many as 86% of the cases could have been due to these other drugs. This highlights one of the major difficulties in attributing a particular toxic effect to an individual drug when no specific test is available for the effect. Further reports of agranulocytosis have, however, accumulated since 1986 and there seems no doubt that the drug does have a tendency to cause this problem. The mechanism is unknown. In two cases studied with monitoring of blood levels of mianserin, high serum levels were present when the patients presented and fell more slowly than expected, suggesting saturable elimination kinetics.[167] Granulocyte recovery occurred 26 days after stopping the drug in one case, and 13 days in the second. Usually recovery occurs within 4–8 days of stopping the drug.[168] This relationship of blood levels to neutropenia raised the possibility of a direct toxic effect on the marrow,[169] but could equally be explained on the basis of slow clearance of the drug in a drug–antibody mediated cytopenia. The bone marrow tends to be hypocellular in these patients[168] which suggests that the destruction of granulocytes begins at an early precursor stage.

Comments on drug-induced neutropenias

Blood dyscrasias produced by drugs are rare but they account for 80% of the fatal drug reactions. Agranulocytosis and aplastic anaemia are the major causes of this mortality. Where the mechanism of drug-induced agranulo-cytosis has been carefully studied, immune mechanisms appear more likely than direct toxic effects upon the marrow, the reverse being true for aplastic anaemia. It should be realized that immune, antibody-mediated responses may also damage granulocytic precursor cells as well as mature neutrophils so that *in vitro* studies of colony forming cells may show a precursor cell deficit if cytotoxic antibodies are present.

Where a drug or group of drugs have a particularly high risk of inducing agranulocytosis, certain risk factors may be identified for patients exposed to the drug. The antithyroid drugs and mianserin tend to affect the older age groups. Agranulocytosis generally occurs within the first 3 months of starting the drug. Renal or hepatic impairment may increase the risk and prolong the agranulocytosis if they inhibit drug elimination. Although special vigilance may be extended to these high-risk groups it has to be realized that agranulocytosis often occurs without warning and in curious settings and that awareness of the problem is necessary for all patients.

DRUG-INDUCED THROMBOCYTOPENIA

The most common cause of isolated thrombocytopenia is autoimmune thrombocytopenia, either idiopathic or associated with systemic lupus or lymphoma. Drug-induced immune thrombocytopenia, although well-described, is rare in comparison with the former which makes the role of drugs in any individual case difficult to determine. An obvious approach is to assume that any drug taken at the time the thrombocytopenia develops is responsible, stop it and see what happens. If the drug is responsible the thrombocytopenia should recover within 2–3 weeks. If corticosteroids have been given during the recovery phase there should be no relapse when they are discontinued if the drug or metabolite is responsible. Challenge with the presumed drug is inadvisable because the fall in platelets may be catastrophic, and bleeding, when it does occur, is most common in the early phase of thrombocytopenia, before the marrow responds.

Drug-induced thrombocytopenia has a special place in the study of adverse reactions to drugs. Quinine was recognized as a cause of purpura in 1865 before platelets were discovered.[169] In one of these cases re-exposure to quinine produced a second attack of purpura. The only other drugs given at the same time were dilute sulphuric acid and tincture of orange peel. These are the first drug-induced blood dyscrasias described. Ackroyd,[170] studying Sedormid-induced thrombocytopenia, first introduced concepts of immune antibody-mediated mechanisms, concepts modified later by Miescher[171] and Shulman,[172] who each studied quinidine-induced thrombocytopenia. Despite this long history it remains unclear precisely what is the nature of the immune attack. Mostly the antibodies involved are IgG and mostly but not inevitably, require the presence of a drug to bind to normal platelets.[173,174] The binding is weak, suggesting that an immune complex is involved. The binding and complement activation are not, however, random. In at least two instances it has been shown that the antigen–antibody complex will not bind to platelets from patients with Bernard

Soulier syndrome,[175] which lack the proteins 1b and IX, and specificity for platelet glycoprotein V has also been suggested.[176]

The incidence of drug-induced thrombocytopenia is not easy to establish. Many drugs have been implicated but, except for quinine, quinidine and heparin, the number of individual cases for each drug is small. Danielson and colleagues[177] studied the incidence of drug-induced cytopenias in a relatively stable hospital population and estimated an overall risk of 1 in 100,000 person years at risk. In a 10 year period with approximately 200,000 patients on the records they found 26 instances of cytopenia, 14 cases of thrombocytopenia of which 9 were related to quinidine, and 7 isolated cases of granulocytopenia, 5 related to sulphonamides.

Drug-induced thrombocytopenia usually appears acutely with clinical features prominent. The bone marrow is cellular with increasing numbers of megakaryocytes. Recovery is swift though the platelets will fall profoundly if the drug is re-introduced because the antibodies persist for many weeks or months.

Table 10.8 shows the most commonly implicated drugs.

Heparin-induced thrombocytopenia

It is perhaps surprising that heparin-induced thrombocytopenia was not recognized earlier or discussed more since its discovery in 1922, as between 1 and 5% of patients receiving the drug are said to develop thrombocytopenia.[178-180] Probably this is because in most patients the thrombocytopenia does not cause clinical problems and resolves rapidly after the drug is withdrawn. The nature of heparin usage means that it is used in short courses and the thrombocytopenia is missed. In a small proportion of patients the thrombocytopenia is accompanied by arterial or venous thrombotic episodes which may lead to myocardial infarction, cerebrovascular accidents, limb ischaemia or pulmonary emboli. In general, the more benign syndrome develops after several days (5–10) of heparin therapy and the fall in platelets is slow, whereas the dangerous syndrome is associated with an early and profound drop in platelets.

The heparin-induced thrombocytopenia is mediated through heparin–antibody immune complexes. Kelton and colleagues have shown that IgG antibodies, dependent on the presence of heparin, which cause serotonin release from platelets, are present in the serum of these thrombocytopenic patients.[181] Both the F(ab')$_2$ and Fc portions of the patients' immunglobulin are required for the release reaction which can be inhibited by normal Fc fractions but only by the patients' F(ab')$_2$ fraction. They suggest that the Fab portion binds to heparin and the complex is bound to platelets through the Fc portion. What determines the severity of the clinical syndrome is not clear, in both instances the immune reaction seems to be identical. It has been suggested that there is binding of immunoglobulin to endothelial cells which may explain the thrombosis[182] but this has not been confirmed in all cases. It would seem prudent to monitor blood counts during the first few days of heparin therapy. It is possible that low molecular weight heparins do not provoke the same response and may be used in the management of heparin-induced thrombotic thrombocytopenia,[183,184] but this is not a

Table 10.8   Drugs Associated with Immune Thrombocytopenia[361-365]

Drug	Representative references
Aminoglutethimide	323
Amiodarone	324
Amphotericin	325
Benzodiazepines	326
Carbamazepine	327, 328
Cephalosporins	329
Cimetidine	330
Danazol	331, 332
Diclofenac	334
Diflunisal	334
Ethambutol	335
Feprazone	336
Frusemide	337
Gold salts	338–340
Hydrochlorthiazide	341
Heparin	see text
Indomethacin	342
α-Interferon	343
Methyl DOPA	344
Mianserin	345
Morphine	346
Nalidixic acid	347
Piroxicam	348
Procainamide	349, 350
Protamine	351
Quinine	see text
Quinidine	see text
Ranitidine	352–354
Rifampicin	355
Sulindac	356
Sulphasalazine	357
Sulphamethoxazolephenazopyridine	358
Valproic acid	359
Vancomycin	360

universal observation.[185] Thrombocytopenia has been seen in patients exposed to small doses of heparin as with intravenous line flushing[186] and subcutaneous administration.[187]

Aplastic anaemia

Aplastic anaemia is the most devastating of the drug-induced blood dyscrasias with a mortality of 30–50% depending on the degree of marrow damage. Fortunately it is rare, with an overall incidence from all causes of about 2 per million per year in Europe and the USA,[188] though it may be higher in the Far East.[189] Drugs are implicated in about 20% of cases. Since the mechanism of drug-induced aplastic anaemia is unknown and there are no tests which confirm that a particular drug or toxin is involved in any individual case, suspicion is based on epidemiology and temporal relationships. The probability that a drug is involved in the aplastic anaemia increases if the drug was the only one administered, if it was taken within 3 months of the onset of the aplasia, if the patient had been exposed to the drug before and if other cases have been reported. Perhaps the best study of drug-related aplasia was that conducted on American soldiers taking atabrine (quinacrine, mepacrine) as malarial prophylaxis during World War 2.[190]

As with other dyscrasias, a large number of drugs have been recorded as causing aplastic anaemia (Table 10.9), but in only a few instances is the relationship firmly established.

Chloramphenicol

It was predicted that chloramphenicol would produce blood dyscrasias because of the similarity of its structure to amidopyrine.[119] The first case of aplastic anaemia was reported in 1950 in a patient who received a prolonged course of the drug.[191] Since then there have been many reports of chloramphenicol-induced aplasia, including patients who have received the drug as eye drops.[192] However, the incidence of aplasia following chloramphenicol eye drops is probably not above the normal background of aplasia. Aplasia is more common in patients who have had previous exposure to the drug[193] and in patients who develop hepatitis subsequent to the chloramphenicol exposure.[194] The subject has recently been reviewed and possible

Table 10.9 Drugs Associated with Aplastic Anaemia

Drug	References
Anticonvulsants	366
Butazones	see text
Chloramphenicol	see text
Dapsone	367
Diclofenac	100, 113
Gold salts	see text
Fenoprofen	368
Ibuprofen	369
Indomethacin	100, 113
Indoprofen	370
Interferon	371
Mianserin	372, 373
Naproxen	374
Piroxicam	375
Quinacrine (atabrine)	190
Sulindac	376, 377
Tocainide	378

mechanisms discussed.[195] Chloramphenicol is a very useful antibiotic and has undoubtedly saved many thousands times more lives than it has destroyed through aplastic anaemia but it would seem appropriate to reserve the drug for specific indications.

Phenylbutazone

Phenylbutazone became the most common cause of drug-induced aplastic anaemia once the dangers of chloramphenicol were recognized.[196] Cases are also reported with oxyphenbutazone. The increased risk of phenylbutazone aplastic anaemia recorded by the IAAAS has already been mentioned.[113]

Other non-steroidal anti-inflammatory agents[116]

Indomethacin and sulindac have both been reported as causing blood dyscrasias, including aplastic anaemia. The former is widely used and it is not possible to determine the real risk of developing aplastic anaemia; it is less than 1:100,000 exposures.

Diclofenac was associated with a surprisingly high risk of aplastic anaemia in a study from Sweden[100] and appears again in the IAAAS[113] study.

Benoxaprofen was associated with at least 20 cases of aplastic anaemia in the UK before its withdrawal from the market.

Gold salts

Gold salts (sodium aurothiomalate, aurothioglucose) are used in the treatment of rheumatoid arthritis. The incidence of blood dyscrasias is low but potentially fatal. Agranulocytosis, thrombocytopenia and aplastic anaemia have been recorded.[197] The first two are reversible when the drug is stopped, aplastic anaemia is prolonged. Blood counts must be monitored in patients receiving gold treatment and the drug stopped if significant cytopenia develops. It is not possible in this way to prevent all cases of aplastic anaemia but there is some suggestion that persisting with the treatment in the face of a reduced neutrophil count is more likely to lead to aplastic anaemia. Many attempts to reverse gold-induced aplasia have been made using dimercaprol (British anti-Lewisite, BAL), which chelates and removes gold. There is no evidence that it is effective. As with other drug-induced aplastic anaemias the prognosis depends entirely on the severity of the bone marrow damage. Elemental gold can be detected in the bone marrow many years after recovery from gold-induced aplastic anaemia and patients respond to bone marrow transplantation in the same way as idiopathic aplastic anaemia,[198] suggesting that the gold itself is not the sole toxic agent.

REFERENCES

1. Dacie, J.V. The hereditary haemolytic anaemias. In *The Haemolytic Anaemias*, Vol. 1. Churchill Livingstone, Edinburgh, 1985.
2. Beutler, E. Energy metabolism and maintenance of erythrocytes. In *Hematology* (eds W.J. Williams, E. Beutler, A.J. Ersler & M.A. Lichtman), pp. 331–44, McGraw-Hill, New York, 1983.
3. Bienze, M. Glucose-6-phosphate dehydrogenase deficiency. Part I: Tropical Africa. *Clin. Haematol.* **10**: 785–99, 1981.
4. Panich, V. Glucose-6-phosphate dehydrogenase deficiency. Part II: Tropical Asia. *Clin. Haematol.* **10**(3): 800–14, 1981.
5. Beutler, E. Glucose-6-phosphate dehydrogenase deficiency. In *Hematology*, 3rd Edn (eds J.W. Williams, E.W. Beutler, A.J. Erslew, & M.A. Lichtman), Chapter 58, pp. 561–74. McGraw-Hill, New York, 1983.
6. Gordon-Smith, E.C. Drug-induced oxidative haemolysis. *Clin. Haematol.* **9**(3): 557–86, 1980.
7. McCaffey, R.P., Halstead, G.H., Wahab, M.F.A. & Robertson, R.P. Chloramphenicol-induced haemolysis in Caucasian glucose-6-phosphate dehydrogenase deficiency. *Ann. Intern. Med.* **74**: 722–6, 1972.
8. Beutler, E. Drug-induced haemolytic anemia. *Pharmacol. Rev.* **21**: 73–103, 1969.
9. Loos, H., Roos, D., Wenning, R. & Houwerzijl, J. Familial deficiency of glutathione reductase in human blood cells. *Blood* **48**: 53, 1976.
10. Necheles, T.F., Steinberg, M.H. & Cameron, D. Erythrocyte gluatatione-peroxidase deficiency. *Br. J. Haematol.* **19**: 605–12, 1970.
11. Hetzog, P. & Feig, S.A. Methaemoglobinaemia in the newborn infant. *Clin. Haematol.* **7**(1): 75–83, 1978.
12. Scott, E.M. Congenital methemaglobinaemia due to DPNH-diaphorase deficiency. In *Heriditary Disorders of Erythrocyte Metabolism* (ed. E. Beutler) pp. 102–10. Grune & Stratton, New York, 1968.
13. Degowin, R.L. A review of the therapeutic and hemolytic effects of dapsone. *Arch. Intern. Med.* **120**: 242–8, 1967.
14. Goodacre, R.L., Ali, M.A., Vanderlinden, B. *et al.* Haemolytic anemia in patients receiving sulfasalazine. *Digestion* **17**: 503–8, 1978.
15. Das, K.M. & Stemlieb, I. Salicylazosulfapyridine in inflammatory bowel disease. *Am. J. Digest. Dis.* **20**: 971–6, 1975.
16. Scott, J.M. & Weir, D.G. Drug induced megaloblastic change. *Clin. Haematol.* **9**(3): 587–606, 1980.
17. Ferone, R., Burchall, J.J. & Hitchings, G.H. *Plasmodium berglei* dihydrofolate reductase: isolation, properties and inhibition by antifolates. *MM Phamacol.* **5**: 49–59, 1969.
18. Shojania, A.M. & Hornady, G.S. Oral contraceptive and folate absorption. *Lab. Clin. Med.* **82**: 869–75, 1973.
19. Chanarin, I. Megaloblastic anaemia due to anticonvulsant drugs. In *The Megaloblastic Anaemias*, 2nd Edn, Chapter 28, pp. 491–503. Blackwell Publications, Oxford, 1979.
20. Herbert, V.L. Hematologic complications of alcoholism. *Semin. Hematol.* **17**: 83–147, 1980.
21. Lieberman, F.L. & Bateman, J.R. Megaloblastic anaemia possibly induced by triamterene in patients with alcoholic cirrhosis: two case reports. *Ann. Intern. Med.* **68**: 168–73, 1969.
22. Dournon, E., Mathcron, S., Rozenbaum, W. *et al.* Effects of zidovudine in 365 consecutive patients with AIDS or AIDS related complex. *Lancet* **ii**: 1297–302, 1988.
23. Mitsuya, H., Weinhold, K.J., Furman, P.A. *et al.* 3' Azido 3' deoxythimidine (BWA509μ) an antiviral agent that inhibits the infectivity and cytopathic effect of

human T-lymphotropic virus type III/lymphadenopathy-associated virus *in vitro. Proc. Natl. Acad. Sci. U.S.A.* **82**: 7096–100, 1985.

24. Richman, D.D., Fische, M.A., Grieco, M.H. *et al.* The toxicity of azidothymidine (AZT) in the treatment of patients with AIDS and AIDS-related complex. A double-blind, placebo-controlled trial. *N. Engl. J. Med.* **317**: 192–7, 1987.

25. Furman, P., Fyfe, J.A., St Clair, M.H. *et al.* Phosphorylation of 3' azido-3' deoxythimidine and selective interaction of the 5' triphosphate with human immunodeficiency virus reverse transciptase. *Proc. Natl. Acad. Sci. U.S.A.* **83**: 8333–7, 1986.

26. Yunis, A.A. & Salem, Z. Drug induced mitochondrial damage and sideroblastic change. *Clin. Haematol.* **9**(3): 607–19, 1980.

27. Werner, R., Kollak, A. & Nierhaus, D. Experiments on the binding sites and the action of some antibiotics which inhibit ribosomal functions. In *Drug Receptor Interactions in Antimicrobial Chemotherapy* (eds J. Drews & F.E. Hahn), Vol. 1, pp. 217–34. Springer-Verlag, New York, 1975.

28. Hahn, F.E. & Gund, P. A structural model of the chloramphenicol receptor site. In *Drug Receptor Interactions and Antimicrobial Chemotherapy* (eds J. Drews & F.E. Hahn), pp. 245–66. Springer-Verlag, New York, 1975.

29. Denslow, N.D. & O'Brien, T.W. Antibiotic susceptibility of the peptide transferase locus of bovine mitochondrial ribosomes. *Eur. J. Biochem.* **91**, 441–8, 1978.

30. Hara, H., Kohsaki, M., Noguchi, K. & Nugai, K. Effect of chloramphenicol on colony formation from erythrocytic precursors. *Am. J. Hematol.* **5**: 123–30, 1978.

31. Mehta, A., Gordon-Smith, E.C. & Luzzato, L. Mitochondrial DNA in patients with aplastic anaemia. *Br. J. Haematol.* **66**: 416–17, 1987.

32. Kearsey, S.E. & Craig, I.W. Altered ribosomal RNA genes in mitochondrial mammal cells with choramphenicol resistance. *Nature* **290**: 607–8, 1981.

33. Chern, C.J. & Beutler, E. Pyridoxal kinase: decreased activity in red blood cells of Afro-Americans. *Science* **187**: 1084–6, 1975.

34. Petz, L.D. Drug-induced immune haemolytic anaemia. *Clin. Haematol.* **9**(3): 455–82, 1980.

35. Petz, L.D. Drug induced immune haemolysis. *N. Engl. J. Med.* **313**: 510–12, 1985.

36. Miescher, P.A. & Gorstein, F. Mechanisms of immunogenic platelet damage. In *Blood Platelets* (eds S.A. Johnson, R.W. Monto, J.W. Reebuck & R.C. Horne), pp. 671–91. J. and A. Churchill, London, 1981.

37. Shulman, N.R. A mechanism of cell destruction in individuals sensitized to foreign antigens and its implications in autoimmunity. *Ann. Intern. Med.* **60**: 506–21, 1964.

38. Salama, A. & Mueller-Eckhardt, C. The role of metabolite-specific antibodies in nomefensine-dependent immune hemolytic anaemia. *N. Engl. J. Med.* **313**: 469–74, 1985.

39. Habibi, B. & Bretagne, Y. Blood group antigens may be the receptors for specific drug-antibody complexes reacting with red blood cells. *C. R. Acad. Sci. Paris* **296**: 693, 1983.

40. Duran Suarez, J.R., Martin-Vega, C., Argelagues, E. *et al.* Red cell I antigen as immune complex receptor in drug-induced hemolytic anemias. *Vox Sang.* **41**: 313–15, 1981.

41. Smith, M.I., Jordan, J. & Reid, D.M. Drug-antibody binding to platelets is mediated by the Fab domain and is Fc-dependent. *Blood* **64** Suppl. 1: 91a, 1984.

42. Carstairs, K.C., Breckenridge, A., Dollery, C.R. & Worlledge, S.M. Incidence of a positive direct Coomb's test in patients on methyl dopa. *Lancet* **ii**: 133–5, 1966.

43. Murphy, W.G. & Kelton, J.C. Methyldopa-induced autoantibodies against red blood cells. *Blood Rev.* **2**: 36–42, 1988.

44. Salama, A. & Mueller-Eckhardt, C. Two types of nomefensine-induced immune

haemolytic anaemia: drug dependent sensitization and/or autoimmunization. *Br. J. Haematol.* **64**: 613–20, 1986.
45. Worlledge, S.M. Immune drug induced hemolytic anemia. *Semin. Hematol.* **6**: 181–200, 1969.
46. Petz, L.D. & Fudenberg, H.H. Coombs' positive hemolytic anemia caused by penicillin administration. *N. Engl. J. Med.* **274**: 171–8, 1966.
47. Yust, I., Frisch, B. & Goldsher, N. Mechanisms of immune haemolysis: cell-dependent destruction of autologous red cells in penicillin-induced haemolytic anaemia. *Scand. J. Haematol.* **28**: 408–16, 1982.
48. Jackson, F.N. & Jaffe, J.P. Fatal penicillin-produced hemolytic anaemia. *J. Am. Med. Assoc.* **242**: 2286–7, 1979.
49. Ries, C.A., Rosenbaum, T.J., Garratty, G. *et al.* Penicillin-induced immune hemolytic anemia. *J. Am. Med. Assoc.* **233**: 432–5, 1975.
50. Yust, I., Frisch, B. & Goldscher, N. Simultaneous detection of two mechanisms of immune destruction of penicillin-treated human red blood cells. *Am. J. Hematol.* **13**: 53–62, 1982.
51. Seldon, M.R., Bain, B., Johnson, C.A. & Lennox, C.S. Ticarcillin-induced immune haemolytic anaemia. *Scand. J. Haematol.* **28**: 455–60, 1982.
52. Gmur, J., Walti, M. & Neftel, K.A. Amoxicillin-induced immune hemolysis. *Acta Haematol. (Basel)* **74**: 230–3, 1985.
53. Gralnick, H., Mcginnis, M., Elton, W. & McCurdy, P. Hemolytic anemia associated with cephalothin. *J. Am. Med. Assoc.* **217**: 1193–7, 1971.
54. Jeannet, M., Bloch, A., Dayer, J.M. *et al.* Cephalothin-induced immune hemolytic anemia. *Acta Haematol.* **55**: 109–17, 1976.
55. Moake, J.L., Butler, C.F., Hewell, G.M. *et al.* Hemolysis induced by cefazolin and cephalothin in a patient with penicillin sensitivity. *Transfusion* **18**: 369–73, 1977.
56. Breckenridge, A., Dollery, C.T., Worlledge, S.M. *et al.* Positive direct Coombs' test and antinuclear factor in patients treated with methyl dopa. *Lancet* **ii**: 1265–8, 1967.
57. Worlledge, S.M. Immune drug induced hemolytic anemias. *Semin. Hematol.* **10**: 327–44, 1973.
58. Issitt, P.D., Pavone, B.G., Goldfinger, D. *et al.* Anti-Wr^b and other auto-antibodies responsible for positive direct antiglobulin tests in 150 individuals. *Br. J. Haematol.* **34**: 5, 1976.
59. Worlledge, S.M. Immune drug induced haemolytic anaemias. In *Blood Disorders due to Drugs and other Agents. Excerpta Medica* (ed R.H. Girdwood), pp. 11–26. Amsterdam, 1973.
60. Henry, R.E., Goldberg, L.S., Sturgeon, P. & Ansel, R.D. Serologic abnormalities associated with l-dopa therapy. *Vox Sang* **20**: 306–16, 1971.
61. Lindstrom, F.D., Lieden, G. & Engstrom, M.S. Dose-related levodopa-induced hemolytic anemia. *Ann. Intern. Med.* **86**: 298–300, 1977.
62. Scott, G.L., Myles, A.B. & Bacon, P.A. Autoimmune haemolytic anaemia and mefenamic acid therapy. *Br. Med. J.* **iii**: 534–5, 1968.
63. Kleinman, S., Nelson, R., Smith, L. & Goldfinger, D. Positive direct antiglobulin tests and immune hemolytic anaemia in patients receiving procainamide. *N. Engl. J. Med.* **311**: 809–12, 1984.
64. Schifman, R.B., Garewal, H. & Shillington, D. Reticulocytopenic, Coombs' positive anemia induced by procainamide. *Am. J. Clin. Pathol.* **80**: 66–8, 1983.
65. Bounerias, F. & Habibi, B. Nomifensine-induced immune haemolytic anaemia and impaired renal function. *Lancet* **ii**: 95–6, 1979.
66. Korsager, S., Sorensen, H., Jensen, O.H. & Falk, J.V. Antiglobulin-tests for detection of auto-immuno-haemolytic anaemia during long-term treatment with ibuprofen. *Scand. J. Rheumatol.* **10**: 174–6, 1981.
67. Guidry, J.B., Ogburn, C.L. & Griffin, F.M. Fatal autoimmune hemolytic anemia

associated with ibuprofen. *J. Am. Med. Assoc.* **242**: 68–9, 1979.
68. Rotoli, B., Formisano, S. & Alfinito, F. Autoimmune haemolytic anaemia associated with cimetidine. *Lancet* **ii**: 583, 1979.
69. Slugg, P.H. & Kunkel, R.S. Complications of methysergide therapy. *J. Am. Med. Assoc.* **213**: 297–8, 1970.
70. Nussey, A.M. Flenfluramine and haemolytic anaemia. *Br. Med. J.* **i**: 177–8, 1973.
71. Sosler, S.D., Behzad, O., Garralty, G. *et al.* Acute hemolytic anemia associated with a chlorpropamide-induced apparent auto-anti-Jka. *Transfusion* **24**: 206–9, 1984.
72. Jain, S. & Seymour, A.E. Mitomycin C associated hemolytic uremic syndrome. *Pathology* **19**: 58–61, 1987.
73. McCarthy, J.T. & Staats, B.A. Pulmonary hypertension, hemolytic anemia, and renal failure. A mitomycin-associated syndrome. *Chest* **89**, 608–11, 1986.
74. Verweij, J., van der Burgh, M.E. & Pinedo, H.M. Mitomycin-induced hemolytic uremic syndrome. Six case reports and review of the literature on renal pulmonary and cardiac side effects of the drug. *Radiother. Oncol.* **8**: 33–41, 1987.
75. Cordonnier, D., Vert-Pre, F.C., Bayle, F. *et al.* La nephrotoxicite de la mitomycin C (a propos de 25 observations). Resultats d'une enquete multi-centrique organisee par la Societe de nephrologie. *Nephrologie* **6**: 19–26, 1985.
76. Bruntsch, U., Groos, G., Tigges, F.J. & Gallmeier, W.M. Microangiopathic hemolytic anemia, a frequent complication of mitomycin therapy in cancer patients. *Eur. J. Cancer Clin. Oncol.* **20**: 950–9, 1984.
77. Price, P.N., Murgo, A.J., Keveney, J.J. *et al.*. Renal failure and hemolytic anemia associated with mitomycin C. A case report. *Cancer* **55**: 51–6, 1985.
78. Verpooten, G.A., Paulus, G.T., Rolls, F. & DeBroe, M.E. De novo occurrence of hemolytic-uremic syndrome in a cyclosporin-treated renal allograft patient. *Transplant-Proc.* **19**: 2943–5, 1987.
79. Van Buren, D., Van, Buren, C.T., Flechner, S.M. *et al.* Do novo hemolytic uremic syndrome in renal transplant recipients immunosuppressed with cyclosporine. *Surgery* **98**: 54–62, 1985.
80. Weinblatt, M.E., Kahn, E., Scimeca, P. & Kochen, J.A. Hemolytic uremic syndrome associated with cisplatin therapy. *Am. J. Pediatr. Hematol. Oncol.* **9**: 295–8, 1987.
81. Powell, A.R., Davidson, P.M., McCredie, D.A. *et al.* Haemolytic-uraemic syndrome after treatment with metronidazole. *Med. J. Aust.* **149**, 222–3, 1988.
82. DeClerk, Y.A., Ettenger, R.B., Ortega, J.A. & Pennisi, A.J. Macrocytosis and pure RBC anemia caused by azathioprine. *Am. J. Dis. Chilh.* **134**: 377–9, 1980.
83. McGrath, B.P., Ibels, L.S., Raik, E. *et al.* Erythroid toxicity of azathioprine: Macrocytosis and selective marrow hypoplasia. *Q. J. Med.* **44**: 57–63, 1975.
84. Medberry, C.A., Pappas, A.A. & Ackerman, B.H. Carbamazepine and erythroid arrest. *Drug. Intell. Clin. Pharm.* **21**: 439–41, 1987.
85. McCulloch, D., Jackson, J.M. & Verneys, J. Drug induced red cell aplasia. *Br. Med. J.* **iv**: 163–4, 1974.
86. Ozer, F.L., Truax, W.E. & Levin, W.C. Erythroid hypoplasia associated with chloramphenicol therapy. *Blood* **16**: 997, 1960.
87. Planas, A.T., Kranwinkel, R.N., Soletsky, H.B. & Pezzimenti, J.F. Chlorpropamide-induced pure red cell aplasia. *Arch. Int. Med.* **140**: 707–8, 1980.
88. Stephens, M.E. Transient erythroid hypoplasia in a patient on long-term co-trimoxazole therapy. *Postgrad. Med. J.* **50**: 235–7, 1974.
89. Unter, C.E. & Abbot, G.D. Co-trimoxazole red cell aplasia in leukaemia. *Arch. Dis. Childh.* **62**: 85–7, 1987.
90. Yune-Gill, J., Jung, Y. & River, G.L. Pure RBC aplasia and diphenylhydantoin. *J. Am. Med. Assoc.* **229**: 314–15, 1974.
91. Dessypris, E.N., Redline, S., Harris, J.W. & Krantz, S.B. Diphenylhydantoin-induced pure red cell aplasia. *Blood* **65**: 789–94, 1985.

92. Michalevicz, R., Baron, S. & Blum, I. Fenbufen induced pure red cell aplasia in rheumatoid arthritis. *J. Rheumatol.* **14**: 1174–6, 1987.
93. Weinberger, K.A. Fenoprofen and red cell aplasia. *J. Rheumatol.* **6**: 475, 1979.
94. Reitz, C.L. & Bottomley, S.S. Pure red cell aplasia associated with fenoprofen. *Am. J. Med. Sci.* **287**: 62–3, 1984.
95. Reid, G. & Patterson, A.L. Pure red cell aplasia after gold treatment. *Br. Med. J.* **ii**: 1457, 1977.
96. Clairborne, R.A. & Dutt, A.K. Isoniazid-induced pure red cell aplasia. *Am. Rev. Respir. Dis.* **131**: 947–9, 1985.
97. Lewis, C.R. & Manoharan, A. Pure red cell hypoplasia secondary to isoniazid. *Postgrad. Med. J.* **63**: 309–10, 1987.
98. Itoh, W., Wong, P., Asai, T. *et al.* Pure red cell aplasia induced by alpha methyl dopa. *Am. J. Med.* **84**: 1088–9, 1988.
99. Bollan, J.L., Hussein, S., Hoffbrand, A.V. & Sherlock, S. Red cell aplasia following prolonged D-penicillamine therapy. *J. Clin. Pathol.* **29**: 135–9, 1976.
100. Arneborn, P. & Palmblad, J. Drug-induced neutropenia – a survey for Stockholm, 1973–1978. *Acta Med. Scand.* **212**: 289–92, 1982.
101. Young, G.A.R. & Vincent, P. Drug induced agranulocytosis. *Clin. Haematol.* **9**(3): 483–504, 1980.
102. Hartl, P.W. Drug induced agranulocytosis. In *Blood Disorders due to Drugs and Other Agents* (ed. R.H. Girdwood, *Excerpta Medica*, pp. 147–86. Amsterdam, 1973.
103. Young, G.A., Croaker, G. & Vincent, P.C. *et al.* The CFU-C assay in patients with neutropenia and, in particular, drug associated neutropenia. *Clin. Lab. Haematol.* **9**: 245–53, 1987.
104. Fibbe, W.E., Claas, P.F.H. & Van Der Star-Dijkstraw. Agranulocytosis induced by propylthiouracil: evidence of a drug dependent antibody reacting with granulocytes, monocytes and haemopoietic progenitor cells. *Br. J. Haematol.* **64**: 363–73, 1986.
105. Editorial. Antibiotic-induced neutropenia. *Lancet* **ii**: 814, 1985.
106. Murphy, M.F., Riordan, T., Minchinton, R.M. *et al.* Demonstration of an immune-mediated mechanism of penicillin-induced neutropenia and thrombocytopenia. *Br. J. Haematol.* **55**: 155–60, 1985.
107. Milsteen, S., Welik, R. & Heyman, M.R. Case report: Prolonged vancomycin-associated neutropenia in a chronic hemodialysis patient. *Am. J. Med. Sci.* **294**, 110–13, 1987.
108. Neftel, K.A., Hauser, S.P. & Muller, M. Inhibition of granulopoiesis in vivo and in vitro by β-lactam antibiotics. *J. Infect. Dis.* **152**, 90–7, 1985.
109. Draper, B.M. & Manoharan, A. Neutropenia with cross intolerance between two tricyclic antidepressant agents. *Med. J. Aust.* **146**: 452–3, 1987.
110. Stamm, O., Siebenmann, R., Bigler, R. & Flury, R. Agranulocytosis in the newborn. *Gynaecologia (Basel)* **159**(5): 266–8, 1965.
111. Huguley, C.M. Drug induced blood dyscrasia II Agranulocytosis. *J. Am. Med. Assoc.* **188**: 817–18, 1964.
112. Discombe, G. Agranulocytosis caused by amidopyrine (aminopyrine): avoidable cause of death. *Br. Med. J.* **i**: 1270–1, 1952.
113. International Agranulocytosis and Aplastic Anaemia Study. Risks of agranulocytosis and aplastic anemia: a first report of their relation to drug use with special reference to analgesics. *J. Am. Med. Assoc.* **256**: 1749–57, 1986.
114. Editorial. Analgesics, agranulocytosis and aplastic anaemia: a major case control study. *Lancet* **ii**: 899–900, 1986.
115. Anon. Phenylbutazone, oxyphenbutazone labeling revised. *FDA Drug Bull.* **14**: 23–4, 1984.
116. Pisciotta, V. Drug-induced agranulocytosis. *Drugs* **15**: 132–43, 1978.
117. Editorial. Dipyrone hearing by the German drug authority. *Lancet* **ii**: 737, 1986.

118. Bharani, A.K., Mehta, R.S. & Sanghvi, V.C. Do we continue to prescribe dipyrone (Analgin)? *J. Assoc. Physician India* **32**: 382–3, 1984.
119. Smadel, J.E. & Jackson, E.B. Chloromycetin, an antibiotic with chemotherapeutic activity in experimental and viral infections: *Science* **106**: 418–19, 1944.
120. O'Brien, W.M. & Bagby, G.F. Rare adverse reactions to nonsteroidal antinflammatory drugs. *J. Rheumatol.* **12**: 347–53, 1985.
121. Hynd, R.F., Klofkorn, R.W., Sholes, C.W. & Moquin, R.B. Neutropenia and pseudomonas septicemia after sulindac therapy: a case report. *Milit. Med.* **147**: 768–9, 1982.
122. Romeril, K.R., Duke, D.A. & Hollings, P.E. Sulindac induced agranulocytosis and bone marrow culture. *Lancet* **ii**: 523, 1981.
123. Mamus, S.W., Burton, J.D., Groat, J.D. *et al.* Ibuprofen-associated pure white cell aplasia. *N. Engl. J. Med.* **314**: 624–5, 1986.
124. Van der Laan, W.P. & Storrie, V.M. A survey of the factors controlling thyroid function with especial reference to newer views on antithyroid substances. *Pharmacol. Rev.* **7**: 301–34, 1955.
125. Cooper, D.S. Antithyroid drugs. *N. Engl. J. Med.* **311**: 1353–62, 1984.
126. International Agranulocytosis and Aplastic Anaemia Study. Risk of agranulocytosis and aplastic anaemia in relation to antithyroid drugs. *Br. Med. J.* **ii**: 262–5, 1988.
127. Cooper, D.A., Goldminz, D., Levin, A.A. *et al.* Agranulocytosis associated with antithyroid drugs. Effects of patients age and drug dose. *Ann. Intern. Med.* **98**: 26–9, 1983.
128. Berkman, E.M., Orlin, J.B. & Wolfsdorf, J. An antineutrophil antibody associated with a propylthiouracil-induced lupus-like syndrome. *Transfusion* **23**: 135–8, 1983.
129. Ascensado, J.L., Flynn, P.J., Slungaard, A. *et al.* Quinidine-induced neutropenia: report of a case with drug-dependent inhibition of granulocyte colony generation. *Acta Haematol. (Basel)* **72**: 349–54, 1984.
130. Alexander, S.J. & Gilmore, R.I. Quinidine induced agranulocytosis. *Am. J. Haematol.* **16**: 95–8, 1984.
131. Chong, B.J., Berndt, M.C., Koutts, J. & Castaldi, P.A. Quinine induced thrombocytopenia and leukopenia: demonstration and characterisation of distinct antiplatelet and antileukocyte antibodies. *Blood* **62**: 1218–25, 1983.
132. Berger, B.E. & Hauser, D.J. Agranulocytosis due to sustained-release procainamide. *Am. Heart J.* **105**: 1035–6, 1983.
133. Ellroat, A.G., Murata, G.H., Predinger, M.S. *et al.* Severe neutropenia associated with sustained-release procainamide. *Ann. Intern. Med.* **100**: 197–201, 1984.
134. Christenen, D.J., Palma, L.F. & Phelps, K. Agranulocytosis, thrombocytopenia and procainamide. *Ann. Intern. Med.* **100**: 918, 1984.
135. Meyers, D.G., Gonzalez, E.R., Peters, L.L. *et al.* Severe neutropenia associated with procainamide: comparison of sustained release and conventional preparations. *Am. Heart J.* **109**: 1393–5, 1985.
136. Volosin, K., Greenberg, R.M. & Greenspon, A.J. Tocainide associated agranulocytosis. *Am. Heart J.* **109**: 1392–3, 1985.
137. Oliphant, L.D. & Goddard, M. Tocainide associated neutropenia and lupus-like syndrome. *Chest* **94**: 427–8, 1988.
138. Dery, C.L. & Schwinghammer, T.L. Agranulocytosis associated with sulfasalazine. *Drug Intell. Clin. Pharm.* **22**: 139–42, 1988.
139. Mitrane, M.P., Singh, A. & Siebold, J.R. Cholestasis and fatal agranulocytosis complicating sulfasalazine therapy: case report and review of the literature. *J. Rheumatol.* **13**: 969–72, 1986.
140. Farr, J., Symmons, D.P., Blake, D.R. & Bacon, P.A. Neutropenia in patients

with inflammatory arthritis treated with sulfasalazine. *Ann. Rheum. Dis.* **45**: 761–4, 1986.

141. Principi, N., Marchisio, P., Biasini, A. *et al.* Early and late neutropenia in children treated with cotrimoxazole (trimethoprim-sulfamethoxazole). *Acta Paediatr. Scand.* **731**: 763–7, 1984.
142. Jaffe, I.A. The adverse effects profile of sulfydryl compounds in man. *Am. J. Med.* **80**: 471–4, 1986.
143. Vmeki, S., Konish, Y., Yasuda, T. *et al.* D-penicillamine and neutrophilic agranulocytosis. *Arch. Intern. Med.* **145**: 2271–2, 1985.
144. Ward, K. & Weir, D.G. Life threatening agranulocytosis and toxic epidermal necrolysis during low dose penicillamine therapy. *Ir. J. Med. Sci.* **150**: 252–3, 1981.
145. Heimpel, J. & Heit, W. Drug induced aplastic anaemia: clinical aspects. *Clin. Haematol.* **9**(3): 41662, 1980.
146. Weiss, A.S., Markenson, J.A., Weiss, M.S. & Kammerer, W.H. Toxicity of D-penicillamine in rheumatoid arthritis. A report of 63 patients including two with aplastic anaemia and one with nephrotic syndrome. *Am. J. Med.* **64**: 114–20, 1978.
147. Irvin, J.D. & Kiav, J.M. Safety profiles of the angiotensin converting enzyme inhibitors captopril and enalapril. *Am. J. Med.* **81**: (suppl. 4C) 46–50, 1986.
148. Suarez, M., Ho, P.W., Johnson, E.S. & Perez, G. Angioneurotic edema agranulocytosis and fatal septicemia following captopril. *Am. J. Med.* **81**: 336–8, 1986.
149. Kirchz, E.J. Angioeneurotic edema, granulocytosis and fatal septicaemia following captopril. *Am. J. Med.* **82**: 576–8, 1987.
150. Murphy, M.F., Metcalf, P., Grant, P.C.A. *et al.* Cephalosporin-induced immune neutropenia. *Br. J. Haematol.* **59**: 9–14, 1985.
151. Adrouny, A., Meguerditchan, S., Koo, Ch. *et al.* Agranulocytosis related to vancomycin therapy. *Am. J. Med.* **81**: 1059–61, 1986.
152. Farwell, A.P., Kendall, L.G., Viki, R.D. and Glen, R.H. Delayed appearance of vancomycin induced neutropenia in a patient with chronic renal failure. *South. Med. J.* **77**: 664–5, 1984.
153. Rouveix, B., Cowlombel, L., Aymard, J.P. *et al.* Amodiaquine-induced immune agranulocytosis. *Br. J. Haematol.* **71**: 7–11, 1989.
154. Hatton, C.S.R., Peto, T.E.A., Bunch, C. *et al.* Frequency of severe neutropenia associated with amodiaquine prophylaxis against malaria. *Lancet* **i**: 411–14, 1986.
155. Carr, R. Neutropenia and prophylactic amodiaquine. *Lancet* **i**: 556, 1986.
156. Rhodes, E.G.H., Ball, J. & Franklin, I.M. Amodiaquine induced agranulocytosis inhibition of colony growth in bone-marrow by anti-malarial agents. *Br. Med. J.* **292**: 717–18, 1986.
157. Notes and News: Amodiaquine and agranulocytosis. *Lancet* **i**: 456, 1986.
158. Bruce-Chwatt, L.J. & Huchinson, D.B.A. Maloprim and agranulocytosis. *Lancet* **ii**: 1487–8.
159. Friman, G., Nystrm-Rosander, C., Jonsell, G. *et al.* Agranulocytosis associated with malaria prophylaxis with maloprim. *Br. Med. J.* **286**: 1244–5, 1983.
160. Ducomb, L. & Baldessarini, R.J. Timing and risk of bone marrow depression by psychotropic drugs. *Am. J. Psychiat.* **134**: 1294–5, 1977.
161. Shabry, F. & Wolk, J.A. Granulocytopenia in children after phenothiazine therapy. *Am. J. Psychiat.* **137**: 374–5, 1980.
162. Clink, H.M. Mianserin and blood dyscrasia. *Br. J. Clin. Pharmacol.* **15**: 291–3 S, 1983.
163. Notes and News: Legal battle over mianserin. *Br. Med. J.* **298**: 479, 1989.
164. Meharg, A.M. & McHare, J. Leucopenia in association with mianserin treatment. *Br. Med. J.* **i**: 623–4, 1979.
165. Curson, D.A. & Hale, A.S. Mianserin and agranulocytosis. *Br. Med. J.* **i**: 378–9, 1979.

166. Organon International BV: Mianserin and blood dyscrasia. A position paper, updated December 1986.
167. O'Donnell, J.L., Sharman, J., Begg, E.J. *et al.* Positive mechanism for mianserin induced neutropenia associated with saturable elimination kinetics. *Br. Med. J.* **ii**: 1375—6, 1985.
168. Adams, P.C., Robinson, A., Reid, M.M. *et al.* Blood dyscrasias and mianserin. *Postgrad. Med. J.* **59**: 31–3, 1983.
169. Vipan, W.H. Quinine as a cause of purpura. *Lancet* **ii**: 37, 1865.
170. Ackroyd, J.F. The pathogenesis of thrombocytopenic purpura due to hypersensitivity to Sedormid. *Clin. Sci.* **7**: 249, 1949.
171. Miescher, P.A. & Graf, J. Drug-induced thrombocytopenia. *Clin. Haematol.* **9**(3): 505–19, 1980.
172. Shulman, N.R. Immunoreactions involving platelets. I. A steric and kinetic model for formation of a complex from a human antibody, quinidine as a haptene, and platelets, and for fixation of complement by the complex. *J. Exp. Med.* **107**: 665, 1958.
173. Van Leevwen, E.F., Engelfreit, C.P. & Von Dem Borne, A.E.G. Studies on quinine- and quinidine-dependent antibodies against platelets and their reaction with platelets in the Bernard-Soulier syndrome. *Br. J. Haematol.* **51**: 551–60, 1982.
174. Lerner, W., Caruso, R, Faig, D. & Karpatkins. Drug-dependent and non-drug-dependent antiplatelet antibody in drug-induced thrombocytopenic purpura. *Blood* **66**: 306–11, 1985.
175. Kunicki, T.J., Johnson, M.M. & Aster, R.H. Absence of the platelet receptor for drug dependent antibodies in the Bernard Soulier Syndrome. *J. Clin. Invest.* **62**: 712–19, 1978.
176. Stricker, R.B. & Shuman, M.A. Quinidine purpura: evidence that glycoprotein V is a target platelet antigen. *Blood* **67**: 1377–81, 1986.
177. Danielson, D.A., Douglas, S.W., Hertzog, P. et al. Drug induced blood disorders. *J. Am. Med. Ass.* **252**: 3257–60, 1984.
178. King, D.J. & Kelton, J.G. Heparin associated thrombocytopenia. *Ann. Intern. Med.* **100**: 535–40, 1984.
179. Bell, W.R., Tomasulo, P.A., Alving, B.N. & Duffy, T.P. Thrombocytopenia occurring during the administration of heparin: a prospective study in 52 patients. *Ann. Intern. Med.* **85**: 155–60, 1976.
180. Bell, W.R. & Royall, R.N. Heparin-associated thrombocytopenia: a comparison of 3 heparin preparations. *N. Engl. J. Med.* **303**: 902–7, 1980.
181. Kelton, J.G., Sheridan, D., Santos, A. *et al.* Heparin-induced thrombocytopenia: laboratory studies. *Blood* **72**: 925–30, 1988.
182. Cines, D.B., Tomaski, A. & Tannenbaum, S. Immune endothelial-cell injury in heparin associated thrombocytopenia. *N. Engl. J. Med.* **316**: 581–9, 1987.
183. Huisee, M.-G., Guillin, M.-C. Bezeaud, A. *et al.* Heparin associated thrombocytopenia: *in vitro* effects of different molcecular weight heparin fractions. *Thromb. Res.* **27**: 485–90, 1982.
184. Leroy, J., Leclerc, M.H., Delahousse, B. *et al.* Treatment of heparin-associated thrombocytopenia and thrombosis with low molecular weight heparin (CY216). *Semin. Thromb. Hemost.* **11**: 326–9, 1985.
185. Horellou, M.H., Conard, J., Lecrubier, C. *et al.* Persistant heparin induced thrombocytopenia despite therapy with low molecular weight heparin. *Thromb. Haemost.* **51**, 134, 1984.
186. Heeger, P.A. & Backstrom, J.T. Heparin flushes and thrombocytopenia. *Ann. Intern. Med.* **105**: 143, 1986.
187. Phillips, Y.Y., Copley, J.B. & Stor, R.A. Thormbocytopenia and low-dose heparin. *South Med. J.* **76**: 526–8, 1983.
188. Szklo, M., Sensenbrenner, L., Markowitz, J. *et al.* Incidence of aplastic anaemia

in metropolitan Baltimore: a population based study. *Blood* **66**: 115–19, 1985.

189. Young, N.S., Issaragrasil, S., Chieh, C.W. & Takaku, F. Annotation: aplastic anaemia in the orient. *Br. J. Haematol.* **62**: 1–6, 1986.

190. Custer, R.P. Aplastic anaemia in soldiers treated with atabrine (quinacrine). *Am. J. Med. Sci.* **212**: 211–24, 1946.

191. Rich, M.L., Ritterhuf, R.J. & Hoffman, R.L. Fatal case of aplastic anaemia following chloramphenicol (choromycetin) therapy. *Ann. Intern. Med.* **33**, 1459–61, 1950.

192. Fraunfelder, F.T., Bagby, G.C. & Kelly, D.J. Fatal aplastic anaemia following topical administration of opthalmic chloramphenicol. *Am. J. Ophthal.* **G3**: 356–60, 1982.

193. Williams, D.M., Lynch, R. & Cartwright, G.F. Drug induced aplastic anaemia. *Semin. Hematol.* **10**: 195–223, 1973.

194. Hagler, L.J., Pastore, R.A. & Bergin, J.J. Aplastic anaemia following virus hepatitis. *Medicine* **54**: 139–63, 1975.

195. Gordon-Smith, E.C. (ed.) Aplastic anaemia. In *Clinical Haematology*, Vol. 2, No. 1. Baillière Tindall, London, 1989.

196. Inman, W.H.W. Para 11. Study of fatal bone marrow depression with special reference to phenylbutazone and oxyphenbutazone. *Br. Med. J.* **i**: 1500–5, 1973.

197. Willame, L.M., Joos, R., Proot, F. & Immesoete, C. Gold induced aplastic anemia. *Clin. Rheumatol.* **6**: 600–5, 1987.

198. Baldwin, J.L., Storb, R., Thomas, E.D. & Mannik, M. Bone marrow transplantation in patients with gold induced marrow aplasia. *Arthr. Rheum.* **20**: 1943–8, 1977.

199. Prchal, J.Y., Huang, S.T., Court, W.S. & Poon, M.L. Immune hemolytic anemia following administration of antithymocyte globulin. *Am. J. Hematol.* **19**: 95–8, 1985.

200. Patmas, M.A., Wilbourn, S.L. & Shankel, S.W. Acute multisystem toxicity associated with the use of non-steroidal anti-inflammatory drugs. *Arch. Intern. Med.* **144**: 519–21, 1984.

201. Duran Suarez, J.R., Martin-Vega, C. & Argelagues, E. The I antigen as an immune complex receptor in a case of haemolytic anaemia induced by an antihistamine agent. *Br. J. Haematol.* **49**: 153–4, 1981.

202. Albazzaz, M.K., Harvey, J.E., Hoffman, J.N. & Siddorn, J.A. Alveolitis and haemolytic anaemia induced by azapropazone. *Br. Med. J.* **293**: 1537–8, 1986.

203. Luderer, J.R., Schoolwerth, A.C., Sinicrope, R.A. *et al.* Acute renal failure, hemolytic anemia and skin rash associated with captopril therapy. *Am. J. Med.* **71**: 493–6, 1981.

204. Stroink, A.R., Skillrud, D.M., Kiely, J.M. & Sundt, T.M. Jr. Carbamazepine-induced haemolytic anaemia. *Acta Haematol. (Basel)* **72**: 356–8, 1984.

205. Salama, A., Northoff, H., Burkhardt, H. & Mueller-Eckhardt, C. Carbimazole induced immune haemolytic anaemia: role of drug–red blood cell complexes for immunization. *Br. J. Haematol.* **68**: 479–82, 1988.

206. Branch, D.R., Berkowitz, L.R., Becker, R.C. *et al.* Extravascular hemolysis following the administration of cefamandole. *Am. J. Hematol.* **18**: 213–19, 1985.

207. Anon. Hemolytic anemia and pancytopenia induced by cefoxitin. *Drug Intell. Clin. Pharm.* **17**: 816–19, 1983.

208. Or, R., Merin, E., Stupp, Y. & Matzner, Y. Chlorpropamide-induced hemolytic anemia. *Drug Intell. Clin. Pharm.* **18**: 981–2, 1984.

209. Susler, S.D., Behzad, O., Garratty, G. *et al.* Acute hemolytic anemia associated with chlorpropamide-induced apparent auto-anti-Jka. *Transfusion* **24**: 206–9, 1984.

210. Saffouri, B., Cho, J.H. & Felber, N. Chlorpropamide-induced haemolytic anaemia. *Postgrad. Med. J.* **57**: 44–5, 1981.

211. Rate, R., Bonnell, M., Chervenak, C. & Paviniuf, G. Cimetidine and

hematologic effects. *Ann. Intern. Med.* **91**: 795, 1979.

212. Petz, L.D., Gitlin, N., Grant, K. *et al.* Cimetidine induced hemolytic anemia: the fallacy of clinical associations. *J. Clin. Gastroenterol.* **5**: 405–9, 1983.

213. Wollheim, F.A., Ljund, G., Gren, H.O. & Blum-Bulow, B. Hemolytic anaemia during cyclofenil treatment of scleroderma. *Acta Med. Scand.* **210**: 429–30, 1981.

214. Russell, M.L. & Schachter, R.K.L Cyclofenil induced hemolytic anaemia in scleroderma. *Acta Med. Scand.* **210**: 431–2, 1981.

215. Kramer, M.R., Levene, C. & Hershko, C. Severe reversible autoimmune haemolytic anaemia and thrombocytopenia associated with diclofenac therapy. *Scand. J. Haematol.* **36**: 118–20, 1986.

216. Samoszuk, M., Reid, M.E. & Toy, P.T. Intravenous dimethylsulfoxide therapy causes severe hemolysis mimicking a hemolytic transfusion reaction. *Transfusion* **23**: 405, 1985.

217. Ribera, A., Monasterio, J., Alebedo, G. *et al.* Dipyrone induced immune haemolytic anaemia. *Vox Sang* **41**: 32–5, 1981.

218. Wong, K.Y., Boose, G.M. & Issitt, C.H. Erythromycin induced hemolytic anemia. *J. Pediatr.* **98**: 647–9, 1981.

219. Martland, T. & Stone, W.D. Haemolytic anaemia associated with fenbufen. *Br. Med. J.* **297**: 921, 1988.

220. Shirley, R.S., Morton, S.J., Lawton, K.B. *et al.* Fenoprofen induced immune hemolysis. Difficulties in diagnosis and complications in compatibility testing. *Am. J. Clin. Pathol.* **89**: 410–14, 1988.

221. Bell, P.M. & Humphrey, C.A. Thrombocytopenia and haemolytic anaemia due to feprazone. *Br. Med. J.* **284**: 17, 1982.

222. Sandvei, P., Nordhagen, R., Michaelsen, T.E. & Wolthuis, K. Fluouracil (5FU) induced acute immune haemolytic anaemia. *Br. J. Haematol.* **65**: 357–9, 1987.

223. Nataas, O.B. & Nesthus, I. Immune haemolytic anaemia induced by glibenclamide in selective IgA deficiency. *Br. Med. J.* **295**: 366–7, 1987.

224. Beck, M.C., Cline, J.F., Hardman, J.T. *et al.* Fatal intravascular immune hemolysis induced by hydrochlorthiazide. *Am. J. Clin. Pathol.* **81**: 791–4, 1984.

225. Shirley, R.S., Bartholomew, J., Bell, W. *et al.* Characterization of antibody and selection of alternative drug therapy in hydrochlorthiazide induced immune hemolytic anemia. *Transfusion* **28**: 70–2, 1988.

226. Garratty, G., Houston, M., Petz, L.D. & Webb, M. Acute immune intravascular hemolysis due to hydrochlorthiazide. *Am. J. Clin. Pathol.* **76**: 73–8, 1981.

227. Korsager, S. Haemolysis complicating ibuprofen treatment. *Br. Med. J.* **i**: 79, 1978.

228. Law, I.P., Wickman, C.J. & Harrison, B.R. Coombs positive hemolytic anemia and ibuprofen. *South Med. J.* **72**: 707–10, 1979.

229. Guidry, J.B., Ogburn, C.L. & Griffin, F.M. Fatal autoimmune hemolytic anemia associated with ibuprofen. *J. Am. Med. Assoc.* **242**: 68–9, 1979.

230. Umstead, G.S., Babiak, L.M. & Teswani, S. Immune hemolytic anemia associated with ketoconazole therapy. *Clin. Pharmacol.* **6**: 499–500, 1988.

231. Wooley, P.V., Sacher, R.A., Priego, V.M. *et al.* Methotrexate induced immune haemolytic anaemia. *Br. J. Haematol.* **54**: 543–52, 1983.

232. Hughes, J.A. & Sudell, W. Hemolytic anemia associated with naproxen. *Arthr. Rheum.* **26**: 1054, 1983.

233. Kickler, T.S., Buck, S., Ness, P. *et al.* Probenecid induced immune hemolytic anemia. *J. Rheumatol.* **13**: 208–9, 1986.

234. Sosler, S.D., Behzad, O., Garratty, G. *et al.* Immune hemolytic anemia associated with probenecid. *Am. J. Clin. Pathol.* **84**: 391–4, 1985.

235. Schifman, R.B., Garewal, H. & Shillington, D. Reticulocytopenic Coombs' positive anemia induced by procainamide. *Am. J. Clin. Pathol.* **80**: 66–8, 1983.

236. Criel, A. & Verwilgehn, R.L. Intravascular haemolysis and renal failure caused by intermittent rifampicin treatment. *Blut* **40**: 147–50, 1980.

237. Mechanik, J.I. Coombs' positive hemolytic anemia following sulfa-salazine therapy in ulcerative colitis; case reports, review and discussion of pathogenesis. *Mt. Sinai J. Med. (N.Y.)* **52**: 667–70, 1985.
238. Kopicky, J.A. & Packman, C.H. The mechanism of sulfonylurea induced immune hemolysis: case report and review of the literature. *Am. J. Hematol.* **23**: 283–8, 1986.
239. Johnson, F.P. Jr, Hamilton, H.E. & Liesch, M.R. Immune hemolytic anemia associated with sulindac. *Arch. Intern. Med.* **145**: 1515–16, 1985.
240. Mintz, P.D., Andreson, G. & Clark, S. Immune hemolytic anemia associated with sulindac. *Arch. Intern. Med.* **146**: 1639, 1986.
241. Habibi, B., Lopez, M., Serdau, M. *et al.* Immune hemolytic anemia and renal failure due to teniposide. *N. Engl. J. Med.* **306**: 1091–3, 1982.
242. Habibi, B., Baumelou, A. & Seradaru, M. Acute intravascular hemolysis and renal failure due to teniposide related antibody. *Lancet* **i**: 1423–4, 1981.
243. Mazza, J.J. & Kryda, M.D. Tetracycline induced hemolytic anemia. *J. Am. Acad. Derm.* **2**: 506–8, 1980.
244. Simpson, M.B., Pryzbylik, J., Innis, B. & Denham, M.A. Hemolytic anemia after tetracycline therapy. *N. Engl. J. Med.* **312**: 840–2, 1985.
245. Habibi, B., Basty, R., Chodez, S. & Prunat, A. Thiopental related immune hemolytic anemia and renal failure. Specific involvement of red cell antigen I. *N. Engl. J. Med.* **312**: 353–5, 1985.
246. Seldon, M.R., Bain, B., Johnson, C.A. & Lennox, C.S. Ticarcillin induced immune haemolytic anaemia. *Scand. J. Haematol.* **28**: 459–60, 1982.
247. Squires, J.E., Mintz, P.D. & Clark, S. Tolmelin induced hemolysis. *Transfusion* **25**: 410–13, 1985.
248. Takahashi, H. & Tsukada, T. Triamterene induced immune haemolytic anaemia with acute intravascular haemolysis and acute renal failure. *Scand. J. Haematol.* **23**: 169–76, 1979.
249. Böttiger, L.E. & Westerholm, B. Drug induced blood dyscrasias in Sweden. *Br. Med. J.* **iii**: 339–43, 1973.
250. Heit, W.F. Hematologic effects of antipyretic analgesics. Drug induced agranulocytosis. *Am. J. Med.* **75**: 65–9, 1983.
251. Yudkin, J.S. Ciba-Geigy, amidopyrine and the Third World. *Lancet* **ii**: 114, 1981.
252. Shinar, E. & Hershko, C. Causes of agranulocytosis in a hospital population – identification of dipyrone as an important causative agent. *Isr. J. Med. Sci.* **19**: 225–9, 1983.
253. Gualda, N. & Malinvaud, G. *In vitro* generation of cytotoxic lymphocytes during noramidopyrine induced agranulocytosis. *Clin. Immunol. Immunopathol.* **24**: 220–6, 1982.
254. McLean, C.A., Begley, C.G. & Harris, R.A. Diflunisal-induced neutropenia. *Aust. NZ J. Med.* **16**: 811–12, 1986.
255. Treusch, P.J., Woelke, B.J., Lechtman, D. *et al.* Agranulocytosis associated with fenoprofen. *J. Am. Med. Assoc.* **241**: 2700–1, 1979.
256. Simon, S.D. & Kosmin, M. Fenoprofen and agranulocytosis. *N. Engl. J. Med.* **299**: 490, 1978.
257. Aaron, S., Davis, P. & Percy, J. Neutropenia occurring during the course of chrysotherapy; a review of 25 cases. *J. Rheumatol.* **12**: 897–9, 1985.
258. Hakala, M., Timonen, T.T., Rossi, O. *et al.* Agranulocytosis in a patient with psoriatic arthritis receiving auranofin and ibuprofen. *Scand. J. Rheumatol.* **16**: 375–6, 1987.
259. Nygard, N. & Starkebaum, G. Naproxen and agranulocytosis. *J. Am. Med. Assoc.* **257**: 1732, 1987.
260. Umeki, S., Konishi, Y., Yasuda, T. *et al.* D-Penicillamine and neutrophilic agranulocytosis. *Arch. Intern. Med.* **145**: 2271–2, 1985.
261. Sheehan, M., Hyland, R.H. & Norman, C. Pentazocine induced agranulo-

cytosis. *Can Med. Assoc. J.* **1232**: 1401, 1985.
262. Haibach, H., Yesus, Y.W. & Doggett, J.J. Pentazocine induced agranulocytosis. *Can. Med. Assoc. J.* **130**: 1165–6, 1984.
263. Marks, A. & Abramson, N. Pentazocine and agranulocytosis. *Ann. Intern. Med.* **92**: 433, 1980.
264. Morris, E.L., Hochberg, M.C. & Dorsch, C.H. Agranulocytosis and sulindac. *Arthr. Rheum.* **24**: 752–3, 1981.
265. Sakai, J. & Joseph, M.W. Tolmetin and agranulocytosis. *N. Engl. J. Med.* **298**: 1203, 1978.
266. Kohler, G.D. Anti-arrhythmic agents and agranulocytosis. *Lancet* **i**: 1415–16, 1980.
267. Opie, L.H. Aprindine and agranulocytosis. *Lancet* **ii**: 689–90, 1980.
268. Pisciotta, A.V. & Cronkite, C. Aprindine induced agranulocytosis. Evidence for immunologic mechanism. *Arch. Intern. Med.* **143**: 241–3, 1983.
269. Samlowski, W.E., Frame, R.N. & Logue, G.L. Flecanide-induced immune neutropenia. Documentation of a hapten mediated mechanism of cell destruction. *Arch. Intern. Med.* **147**: 383–4, 1987.
270. Dover, D. & Eisensten, Z. Methimazole induced agranulocytosis: growth inhibition of myeloid progenetor cells by the patient's serum. *Eur. J. Haematol.* **40**: 91–4, 1988.
271. Heimpel, H. The potential immune mechanism in a case of methimazole induced agranulocytosis. *Eur. J. Haematol.* **41**: 302, 1988.
272. Fincher, M.E., Fariss, B.L., Plymate, S.R. *et al.* Agranulocytosis and a small dose of methimazole. *Ann. Intern. Med.* **101**: 404, 1984.
273. Cooper, D.S., Daniels, E.H. & Ridgeway, E.C. Agranulocytosis and dose of methimazole. *Ann. Intern. Med.* **101**: 283, 1984.
274. Toth, E.L., Mant, M.J., Shivji, S. & Ginsberg, J. Propylthiouracil induced agranulocytosis: an unusual presentation and a possible mechanism. *Am. J. Med.* **85**: 725–7. 1988.
275. Guffy, N.M., Goeken, N.E. & Burns, C.P. Granulocytotoxic antibodies in a patient with propylthiouracil induced agranulocytosis. *Ann. Intern. Med.* **101**: 404–5, 1984.
276. Scmid, L., Heit, W. & Flury, R. Agranulocytosis associated with semi-synthetic penicillins and cephalosporins. Report of 7 cases. *Blut* **48**: 11–18, 1984.
277. Rouveiz, B., Lassoued, K., Vittecoq, D. & Regnier, B. Neutropenia due to beta lactamine antibodies. *Br. Med. J.* **287**: 1832–4, 1983.
278. Kirwood, C.F., Smith, L.L., Rustagi, P.K. & Schentag, J.J. Neutropenia associated with beta-lactam antibiotics. *Clin. Phamacol.* **2**: 569–78, 1983.
279. Ohsawa, T. & Furukawa, F. Neutropenia associated with cefotoxime. *Drug Intell. Clin. Pharm.* **17**: 739–41, 1983.
280. Thomas, M.C., Peat, B. & Lang, S.D. Neutropenia during therapy with ceftriaxone. *NZ Med. J.* **98**: 23–4, 1985.
281. Lawson, A.A., McArdle, T. & Ghosh, S. Cephradine associated immune neutropenia. *N. Engl. J. Med.* **312**: 651, 1985.
282. Revell, P., Nicholson, F. & Pearson, T.C. Granulocytopenia due to fusidic acid. *Lancet* **ii**: 454–5, 1988.
283. Evans, D.I. Granulocytopenia due to fusidic acid. *Lancet* **ii**: 851, 1988.
284. Patoia, L., Guerciolini, R., Menichetti, F. *et al.* Norfloxacin and neutropenia. *Ann. Intern. Med.* **107**: 788–9, 1984.
285. Kumar, K. & Kumar, A. Reversible neutropenia associated with ampicillin therapy in pediatric patients. *Drug Intell. Clin. Pharm.* **15**: 802–6, 1981.
286. Desgrandchamps, D. & Schnyder, C. Severe neutropenia in prolonged treatment with orally administered augmentin (amoxicillin/clavulanic acid). *Infection* **15**: 260–1, 1987.
287. Snavely, S.R., Helzberg, J.H., Bodensteiner, D.C. *et al.* Profound neutropenia

associated with benzyl penicillin. *South Med. J.* **76**: 1299–302, 1983.

288. Corbett, G.M., Perry, D.J. & Shaw, T.R.D. Penicillin-induced leukopenia. *N. Engl. J. Med.* **307**: 1642–3, 1982.

289. Gatell, J.M., Rello, J., Miro, J.M. *et al.* Cloxacillin induced neutropenia. *J. Infect. Dis.* **154**: 372, 1986.

290. Mallouh, A.A. Methicillin induced neutropenia. *Pediatr. Infect. Dis.* **4**: 262–4, 1985.

291. Kirkwood, C.F. & Lasezkay, G.M. Neutropenia associated with mezlocillin and piperacillin. *Drug Intell. Clin. Pharm.* **19**: 112–14, 1985.

292. Ohning, B.L., Reed, M.D., Doershuk, C.F. & Bwmer, J.L. Ticarcillin associated granulocytopenia. *Am. J. Dis. Childh.* **136**: 645–6, 1982.

293. Irvine, A.E., Morris, T.C., Kelly, A.J. & McCracken, N. Ticarcillin-induced neutropenia corroborated by *in vitro* CFU-C toxicity. *Acta Haematol. (Basel)* **70**: 364–8, 1983.

294. Wilson, P., George, R. & Raine, P. Topical silver sulphadiazine and profound neutropenia in a burned child. *Burns Incl. Therm. Inj.* **12**: 295–6, 1986.

295. Don, P.C., Kahn, T.A. & Bickers, D.L. Chloroquine induced neutropenia in a patient with dermatomyositis. *J. Am. Acad. Dermatol.* **16**: 629–30, 1987.

296. Olsen, V.V., Loft, S. & Christensen, K.D. Serious reactions during malaria prophylaxis with pyrimethamine-sulphadoxine. *Lancet* **ii**: 994, 1982.

297. Bonadonna, A., Bisetto, F., Munaretto, G. *et al.* Agranulocytosis during nifedepine treatment in a hemodialysis patient. *Nephron* **47**: 306–7, 1987.

298. Luchins, D.J. Fatal agranulocytosis in a chronic schizophrenic patient treated with carbamazepine. *Am. J. Psychiatry* **141**: 687–8, 1984.

299. Rush, J.A. & Beran, R.G. Leucopenia as an adverse reaction to carbamazepine therapy. *Med. J. Aust.* **140**: 426–8, 1984.

300. Burckart, G.J., Snidow, J. & Bruce, W. Neutropenia following acute chlorpromazine ingestion. *Clin. Toxicol.* **18**: 797–801, 1981.

301. Hardin, T.C. & Conrath, F.C. Desimipramine induced agranulocytosis. A case report. *Drug Intell. Clin. Pharm.* **16**: 62–3, 1982.

302. Doery, J.C., Meredith, H.A. & Mashford, M.L. Agranulocytosis associated with dothiepin. *Med. J. Aust.* **2**: 389–90, 1982.

303. Shabry, F. & Wolk, J.A. Granulocytopenia in children after phenothiazine therapy. *Am. J. Psychiatry* **137**: 374–5, 1980.

304. Yassa, R. Agranulocytosis in the course of phenothiazine therapy: case reports. *J. Clin. Psychiatry* **46**: 341–3, 1985.

305. Hardin, A.S. Chlorpheniramine and agranulocytosis. *Ann. Intern. Med.* **108**: 770, 1988.

306. Anger, B., Reichert, S. & Heimpel, H. Clozapine induced agranulocytosis. *Blut* **54**: 63–4, 1987.

307. Lieberman, J.A., Johns, C.H., Kane, J.M. *et al.* Clozapine induced agranulocytosis: non-cross-reactivity with other psychotropic drugs. *J. Clin. Psychiatry* **49**: 271–2, 1988.

308. Ward, S. & Meecham, J. Reversible agranulocytosis due to meprobamate. *Postgrad. Med. J.* **62**: 499–500, 1986.

309. Harvey, R.L. & Luzar, M.J. Metoclopramide induced agranulocytosis. *Ann. Intern. Med.* **108**: 214–15, 1988.

310. Lewis, D.S. & Beck, E.R. Reversible agranulocytosis in association with cimetidine and hepatic failure. *Postgrad. Med. J.* **58**: 443–4, 1982.

311. Seville, P. Cimetidine and agranulocytosis. *Med. J. Aust.* **1**: 250, 1982.

312. Fitchen, J.H. & Koeffler, H.P. Cimetidine and granulopoiesis: bone marrow culture studies in normal man and patients with cimetidine associated neutropenia. *Br. J. Haematol.* **46**: 361–6, 1980.

313. Brenner, L.D. Agranulocytosis and ranitidine. *Ann. Intern. Med.* **104**: 896–7, 1986.

314. List, A.F., Beaird, D.H. & Kismmett, T. Ranitidine induced granulocytopenia: recurrence with cimetidine administration. *Ann. Intern. Med.* **108**: 567–7, 1988.
315. Stricker, B.H., Meyboom, R.H., Bleeker, P.A. & Van Wieringen, K. Blood disorders associated with pirenzepine. *Br. Med. J.* **293**: 1074, 1986.
316. Levitt, L.J. Chlorpropamide induced pure white cell aplasia. *Blood* **69**: 394–400, 1987.
317. Kanefsy, T.M. & Medoff, S.J. Stevens-Johnson syndrome and neutropenia with chlorpropamide therapy. *Arch. Intern. Med.* **140**: 1543, 1980.
318. Liegener, K.B., Beck, E.M. & Rosenberg, A. Laetrile induced agranulocytosis. *J. Am. Med. Assoc.* **246**: 2841–2, 1981.
319. Anon. Severe neutropenia during pentamidine treatment of *Pneumocystis carinii* pneumonia in patients with acquired immunodeficiency syndrome – New York City. *Morbidity Mortality Weekly Rep.* **33**; 65–7, 1984.
320. Woodbury, D.M., Penry, J.K. & Schmidt, R.P. (eds) Symposium: *Anti-epileptic Drugs*. Raven Press, New York, 1972.
321. Symon, D.N. & Russell, G. Sodium valproate and neutropenia. *Arch. Dis. Childh.* **58**: 235, 1983.
322. Stricker, B.H. & Oei, T.T. Agranulocytosis caused by spironolactone. *Br. Med. J.* **289**: 731, 1984.
323. Buzdar, A.U., Fraschini, G. & Blumenschein, G.R. Hematologic adverse effects of aminoglutethimide. *Ann. Intern. Med.* **100**: 159, 1984.
324. Weinberger, I., Rotenberg, Z., Fuchs, J. *et al.* Amiodarone induced thrombocytopenia. *Arch. Intern. Med.* **147**: 735–6, 1987.
325. Chan, C.S., Tuazon, C.V. & Lessin, L.S. Amphotericin B induced thrombocytopenia. *Ann. Intern. Med.* **96**: 332–3, 1982.
326. Conti, L. & Gandolfo, G.M. Benzodiazepine induced thrombocytopenia. Demonstration of drug dependent platelet antibodies in two cases. *Acta Haematol. (Basel)* **70**: 386–8, 1983.
327. Baciewicz, G. & Yerevanian, B.I. Thrombocytopenia associated with carbamazepine: case report and review. *J. Clin. Psychiatry* **45**: 315–16, 1984.
328. Drury, I. & Vanderzant, C.W. Carbamazepine-induced isolated thrombocytopenia. *Am. J. Psychiatry* **145**: 1034, 1988.
329. Lown, J.A. & Barr, A.L. Immune thrombocytopenia induced by cephalosporins specific for thiomethyltetrozole side chain. *J. Clin. Pathol.* **40**: 700–10, 1987.
330. Mann, H.J, Schneider, J.R., Miller, J.B. & Delaney, J.P. Cimetidine associated thrombocytopenia. *Drug Intell. Clin. Pharm.* **17**: 126–8, 1983.
331. Rabinowe, S.N. & Miller, K.B. Danazol induced thrombocytopenia. *Br. J. Haematol.* **65**: 383–4, 1987.
332. Arrowsmith, J.B. & Dreis, M. Thrombocytopenia after treatment with danazol. *N. Engl. J. Med.* **315**: 585, 1986.
333. Kramer, M.R., Levene, R.C. & Hershko, C. Severe reversible autoimmune haemolytic anaemia and thrombocytopenia associated with diclofenac therapy. *Scand. J. Haematol.* **36**: 118–20, 1986.
334. Bobrove, A.M. Diflusinal associated thrombocytopenia in a patient with rheumatoid arthritis. *Arthr. Rheum.* **31**: 148–9, 1988.
335. Rabinovitz, M., Pitlik, S.D., Halevy, J. & Rosenfeld, J.B. Ethambutol induced thrombocytopenia. *Chest* **81**: 765–6, 1982.
336. Bell, P.M. & Humphrey, C.A. Thrombocytopenia and haemolytic anaemia due to feprazone. *Br. Med. J.* **i**: 17, 1982.
337. Duncan, A., Moore, S.B. & Barker, P. Thormbocytopenia caused by frusemide-induced platelet antibody. *Lancet* **i**: 1210, 1981.
338. Cicuttini, F.M., Wiley, J.S. & Fraser, K.J. Immune thrombocytopenia in association with oral gold treatment. *Arthr. Rheum.* **31**: 299–300, 1988.
339. Adachi, J.D., Bensen, W.G., Kassam, Y. *et al.* Gold induced thrombocytopenia. 12 cases and a review of the literature. *Semin. Arthr. Rheum.* **16**: 287–93, 1987.

340. Von dem Borne, A.E., Pegels, J.G., Van der Stadt, R.J. *et al.* Thrombocytopenia associated with gold therapy – a drug induced autoimmune disease? *Br. J. Haematol.* **63**: 509–16, 1986.
341. Okafor, K.C., Griffin, C. & Ngole, P.M. Hydrochlorthiazide induced thrombocytopenic purpura. *Drug Intell. Clin. Pharm.* **20**: 60–1, 1986.
342. Camba, L. & Joyner, M.V. Acute thrombocytopenia following ingestion of indomethacin. *Acta Haematol. (Basel)* **71**: 350–2, 1984.
343. Abdi, E.A. & Venner, P.M. Immune thrombocytopenia after alpha interferon therapy in patients with cancer. *J. Am. Med. Assoc.* **255**: 1878–9, 1986.
344. Pai, R.G. & Pai, S.M. Methyl-dopa-induced reversible immune thrombocytopenia. *Am. J. Med.* **85**: 123, 1988.
345. Stricker, B.J., Barendregt, J.N. & Claas, F.H. Thrombocytopenia and leucopenia with mianserin dependent antibodies. *Br. J. Clin. Pharmacol.* **19**: 102–4, 1985.
346. Cimo, P.L., Hammond, J.J. & Moake, J.L. Morphine induced immune thrombocytopenia. *Arch. Intern. Med.* **142**: 832–4, 1982.
347. Mayboom, R.H. Thrombocytopenia induced by nalidixic acid. *Br. Med. J.* **289**: 962, 1984.
348. Bjornstad, H. & Vik, O. Thrombocytopenic purpura associated with piroxicam. *Br. J. Clin. Pract.* **40**: 42, 1986.
349. Meisner, D.J., Carlson, R.J. & Gottlieb, A.S. Thrombocytopenia following sustained release procainamide. *Arch. Intern. Med.* **145**: 700–2, 1985.
350. Rosenstein, R., Kosfeld, R.E., Leight, L. & Liu, Y.K. Procainamide induced thrombocytopenia. *Am. J. Hematol.* **16**: 181–3, 1984.
351. Al Mondhiry, H., Pierce, W.S. & Basarab, R.M. Protamine induced thrombocytopenia and leukopenia. *Thromb. Haemost.* **53**: 60–4, 1985.
352. Gafter, U., Komlos, L., Weinstein, T. *et al.* Thrombocytopenia, eosinophilia and ranitidine. *Ann. Intern. Med.* **106**: 477, 1987.
353. Gibson, P.R. & Pidcock, M.E. Immune-mediated thrombocytopenia associated with ranitidine therapy. *Med. J. Aust.* **145**: 661–2, 1986.
354. Spychal, R.T. & Wickham, N.W. Thrombocytopenia associated with ranitidine. *Br. Med. J.* **291**: 1687, 1985.
355. Pau, A.K. & Fischer, M.A. Severe thrombocytopenia associated with once-daily rifampicin therapy. *Drug Intell. Clin. Pharm.* **21**: 882–4, 1987.
356. Karachalios, G.N. & Parigorakis, J.G. Thrombocytopenia and sulindac. *Ann. Intern. Med.* **104**: 128, 1986.
357. Pena, J.M., Gonzalez-Garga, J.J., Garga-Alegria, J. *et al.* Thrombocytopenia and sulfasalazine. *Ann. Intern. Med.* **102**: 277–8, 1985.
358. Wilde, J.T. & Prentice, A.G. Sulfamethoxazole-phenazopyridine and thrombocytopenia. *Ann. Intern. Med.* **104**: 128–9, 1986.
359. Barr, R.D., Copeland, S.A., Stockwell, M.L. *et al.* Valproic acid and immune thrombocytopenia. *Arch. Dis. Childh.* **57**: 681–4, 1982.
360. Walker, R.W. & Heaton, A. Thrombocytopenia due to vancomycin. *Lancet* **i**: 932, 1985.
361. McVie, S.G. Drug induced thrombocytopenia. In *Blood Disorders due to Drugs and other Agents* (ed. R.H. Girdwood), pp. 187–208. Excerpta Medica, Amsterdam, 1973.
362. Miescher, P.A. & Graf, J. Drug induced thrombocytopenia. *Clin. Haematol.* **9**: 505–19, 1980.
363. Hackett, T., Kelton, J.G. & Powers, P. Drug induced platelet destruction. *Semin. Thromb. Hemost.* **8**: 116–37, 1982.
364. Moss, R.A. Drug induced immune thrombocytopenia. *Am. J. Hematol.* **9**: 439–46, 1980.
365. Berndt, M.C. & Castaldi, P.A. Drug mediated thrombocytopenia. *Blood Rev.* **1**: 111–8, 1987.
366. Gerson, W.I., Fine, D.G., Spielberg, S.P. & Sensenbrenner, L.L. Anti-

convulsant induced aplastic anemia: increased susceptibility to toxic drug metabolites *in vitro*. *Blood* **61**: 889–93, 1983.

367. Foucauld, J., Uphouse, W. & Berenberg, J. Dapsone and aplastic anaemia. *Ann. Intern. Med.* **102**: 139, 1985.

368. Ashraf, M., Pearson, R.M. & Ninfield, D.A. Aplastic anaemia associated with fenoprofen. *Br. Med. J.* **i**: 1301–2, 1982.

369. Gryfe, C.I. & Rubenzahl, S. Agranulocytosis and aplastic anemia possibly due to ibuprofen. *Can. Med. Assoc. J.* **114**: 877, 1976.

370. Saal, J.G., Daniel, P.T., Berg, P.A. & Waller, H.D. Indoprofen-induced aplastic anaemia in systemic lupus, diagnosed by lymphocyte transformation tests. *Lancet* **i**: 1450–1, 1985.

371. Mangan, K.F., Ziadar, B., Shadduck, R.K. *et al.* Interferon induced aplastic anemia: evidence for T-cell mediated suppression of hematopoiesis and recovery after treatment with horse antihuman thymocyte globulin. *Am. J. Hematol.* **19**: 401–13, 1985.

372. Adams, P.C., Robinson, A., Reid, M.M. *et al.* Blood dyscrasias and mianserin. *Postgrad. Med. J.* **59**: 51–3, 1983.

373. Durrant, S. & Read, D. Fatal aplastic anaemia associated with mianserin. *Br. Med. J.* **ii**: 437, 1982.

374. McNeil, P., Mackenzie, I. & Manoharan, A. Naproxen associated aplastic anaemia. *Med. J. Aust.* **145**: 53–5, 1986.

375. Lee, S.J., Fawcett, P.V. & Preece, J.M. Aplastic anaemia associated with piroxicam. *Lancet* **i**: 1186, 1982.

376. Miller, J.L. Marrow aplasia and sulindac. *Ann. Intern. Med.* **92**: 129, 1980.

377. Sanz, M.A., Martinez, J.A., Gomis, F. *et al.* Sulindac induced bone marrow toxicity. *Lancet* **ii**: 802, 1980.

378. Gertz, M.A., Garton, J.P. & Jennings, W.H. Aplastic anemia due to tocainide. *N. Engl. J. Med.* **314**: 583–4, 1986.

11

Viral-induced cytopenias and immune deficiencies

R.P. Brettle
Consultant Physician, City Hospital, Edinburgh, UK

INTRODUCTION

The pathology of viral infections is dependent upon the direct effect of viruses on cells as well as the direct or indirect effects of the immune system in trying to deal with the virus infection. Viral infections may be local or systemic and it depends upon the site of infection generally whether or not haematological or immune effects are seen. The spectrum of viral infection extends from almost purely local infections, such as rhinoviruses, to actual infection of the immune cells themselves, as in human immune deficiency virus (HIV) infection.

Viruses are able to attack a variety of cells depending upon the presence or absence of critical receptors but they can often only replicate in specific cell lines. Viruses can produce damage by persistent infection, alteration of cell receptors, cell lysis or even purely attachment. It has recently been shown that HIV can exert profound effects upon the T_4-lymphocyte even at the stage of initial attachment prior to penetration.[1] The immune system, in coping with viral attack, may use interferons, lymphokines or cell-dependent cytotoxicity. In assessing the haematological or immune effects of viral infections it is difficult to decide on the exact underlying pathophysiology.

Probably the commonest known haematological effect of viral infection is a normal or low white cell count. The white cell abnormalities of common viral infections, i.e. neutropenia, may be due to redistribution, accelerated removal or defective production. In the latter case the granulocytic hypoplasia may be due to direct viral infection or T-cell suppression. In the vast majority of cases recovery is uneventful and the patient or doctor is unaware of the problem. Similarly with the advent of the clinical use of interferons it has been realized that many of the effects of viral infections are in fact those of interferon.[2] The fatigue, malaise, etc. of influenza can be replicated by the use of interferon, and common haematological side-effects, such as leucopenia, occurred in one-third whilst thrombocytopenia occurred in up to 20% of patients.[2] Leucopenia can, however, also occur in a number of bacterial infections such as typhoid, brucella or endotoxaemia and care is therefore needed in diagnosing a viral infection on a low white count alone.

COMMON VIRAL INFECTIONS

Measles

Measles is a common endemic and epidemic viral infection usually affecting children and characterized by a skin rash or exanthem. The illness begins with a 4 day prodromal period consisting of high fever of up to 40°C, bright red conjunctivitis, a harsh cough and coryza, followed by the development of a maculopapular eruption. This starts behind the ears and spreads onto the face, arms, trunk and legs. It becomes confluent and fades by desquamation and staining. It is usually an uneventful illness but may be complicated by viral pneumonia or secondary bacterial infections such as otitis media. Leucopenia is common and thrombocytopenia can also occur. Haemorrhagic measles in most cases is due to thrombocytopenia. The onset usually occurs within 14 days and lasts approximately 2 weeks. The platelet count, when abnormal, is usually back to within the normal range within one month. Bleeding may occur into the skin and also from the gastrointestinal and genito-urinary tracts. Occasionally a fatal intracerebral haemorrhage may occur. When severe, such patients require general supportive measures such as the use of steroids or platelet transfusions.[3]

Measles infection can also produce immunosuppression. Cell-mediated immunity, as determined by delayed type hypersensitivity skin reactions with *Candida* and tuberculin protein, are depressed not only by the illness but also by measles vaccination.[4,5] This depression of skin reactivity occurs because measles antigen competes for receptors on lymphocytes and the virus interferes with DNA synthesis after infecting transforming lymphocytes.[6,7]

Controversy exists, however, as to whether measles immunosuppression has any clinical relevance. One study of an epidemic of measles in children with tuberculosis failed to reveal any deterioration, but another suggested the opposite.[8,9] An increase in the incidence of tuberculosis was noted, however, during one epidemic of measles.[10]

Rubella

Rubella is a mild infection of little consequence unless contracted during pregnancy. It occurs as an endemic and epidemic infection and is characterized by malaise, headaches, conjunctivitis and fever. On the second day a rash of rose-pink or macular spots appears on the face, spreads rapidly to the trunk and extremities and then fades within 1–3 days. There is accompanying lymphadenopathy. In adults arthralgia may be a prominent feature of the illness. In a series of 200 patients with congenital rubella, 70 or 35% had complicating thrombocytopenia.[11] They presented with purpuric eruption within 24 h of delivery. The rash was most prominent on the face and upper trunk. Enlargement of the liver and spleen was noted in about 70% of cases and lymphadenopathy occurred in around 20% of cases. Of 58 which could be studied more extensively, over 80% had a platelet count <90 × 10^9 per litre but only 20% were as low as 20 × 10^9 per litre. The platelet count was usually back to normal within one month and in the majority was back to normal within 4 months. Steroids appeared to have little value.

In those patients in whom bone marrow examinations were available a paucity of megakaryocytes was noted, although those that were seen were normal in appearance. The fatality rates were low as far as bleeding was concerned, only one patient out of 200 having a fatal outcome. However, many had more minor problems such as haematomas at the sites of injections.[11]

The virus was disseminated in these patients and often isolated from many sites such as endocrine glands, bone, cerebrospinal fluid, the major organs, skin and lymphoid tissue. Persistence of virus for up to one year was noted in the study, despite the presence of neutralizing antibodies. An associated 17% of patients had anaemia and 22% hepatitis.[11]

As far as adult patients are concerned, symptomatic thrombocytopenia appears to be fairly rare although low counts are fairly common. There is an associated increase in capillary fragility which presumably can account for the occasional cases of non-thrombocytopenic purpura. The predisposition to thrombocytopenia is not generalized in childhood illnesses since there is one case described of haemorrhage associated with rubella in which prior infection with mumps and varicella produced no bleeding diathesis.[12]

Mumps

Mumps is an endemic and epidemic viral infection usually contracted in childhood, which in up to one-third may be asymptomatic or associated with only fever and malaise. It is characteristically associated with parotitis but can additionally cause pancreatitis, oophoritis, orchitis and lymphocytic meningitis. Rarer complications include thyroiditis, nerve palsies and meningo-encephalitis. A leucopenia is the norm except in the case of orchitis when a leucocytosis can occur. Thrombocytopenia is uncommon with mumps and only sporadic cases have been described.[13,14]

Herpes varicella zoster virus

Varicella or chickenpox is an endemic and epidemic viral infection usually contracted in childhood. The initial or primary infection is characterized by fever and an eruption. There is a prodromal period of 1–2 days consisting of malaise, fever and vomiting, which is followed by the appearance of an eruption. This begins as a macule which rapidly progresses through papule, vesicle, pustule and crust within 48 h. The fever continues for about 5 days, during which time further viraemia produces fresh lesions or crops. Complications in childhood are rare and consist of secondary bacterial infections usually of the skin, but occasionally pneumonia is seen. Primary viral pneumonia, usually in adults, can occur, as can meningitis, encephalitis and nerve palsies.

A bleeding diathesis has been described for many years in children as well as adults.[15–18] Bleeding may occur as early as the third day but usually about one week after the appearance of the vesicle eruption.[15] Although most cases are associated with thrombocytopenia alone, accompanying disseminated intravascular coagulation (DIC) has been reported and may explain some of the more severe cases.[19] Prior to supportive treatment being available the mortality was high.[20] There is usually an increased number of megakaryocytes in the bone marrow and the thrombocytopenia appears to be due to reduced platelet survival time secondary to immune-mediated platelet destruction.[21]

Varicella then becomes a latent viral infection and reactivation may occur 40–50 years later as varicella zoster or shingles. This manifests itself usually by recurrence in the skin, although recurrence in motor nerves can also occur. A recurrence is characterized by the onset of severe pain and hyperaesthesia in the area affected, together with malaise and slight fever. After 3–4 days the area affected develops an erythematous rash which is followed by the appearance of closely grouped vesicles. These vesicles rapidly progress to pustules and crusts.

There is usually an accompanying viraemia with sparse dissemination to other areas. In the immunocompromised, however, this viraemia may be prolonged or severe, producing disseminated varicella which looks the same as primary chickenpox. Haematological complications usually do not occur in uncomplicated shingles.

Influenza

There are three types of influenza: A, B and C. Type C influenza is relatively uncommon and type B produces endemic and small epidemics of influenza. By contrast, type A virus produces endemic, epidemic and pandemics of influenza. Influenza is characterized by a short incubation period of 1–4 days, followed by the sudden onset of fever, headaches, myalgia and a cough. The fever usually settles by the third day and the illness by about one week. The illness may be complicated by a viral or secondary bacterial pneumonia. If fatal, *Staphylococcus aureus* is implicated in 60% of cases but *Haemophilus influenzae* and *Streptococcus pneumoniae* are also involved. Whilst a leucopenia is common, a neutrophilia is seen in secondary bacterial infections.

The susceptibility to bacterial pneumonia is, in part, due to damage to the bronchial epithelium and 'mucociliary escalator'.[22] There is evidence, however, that the influenza virus either directly or indirectly is also able to affect immune function. Human neutrophils and monocytes exposed *in vitro* to influenza virus show impaired chemotaxis oxidative metabolism and bacteriocidal capacity,[23,24] and the same is true for circulating neutrophils in both natural and experimental influenza.[22] Influenza has also been shown in both *in vitro* and *in vivo* systems to induce abnormalities of neutrophil and macrophage function, including depression of oxidative, phagocytic and bacteriocidal activities. Influenza also depresses T-cell function as seen by diminished delayed cutaneous sensitivity in patients recovering from influenza and reduced production of diptheria antitoxin by human tonsillar cells exposed to influenza virus.[22]

Interferon can often be found in the circulation in influenza and may have some role in the immune abnormalities described since it can produce diminished T-cell and macrophage function as well as modulating B-cell function. Bacterial adherence may also be important in explaining susceptibility since it has been demonstrated that certain bacteria adhere to viral infected cells.[22]

Hepatitis

Type A viral hepatitis is an endemic and epidemic infection which usually spreads among children. The illness has a short incubation period of 2–6 weeks and in 90% of the cases it is non-icteric. Clinically apparent hepatitis is manifest by a prodrome of anorexia, malaise and lassitude. Occasionally there is fever, a skin rash, arthralgia and abdominal pain before the onset of jaundice.

Type B hepatitis is essentially a sporadic infection, although in the special circumstances often associated with modern technological medicine such as dialysis units, it may assume epidemic proportions unless procedures are introduced to prevent its transmission. It is spread by blood and blood products, and to a lesser degree by saliva, vomit, urine, semen and cervical secretions. Intact skin is a sufficient barrier against the virus and therefore most cases are associated with some form of inoculation, for instance surgery, tattooing and acupuncture needles. Additionally, the sharing of equipment by intravenous drug abusers is a potent method of spreading the virus. Broken skin or mucous membranes are unable to prevent infection and therefore transmission may also be associated with splashed or aerosolized virus in vomit or saliva etc. via the oral or conjunctival membranes as well as via the genito-urinary mucous membranes as a result of semen or cervical secretions.

The incubation period is relatively long from 6 weeks to 6 months. The illness is not particularly different clinically from other forms of hepatitis except for, perhaps, a more severe prodrome. The acute illness may be complicated by rapid progression to liver failure and death. The infection may also be complicated by the eventual development of chronic liver disease or a chronic carrier state.

Whilst most patients with chronic active hepatitis of unknown origin should be treated with immunosuppressant drugs, there is little to support the use of immunosuppressive drugs in chronic active hepatitis secondary to hepatitis B.[25–28] The antiviral agents α-interferon and vidarabine have been used in patients with chronic active hepatitis and suppression of viral replication occurred but no therapeutic benefit has been shown to date in randomized trials.[29–31] However, in a randomized trial, loss of hepatitis B 'e' antigen occurred in 6 out of 23 treated patients but in none of the untreated group. Seroconversion to the immune state was preceded in all cases by a hepatitis-like illness.[32]

Hepatitis may also be associated with a glandular fever syndrome caused by either Epstein–Barr virus (EBV) or cytomegalovirus (CMV). Non-A, non-B hepatitis is a term used for episodes of hepatitis in which other pathogens cannot be demonstrated. It is the commonest form of hepatitis in developed countries which follows a transfusion of blood. Unfortunately, because of the lack of a serological marker, the diagnosis currently has to be one of exclusion. There are, almost certainly, a number of different pathogens involved in non-A, non-B hepatitis.

On clinical grounds the illness can be broadly divided into two forms. Firstly, that associated with parenteral exposure, usually blood transfusion or blood products. In the USA this form accounts for 80–90% of post-transfusion hepatitis and 12–25% of the sporadic forms of non-A, non-B.[33] The incubation period varies from 21 to 84 days and 10–40% may go on to develop chronic liver disease. There is at least one, if not more, blood-borne pathogen and because of the presence of reverse transcriptase activity in the serum of some patients with non-A, non-B hepatitis it has been suggested that at least one form is a retrovirus.[34,35]

In contrast, the non-parenteral form has an incubation period of 10–56 days, is not associated with chronic liver disease and maybe transmitted faeco-orally like hepatitis A.[36] The current estimated risk of post-transfusion non-A, non-B hepatitis is approximately 10% but increases with the amount of blood transfused, the use of commercial blood, the presence of hepatitis B core antibody in the donor or the presence of elevated liver transaminase levels.[37,38] With 1–14 units transfused the risk is around 5% but this rises sharply to 29% with 40–59 units transfused and 45% if over 60 units are transfused. Whilst albumin and immunoglobulin are generally safe, pooled plasma clotting concentrates and even washed red cells can contain virus.[39,40]

One form of non-A, non-B hepatitis that has been recently characterized is hepatitis D virus, also known as delta virus or delta agent. This is a defective RNA virus which requires hepatitis B virus to be present before replication can occur.[41] The delta virus RNA and the delta antigen are contained within an external coat made up of the hepatitis B surface antigen. Its importance appears to be in the fact that a simultaneous infection with both agents may produce a more severe form of acute hepatitis.[42,43]

Marrow aplasia is a well-recognized complication of hepatitis which is not usually severe. Typically aplasia occurs nearly twice as commonly in males although the prognosis appears to be worse with females. There is a high fatality rate of around 80%.[45–46] The illness usually comes on within 2 months of an episode of hepatitis and 75% of the patients are less than 20 years of age. There is, unfortunately, a lack of serological data and many of the patients have also had other hepato-toxic drugs such as halothane and chloramphenicol. Whilst the hepatitis is assumed to be viral in origin there is little convincing proof. Hepatitis B surface antigen is usually not detected but this does not exclude hepatitis B infection since surface antigen may be cleared rapidly. It is possible that this is a complication of non-A, non-B hepatitis, especially as some of the patients were noted to have chronic hepatitis. With the description of parvovirus which is now associated with the aplasia of chronic haemolytic anaemias it is quite possible that post-hepatic aplasia will eventually be found to be associated with one particular viral aetiology which will explain its sporadic nature. It has been suggested that some form of sporadic marrow aplasia could be associated with non-icteric hepatitis.[44] Management is by general supportive measures including the use of immunosuppression with anti-lymphocyte globulin. Bone marrow transplantation has been tried but without much success.[45]

Epstein–Barr virus infection

This is an endemic viral infection which commonly affects young people between the ages of 15 and 25 years and is characterized by fever, sore throat, lymphadenopathy and abnormal lymphocytes in the peripheral blood. It was initially described in the late part of the nineteenth century as glandular fever, and then again in the 1920s as infectious mononucleosis because of the atypical mononuclear cells in the blood. A serological test, the heterophil antibody, was described in 1932 and was the diagnostic test until the association with the Epstein–Barr virus was made in 1968.[47] Serological surveys have shown that by the age of 50 some 90% of the population have experienced this virus, although in large numbers the typical clinical illness does not occur.[47]

Eighty per cent of those that present with a clinical illness present with 'anginose glandular fever' or acute pharyngitis. There is often a prodromal illness consisting of malaise, headaches and fatigue followed by high fevers, pharyngitis with generalized lymphadenopathy. Many of the remainder present with a more chronic form once known as 'typhoidal glandular fever'. This consists of fever, night sweats and fatigue which may be excessive. Approximately 5% present with mild hepatitis.[47]

The heterophil antibody is an IgM antibody that will agglutinate sheep red cells and, if still present after absorption with beef or guinea-pig red cells, is diagnostic of infectious mononucleosis (the Paul Bunnell antibody). A commercial system is now used called the 'monospot test' and utilizes the agglutination of horse red cells after removal of non-specific heterophil antibodies by a homogenate of guinea-pig kidney. This system of diagnosing infectious mononucleosis is frequently used but a more specific result is now available using Epstein–Barr serology. This has shown that EBV infection is the cause of infectious mononucleosis in 91% of cases and that 76% of the non-EBV cases are due to CMV infection.[47]

The classic peripheral blood appearance in infectious mononucleosis is an absolute lymphocytosis (> 50% or more than 5×10^9 per litre), together with an abundance of atypical lymphocytes. In addition to heterophil antibodies a wide variety of other serological abnormalities may be detected, mostly IgM antibodies. These include antinuclear antibody, rheumatoid factor, smooth muscle antibody and weakly positive syphilis serology. The patients also have transiently depressed cell-mediated immunity as evidenced by skin anergy and decreased lymphoproliferative response to mitogens. The underlying pathophysiology seems to be that EBV specifically infects B-cells and then incites a T-cell response (atypical lymphocytes).

Complications are unusual but consist of splenic rupture, pharyngeal obstruction, nerve palsies and encephalitis. The haematological complications that have been described include thrombocytopenia, aplastic anaemia and haemolytic anaemia.

Haemorrhagic complications in infectious mononucleosis, notably epistaxis and haematuria, were reported soon after the original clinical description, as was uncomplicated thrombocytopenia.[48] The incidence of haemorrhage associated with infectious mononucleosis is reported as 6.9% of 450 patients and the majority were not associated with thrombocytopenia.[49] Uncomplicated cases of infectious mononucleosis show a consistent mild reduction in platelet count during the first 4 weeks of the illness; only 5 of 47 patients had counts below 100,000, the lowest being 63,000.[50] Severe thrombocytopenia occurred in only 2 (0.6%) of 300 patients requiring hospitalization for infectious mononucleosis.[51]

The average age of those suffering from thrombocytopenia was, not surprisingly, 18 years but, unusually, there was an excess of males, the male to female ratio being just over 2:1. By comparison, there is usually an excess of females in idiopathic thrombocytopenia. The thrombocytopenia usually presents within 6 days although it can occur up to 3 weeks after the onset of the acute illness. Approximately one-third had haemorrhagic presenting features which included epistaxis, gingival bleeding or haematuria. In post-puerperal females menorrhagia was also common.[52] The mechanism of thrombocytopenia is possibly splenic pooling as a consequence of anti-platelet antibodies.[47,50–52]

There was often an associated anaemia although this was usually proportional to the blood loss that had occurred. In 9 of 15 patients in whom a bone marrow examination was available, an increase in the number of megakaryocytes was observed although they were immature and suggestive of decrease in production. In two patients the bone marrow appeared to be entirely normal.[52]

Anaemia in infectious mononucleosis is relatively unusual but is one of the features that is used to distinguish infectious mononucleosis from acute leukaemia. Of a series of 300 patients with infectious mononucleosis only 6 were anaemic and half of these were associated with pancytopenia.[53] Acute haemolytic anaemia is relatively rare and its description relies on case reports.[54–56] The exact aetiology remains obscure although hypersplenism and cold agglutinins have both been put forward as possible causes. In most cases of infectious mononucleosis-related haemolytic anaemia the Coombs test is positive but the antibody specificity is unknown. It is a self-limiting process which rapidly recovers and requires only general supportive measures including, occasionally, steroids.[55]

As with other common viral infections, a mild neutropenia is common but agranulocytosis is rare. The exact mechanisms involved in neutropenia are unknown but splenic pooling, reduced formation in the marrow or peripheral destruction are all possible.

Aplastic anaemia is similarly rare with only a handful of case reports in the literature.[57,58] Pancytopenia occurred within 21 days of the acute illness, the range being from 7–49 days.[57] Bone marrow examinations were available in 5 patients and of these, 2 were hypercellular and 3 truly aplastic.[58] Fifty per cent of the cases recovered. Where this occurred the recovery was rapid, occurring between 4 and 8 days. The outlook appears to be not as pessimistic as with post-hepatitic pancytopenia.[58] The cause appears to be bone marrow damage secondary to an EBV-associated haemophagocytic syndrome caused by an aberrant immune response[59] (see below).

Infectious mononucleosis is not normally a fatal disease and only 20 cases had been described by 1970.[59] A close study of these fatalities, however, has increased our understanding not only of EBV infection but also of immune mechanisms. In 1975 the Duncan family were described with a form of immunodeficiency with respect to EBV infection. It was initially reported that of 18 related boys, 6 had died of a lymphoproliferative disease.[60,61] In 3 of 5 boys, EBV had been involved as a terminal event. It was reported that in 3 the fatal EBV infection had been associated with either agammaglobulinaemia or hypergammaglobulinaemia. In the 2 others lymphohistiocytic proliferation was present as well as either hypergammaglobulinaemia or a subclinical EBV infection. This immunodeficiency with reference to EBV infection appeared to be inherited as a sex-linked recessive disorder with differing phenotypic expression.

By 1978, more of the family had been studied and the term X-linked recessive lymphoproliferative syndrome or XLRLS was coined.[62] This disorder appeared to have three expressions: (1) hypergammaglobulinaemia and subclinical EBV infection, (2) a defective immune response to EBV which was fatal, and (3) a history of histiocytic lymphoma.

A recent review of fatal infectious mononucleosis compared those fatalities due to the XLRLS with spontaneous fatal infectious mononucleosis (SIM).[59] The mean age of SIM was 5.5 years versus 2.5 years for XLRLS. Interestingly, the male to female ratio in the SIM was 1:1. Median time to death after infection was 6 weeks (range 2 days to 600 weeks). The causes of death were fatal acute haemorrhage in 18 patients and an opportunistic infection in 23 patients. Contributing factors to death were fulminant hepatitis in 23 patients and a meningo-encephalitis in 16 patients. Eighty per cent of the patients exhibited the findings on bone marrow of viral-associated haemophagocytic syndrome (VAHS). A pancytopenia occurred precipitously and bone marrow examination showed infiltration by atypical lymphoid cells and cellular necrosis. Terminally the bone marrows were found to be hypocellular. The necrosis appears to be secondary to invasion by EBV-infected B-cells. The normal bone marrow seems to be innocently killed by unregulated natural killer activity against EBV-infected cells. The unique vulnerability of males with XLRLS to EBV is due to an inherited defect on the X chromosome that results in a failure of regulation of cytotoxic and cellular responses to EBV-induced B-cell proliferation. Those patients with XLRLS that survive an attack of EBV are left with combined variable immunodeficiency as manifest by hypogammaglobulinaemia and inverted T_4/T_8 ratios. They are left with a secondary immune deficiency as a consequence of the bone marrow necrosis. The predisposition to lymphoma is as a consequence of this secondary immune deficiency. By 1987, 161 patients with XLRLS had been reported. Fifty-seven per cent died of infectious mononucleosis, 29% developed hypogammaglobulinaemia and 24% a malignant lymphoma. The overall mortality was 80%, 70% by 10 years of age and 100% by 40 years of age.[63]

The similarity of SIM to XLRLS would suggest that vulnerability to EBV can occur as a consequence of a spontaneous failure of regulation of cytotoxic and cellular responses to virus infections.

Cytomegalovirus

CMV is a herpes virus with a propensity for latent and recurrent infections similar to other herpes viruses such as herpes simplex and varicella zoster virus. The clinical spectrum of a primary infection was first described in 1965 but tends to vary with the age of the patient.[64]

Infection as an adult is characterized by fever, lethargy, malaise, hepatosplenomegaly and transaminase abnormalities but rarely icterus.[65,66] The haematological changes are similar to infectious mononucleosis except that the heterophile antibody response is absent.[65] It is responsible for 50–76% of non-EBV mononucleosis and is often subclinical since by the age of 60, 90% of adults have been exposed to the virus.[47,65,66]

In contrast, CMV infection as a child, while associated with similar symptoms, is more often associated with cervical lymphadenopathy which occurs in over 80% of cases compared with only 6% of adults. Hepatomegaly occurs in 100% of cases and splenomegaly in 60% of cases by comparison to 53% of cases as adults. The most striking difference, however, is the fact that in 21% of children's cases an exudative tonsillitis similar to EBV mononucleosis occurs, but this is rare in adults, occurring in only 1 out of 17.[67]

The most common haematolgial abnormality is lymphocytosis ($>5 \times 10^9$ per litre) which occurred in 93% of children and 53% of adults. Atypical lymphocytes ($>1 \times 10^9$ per litre) occurred in 93% of children and 71% of adults.[67] The lymphocytosis may persist for months after clinical recovery and a thrombocytopenia or haemolytic anaemia may also readily occur.[67]

Infection with CMV has been implicated as a complication of blood transfusion. The post-perfusion syndrome or mononucleosis-like syndrome consists of fever, atypical lymphocytosis and splenomegaly. It was first associated with open heart surgery. CMV being isolated from urine 7–25 weeks after surgery together with positive serology. In a prospective study of post-transfusion CMV, infection occurred in 7% of patients receiving 1 unit of blood, 21% of those receiving multiple units and in 52% of multiply transfused immunocompromised patients. The risk appears to be directly proportional to the volume transfused and the presence of immunosuppression but not with the use of fresh blood. It only occurs in patients receiving blood products containing leucocytes. It has also been observed that re-infection after transfusion can cause reactivation of CMV in those already infected.[68]

Between 0.5% and 2% of newborn infants are infected with CMV but clinical illness occurs in less than 5% of those infected.[66] The clinical syndrome consists of intrauterine growth retardation, jaundice, hepatosplenomegaly, microcephaly, choroidoretinitis and other congenital abnormalities. Purpuric skin lesions occur soon after birth, thrombocytopenia or haemolytic anaemia are common haematological abnormalities and DIC occasionally occurs.[66] Post-transfusion CMV can also be one cause of neonatal CMV and occurred in 33% of children having exchange transfusions for hyperbilirubinaemia although few were symptomatic. In contrast prematurity, which is one form of immunosuppression, and transfusion is associated with an increased risk. The risk of acquiring symptomatic post-transfusion CMV was associated with a seronegative mother, a birth weight of less than 1200 g, a stay in an intensive care unit for longer than 28 days and a transfusion of more than 50 ml of blood.[68]

CMV infection is known to affect patients with cellular immunodeficiency such as severe combined immunodeficiency, but with the advent of powerful iatrogenic immunosuppressive drugs for use in transplantation, CMV has become an important pathogen in the immunocompromised host.

Between 60 and 90% of renal transplants excrete CMV within the first year after transplantation.[66] This may occur because of reactivation or because of a primary infection as a consequence of receiving infected blood or organs. Clinical symptoms appear to be more common with a primary infection and this is usually manifest as fever, pneumonitis, hepatitis, choroidoretinitis, encephalitis or colitis. The illness may be associated with a leucopenia and the appearance of atypical lymphocytes. As immunosuppression increases the illness is often associated with other infections such as *Pneumocystis carinii* pneumonia.[66]

As with EBV infection some patients with CMV exhibit a severe infection of the bone marrow known as virus-associated haemophagocytic syndrome (VAHS). EBV can cause spontaneous VAHS probably associated with a sporadic immunodeficiency, whereas CMV VAHS is usually associated with iatrogenic immunosuppression.[59,69] The pathology appears to be histiocytic hyperplasia with prominent phagocytosis of red cells and granulocytes. The exact reason is unknown but may be because of membrane changes associated with the viral infection and an excessive T-cell response.[59,69]

The clinical picture consists of high fever, constitutional symptoms, hepatosplenomegaly, enlarged lymph nodes, deranged liver function tests, DIC, anaemia and leucopenia which may be severe. Atypical lymphocytes are always present in the peripheral blood. The bone marrow examinations showed hypocellularity with decreased granulopoiesis and erythropoiesis. The essential step in management is to distinguish the illness from malignancy, to reduce the immunosuppression when present and to avoid it if not present.[69]

The treatment of CMV infection is currently with experimental drugs such as gancyclovir (9,2-hydroxy-1-hydroxymethyl ethoxymethyl guanine or DHPG) and there is varying success depending on the site. For instance, choroidoretinitis appears to respond better than pneumonitis. The use of gammaglobulin is not yet of proven efficacy although post-transfusion CMV seems to be less severe in the presence of pre-existing antibodies. The major strategy at present is prevention, utilizing where possible, seronegative donors.[68,70] Alternatively it is possible in certain circumstances to use only frozen deglycerolized red cells. After freezing and before use, these cells are washed extensively and this removes 99% of the leucocytes. This has been shown to reduce CMV mononucleosis following cardiac surgery.[68] Other CMV preventative strategies recently shown to be of value include the use of CMV immune globulin in renal transplant recipients and intravenous acyclovir for 30 days after bone marrow transplantation.[71,72]

Parvovirus and erythema infectiosum

The first human infection with parvovirus was reported by Dr Cossart in 1975.[73] During the screening of blood donors' sera for hepatitis B, nine donors were noted to have a particulate antigen in their sera which was distinct from hepatitis B and had the morphology and density of a parvovirus. The donors were totally well and thus the associated clinical picture was, at that time, unknown. At that time the prevalence of antibody to the new antigen was shown to rise steadily throughout childhood to 30% in adults.[73]

In 1981 it was demonstrated that antibodies to this particulate antigen were usually acquired between the ages of 4 and 10 and that 61% of adults had IgG antibodies.[74,75] By that time the only known clinical illness associated with parvovirus was a mild febrile illness that had been noted in two soldiers following tattooing in Africa.[76] Between 1981 and 1983 it was noted that acute infection with parvovirus was the principal cause of acute anaemic episodes in chronic haemolytic anaemias such as sickle cell disease, hereditary spherocytosis and pyruvate kinase deficiency.[77-79] Laboratory studies demonstrated that the pathophysiology was inhibition of colony formation but the common childhood presentation remained unknown.[80] In 1983 outbreaks of erythema infectiosum or fifth disease were associated with acute parvovirus in outbreaks that occurred in London.[81]

The clinical picture is of a mild febrile illness associated with headaches, anorexia, arthralgia and a rash. There may be the characteristic slapped cheek appearance followed by a macular papular eruption on the trunk and extremities which coincides with the appearance of antibodies.[81,82]

More recently infection with parvovirus in pregnancy has been shown to be associated in a few cases with hydrops fetalis.[73,83,84] The problem appears to be similarly associated with a shortened red cell survival and hyperplastic erythropoiesis. In this situation the erythroid progenitor cells appear to be particularly vulnerable to agents such as parvovirus.[85]

Viral haemorrhagic fevers

Haemorrhagic syndromes associated with viral infections such as smallpox and yellow fever have been known and described for centuries. During the past 40 years a number of 'new viral haemorrhagic fevers' have been detailed. The majority are almost certainly not new and all have existed unnoticed for many years. Examples are:

1. Rift Valley fever,
2. Congo/Crimea haemorrhagic fever,
3. Argentinian/Bolivian haemorrhagic fever,
4. Lassa fever,
5. Marburg virus disease,
6. Ebola virus disease,
7. Korean haemorrhagic fever,
8. Dengue haemorrhagic fever.

Transmission varies from mosquito bites (yellow fever, Rift Valley fever, dengue haemorrhagic fever) to tick bites (Crimean/Congo haemorrhagic fever) to contact with animals (Lassa fever, Argentinian fever/Bolivian haemorrhagic fever).

The cause of the haemorrhagic shock syndrome seen in these diseases varies and in many cases is still unknown. Abnormalities described include arteriolar and capillary endothelial damage leading to hypotension and capillary leakage, e.g. dengue haemorrhagic fever, Korean haemorrhagic fever and Lassa fever. Thrombocytopenia is seen in Argentinian/Bolivian haemorrhagic fever, Marburg virus disease and Ebola virus disease. DIC and clotting abnormalities have been noted in yellow fever, Marburg/Ebola virus disease and dengue haemorrhagic fever. A leucopenia has been noted in Congo/Crimean haemorrhagic fever, Argentinian/Bolivian haemorrhagic fever, Lassa fever, Marburg virus disease, Ebola virus disease and a leucocytosis in some cases of Marburg/Ebola virus disease.[86-88]

Human immunodeficiency virus

The original description of AIDS, or the acquired immune deficiency syndrome, appeared in 1981. This described 26 patients with Kaposi's sarcoma, a skin tumour which until then was seen only in elderly men, in African races, and in those with considerable iatrogenic immunosuppression, and five men with oral thrush and pneumocystis pneumonia which again, was usually associated with iatrogenic immunosuppression. The connection between the two groups was that they were all young male homosexuals with a mean age of 32 years.[89] However, before long other 'high risk groups' were recognized and included injection drug users, haemophiliacs, transfusion recipients, the heterosexual partners of patients with AIDS and children.[90-100]

Between 1983 and 1984 a virus was isolated from patients and characterized.[101-103] There was initially a profusion of names but recently the term human immunodeficiency virus or HIV was adopted.[104]

The isolation of the virus led to the development of a variety of antibody tests and as a consequence we now have a better idea of the spectrum of HIV infection. The Centers for Disease Control (CDC) introduced a definition to help collate accurate information about the condition. This definition initially only required the clinical diagnosis of conditions that were moderately predictive of cellular immunodeficiency without an underlying cause. The definition was revised in 1987 to take into account serological evidence of HIV infection.[105]

The following conditions, diagnosed definitively in association with evidence of HIV infection, are used currently for the diagnosis of AIDS.

1. Bacterial infections, multiple or recurrent (any combination of at least two within a 2 year period), of the following types affecting a child <13 years of age:
   septicaemia, pneumonia, meningitis, bone or joint infection, or abscess of an internal organ or body cavity (excluding otitis media or superficial skin or mucosal abscesses), caused by *Haemophilus*, *Streptococcus* (including *Pneumococcus*), or other pyogenic bacteria.
2. Coccidioidomycosis, disseminated (at a site other than or in addition to lungs or cervical or hilar lymph nodes).
3. HIV encephalopathy (also called 'HIV dementia', 'AIDS dementia', or 'subacute encephalitis due to HIV').
4. Histoplasmosis, disseminated (at a site other than or in addition to lungs or cervical or hilar lymph nodes).
5. Isosporiasis with diarrhoea persisting >1 month.
6. Kaposi's sarcoma at any age.

7. Lymphoma of the brain (primary) at any age.
8. Other non-Hodgkin's lymphoma of B-cell or unknown immunological phenotype and the following histologic types:
   (a) small, non-cleaved lymphoma (either Burkitt or non-Burkitt type);
   (b) immunoblastic sarcoma (equivalent to any of the following, although not necessarily all in combination: immunoblastic lymphoma, large-cell lymphoma, diffuse histiocytic lymphoma, diffuse undifferentiated lymphoma, or high-grade lymphoma).
   Note: Lymphomas are not included here if they are of T-cell immunological phenotype or their histological type is not described or is described as 'lymphocytic', 'lymphoblastic', 'small cleaved' or 'plasmacytoid lymphocytic'.
9. Any mycobacterial disease caused by mycobacteria other than *M. tuberculosis*, disseminated (at a site other than or in addition to lungs, skin or cervical or hilar lymph nodes).
10. Disease caused by *M. tuberculosis*, extrapulmonary (involving at least one site outside the lungs, regardless of whether there is concurrent pulmonary involvement.
11. *Salmonella* (non-typhoid) septicaemia, recurrent.
12. HIV wasting syndrome (emaciation, 'slim disease').

By 31 May 1988 over 96,000 cases had been notified worldwide, more than 70,000 from the USA, 12,000 from Europe and more than 1500 from the UK.[106]

In addition to AIDS there are a number of other conditions related to HIV. The exact interrelationship is not known but in an attempt to ease the problem of definition the CDC recently developed a classification system which is descriptive and does not attempt to map out any interconnections.[107] It essentially details four categories of HIV infection as shown in Table 11.1

For a more detailed description of the classification system see Appendix.

AIDS and HIV infections are associated with a variety of risk activities. In the USA 70% are associated with homosexual intercourse, 24% with drug misuse and/or homosexual intercourse, 2% with heterosexual intercourse, 2% with receiving blood transfusions, and 1% with haemophilia.[108] By comparison, in the UK to date 84% of the cases have been associated with

Table 11.1   Classification of Effects of HIV Infection

I	Acute infection with seroconversion	
II	Asymptomatic infection	
III	Persistent generalized lymphadenopathy	
IV	A	Constitutional disease
	B	Neurological disease
	C	Immunodeficiency
		C1 CDC definition of AIDS
		C2 infections outwith definition
	D	Tumours in CDC definition of AIDS
	E	Other, e.g. Hodgkin's, carcinoma, lymphoid interstitial pneumonia

homosexual intercourse, 3.5% with heterosexual intercourse, 3% with injection drug misuse, but 6% with haemophilia and 2% with blood transfusion.[108] However, in Europe as a whole, injection drug misuse is the fastest growing risk activity.[109] There is a small but increasing number of paediatric cases, the majority of which are associated with HIV infection in the mother.[108]

The distribution of cases is characteristic of a blood-associated virus when transmission occurs via blood contact, from sexual intercourse and perinatally. Consequently, the patients likely to be affected are:

1. homosexuals/bisexuals;
2. injection drug misusers;
3. the recipients of blood products either coagulation products or blood itself, especially prior to 1985 when testing became available in the UK and the USA;
4. the children of infected women; and
5. sexual contacts of infected patients.

Whilst this latter group is currently small, this may change in the future and certainly in Africa, although reporting is difficult, there appears no doubt that the disease is now heterosexually spread in the majority of cases.

At any one time, approximately 50% of the cumulative number of cases have died.[108] The mortality depends upon the presentation. Those presenting with an opportunistic infection have a current case mortality rate of over 50% whereas those with Kaposi's sarcoma have a case mortality rate of only 33%. Those patients presenting with both an opportunistic infection and Kaposi's sarcoma have a current case mortality rate of 63%.[108] The survival time also varies with the type of presentation in AIDS; the median survival time for those patients with Kaposi's sarcoma in the absence of opportunistic infections varies between 20 and 30 months whereas the median survival time for patients with opportunistic infections varies between 4 and 11 months.[110,111]

The seroprevalence of HIV amongst haemophiliacs depends very much upon the blood product that was used and varies from 14 to 31% for cryoprecipitate and from 71 to 86% for Factor VIII concentrate.[112–115] Additionally, the incidence varies with the severity of the illness, reflecting presumably the increased use made of blood products. For instance, the incidence of AIDS is tenfold greater for haemophiliac type A, that is 345.7 per 100,000 versus 34.5 per 100,000 for haemophiliac type B.[116] It appears that the majority of haemophiliac patients seroconverted in the USA between 1981 and 1982 but some seroconversions occurred as early as 1979. Currently about 2% of these individals develop AIDS per year.[117]

As previously mentioned, the first case of transfusion-associated AIDS occurred in a young child who had a platelet transfusion.[96] Between 1978 and 1983 in the USA the risk of acquiring HIV via blood transfusion was estimated at 0.6 cases of AIDS per 100,000 adults transfused and 2.8 cases of AIDS per 100,000 children transfused.[116] The risk was increased by a factor of 32 for adults given more than 10 units of blood and by a factor of 27 for children given more than 10 units of blood.[118] The risk occurs with whole blood, packed cells, platelets or frozen plasma and the mean incubation period from transfusion to the development of AIDS is 21 months for children and 31 months for adults.[119] This incubation period is considerably shorter than, let us say, for haemophiliacs and there is therefore some suggestion that the virus given to haemophiliacs may have been altered in some way.

The risk of acquiring HIV from an infected blood product appears to be about 66% and infection appears more likely the closer the donor is to developing AIDS.[120] This does rather suggest that infectivity in donors rises as they develop symptoms. Antibody screening for HIV was introduced to the Blood Transfusion Service in 1985 in the USA[121] and taken together with heat treatment of Factor VIII concentrates and attempts to exclude high-risk donors, the risk for transfusion is now between 1 in 100,000 to 1 in 1,000,000.[121–123] Isolated cases of HIV antibody negative donors transmitting infection in the incubation period prior to seroconversion have been reported and further emphasizes the importance of persuading high-risk donors not to donate.[124]

Currently the exact explanation for progression from HIV infection to AIDS is unknown. Almost certainly a number of factors will be involved, including genetic susceptibility, gender, pregnancy and continued risk activity. Additional immunosuppressive factors might be the use of opiates, stimulation of the immune system via soluble antigens and DNA viruses and the acquisition of differing strains of HIV.[1,111,125–127] A number of markers of this progression have been noted, including age of the patient, low numbers of T_4-lymphocytes (a figure of less than 200 suggests that 50% will progress in 2 years), immune thrombocytopenic purpura, the presence of HIV antigen in serum and rising levels of β_2-microglobulin.[128–133]

The causative virus involved in AIDS was first isolated in 1983 by Dr Luc Montagnier and it was propagated in a cell line by Dr Robert Gallo in 1984.[101,102] A variety of names were used for the virus initially, including LAV, ARV, HTLV-III but these have all now been replaced by HIV.[105] HIV is a retrovirus, i.e. an RNA virus which utilizes an enzyme known as DNA polymerase or reverse transcriptase to produce a DNA provirus that is able to insert itself into the host DNA. It contains three major genes: *gag*, *pol* and *env*.[134]

The *gag* gene codes for core or shell proteins that enclose the RNA. These proteins are also known as p24, p18 and p15. The *pol* gene codes for at least three enzymes: protease, reverse transcriptase and an endonuclease. The *env* gene codes for the outer spike glycoproteins and transmembrane glycoproteins. These are also known as gp120 and gp41. Before leaving a host cell a newly assembled virus takes with it part of the host cell membrane into which the gp120 and gp41 viral proteins have been inserted.

HIV preferentially infects lymphocytes that function as T-helper cells. These cells are distinguished by the presence of a specific receptor molecule known as CD4 or T_4 after the monoclonal antibodies that specifically recognized the molecule. The gp120 viral protein appears to specifically bind to the T_4 receptor molecule before penetrating into the cell. In addition to helper lymphocytes this receptor molecule may be found on 10–20% of monocytes or macrophages, Langerhans cells in the dermis and microglial cells in the central nervous system.[134]

AIDS is characterized by a marked depletion of T_4-lymphocytes in the peripheral blood. Exactly how this depletion takes place is as yet unknown but a number of possible mechanisms have been suggested, including a direct cytopathic effect of HIV, syncytia or giant cell formation with subsequent cell death and a form of autoimmunity against lymphocytes using either cytotoxic T-cells or other antilymphocytic factors.

The various viral proteins produced by HIV infection stimulate an immune response although in many individuals this immune response does not neutralize or protect against the virus. The major antibody response is against the *env* gene products or outer glycoproteins, notably gp120. Antibodies against gp120 appear about 6 weeks after infection and persist until the terminal stages of AIDS. Soon after this, antibodies against the *gag* or core proteins, notably p24, appear. High levels of anti-p24 may be protective since low levels predispose to the development of AIDS.[134] The commercial assays available for screening purposes detect gp120 antibodies. Commercial assays are now available to detect anti-p24 antibody as well as antigen. The appearance of HIV p24 antigen in the circulation together with the loss of anti-p24 antibody is thought to be predictive of progression to AIDS.[134–137]

The major effect of HIV infection appears to be damage to the cell-mediated immune mechanism, resulting in characteristic susceptibility to opportunistic infections. This susceptibility is usually to intracellular organisms such as latent viruses, fungi or protozoa. Such organisms require the presence of an intact cell-mediated immune system which relies on T-lymphocytes and macrophages. This susceptibility is associated with a marked depletion of peripheral blood T_4-lymphocytes. These lymphocytes play a key role in initiating and promoting immune responses including the initiation of a de novo humoral response. Most adults with HIV infection seem to have reasonable B-cell memory although recurrent bacterial infections can occur in HIV infection. This humoral defect is worst in children where B-cell memory is limited and the patient may be rendered effectively hypogammaglobulinaemic. The humoral defect also limits the usefulness of serology in the diagnosis of many disorders, for instance latent viruses may exhibit persistent and stable levels of antibodies and other organisms produce little in the way of an antibody response.[138]

The marked loss of T-cell immunity results in a susceptibility to reactivation of latent or controlled infections such as CMV, toxoplasmosis or tuberculosis or attack by relatively non-pathogenic organisms which may be endogenous or common in the patient's environment. Examples of this type of infection are *Pneumocystis carinii* pneumonia (PCP), candidiasis or atypical mycobacteria.

The loss of T-cell function also results in only limited macrophage activity. Infection in these patients often produces little in the way of an inflammatory response and consequently little in the way of clinical signs. A number of immunological abnormalities have been described, including:

1. leucopenia and lymphopenia,
2. loss of T_4-lymphocytes from the peripheral blood,
3. hypergammaglobulinaemia,
4. skin anergy,
5. decreased *in vitro* lymphocyte proliferation, cytotoxic T-cell response and

antibody production to new antigens, and
6. elevated levels of immune complexes, interferon and β_2 microglobulin.[138]

Haematological abnormalities

The haematological abnormalities associated with HIV infection vary with the clinical state of the patient. In a series of patients within 4 years of HIV infection in Edinburgh 33% had a normal total white cell count but a depressed lymphocyte count ($<1.5 \times 10^9$ per litre) and 67% had a normal total white cell count and lymphocyte count but a depressed T_4-lymphocyte sub-set count ($<1.0 \times 10^9$ per litre). At this time, only 4% of the patients examined had progressed to CDC stage 4, 65% were at CDC stage 3 and 31% stage 2. None were anaemic but 12% had a leucopenia ($<4.0 \times 10^9$ per litre), 38% a lymphopenia, 43% a T_4 count of $<0.5 \times 10^9$ per litre and 13% a T_4 count of $<0.25 \times 10^9$ per litre.

Haematological abnormalities are commoner as HIV infection progresses. For instance 12% of AIDS/AIDS-related complex (ARC) patients were leucopenic, 20% were neutropenic, 75% were lymphopenic and 93% were anaemic.[139,140] The reasons for these abnormalities are multifactorial and involve the effects of HIV infection, drug effects, chronic infection and the effects of opportunistic infections. In a series of patients who underwent bone marrow examination a number of abnormalities were noted including:

1. reticulo-endothelial iron blockade – ?secondary to opportunistic infection,
2. dyserythropoiesis and megaloblastic change – ?secondary to co-trimoxazole treatment,
3. erythroid hypoplasia – ?secondary to mycobacteria infection,
4. excess histiocytes and viral-associated haemophagocytic syndrome – ?secondary to HIV or CMV.[139]

Despite the peripheral lymphopenia, bone marrow lymphopenia is uncommon, perhaps because T-cells predominate in the peripheral blood whereas B-cells predominate in the bone marrow.

Immune thrombocytopenia (ITP) is usually associated with children and middle-aged women. An ITP syndrome was noted early on to be an AIDS-related condition in homosexuals, injection drug misusers, and haemophiliacs.[141–144] In patients with AIDS about 30% have a depressed platelet count and it often falls further with treatment for PCP.[141,145] The reason for this is not clear but it has been suggested that the treatment effectively clears blockade of the RES by opportunistic infection and allows platelets to be removed.[141,145]

The platelet count is generally depressed in HIV infection and ITP has been noted to occur in HIV infection before the advent of AIDS.[141–143] In Edinburgh 23% of patients had a platelet count $<150 \times 10^9$ per litre but ony 4% had symptoms of excessive bruising or bleeding with counts of $<20 \times 10^9$ per litre. In other studies about 5–10% of PGL patients have mildly depressed platelet counts.[145] Our experience that this is a relatively benign condition supports the USA experience. The commonest symptoms are excessive bruising, epistaxis, gingival and rectal bleeding. Major life-threatening haemorrhage is rare. Platelet-associated immunoglobulin has been demonstrated in the majority of patients studied.[145]

HIV-related ITP usually runs a benign course and, of course, progression to AIDS may occur. It has been reported that this is heralded by a rise in the platelet count and this has been interpreted as further evidence that the ITP is related to RES dysfunction. As AIDS develops and RES blockade by pathogens occurs, the immune-mediated removal of platelets by the RES can no longer occur.[145]

Despite the minor nature of the condition a number of therapeutic options have been tried. Essentially all the treatment modalities used in non-HIV ITP appear to work and this includes steroids, high-dose intravenous gammaglobulin, splenectomy and danazol.

Management of HIV infection

Until recently, the management of HIV infection was based on: (1) the prevention of spread, (2) the prevention of progression to AIDS once infected with HIV, and (3) the treatment of opportunistic cancers and infections.

The particular measures which have been suggested to reduce transmission are: (1) a reduction in the number of sexual partners, (2) avoidance of anal intercourse for homosexuals and heterosexuals, (3) use of barrier contraceptives, especially condoms or sheaths combined with spermicides, (4) avoidance of needle and syringe sharing, and (5) avoidance of pregnancy with the increased chance of infecting the child.

The particular measures which have been suggested to reduce the progression to AIDS once infected are: (1) avoidance of needle sharing to reduce further HIV infection, (2) avoidance of needle drug abuse, (3) avoidance of pregnancy, (4) avoidance of anal intercourse for heterosexuals and homosexuals, (5) avoidance of recurrent infections such as venereal disease etc., (6) use of barrier contraceptives to reduce any immunosuppressive effect of semen or further infection with HIV.

The majority of these measures are not contentious except, perhaps, in the methods of informing the population at large and many of the measures such as prevention of pregnancy and barrier contraception are effective for both aims and are particularly important for a heterosexual population.

The prevention of pregnancy is important on the grounds of progression to AIDS in the mother as well as the prevention of transmission to the child. The risk of transmission from mother to child may be as low as 0% if HIV infection occurs during the pregnancy.[146] Reports which unfortunately rely upon the identification of a symptomatic child, will suggest high rates of perinatal transmission and these may not be widely applicable. Preliminary reports of prospective surveys suggest a risk of between 22 and 51%.[147–151] Of more importance may be the immunological status of the mother. The risk of transmission from a haemophiliac to his spouse seems to depend upon low numbers of T_4-lymphocytes, the presence of thrombocytopenia and HIV antigenaemia.[129,136] One report from Africa suggested a similar correlation between low numbers of T_4-lymphocytes in the mother and transmission to the child.[152]

In the USA only about 25% of HIV-infected mothers were well 2.5 years after delivery.[153] In one series of 16 mothers identified by the birth of a child with AIDS only 4 remained asymptomatic at a mean follow-up time of 2.5 years after delivery of the child. However, 11 of 16 women had a subsequent pregnancy during this time and we know nothing of their total parity. Additionally, in 5 of these 11 subsequent pregnancies the mothers developed AIDS or ARC during that pregnancy.[153] A second study in New York looked at 34 mothers, again identified by the birth of an affected child, after a mean of 27.8 months. Fifteen or 44% of the mothers had become symptomatic with AIDS or ARC. Fourteen mothers had gone on to have subsequent pregnancies.[154] The problem with both these studies was that the patients were identified by the ill-health of a child and if there is a link between maternal and child ill-health then it will be exaggerated by this form of selection.

In Edinburgh, to date, we have followed over 80 females selected only by the fact that they are HIV seropositive. In 21 non-pregnant and 67 pregnant females there is currently no association between parity and clinical or immunological status. Despite what seemed to be adequate counselling, unwanted pregnancies have occurred and mothers have elected to continue with the pregnancy despite the risks to themselves and their child.

The management of drug misusers at risk of, or infected with, HIV has a number of particular problems not often seen with other high-risk groups, and perhaps the most important problem is tackling the clients' drug use and above all trying to achieve harm reduction.

There are a number of reasons to persuade parenteral drug misusers to cease injection drug misuse (IDM). Dr Don De Jarlais in New York has recently demonstrated a relationship between the frequency of IDM and the loss of T_4-lymphocytes from the peripheral blood.[155] The drift in molecular composition demonstrated in different HIV isolates might result in the acquisition of differing strains of HIV.[127] These additional doses of HIV acquired as a consequence of persistent needle-sharing, might be expected to hasten disease progression. Opiates themselves depress the immune system. Morphine given to mice reduced the numbers of neutrophils and macrophages as well as their efficiency in phagocytosing and killing *Candida albicans*. Morphine-treated mice succumbed more rapidly to *Klebsiella* pneumonia peritonitis. There was a depressed lymphoproliferative response to mitogens in the presence of opiates.[125,126]

Abstinence has, until now, been the major goal of dealing with misusers but with the appearance of HIV these goals need to be adjusted to one of 'risk or harm reduction'. The *eventual* goal is still one of abstinence but initially it is important to start with a more realistic goal identified for each patient. Depending upon the individual, this may encompass substitution therapy on a long- or short-term basis in order to avoid needles drug abuse, or the provision of needles and syringes to reduce sharing.

Of more importance is the fact that specific anti-HIV chemotherapy is now becoming available. The most well known is azidothymidine (AZT) also known as Zidovidine or Retrovir. It was discovered in 1964 and was briefly investigated as an anti-cancer agent but in 1985 it was noted to inhibit HIV *in vitro*. A double-blind placebo controlled clinical trial of AZT therapy was begun in 282 patients with AIDS or ARC in January 1986. The trial was discontinued in September 1986 because preliminary analysis demonstrated a significant advantage for the AZT-treated group.

There were significant differences between the two groups with respect to mortality, the frequency of opportunistic infections, weight gain and symptomatic improvement. Nineteen placebo patients died, compared to only one AZT patient. Side-effects did occur but significantly they were less likely if the patients started with more than 0.1×10^9 T_4-lymphocytes per litre. Twenty-four per cent of the AZT-treated patients developed anaemia (<7.5 g/dl), 16% developed significant neutropenia (<0.5×10^9 per litre) and 21% required multiple blood transfusions. The concurrent use of paracetamol was associated with a higher frequency of haematological side-effects. About 10% of the patients developed minor side-effects such as headaches, nausea, abdominal pain, skin rashes, a fever or diarrhoea.[156,157]

Numerous other agents are undergoing extensive evaluation such that there is now a 90 page directory detailing the trials.[158] As yet, however, few of these compounds have been shown to have an effect in well-controlled trials. Another nucleoside analogue, dideoxycytidine has recently completed Phase I trials but was complicated by serious side-effects such as a painful neuropathy.[159] The recent demonstration of neutralization of HIV by anti-idiotypic antibodies against the T_4 molecule raises the possibility of some form of immunological modulation in the future.[160] The possibility remains that a large number of well-known compounds may be active against HIV.

REFERENCES

1. Fauci, A. Immunopathogenesis of HIV. *IIIrd International Conference on AIDS*, Washington DC, 1–5 June, 1987.
2. Linder-Ciccolunghi, S.N. Improving the acceptability and tolerability of interferon therapy in cancer patients – A review. In Brookes, L.J. (ed.). *Proceedings of Satellite Symposium, 3rd European Conference on Clinical Oncology on Cancer Nursing* (ECCO), 19 June 1985.
3. Hudson, J.B., Weinstein, L. & Chang, T.-W. Thrombocytopenic purpura in measles. *J. Pediatr.* **48**: 48–58, 1956.
4. Von Pirquet cited by Dunmire, C., Ruckdeschel, J.C., Mardiney, M.R., Jr. Suppression of *in vitro* lymphocyte responsiveness to purified protein derivative by measles virus. *Cell Immunol.* **20**: 205–17, 1975.
5. Fireman, P., Friday, G. & Kumate, J. Effect of measles vaccine on immunological responsiveness. *Pediatrics* **43**: 264–72, 1969.
6. Dunmire, C., Ruckdeschel, J.C., Mardiney, M.R., Jr. Suppression of *in vitro* lymphocyte responsiveness to purified protein derivative by measles virus. *Cell Immunol.* **20**: 205–17, 1975.
7. Sullivan, J.L., Barry, D.W., Lucas, S.J. *et al.* Measles infection of human mononuclear cells – I. Acute infection of peripheral blood lymphocytes and monocytes. *J. Exp. Med.* **142**: 773–84, 1985.
8. Mascia, A.V., Chick, F.E. & Levy, W.E. Effects of rubeola on tuberculosis. *J. Pediatr.* **43**: 294–6, 1953.
9. Kohn, J.L. & Koiransky, H. Relation of measles and tuberculosis in young children. *Am. J. Dis. Childh.* **44**: 1187–210, 1932.
10. Bech, V. Measles epidemic in Greenland. *Am. J. Dis. Childh.* **103**: 252–3, 1962.
11. Cooper, L.Z., Green, R.H., Krugman, S., Giles, J.P. & Mirick, G.S. Neonatal thrombocytopenic purpura and other manifestations of rubella contracted in utero. *Am. J. Dis. Chilh.* **110**: 416–27, 1965.

12. Ackroyd, J.F. Three cases of thrombocytopenic purpura occurring after rubella. Q. J. Med. **XVIII**: 299–318, 1949.
13. Kolars, C.P. & Spink, W.W. Thrombopenic purpura as a complication of mumps. J. Am. Med. Assoc. **168**: 2213–15, 1958.
14. Famma, P.G., Paton, W.B. & Bostock, M.I. Thrombocytopenic purpura complicating mumps. Br. Med. J. **1**: 1244, 1964.
15. Whitaker, A.G. Haemorrhagic chicken-pox. Br. Med. J. **1**: 14, 1915.
16. Marsden, J.P. & Coughlan, W.J. A case of confluent chicken-pox with haemorrhagic symptoms. Br. Med. J. **1**: 1066–7, 1952.
17. Stoesser, A.V. & Lockwood, W.W. Varicella complicated with acute thrombocytopenic purpura and gangrene. J. Pediatr. **12**: 641–7, 1938.
18. Welch, R.G. Thrombocytopenic purpura and chickenpox. Arch. Dis. Childh. **31**: 38–41, 1956.
19. Hattersley, P.G. Purpura fulminans. Am. J. Dis. Childh. **120**: 467–71, 1970.
20. Cohen, J.J. & Bansmer, C. Chicken-pox with simultaneous idiopathic thrombocytopenic purpura. N. Engl. J. Med. **237**: 222–4, 1947.
21. Feusner, J.H., Slichter, S.J. & Harker, L.A. Mechanisms of thrombocytopenia in varicella. Am. J. Hematol. **7**: 255–64, 1979.
22. Editorial. How does influenza virus pave the way for bacteria? Lancet **1**: 485–6, 1982.
23. Abramson, J.S., Mills, E.I., Giebink, G.S. & Quie, P.G. Depression of monocyte and polymorphonuclear leukocyte oxidative metabolism and bactericidal capacity by influenza A virus. Infect. Immun. **35**: 350–5, 1982.
24. Verhoef, J., Mills, E.L., Debets-Ossenkopp, Y. & Verbrugh, H.A. The effect of influenza virus on oxygen-dependent metabolism of human neutrophils. Adv. Exp. Med. Biol. **141**: 647–54, 1982.
25. Soloway, R.D., Summerskill, W.H.J., Baggenstoss, A.J. et al. Clinical, biochemical, and histological remission of severe chronic active liver disease; a controlled study of treatments and early prognosis. Gastroenterology **63**: 820, 1972.
26. Cook, G.C., Mulligan, R. & Sherlock, S. Controlled prospective trial of corticosteroid therapy in active chronic hepatitis. Q. J. Med. **40**: 160, 1971.
27. Lam, K.C., Lai, C.L., Ng, R.P. et al. Deleterious effect of prednisolone in HBsAg-positive chronic active hepatitis. N. Engl. J. Med. **304**: 380, 1981.
28. Wu, P.L., Laid, C.L., Lam, K.C. et al. Prednisolone in HBsAg-positive chronic active hepatitis, histologic evaluation in a controlled prospective study. Hepatology **2**: 777, 1982.
29. Hoofnagle, J.H., Hanson, R.G., Minuk, G.Y. et al. Randomized controlled trial of adenine arabinoside monophosphate for chronic type B hepatitis. Gastroenterology **86**: 150, 1984.
30. Weimar, W., Heijtink, R.A., Ten Kate, F.J.P. et al. Double-blind study of leukocyte inteferon administration in chronic HBsAg-positive hepatitis. Lancet **1**: 336, 1980.
31. Lai, C.L., Lok, A.S.F., Lin, H.J. et al. Placebo-controlled trial of recombinant α_2-interferon Chinese HBsAg-carrier children. Lancet **2**: 877–80, 1987.
32. Alexander, G.J.M., Brahm, J., Fagan, E.A. et al. Loss of HBsAg with interferon therapy in chronic hepatitis B virus infection. Lancet **2**: 66–9, 1987.
33. Seeff, L.B., Zimmerman, H.J., Wright, E.C. et al. A randomized, double-blind controlled trial of the efficacy of immune serum globulin for the prevention of post-transfusion hepatitis: a Veterans Administration cooperative study. Gastroenterology **72**: 111, 1977.
34. Brotman, B., Prince, A.M. & Huima, T. Non-A, non-B hepatitis: is there more than a single blood-borne strain? J. Infect. Dis. **151**: 618, 1985.
35. Seto, B., Coleman, W.G., Iwarson, S. et al. Detection of reverse transcriptase activity in association with the non-A, non-B hepatitis agent(s). Lancet **2**: 941, 1984.

36. Tabor, E. The three viruses of non-A, non-B hepatitis. *Lancet* **1**: 743, 1985.
37. Aach, R.D., Szmuness, W., Mosley, J.W. *et al.* Serum alanine aminotransferase of donors in relation to the risk of non-A, non-B hepatitis in recipients: the transfusion-transmitted viruses study. *N. Engl. J. Med.* **304**: 989, 1981.
38. Stevens, C.E., Aach, R.D., Hollinger, F.B. *et al.* Hepatitis B virus antibody in blood donor and the occurrence of non-A, non-B hepatitis in transfusion recipients; an analysis of the Transfusion-Transmitted Viruses Study. *Ann. Intern. Med.* **101**: 733, 1984.
39. Kingdon, H.S. Hepatitis after Konyne (letter). *Ann. Intern. Med.* **73**: 656, 1970.
40. Haugen, R.K. Hepatitis after the transfusion of frozen red cells and washed red cells. *N. Engl. J. Med.* **301**: 393, 1979.
41. Nicholson, K.G. Hepatitis delta infections. *Br. Med. J.* **290**: 1370, 1985.
42. Shattock, A.G., Irwin, F.M., Morgan, B.M. *et al.* Increased severity and morbidity of acute hepatitis in drug abusers with simultaneously acquired hepatitis B and hepatitis D virus infections. *Br. Med. J.* **290**: 1377, 1985.
43. Rosina, F., Saracco, G. & Rizetto, M. Risk of post-transfusion infection with the hepatitis delta virus: a multicenter study. *N. Engl. J. Med.* **312**: 1488, 1975.
44. Barrett-Connor, E. Anaemia and infection. *Am. J. Med.* **52**: 242–53, 1972.
45. Camitta, B.M., Nathan, D.G., Forman, E.N. *et al.* Posthepatitic severe aplastic anemia – An indication for early bone marrow transplantation. *Blood* **43**: 473–83, 1974.
46. Hagler, L., Pastore, R.A., Bergin, J.J. & Wrensch, M.R. Aplastic anemia following viral hepatitis: Report of two fatal cases and literature review. *Medicine* **54**: 139–64, 1975.
47. Shurin, S.B. Infectious mononucleosis. *Pediatr. Clin. North Am.* **26**: 315–26, 1979.
48. Clarke, B.F. & Davies, S.H. Severe thrombocytopenia in infectious mononucleosis. *Am. J. Med. Sci.* **248**: 703–8, 1964.
49. Schumacher, H.R. & Barcay, S.J. Hemorrhagic phenomena in infectious mononucleosis. *Am. J. Med. Sci.* **243**: 175–82, 1962.
50. Carter, R.L. Platelet levels in infectious mononucleosis. *Blood* **25**: 817–21, 1965.
51. Pader, E. & Grossman, H. Thrombocytopenic purpura in infectious mononucleosis. *N. Y. J. Med.* **56**: 1905–10, 1956.
52. Radel, E.G. & Schorr, J.B. Thrombocytopenic purpura with infectious mononucleosis. *J. Pediatr.* **63**: 46–60, 1963.
53. Read, J.T. & Helwig, F.C. Infectious mononucleosis. *Arch. Intern. Med.* **75**: 376–80, 1945.
54. Hall, B.D. & Archer, F.C. Acute hemolytic anemia associated with infectious mononucleosis. *N. Engl. J. Med.* **249**: 973–6, 1953.
55. Fekete, A.M. & Kerpelman, E.J. Acute hemolytic anemia complicating infectious mononucleosis. *J. Am. Med. Assoc.* **194**: 1326–7, 1965.
56. Mengel, C.E., Wallace, A.G. & McDaniel, H.G. Infectious mononucleosis, hemolysis, and megaloblastic arrest. *Arch. Intern. Med.* **114**: 333–5, 1964.
57. Koziner, B., Hadler, N., Parrillo, J. & Ellman, L. Agranulocytosis following infectious mononucleosis. *J. Am. Med. Assoc.* **225**: 1235–6, 1973.
58. Lazarus, K.H. & Baehner, R.L. Aplastic anemia complicating infectious mononucleosis: A case report and review of the literature. *Pediatrics* **67**: 907–10, 1981.
59. Mroczek, E.C., Weisenburger, D.D., Grierson, H.L., Markin, R. & Purtilo, D.T. Fatal infectious mononucleosis and virus-associated hemophagocytic syndrome. *Arch. Pathol. Lab. Med.* **111**: 530–5, 1987.
60. Purtilo, D.T., Cassel, C. & Yang, J.P.S. Fatal infectious mononucleosis in familial lymphohistiocytosis. *N. Engl. J. Med.* **291**: 736, 1974.
61. Purtilo, D.T., Cassel, C.K., Yang, J.P.S. *et al.* X-Linked recessive progressive combined variable immunodeficiency (Duncan's disease). *Lancet* **i**: 935–40, 1975.
62. Purtilo, D.T., Szymanski, I., Bhawan, J. *et al.* Epstein–Barr virus infections in

the X-linked recessive lymphoproliferative syndrome. *Lancet* **i**: 798–801, 1978.

63. Grierson, H. & Purtilo, D.T. Epstein–Barr virus infections in males with the X-linked lymphoproliferative syndrome. *Ann. Intern. Med.* **106**: 538–45, 1987.

64. Klemola, E. & Kariainen, L. Cytomegalovirus as a possible cause of a disease resembling infectious mononucleosis. *Br. Med. J.* **2**: 1099–1102, 1965.

65. Editorial. Cytomegalovirus infection in previously healthy adults. *Ann. Intern. Med.* **79**: 267–8, 1973.

66. Starr, S.E. Cytomegalovirus. *Pediatr. Clin. North Am.* **26**: 283–93, 1979.

67. Pannuti, C.S., Vilas Boas, L.S., Angelo, M.J. *et al.* Cytomegalovirus mononucleosis in children and adults: differences in clinical presentation. *Scand. J. Infect. Dis.* **17**: 153–6, 1985.

68. Simon, T.L. Cytomegaloviruses and blood transfusion. *Plasma Ther. Transfusion Technol.* **6**: 69–79, 1985.

69. Risdall, R.J., McKenna, R.A., Nesbit, M.E. *et al.* Virus-associated hemophagocytic syndrome. *Cancer* **44**: 993–1002, 1979.

70. Bowden, R.A., Sayers, M., Flournoy, N. *et al.* Cytomegalovirus immune globulin and seronegative blood products to prevent primary cytomegalovirus infection after marrow transplantation. *N. Engl. J. Med.* **314**: 1006–10, 1986.

71. Snydman, D.R., Werner, B.G., Heinze-Lacey, B., Berardi, V.P. *et al.* Use of cytomegalovirus immune globulin to prevent cytomegalovirus disease in renal-transplant recipients. *N. Engl. J. Med.* **317**: 1049–54, 1987.

72. Meyers, J.D., Reed, E.C., Shepp, D.H., Thornquist, M. *et al.* Ayclovir for prevention of cytomegalovirus infection and disease after allogeneic marrow transplantation. *N. Engl. J. Med.* **318**: 70–5, 1988.

73. Cossart, Y.E., Field, A.M., Cant, B. & Widdows, D. Parvovirus-like particles in human sera. *Lancet* **1**: 72–3, 1975.

74. Edwards, J.M.B., Kessel, I., Gardner, S.D. *et al.* A search for a characteristic illness in children with serological evidence of viral or toxoplasma infection. *J. Infect.* **3**: 316–23, 1981.

75. Cohen, B.J., Mortimer, P.P. & Pereira, M.S. Diagnostic assays with monoclonal antibodies for the human serum parvovirus-like virus (SPLV). *J. Hyg. (Lond.)* **91**: 113–30, 1983.

76. Shneerson,, J.M., Mortimer, P.P. & Vandervelde, E.M. Febrile illness due to a parvovirus. *Br. Med. J.* **2**: 1580, 1980.

77. Serjeant, G.R., Topley, J.M., Mason, K. *et al.* Outbreak of aplastic crises in sickle cell anaemia associated with parvovirus like agent. *Lancet* **ii**: 595–7, 1981.

78. Kelleher, J.F., Luban, N.L., Mortimer, P.P. & Kamimura, T. Human serum "Parvovirus": a specific cause of aplastic crisis in children with hereditary spherocytosis. *J. Pediatr.* **102**: 720–2, 1983.

79. Duncan, J.R., Potter, C.B., Cappellini, M.D., Kurtz, J.B., Anderson, M.J. & Weatherall, D.J. Aplastic crisis due to parvovirus infection in pyruvate kinase deficiency. *Lancet* **ii**: 14–16, 1983.

80. Mortimer, P.P., Humphries, R.K., Moore, J.G., Purcell, R.H. & Young, N.S. A human parvovirus like virus inhibits haematopoietic colony formation *in vitro*. *Nature* **302**: 426–9, 1983.

81. Anderson, M.J., Jones, S.E., Fisher-Hoch, S.P. *et al.* Human parvovirus, the cause of erythema infectiosum (fifth disease)? *Lancet* **i**: 1378, 1983.

82. Cohen, B.J. Update on the human parvovirus. *Communicable Dis. Scot.* **84/10a**: VII–IX, 1984.

83. Anand, A., Gray, E.S., Brown, T., Clewley, J.P. & Cohen, B.J. Human parvovirus infection in pregnancy and hydrops fetalis. *N. Engl. J. Med.* **316**: 183–6, 1987.

84. Carrington, D., Gilmore, D.H., Whittle, M.J. *et al.* Maternal serum α-fetoprotein – A marker of fetal aplastic crisis during intrauterine human parvovirus infection. *Lancet* **i**: 433–5, 1987.

85. Gray, E.S., Davidson, R.J.L. & Anand, A. Human parvovirus and fetal anaemia. *Lancet* **i**: 1144, 1987.
86. Bowen, E.T.W. & Simpson, D.I.H. Dangerous virus diseases. *Hospital Update* **7**(2): 175–83, 1981.
87. Simpson, D.I.H. Arbovirus diseases. *Med. Intern.* **2**: 161–5, 1984.
88. Isaacson, M. Viral haemorrhagic fevers. *Med. Intern.* **2**: 166–70, 1984.
89. Centers for Disease Control. Kaposi's sarcoma and pneumocystis pneumonia among homosexual men – New York and California. *Morbidity Mortality Weekly Rep.* **30**: 305, 1981.
90. Zinkernagel, R.M. & Doherty, P.C. H-2 compatibility requirement for T-cell-mediated lysis of target cells infected with lymphocytic choriomeningitis virus: different cytotoxic T-cell specificities are associated with structures coded for in H-2K or H-2D. *J. Exp. Med.* **141**: 1427–36, 1975.
91. Meuer, S.C., Acuto, O., Hussey, R.E. *et al.* Evidence for the T3-associated 90K heterodimer as the T-cell antigen receptor. *Nature* **303**: 808–10, 1983.
92. Davis, K.C., Horsburgh, C.R. Jr., Hasiba, U., Schocket, A.L. & Kirkpatrick, C.H. Acquired immunodeficiency syndrome in a patient with hemophilia. *Ann. Intern. Med.* **98**: 284–6, 1983.
93. Elliott, J.L., Hoppes, W.L., Platt, M.S., Thomas, J.G., Patel, I.P. & Gansar, A. The acquired immunodeficiency syndrome and *Mycobacterium avium-intracellulare* bacteremia in a patient with hemophilia. *Ann. Intern. Med.* **98**: 290–3, 1983.
94. Poon, M.C., Landay, A., Prasthofer, E.F. & Stagno, S. Acquired immuno-deficiency syndrome with *Pneumocystis carinii* pneumonia and *Mycobacterium avium-intracellulare* infection in a previously healthy patient with classic hemophilia: clinical, immunologic, and virologic findings. *Ann. Intern. Med.* **98**: 287–90, 1983.
95. Ragni, M.V., Spero, J.A., Lewis, J.H. & Bontempo, F.A. Acquired immuno-deficiency-like syndrome in two haemophiliacs. *Lancet* **1**: 213–14, 1983.
96. Centers for Disease Control. Possible transfusion-associated acquired immune deficiency syndrome (AIDS): California. *Morbidity Mortality Weekly Rep.* **31**: 652–4, 1982.
97. Samelson, L.E., Harford, J.B. & Klausner, R.D. Identification of the components of the murine T cell antigen receptor complex. *Cell* **43**: 223–31, 1985.
98. Reinherz, E.L., Meuer, S., Fitzgerald, K.A., Hussey, R.E., Levine, H. & Schlossman, S.F. Antigen recognition by human T lymphocytes is linked to surface expression of the T3 molecular complex. *Cell* **30**: 735–43, 1982.
99. Harris, C., Small, C.B., Klein, R.S. *et al.* Immunodeficiency in female sexual partners of men with the acquired immunodeficiency syndrome. *N. Engl. J. Med.* **308**: 1181–4, 1983.
100. Oleske, J., Minnefor, A., Cooper, R. *et al.* Immune deficiency syndrome in children. *J. Am. Med. Assoc.* **249**: 2345–9, 1983.
101. Barré-Sinoussi, F., Chermann, J.C., Rey, F. *et al.* Isolation of a T-lymphotropic retrovirus from a patient at risk for the acquired immune deficiency syndrome (AIDS). *Science* **220**: 868–71, 1983.
102. Gallo, R.C., Salahuddin, S.Z., Popovic, M. *et al.* Frequent detection and isolation of cytopathic retrovirus (HTLV-III) from patients with AIDS and at risk for AIDS. *Science* **224**: 500–3, 1984.
103. Levy, J.A., Hoffman, A.D., Kramer, S.M., Landis, J.A., Shimabukuro, J.M. & Oshiro, L.S. Isolation of lymphocytopathic retroviruses from San Francisco patients with AIDS. *Science* **225**: 840–2, 1984.
104. Coffin, J., Haase, A., Levy, J.A. *et al.* Human immunodeficiency viruses. *Science* **232**: 697, 1986.
105. Revision of the CDC Surveillance Case Definition for Acquired Immuno-deficiency Syndrome. *Morbidity Mortality Weekly Rep.* **36**(1S), 1987.

106. Answer. (AIDS News Supplement, CDS Weekly Report). *Communicable Dis. Scotl.* **88/22**: 1–2, 1988.
107. Centers for Disease Control. Classification system for HTLV-III/LAV infections. *Ann. Intern. Med.* **105**: 234–7, 1986.
108. Statistics from the World Health Organization and the Centers for Disease Control. *AIDS* **2**: 145–9, 1988.
109. AIDS Surveillance in Europe: Update to 30 June 1987 (part 2). *Communicable Dis. Scotl.* **87/47**(A34): 1–25, 1987.
110. Moss, A., McCallum, G., Volberding, P., Bacchetti, P. & Dritz, S. Mortality associated with mode of presentation in AIDS. *J. Natl. Cancer Inst.* **73**: 1281–4, 1984.
111. Rivin, B., Monroe, J. Hubschuman, B. & Thomas, P. AIDS outcome: a first follow-up. *N. Engl. J. Med.* **311**: 857, 1984.
112. Evatt, B., Gomperts, E., McDougal, J. & Ramse, R. Coincidental appearance of LAV/HTLV-III antibodies in hemophiliacs and the onset of the AIDS epidemic. *N. Engl. J. Med.* **312**: 483–6, 1985.
113. Jason, J., McDougal, J., Holman, R. *et al.* Human T-lymphotrophic retrovirus type III/lymphadenopathy associated virus antibody: association with hemophiliacs' immune status and blood component usage. *J. Am. Med. Assoc.* **253**: 3409–15, 1985.
114. Koerper, M.A., Kaminsky, L.S. & Levy, J.A. Differential prevalance of antibody to AIDS-associated retrovirus in haemophiliacs treated with factor VIII concentrate versus cyroprecipitate. *Lancet* **ii**: 275, 1985.
115. McGrady, G., Gjerset, G. & Kennedy, S. Risk of exposure to HTLV-III/LAV and the type of clotting factor used in hemophilia. Abstracts of the *International Conference on Acquired Immunodeficiency Syndrome*, Atlanta, 1985, p. 48.
116. Curran, J., Morgan, W., Hardy, A. *et al.* The epidemiology of AIDS: current status and future prospects. *Science* **299**: 1352–7, 1985.
117. Hilgartner, M.W. AIDS and hemophilia. *N. Engl. J. Med.* **317**: 1153–4, 1987.
118. Hardy, A., Allen, J., Morgan, W. & Curran, J. The incidence rate of acquired immunodeficiency syndrome in selected populations. *J. Am. Med. Assoc.* **253**: 215–20, 1985.
119. Peterman, T., Jaffe, H., Feorino, P. *et al.* Transfusion associated acquired immunodeficiency syndrome in the United States. *J. Am. Med. Assoc.* **254**: 2913–17, 1985.
120. Yanagi, Y., Yoshikai, Y., Leggett, K., Clark, S.P., Aleksander, I. & Mak, T.W. A human T cell-specific cDNA clone encodes a protein having extensive homology to immunoglobulin chains. *Nature* **308**: 145–9, 1984.
121. Hannum, C.H., Kappler, J.W., Trowbridge, I.S., Marrack, P. & Freed, J.H. Immunoglobulin-like nature of the α-chain of a human T-cell antigen/MHC receptor. *Nature* **312**: 65–7, 1984.
122. Saito, H., Kranz, D.M., Takagaki, D., Hayday, A.C., Eisen, H.N. & Tonegawa, S. A third rearranged and expressed gene in a clone of cytotoxic T lymphocytes. *Nature* **312**: 36–40, 1984.
123. Friedland, G.H. & Klein, R.S. Transmission of the human immunodeficiency virus. *N. Engl. J. Med.* **317**: 1125–35, 1987.
124. Editorial Note. Transfusion associated human T lymphotrophic virus 3/lymphadenopathy associated virus infection from seronegative donor – Colorado. *Morbidity Mortality Weekly Rep.* **35**: 389–90, 1986.
125. Tubaro, E., Borelli, G., Croce, C., Cavallo, G. & Santiangeli, C. Effect of morphine on resistance to infection. *J. Infect. Dis.* **148**: 656–6, 1983.
126. Editorial. Opiates, opioid peptides, and immunity. *Lancet* **i**: 774–5, 1984.
127. Hahn, B.H., Shaw, G.M., Taylor, M.E. *et al.* Genetic variation in HTLV-III/LAV over time in patients with AIDS or at risk for AIDS. *Science* **232**: 1548–53, 1986.
128. Polk, B.F., Fox, R., Brookmeyer, R. *et al.* Predictors of the acquired

immunodeficiency syndrome developing in a cohort of seropositive homosexual men. *N. Engl. J. Med.* **316**: 61–6, 1987.

129. Eyster, M.E., Gail, M.H., Ballard, J.O., Al-Mondhiry, N. & Goerdert, J.J. Natural history of human immunodeficiency virus infection in haemophiliacs: effects of T-cell subsets, platelet counts and age. *Ann. Intern. Med.* **107**: 1–6, 1987.

130. Lacey, C.J.N., Forbes, M.A., Waugh, M.A., Cooper, E.H., Cooper, J. & Hambling, M.H. Serum β_2-microglobulin and HIV infection. *IV International Conference on AIDS*, Stockholm, Sweden, 12–16 June, 1988.

131. Anderson, R.E., Lang, W., Geyer, J., Royce, R., Jewell, N. & Winkelstein, W. Beta-2 microglobulin level predicts AIDS. *IV International Conference on AIDS*, Stockholm, Sweden, 12–16 June, 1988.

132. Gold, J., Morlet, A., Nicolas, T., Guinan, J.J. & Stevens, M. Elevation of serum beta-2 microglobulin associated with decreased CD4 lymphocyte count in HIV infection. *IV International Conference on AIDS*, Stockholm, Sweden, 12–16 June, 1988.

133. Lambin, P., Lefrère, J.J., Doinel, C., Fine, J.M. & Salmon, C. Neopterin and beta 2 microglobulin in sera of HIV seropositive subjects during a two year follow-up. *IV International Conference on AIDS*, Stockholm, Sweden 12–16 June, 1988.

134. Weber, J.N. & Weiss, R.A. The virology of human immunodeficiency viruses. *Br. Med. Bull.* **44**: 20–37, 1988.

135. Forster, S.M., Osborne, L.M., Cheingsong-Popov, R. *et al.* Decline of anti-p24 antibody precedes antigenaemia as correlate of prognosis in HIV-1 infection. *AIDS* Vol. **1**(4): 235–40, 1987.

136. Lange, J.M.A.A., Paul, D.A., Huismaan, H.G. *et al.* Persistent HIV anti-genaemia and decline of HIV core antibodies associated with transition to AIDS. *Br. Med. J.* **293**: 1459–62, 1986.

137. Allain, J.P., Laurian, Y., Paul, D.A. *et al.* Long term evaluation of HIV antigen and antibodies to p24 and gp41 in patients with haemophilia. Potential clinical importance. *N. Engl. J. Med.* **317**: 1114–1, 1987.

138. Eales, L.J. & Parkin, J.M. Current concepts in the immunopathogenesis of AIDS and HIV infection. *Br. Med. Bull.* **144**: 38–55, 1988.

139. Treacy, M., Lai, L., Costello, C. & Clark, A. Peripheral blood and bone marrow abnormalities in patients with HIV related disease. *Br. J. Haematol.* **65**: 289–94, 1987.

140. Murphy, M.F., Metcalfe, P., Waters, A.H. *et al.* Incidence and mechanism of neutropenia and thrombocytopenia in patients with human immunodeficiency virus infection. *Br. J. Haematol.* **66**: 337–40, 1987.

141. Jaffe, H.S., Abrams, D.I., Anmann, A.J., Lewis, B.J. & Golden, J.A. Complica-tions of co-trimoxazole in treatment of AIDS associated *Pneumocystis carinii* pneumonia in homosexual men. *Lancet* **2**: 1109–11, 1983.

142. Morris, L., Distenfeld, A., Amorosi, E. & Karpatkin, S. Autoimmune thrombocytopenic purpura in homosexual men. *Ann. Intern. Med.* **96**: 714–17, 1982.

143. Savona, S., Nardi, M., Lennette, E.T. & Karpatkin, S. Thrombocytopenic purpura in narcotic addicts. *Ann. Intern. Med.* **102**: 737–41, 1985.

144. Ratnoff, O.D., Menitove, J.E., Aster, R.H. & Lederman, M.M. Coincident classic hemophilia and 'idiopathic' thrombocytopenic purpura in patients under treatment with concentrates of antihemophilic factor (factor VIII). *N. Engl. J. Med.* **308**: 439–42, 1983.

145. Abrams, D. AIDS related conditions. *Clin. Immunol. Allergy* **6**: 581–99, 1986.

146. Stewart, G.J., Tyler, J.P.P., Cunningham, A.L. *et al.* Transmission of HTLV-III by artificial insemination by donor. *Lancet* **2**: 581–5, 1985.

147. Selwyn, P.A., Schoenbaum, E.E., Feingold, A.R. *et al.* Perinatal transmission of

HIV in Intravenous Drug Abusers. *IIIrd International Conference on AIDS*, Th. 7.2, Washington, DC, 1–5 June, 1987.

148. Mok, J.Q., Giaquinto, C., de Rossi, A., Grosch-Worner, I., Ades, A.E. & Peckham, C.S. Infants born to mothers seropositive for human immuno-deficiency virus. *Lancet* **1**: 1164–7, 1987.

149. Willoughby, A., Mendez, H., Minkoff, H. *et al.* HIV in pregnant women and their offspring. *IIIrd International Conference on AIDS*, Th. 7.3, Washington, DC, 1–5 June, 1987.

150. Blanche, S., Rouzioux, C., Veber, F. *et al.* Prospective study of HIV seropositive women. *IIIrd International Conference on AIDS*, Th. 7.4, Washington, DC, 1–5 June, 1987.

151. Bradick, M., Kreiss, J.K., Quin, T. *et al.* Congenital transmission of HIV in Nairobi, Kenya. *IIIrd International Conference on AIDS*, Th. 7.5, Washington, DC, 1–5 June, 1987.

152. Nzila, N., Ryden, R.W., Behets, F., Francis, H., Bayende, E., Nelson, A. & Mann, J.M. *et al.* Perinatal HIV transmission in two African hospitals. Abstract TJ 7.6. *IIIrd International Conference on AIDS*, Th. 7.6, Washington, DC, 1–5 June, 1987. Quoted by Piot, P., Kreiss, J.K., Ndinya-Achola, J.O., Ngugi, E.N., Simonsen, J.N., Cameron, D.W., Taelman, H. & Plummer, F.A. Heterosexual transmission of HIV. *AIDS* **1**: 199–206, 1987.

153. Scott, G.B., Fischl, M.A., Klimas, N. *et al.* Mother of infants with the Acquired Immune Deficiency Syndrome. *J. Am. Med. Assoc.* **253**: 363–6, 1985.

154. Minkoff, H., Nanda, D., Menez, R. & Fikeig, S. Pregnancies resulting in infants with AIDS or AIDS related complex. *Obstet. Gynecol.* **69**: 285–7, 1987.

155. Des Jarlais, D.C., Friedman, S.R., Marmor, M., Cohen, H., Mildvan, D., Yancovitz, S. *et al.* Development of AIDS, HIV seroconversion, and potential co-factors for T4 cell loss in a cohort of intravenous drug users. *AIDS* **1**: 105–11, 1987.

156. Fischl, M.A., Richman, D.D., Grieco, M.H. *et al.* The efficacy of Azido-thymidine (AZT) in the treatment of patients with AIDS and AIDS-related complex. *N. Engl. J. Med.* **317**: 185–91, 1987.

157. Richman, D.D., Fischl, M.A., Grieco, M.H., Gottlieb, M.S., Volberding, P.A., Laskin, O.L. *et al.* The toxicity of azidothymidine (AZT) in the treatment of patients with AIDS and AIDS-related complex. *N. Engl. J. Med.* **317**: 192–7, 1987.

158. Abrams, D., Gottlieb, M., Grieco, M., Speer, M. & Bernstien, S. (eds) *AmFAR Directory of Experimental Treatments for AIDS and ARC*. Vol. I, Revised and Expanded October, 1987. Mary Ann Liebert, Inc., New York.

159. Yarchoan, R., Perno, C.F., Thomas, R.V. *et al.* Phase 1 Studies of 2',3'-dideoxycytidine in severe human immunodeficiency virus infection as a single agent and alternating with zidovudine (AZT). *Lancet* **1**: 76–80, 1988.

160. Dalgleish, A.G., Thomson, B.J., Chanh, T.C., Malkovsky, M. & Kennedy, R.C. Neutralisation of HIV isolates by anti-idiotypic antibodies which mimic the T4 (CD4) epitope: a potential AIDS vaccine. *Lancet* **2**: 1047–9, 1987.

161. Faber, V., Dalgleish, A.G., Newell, A. & Malkovsky, M. Inhibition of HIV replication *in vitro* by fusidic acid. *Lancet* **2**: 827–8, 1987.

APPENDIX: CLASSIFICATION SYSTEM FOR HUMAN T-LYMPHOTROPIC VIRUS TYPE III/LYMPHADENOPATHY-ASSOCIATED VIRUS INFECTIONS
(From *Morbidity and Mortality Weekly Report*, Vol. 35(20), 1986.

Introduction

Persons infected with the etiologic retrovirus of acquired immunodeficiency syndrome (AIDS) (1–4)* may present with a variety of manifestations ranging from asymptomatic infection to severe immunodeficiency and life-threatening secondary infectious diseases or cancers. The rapid growth of knowledge about human T-lymphotropic virus type III/lymphadenopathy-associated virus (HTLV-III/LAV) has resulted in an increasing need for a system of classifying patients within this spectrum of clinical and laboratory findings attributable to HTLV-III/LAV infection (5–7).

Various means are now used to describe and assess patients with manifestations of HTLV-III/LAV infection and to describe their signs, symptoms, and laboratory findings. The surveillance definition of AIDS has proven to be extremely valuable and quite reliable for some epidemiologic studies and clinical assessment of patients with the more severe manifestations of disease. However, more inclusive definitions and classifications of HTLV-III/LAV infection are needed for optimum patient care, health planning, and public health control strategies, as well as for epidemiologic studies and special surveys. A broadly applicable, easily understood classification system should also facilitate and clarify communication about this disease.

In an attempt to formulate the most appropriate classification system, CDC has sought the advice of a panel of expert consultants† to assist in defining the manifestations of HTLV-III/LAV infection.

---

* The AIDS virus has been variously termed human T-lymphotropic virus type III (HTLV-III), lymphadenopathy-associated virus (LAV), AIDS-associated retrovirus (ARV), or human immunodeficiency virus (HIV). The designation human immunodeficiency virus (HIV) has recently been proposed by a subcommittee of the International Committee for the Taxonomy of Viruses as the appropriate name for the retrovirus that has been implicated as the causative agent of AIDS (4).

† The following persons served on the review panel: D.S Burke, MD, R.R Redfield, MD, Walter Reed Army Institute of Research, Washington, DC; J. Chin, MD, State Epidemiologist, California Department of Health Services; L.Z. Cooper, MD, St Luke's-Roosevelt Hospital Center, New York City; J.P. Davis, MD, State Epidemiologist, Wisconsin Division of Health; M.A. Fischl, MD, University of Miami School of Medicine, Miami, Florida; G. Friedland, MD, Albert Einstein College of Medicine, New York City; M.A. Johnson, MD, D.I. Abrams, MD, San Francisco General Hospital; D. Mildvan, MD, Beth Israel Medical Center, New York City; C.U. Tuazon, MD, George Washington University School of Medicine, Washington, DC; R.W. Price, MD, Memorial Sloan-Kettering Cancer Center, New York City; C. Konigsberg, MD, Broward County Public Health Unit, Fort Lauderdale, Florida; M.S. Gottlieb, MD, University of California–Los Angeles Medical Center; representatives of the National Institute of Allergy and Infectious Diseases, National Cancer Institute, National Institutes of Health; Center for Infectious Diseases, CDC.

Goals and objectives of the classification system

The classification system presented in this report is primarily applicable to public health purposes, including disease reporting and surveillance, epidemiologic studies, prevention and control activities, and public health policy and planning.

Immediate applications of such a system include the classification of infected persons for reporting of cases to state and local public health agencies, and use in various disease coding and recording systems, such as the forthcoming 10th revision of the International Classification of Diseases.

Definition of HTLV-III/LAV infection

The most specific diagnosis of HTLV-III/LAV infection is by direct identification of the virus in host tissues by virus isolation; however, the techniques for isolating HTLV-III/LAV currently lack sensitivity for detecting infection and are not readily available. For public health purposes, patients with repeatedly reactive screening tests for HTLV-III/LAV antibody (e.g. enzyme-linked immunosorbent assay) in whom antibody is also identified by the use of supplemental tests (e.g., Western blot, immunofluorescence assay) should be considered both infected and infective (8–10).

Although HTLV-III/LAV infection is identified by isolation of the virus or, indirectly, by the presence of antibody to the virus, a presumptive clinical diagnosis of HTLV-III/LAV infection has been made in some situations in the absence of positive virologic or serologic test results. There is a very strong correlation between the clinical manifestations of AIDS as defined by CDC and the presence of HTLV-III/LAV antibody (11–14). Most persons whose clinical illness fulfills the CDC surveillance definition for AIDS will have been infected with the virus (12–14).

Classification system

This system classifies the manifestations of HTLV-III/LAV infection into four mutually exclusive groups, designated by Roman numerals I through IV (Table 11.1A). *The classification system applies only to patients diagnosed as having HTLV-III/LAV infection (see previous section, **DEFINITION OF HTLV-III/LAV INFECTION**).* Classification in a particular group is not explicitly intended to have prognostic significance, nor to designate severity of illness. However classification in the four principal groups, I–IV, is hierarchical in that persons classified in a particular group should not be reclassified in a preceding group if clinical findings resolve, since clinical improvement may not accurately reflect changes in the severity of the underlying disease.

Group I includes patients with transient signs and symptoms that appear at the time of, or shortly after, initial infection with HTLV-III/LAV as identified by laboratory studies. All patients in Group I will be reclassified in another group following resolution of this acute syndrome.

Table 11.1A Summary of Classification System for Human T-Lymphotropic
Virus Type III/Lymphadenopathy-Associated Virus

Group I. Acute infection

Group II. Asymptomatic infection[a]

Group III. Persistent generalized lymphadenopathy[a]

Group IV. Other disease
  Subgroup A. Constitutional disease
  Subgroup B. Neurologic disease
  Subgroup C. Secondary infectious diseases
    Category C-1. Specified secondary infectious diseases listed in the CDC
      surveillance definition for AIDS[b]
    Category C-2. Other specified secondary infectious diseases
  Subgroup D. Secondary cancers[b]
  Subgroup E. Other conditions

---

[a] Patients in Groups II and III may be subclassified on the basis of a laboratory
evaluation.
[b] Includes those patients whose clinical presentation fulfills the definition of AIDS
used by CDC for national reporting.

Group II includes patients who have no signs or symptoms of HTLV-III/LAV infection. Patients in this category may be subclassified based on whether hematologic and/or immunologic laboratory studies have been done and whether results are abnormal in a manner consistent with the effects of HTLV-III/LAV infection.

Group III includes patients with persistent generalized lymphadenopathy, but without findings that would lead to classification in Group IV. Patients in this category may be subclassified based on the results of laboratory studies in the same manner as patients in Group II.

Group IV includes patients with clinical symptoms and signs of HTLV-III/LAV infection other than or in addition to lymphadenopathy. Patients in this group are assigned to *one or more* subgroups based on clinical findings. These subgroups are: A. constitutional disease; B. neurologic disease; C. secondary infectious diseases; D. secondary cancers; and E. other conditions resulting from HTLV-III/LAV infection. There is no *a priori* hierarchy of severity among subgroups A through E, and these subgroups are not mutually exclusive.

Definitions of the groups and subgroups are as follows:

Group I. Acute HTLV-III/LAV Infection. Defined as a mononucleosis-like syndrome, with or without aseptic meningitis, associated with sero-conversion for HTLV-III/LAV antibody (*15–16*). Antibody seroconversion is required as evidence of initial infection; current viral isolation procedures are not adequately sensitive to be relied on for demonstrating the onset of infection.

Group II. Asymptomatic HTLV-III/LAV Infection. Defined as the absence of signs or symptoms of HTLV-III/LAV infection. To be classified in Group II, patients must have had no previous signs or symptoms that would have led to classification in Groups III or IV. Patients whose clinical findings caused them to be classified in Groups III or IV should not be reclassified in Group II if those clinical findings resolve.

Patients in this group may be subclassified on the basis of a laboratory evaluation. Laboratory studies commonly indicated for patients with HTLV-III/LAV infection include, but are not limited to, a complete blood count (including differential white blood cell count) and a platelet count. Immunologic tests, especially T-lymphocyte helper and suppressor cell counts, are also an important part of the overall evaluation. Patients whose test results are within normal limits, as well as those for whom a laboratory evaluation has not yet been completed, should be differentiated from patients whose test results are consistent with defects associated with HTLV-III/LAV infection (e.g., lymphopenia, thrombocytopenia, decreased number of helper [T_4]T-lymphocytes).

Group III. Persistent Generalized Lymphadenopathy (PGL). Defined as palpable lymphadenopathy (lymph node enlargement of 1 cm or greater) at two or more extra-inguinal sites persisting for more than 3 months in the absence of a concurrent illness or condition other than HTLV-III/LAV infection to explain the findings. Patients in this group may also be subclassified on the basis of a laboratory evaluation, as is done for asymptomatic patients in Group II (see above). Patients with PGL whose clinical findings caused them to be classified in Group IV should not be reclassified in Group III if those other clinical findings resolve.

Group IV. Other HTLV-III/LAV Disease. The clinical manifestations of patients in this group may be designated by assignment to one or more subgroups (A–E) listed below. Within Group IV, subgroup classification is independent of the presence or absence of lymphadenopathy. Each subgroup may include patients who are minimally symptomatic, as well as patients who are severely ill. Increased specificity for manifestations of HTLV-III/LAV infection, if needed for clinical purposes or research purposes or for disability determinations, may be achieved by creating additional divisions within each subgroup.

Subgroup A. Constitutional disease. Defined as one or more of the following: fever persisting more than 1 month, involuntary weight loss of greater than 10% of baseline, or diarrhoea persisting more than 1 month; and the absence of a concurrent illness or condition other than HTLV-III/LAV infection to explain the findings.

Subgroup B. Neurologic disease. Defined as one or more of the following: dementia, myelopathy, or peripheral neuropathy; and the absence of a concurrent illness or condition other than HTLV-III/LAV infection to explain the findings.

Subgroup C. Secondary infectious diseases. Defined as the diagnosis of an infectious disease associated with HTLV-III/LAV infection and/or at least moderately indicative of a defect in cell-mediated immunity. Patients in this subgroup are divided further into two categories:

> **Category C-1.** Includes patients with symptomatic or invasive disease due to one of 12 specified secondary infectious diseases listed in the surveillance definition of AIDS[§]: *Pneumocystis carinii* pneumonia, chronic

[§]This subgroup includes patients with one or more of the specified infectious diseases listed whose clinical presentation fulfils the definition of AIDS as used by CDC for national reporting.

cryptosporidiosis, toxoplasmosis, extra-intestinal strongyloidiasis, isosporiasis, candidiasis (esophageal, bronchial, or pulmonary), crypto-coccosis, histoplasmosis, mycobacterial infection with *Mycobacterium avium* complex or *M. kansasii*, cytomegalovirus infection, chronic muco-cutaneous or disseminated herpes simplex virus infection, and progressive multifocal leukoencephalopathy.

Category C-2. Includes patients with symptomatic or invasive disease due to one of six other specified secondary infectious diseases: oral hairy leukoplakia, multidermatomal herpes zoster, recurrent *Salmonella* bacteremia, nocardiosis, tuberculosis, or oral candidiasis (thrush).

Subgroup D. Secondary cancers. Defined as the diagnosis of one or more kinds of cancer known to be associated with HTLV-III/LAV infection as listed in the surveillance definition of AIDS and at least moderately indicative of a defect in cell-mediated immunity[¶]: Kaposi's sarcoma, non-Hodgkin's lymphoma (small, noncleaved lymphoma or immunoblastic sarcoma), or primary lymphoma of the brain.

Subgroup E. Other conditions in HTLV-III/LAV infection. Defined as the presence of other clinical findings or diseases, not classifiable above, that may be attributed to HTLV-III/LAV infection and/or may be indicative of a defect in cell-mediated immunity. Included are patients with chronic lymphoid interstitial pneumonitis. Also included are those patients whose signs or symptoms could be attributed either to HTLV-III/LAV infection or to another coexisting disease not classified elsewhere, and patients with other clinical illnesses, the course or management of which may be complicated or altered by HTLV-III/LAV infection. Examples include: patients with constitutional symptoms not meeting the criteria for subgroup IV-A; patients with infectious diseases not listed in subgroup IV-C; and patients with neoplasms not listed in subgroup IV-D.

Reported by Center for Infectious Diseases, CDC.

Editorial Note: The classification system is meant to provide a means of grouping patients infected with HTLV-III/LAV according to the clinical expression of disease. It will require periodic revision as warranted by new information about HTLV-III/LAV infection. The definition of particular syndromes will evolve with increasing knowledge of the significance of certain clinical findings and laboratory tests. New diagnostic techniques, such as the detection of specific HTLV-III/LAV antigens or antibodies, may add specificity to the assessment of patients infected with HTLV-III/LAV.

The classification system defines a limited number of specified clinical presentations. Patients whose signs and symptoms do not meet the criteria for other groups and subgroups, but whose findings are attributable to HTLV-III/LAV infection, should be classified in subgroup IV-E. As the classification system is revised and updated, certain subsets of patients in subgroup, IV-E may be identified as having related groups of clinical findings that should be separately classified as distinct syndromes. This

¶This subgroup includes those patients with one or more of the specified cancers listed whose clinical presentation fulfils the definition of AIDS as used by CDC for national reporting.

could be accomplished either by creating additional subgroups within Group IV or by broadening the definitions of the existing subgroups.

Persons currently using other classification systems (6–7) or nomenclatures (e.g., AIDS-related complex, lymphadenopathy syndrome) can find equivalences with those systems and terminologies and the classification presented in this report. Because this classification system has only four principal groups based on chronology, presence or absence of signs and symptoms, and the type of clinical findings present, comparisons with other classifications based either on clinical findings or on laboratory assessment are easily accomplished.

This classification system does not imply any change in the definition of AIDS used by CDC since 1981 for national reporting. Patients whose clinical presentations fulfil the surveillance definition of AIDS are classified in Group IV. However, not every case in Group IV will meet the surveillance definition.

Persons wishing to comment on this material are encouraged to send comments in writing to the AIDS Program, Center for Infectious Diseases, CDC.

REFERENCES

1. Gallo, R.C., Salahuddin, S.Z., Popovic, M. *et al.* Frequent detection and isolation of cytopathic retroviruses (HTLV-III) from patients with AIDS and at risk for AIDS. *Science* **224**: 500–3, 1984.
2. Barré-Sinoussi, F., Chermann, J.C., Rey, F. *et al.* Isolation of a T-lymphotropic retrovirus from a patient at risk for acquired immune deficiency syndrome (AIDS). *Science* **220**: 868–71, 1983.
3. Levy, J.A., Hoffman, A.D., Kramer, S.M., Landis, J.A., Shimabukuro, J.M., Oshiro, L.S. Isolation of lymphocytopathic retroviruses from San Francisco patients with AIDS. *Science* **225**: 840–2, 1984.
4. Coffin, J., Haase, A., Levy, J.A. *et al.* Human immunodeficiency viruses (Letter). *Science* **232**: 697, 1986.
5. CDC. Revision of the case definition of acquired immunodeficiency syndrome for national reporting – United States. *M.M.W.R.* **34**: 373–5, 1985.
6. Haverkos, H.W., Gottlieb, M.S., Killen, J.Y., Edelman, R. Classification of HTLV-III/LAV-related diseases (Letter). *J. Infect. Dis.* **152**: 1095, 1985.
7. CDC. Antibodies to a retrovirus etiologically associated with acquired immunodeficiency syndrome (AIDS) in populations with increased incidences of the syndrome. *M.M.W.R.* **33**: 377–9, 1984.
9. CDC. Update: Public Health Service Workshop on Human T-Lymphotropic Virus Type III Antibody Testing – United States. *M.M.W.R.* **34**: 477–8, 1985.
10. CDC. Additional recommendations to reduce sexual and drug abuse-related transmission of human T-lymphotropic virus type III/lymphadenopathy-associated virus. *M.M.W.R.* **35**: 152–5, 1986.
11. Selik, R.M., Haverkos, H.W., Curran, J.W. Acquired immune deficiency syndrome (AIDS) trends in the United States, 1978–1982. *Am. J. Med.* **76**: 493–500, 1984.
12. Sarngadharan M.G., Popovic, M., Bruch, L., Schüpbach, J., Gallo, R.C. Antibodies reactive with human T-lymphotropic retroviruses (HTLV-III) in the serum of patients with AIDS. *Science* **224**: 506–8, 1984.
13. Safai, B., Sarngadharan, M.G., Groopman, J.E. *et al.* Seroepidemiological studies of human T-lymphotropic retrovirus type III in acquired immunodeficiency

syndrome. *Lancet* **1**: 1438–40, 1984.

14. Laurence, J., Brun-Vezinet, F., Schutzer, S.E. *et al.* Lymphadenopathy associated viral antibody in AIDS. Immune correlations and definition of a carrier state. *N. Engl. J. Med.* **311**: 1269–73, 1984.

15. Ho, D.D., Sarngadharan, M.G., Resnick, L., Dimarzo-Vcronese F., Rota, T.R., Hirsch, M.S. Primary human T-lymphotropic virus type III infection. *Ann. Intern. Med.* **103**: 880–3, 1985.

16. Cooper, D.A., Gold, J., Maclean, P. *et al.* Acute AIDS retrovirus infection. Definition of a clinical illness associated with seroconversion. *Lancet* **1**: 537–40, 1985.

12

Monitoring the acute-phase response – laboratory tests and clinical application

J. Stuart
Professor of Haematology, Medical School, University of Birmingham, Birmingham, UK

J.T. Whicher
Professor of Chemical Pathology, Old Medical School, University of Leeds, Leeds, UK

The acute-phase response is a systemic adaptive response, generally considered to be protective in nature, that follows any form of tissue injury. It comprises fever, a leucocytosis, muscle proteolysis, hormonal changes, and an increase in serum concentration of a number of liver-derived plasma proteins, the acute-phase proteins.[1] A complex array of cytokines, predominantly derived from macrophages, have been shown to mediate the above effects. The best known of these cytokines, interleukin-1, mediates all of these systemic responses and has a number of local effects also, particularly on B- and T-cells. Recent evidence has shown that tumour necrosis factor and interleukin-6 are also mediators of acute-phase protein production and that these cytokines may have synergistic effects. It is also probable that individual acute-phase proteins are regulated by different cytokines and hormones.[2]

The major acute-phase proteins are shown in Table 12.1; they belong to several functional families of plasma proteins but probably all have a role to play in inflammation.[4] They function as mediators of inflammation, as inhibitors of mediator pathways, as inhibitors of proteases released from phagocytosing leucocytes, and as scavengers of the molecular debris of tissue damage. The acute-phase increase in liver synthesis, and thus in plasma concentration, of acute-phase proteins is a physiological mechanism which increases their concentration in tissue fluid at the inflammatory site. Increased synthesis maintains the plasma concentration of proteins, such as those of the coagulation cascade and complement pathways, that would otherwise be rapidly catabolized as they fulfil their individual functions. In addition, the possibility of differential induction of proteins in different forms of inflammation suggests that acute-phase proteins may modulate the nature of the inflammatory lesion.

The hepatocyte is the major site of synthesis of the acute-phase proteins, all of which can be synthesized by a single cell.[5] Following induction of inflammation, recruitment of hepatocytes to the synthesis of acute-phase proteins proceeds from the periphery of the hepatic lobule inwards and

Table 12.1   The Acute-phase Proteins of Inflammation (After Whicher & Dieppe[3])

Protein	Function
Mediators	
C-Reactive protein	Ligand binding, complement activation
Complement components C1s, C2, C3, C4, C5, C9, Factor B	Opsonization, chemotaxis, mast cell degranulation
Kininogenase (kallikrein) Kinin	Vascular permeability and dilatation
Factor VIII Fibrinogen Prothrombin	Clotting, formation of a fibrin matrix for repair
Plasminogen	Proteolytic activation of complement and fibrinolysis
Inhibitors	
Antithrombin III C1 1NH Factor 1 Factor H	Control of mediator pathways
α_1-Antitrypsin α_1-Antichymotrypsin Haptoglobin Cysteine protease inhibitor Inhibitor of tissue plasminogen activator	Collagenase, elastase Cathepsin G Cathepsin B, H, L? Cysteine proteases Plasminogen activator ⎫ Inhibited
Scavengers	
Haptoglobin Serum amyloid A protein Ceruloplasmin C-Reactive protein	Haemoglobin Cholesterol? Oxygen free radicals? DNA? ⎫ Scavenged
Immune regulation	
C-Reactive protein Orosomucoid	Interactions with T- and B-cells Expressed on lymphocyte surface; T-cell inhibitor
Repair and resolution	
Orosomucoid	Promotes fibroblast growth and interacts with collagen
α_1-Antitrypsin α_1-Antichymotrypsin C1-1NH	? Control remodelling of connective tissue; bound to surface of new elastic fibres

30–40% of liver protein synthesis becomes committed to it.[6] There is a concomitant decrease in hepatic messenger RNA and the synthesis of several transport proteins such as albumin, pre-albumin, retinol-binding protein, and some apo-lipoproteins. Although this reduction is cytokine mediated, it is a matter of speculation as to whether it has a functional role in inflammation. There is evidence that some acute-phase proteins may be synthesized outside the liver, by cells such as macrophages or lymphocytes, and this may be of local importance at the site of inflammation while making little or no contribution to the plasma protein concentration.[7,8]

It is uncertain whether other proteins that are increased in inflammation, by mechanisms distinct from cytokine-induced liver synthesis, should be termed acute-phase proteins. Ferritin, alkaline phosphatase and β_2-microglobulin may all increase in inflammation and, while ferritin may have a role to play in inflammation, there is no evidence that the others do. Cytokines, such as interleukin-1, may also induce release of proteins from non-hepatic tissue, such as von Willebrand factor from human vascular endothelial cells.[9] To consider these as acute-phase proteins only serves to confuse the issue as they may increase markedly in conditions in which inflammation is absent. It is also important to appreciate that some acute-phase proteins may respond to entirely different inductive stimuli (e.g. fibrinogen synthesis induced by fibrin degradation products).[10] Thus plasma fibrinogen may increase independently from other acute-phase proteins in response to, for example, endothelial injury and fibrin deposition. Also, α_1-antitrypsin and ceruloplasmin show significant increases in pregnancy and α_2-pregnancy-associated glycoprotein may show acute-phase behaviour in the non-pregnant state.[11]

The kinetics of the acute-phase response in acute inflammation vary considerably between different proteins but show a fairly constant hierarchy, as in the post-operative response (Fig. 12.1).[12] This may reflect the degree to which cytokines induce liver synthesis as well as the effects of molecular characteristics on the distribution and catabolism of individual proteins. In chronic inflammation, the situation is less well understood and this constant hierarchical pattern does not hold true, the pattern of plasma protein increase varying from disease to disease. This may reflect differential cytokine induction or changes in fractional catabolic rate of proteins in different forms of inflammation. Notable examples of altered protein catabolism include fibrinogen (which may be consumed in intravascular coagulation), haptoglobin (consumed in the presence of haemolysis) and α_1-antitrypsin (consumed in vasculitis). The plasma concentration of these proteins may thus be inappropriately low compared with other acute-phase proteins. This disharmonic response may indicate the presence of one or more of the above complications in a patient with inflammatory disease.[13]

In acute inflammation, C-reactive protein (CRP), serum amyloid A protein (SAA), α_1-antichymotrypsin, and orosomucoid are apparently unaffected by such changes in catabolism. They vary in their sensitivity to minimal inflammation, SAA being the most sensitive, followed closely by CRP and α_1-antichymotrypsin; orosomucoid is considerably less sensitive. At the present time practical constraints make CRP the most useful measure of acute inflammation. In chronic inflammation, more complex and variable changes in acute-phase proteins occur so that tests, such as the erythrocyte

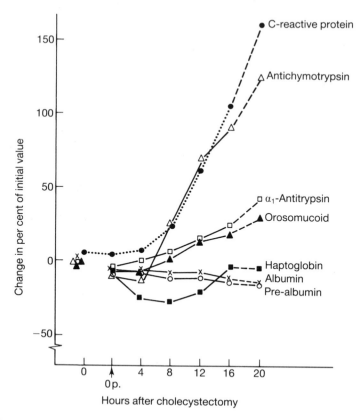

Fig. 12.1. Quantitative changes in acute-phase reactants during the first day after cholecystectomy. The results are given as means for blood samples from 6 patients taken every fourth hour after the operation. C-Reactive protein is given as mg/litre while the percentage deviation from the initial level has been used for the other variables. The broken line between 16 and 20 h denotes that samples were obtained from 4 of the 6 patients at 20 h. (Courtesy of Aronsen *et al.*[12])

sedimentation rate (ESR) or plasma viscosity, that integrate the effects of multiple plasma proteins, are often used to monitor the acute-phase response.

LABORATORY METHODS FOR MEASURING THE ACUTE-PHASE RESPONSE

Assay of individual proteins

In common with other plasma proteins, acute-phase proteins may be measured by any immunochemical assay using specific antisera. Commercial antisera are available to all the acute-phase proteins of clinical interest which we would define as CRP, SAA, α_1-antichymotrypsin, orosomucoid (α_1-acid glycoprotein), α_1-antitrypsin, haptoglobin and fibrinogen.

C-Reactive protein

CRP has a very wide normal range from 0.1 to 8.0 mg/litre, mild or even trivial inflammation causing increases of up to 40 mg/litre.[14] Many assays for CRP are available but sensitive assays such as radioimmunoassay, fluoro-immunoassay,[15] or enzyme immunoassay[16] are necessary to measure serum concentrations within the normal range. This may be important in neonates (who have low levels) and when following the progress of mild inflammation. In practice, most commercial assay kits (using enzyme immunoassay, radial immunodiffusion, nephelometry, or immunoturbidimetry) have a lower limit of detection of between 6 and 10 mg/litre but provide quantitative results at higher concentrations and are adequate for most purposes. Problems of interlaboratory comparison have arisen from the lack of an agreed reference material although a World Health Organization international standard[17] is now available and should improve comparability. Latex agglutination techniques are widely used and are fast but semi-quantitative.[18] They are satisfactory for detecting high levels of CRP (above about 100 mg/litre) in an emergency but should not be used to attempt quantitative measurements on diluted sera. A raised result should always be confirmed by an appropriate quantitative assay.

Serum amyloid A protein

SAA is an apo-lipoprotein of high-density lipoprotein and this property causes problems in comparability between assays owing to the variable influence of the lipid moiety. For example, radial immunodiffusion assays suggest a normal range, based on a calibrant derived from tissue amyloid, of 1–30 mg/litre,[19] whereas radioimmunoassay, using purified SAA, suggests a normal range of <200 mg/litre.[20] No internationally agreed reference material exists and antisera are difficult to raise (at the present time only one is available commercially), possibly due to an immunosuppressive role of SAA. This is an interesting and sensitive acute-phase protein and will be of interest to many workers undertaking clinical studies of inflammation. Enzyme immunoassays for SAA protein are the easiest assays to establish but calibration is arbitrary and assays for this protein are not yet suitable for routine clinical practice.

α_1-Antichymotrypsin

This much neglected protein is present in serum at a reasonably high concentration of 0.2–0.5 g/litre.[21] Antisera are easily raised and the protein may be measured by immunonephelometry, immunoturbidimetry, radial immunodiffusion, or by Laurell 'rocket'. It thus has much to commend it as a simple protein to measure. There is no agreed reference material although published normal ranges vary little suggesting that calibration of the available reference materials is in reasonably good agreement. We agree with Laurell[13] that this is an attractive protein which deserves more attention, although its clinical use is somewhat limited by the lack of published data concerning its modification in different inflammatory diseases. It is of some interest in having a longer half-time than CRP and thus makes a useful partner if more than one protein is to be measured.

Haptoglobin

The disharmonic response of this protein to inflammation associated with haemolysis makes it unsuitable as a general purpose acute-phase reactant. It is, however, useful as a measure of intravascular haemolysis. Common genetic allotypes in the population affect gel-based assays such as radial immunodiffusion or the Laurell 'rockets', though not nephelometry or immunoturbidimetry.[22]

α_1-Antitrypsin

This important protein is widely used to detect individuals with a genetic deficiency, which is relatively common. Heterozygotes occur in about 15% of Caucasians, rendering the protein useless as a measure of the acute-phase response.[23] The plasma concentration in the normal MM phenotype ranges between 1.1 and 2.1 g/litre[24] and, with the availability of a World Health Organization reference preparation,[25] it may be measured by techniques such as radial immunodiffusion, nephelometry, and immunoturbidimetry.

Fibrinogen

Unlike the other acute-phase proteins, fibrinogen must be measured in plasma rather than serum. It is unstable on storage and, particularly when levels are raised as in the acute-phase response, it shows a marked tendency to cryoprecipitate at 4°C within 1 or 2 days. Measurements should thus be made on fresh plasma anticoagulated with EDTA, oxalate or citrate; heparin is undesirable owing to the formation of complexes with fibronectin and fibrinogen. Immunoassays using gel techniques are unsuitable owing to the tendency of the protein to precipitate. Standardization also presents problems owing to the instability of reference materials.

Orosomucoid

This protein is a rather insensitive acute-phase reactant. It is catabolized in the renal tubule and the serum concentration is thus increased in renal impairment.[13]

Erythrocyte sedimentation

The erythrocyte sedimentation rate (ESR)[26] remains the most widely used method for detecting and monitoring the acute-phase response. The selected method of the International Committee for Standardization in Haematology[27] is based on that of Westergren,[28] using blood diluted in sodium citrate. The Westergren ESR is a measure of the rate of sedimentation of erythrocytes in a vertical tube (200 mm column of blood; British Standards Institution[29]) over a standard period of 1 h. Sedimentation is a consequence of erythrocyte aggregation induced by plasma proteins of large molecular size (fibrinogen, α_2-macroglobulin and some immunoglobulins). Of these, fibrinogen is particularly important because of the combination of its asymmetric shape (high frictional ratio), large molecular size and high plasma concentration.[30]

There have been minor modifications to the ESR test over the years (disposable plastic Westergren tubes, vacuum aspiration of the blood sample into the ESR tube, automated methods for reading the end-point at 1 h, combined blood sample tube and ESR tube) but these have been primarily aimed at reducing biohazard risks and the limitations of the test remain.

Erythrocyte aggregation is influenced by the number, shape, density and deformability of erythrocytes. There is no satisfactory method of adjusting the Westergren ESR for the number of erythrocytes and the coexistence of anaemia severely limits the value of the test, the ESR being falsely increased by a small fall in haematocrit within two standard deviations below the normal mean.[31] When anaemia is secondary to the primary disease it increases the apparent sensitivity of the ESR[32] but, when due to other causes, anaemia reduces the specificity of the ESR. A second limitation of the test is its slow response to changes in the inflammatory stimulus, as the plasma fibrinogen concentration usually does not increase by much until 24 h or more after the onset of inflammation and falls with a long half-time of 96–144 h on resolution of inflammation.[33] The ESR is also insensitive to small changes in the degree of inflammation, is influenced by plasma proteins (e.g. immunoglobulins) that are not acute-phase reactants, is often not subjected to laboratory quality control procedures, should be performed within 2 h of venepuncture, and may be influenced by time of venepuncture in relation to feeding.[34]

Furthermore, the sensitivity and specificity of the ESR are highly dependent on the reference (normal) range that is used.[32] This should always be based on the local population under study but approximate upper limits of the reference range in mm/1 h[32,35] are shown in Table 12.2.

Advantages of the ESR include its technical simplicity, low cost and independence from an electrical power supply. As the test is sensitive to several acute-phase proteins, as well as immunoglobulins and immune complexes, it provides a wider screen for the detection of disease than does the measurement of any one acute-phase protein alone. As the hyperproteinaemia of chronic disease is more complex than in the first 24 h of acute illness, the ESR is more suited to monitoring fluctuations in the activity of chronic disorders. The main reason, however, for the continuing popularity of the test has been the lack of an alternative test of equal technical simplicity.

Table 12.2 Approximate Upper Limits of Reference Range of ESR (mm/1 h)

Age	Male	Female
17–50	10	12
51–60	12	19
> 60[a]	14	20

[a] But see section on acute-phase response in the elderly.

Other tests of erythrocyte aggregation

Aggregation of erythrocytes can be measured by techniques other than sedimentation. These include microscopic counting of aggregates, measurement of whole-blood viscosity at a low-shear rate (~ 1 s^{-1}), alteration in either the transmission or back-scattering of light as erythrocytes aggregate, and the aggregation of cells when subjected to a low (7–8 g) and intermittent centrifugal force (zeta sedimentation). Guidelines on the measurement of whole-blood viscosity and other tests of erythrocyte aggregation have recently been prepared by the International Committee for Standardization in Haematology[36,37] and experimental methods for measuring erythrocyte aggregation have been reviewed.[38]

In all such methods, the presence of erythrocytes causes dependency on packed cell volume (PCV) so that adjustment for anaemia is essential. Of the above methods, measurement of zeta sedimentation using a Zetafuge[39] with adjustment for PCV has been shown to be of clinical value in monitoring disease activity.[40–42] Measurement of whole-blood viscosity at low shear (0.2 s^{-1}) has shown poor sensitivity, in comparison with the ESR and plasma viscosity, for monitoring protein changes in patients with rheumatoid arthritis, infection or old age.[32] Measurement of erythrocyte aggregation, measured photometrically in a cone-plate rheoscope, was found to correlate more closely than did the ESR with the plasma concentration of several acute-phase proteins, in particular fibrinogen.[43]

Plasma viscosity

As in the case of the ESR, plasma viscosity is primarily determined by the plasma concentration of proteins of large molecular size, particularly those, such as fibrinogen, with axial asymmetry. Plasma viscosity has been shown to correlate more closely ($r = 0.81$) than the Westergren ESR ($r = 0.55$) with the plasma fibrinogen concentration of non-anaemic patients.[31] When anaemic patients were included, the correlation between ESR and fibrinogen fell further to an r value of 0.25. α_2-Macroglobulin and the immunoglobulins also contribute significantly to plasma viscosity which correlates more closely with total globulin, in both anaemic and non-anaemic patients, than does the Westergren ESR.[31]

Measurement of plasma viscosity is technically simple because plasma is a

Newtonian fluid whose viscosity is independent of the shear rate at which it is measured. Thus a relatively low-cost capillary, rotational or falling-ball viscometer can be used. Until recently, viscometers have not been designed primarily for rheological measurements on blood or plasma but, with the introduction of automated methods for measuring plasma viscosity,[44] the popularity of the test is likely to increase in diagnostic laboratories.[45]

Advantages of measuring plasma viscosity rather than the ESR, include independence from the effects of erythrocytes, low running costs, speed of assay, a reference range that is independent of gender and much less dependent on age, ease of quality control checks, and the facility to test stored specimens. Like the ESR, its disadvantages include sensitivity to proteins that are relatively slow-responding acute-phase proteins (e.g. fibrinogen) or are not acute-phase proteins (e.g. immunoglobulins and immune complexes). Thus its primary value lies in monitoring changes in the activity of chronic disease or in acute disorders at least 24 h after the onset of inflammation. Unlike the ESR, which increases as serum albumin falls, plasma viscosity may be falsely low in hypoalbuminaemic patients.

Which laboratory test to select?

An increase in the blood concentration of acute-phase proteins indicates the presence of an acute or chronic inflammatory response to tissue damage whether caused by infection, ischaemia, trauma, immune damage, malignancy or other pathology. A wide range of pathologies can therefore initiate the response and it is essential to interpret laboratory test results against full knowledge of the clinical picture.

Tests of the acute-phase response may be used to detect tissue damage, assess the size of the inflammatory response and its prognostic implications, and monitor the response to treatment. In the early stages (<24 h) of the onset or resolution of an inflammatory response, a fast-reacting test is required and measurement of serum CRP is the test of choice. It is important to avoid an oversensitive acute-phase protein, such as SAA, which may respond to trivial viral infections such as the common cold.

After 24 h, the nature of the acute-phase hyperproteinaemia becomes more complex and may be complicated by anaemia and a fall in some serum proteins such as albumin. No one acute-phase protein is representative of this stage of the response and, rather than assay multiple individual proteins, it is usually more cost-effective to use a less specific test that is sensitive to the combined effect of several plasma proteins. Hence the value of measuring the ESR or plasma viscosity. These tests are complementary to measurement of CRP and should be used for different purposes.

The limitations of the ESR, particularly its dependence on quantitative and qualitative changes in erythrocytes, are obvious. It is intrinsically unsound to use a test that has, as its visual end-point, the sedimentation of a component that is itself an independent variable. This criticism will also require to be addressed if one of the newer tests of erythrocyte aggregation is developed as an alternative.

Measurement of plasma viscosity has several theoretical and practical advantages over the ESR and is likely to be used increasingly in larger laboratories as instrument manufacturers develop automated instruments.[44] While the reference (normal) range of 1.50–1.72 mPa s at 25°C[46] is independent of gender, and largely independent of age until late middle age, it has proved difficult for clinicians to appreciate the significance of small changes as very small increases (0.03–0.05 mPa s) may be meaningful. The potential of the test is considerable, however, and difficulties in interpretation are likely to be overcome as familiarity with it increases.

More detailed guidelines on the selection of tests for monitoring the acute-phase response have recently been prepared by the International Committee for Standardization in Haematology.[37]

CLINICAL APPLICATIONS OF THE ACUTE-PHASE RESPONSE

The demonstration of an acute-phase protein response provides unequivocal evidence of the presence of inflammation and bears some quantitative relationship to the activity and mass of inflamed tissue. A normal blood concentration of acute-phase proteins does not exclude inflammation, however, as inflammatory activity is occasionally too low to elicit a response. Apart from this example, quantitative assessment of the acute-phase response is of value for monitoring inflammation in a wide range of clinical disorders.

Infection

Bacterial infection is a potent stimulus to acute-phase protein synthesis with marked elevations in CRP of up to 200 mg/litre in bacterial infection and up to 500 mg/litre in severe infection. Viral and parasitic infections may also elicit a response but it is much less marked, rarely more than 100 mg/litre.[47]

Measurement of acute-phase proteins may be of value as an indicator of bacterial infection in certain clinical settings where microbiological diagnosis may be slow, difficult, or impossible owing to inaccessibility of the infected organ or tissue.[48] Bacterial, as opposed to viral, infection may be suspected if the serum CRP concentration is above 100 mg/litre. A satisfactory response of infection to antibiotics may be inferred from a fall in the concentration of acute-phase proteins to normal.[49]

Infection in the neonate

The CRP concentration is raised in neonates with bacterial or fungal infection and a number of workers have suggested that measurement of CRP may be useful in diagnosing infection at birth or soon after.[50–54] In premature rupture of the membranes, a CRP concentration of greater than 125 mg/litre was shown by Hawrylyshyn *et al.*[55] to have a positive predictive value of 96% and a negative predictive value of 89% for diagnosing chorioamnionitis and, owing to the difficulty of amniocentesis, it was felt to be a more useful diagnostic test. The ESR was also useful, with a positive predictive value of 100% and a negative predictive value of 67%. It is clear that the 'high action limit' of 125 mg/litre for CRP, used by Hawrylyshyn *et al.*,[55] is important in the neonate as a raised serum concentration may be caused by maternal fever and by foetal asphyxia, distress, shock or meconium aspiration. Ainbender *et al.*[56] argued that, because of the frequency of these conditions, the CRP concentration may often be raised above normal for reasons other than infection. Dyck *et al.*[57] demonstrated that the median CRP level of 2 mg/litre in serum taken during the first 96 h in neonates is unaltered in the respiratory distress syndrome, while neonates with other problems (including pneumonia, aspiration and extrapulmonary sepsis) had significantly elevated levels (median 24 mg/litre). They concluded that the CRP measurement provided a reliable means of distinguishing infants with uncomplicated respiratory distress syndrome from those with severe pulmonary or extrapulmonary disease.

Infection in childhood

Assay of CRP is useful in distinguishing invasive bacterial infection from the many other causes of the non-specific symptoms that may arise in this age group. Its sensitivity for diagnosis of bacterial infection varies with the level of CRP considered and the time at which blood is taken during the course of the disease.[58] In older children, Putto *et al.*[59] showed that, in those who had been febrile for more than 12 h, a serum CRP level of 40 mg/litre on admission had a sensitivity of 79% and a specificity of 90% for the detection of bacterial infection, while an ESR of 30 mm/h had a sensitivity of 91% and a specificity of 89%. In a study of children with suspected meningitis, a serum CRP concentration of 20 mg/litre or more indicated a bacterial rather than a viral origin.[60] Serum CRP measurement is most useful if serial quantitative measurements are made and a progressive increase can be shown in the first 24 h. In general, the ESR is of limited value in neonates and children owing to the complicating effects of anaemia and the difficulty of obtaining a large enough blood sample.

Measurement of CRP in cerebrospinal fluid has been shown in a prospective study to be more sensitive in distinguishing bacterial from non-bacterial meningitis than measuring cerebrospinal fluid leucocytes, glucose or protein, or performing a Gram stain.[61] Others have suggested that measurement of CRP in the serum may be more useful.[62]

Infection in adults

Infection is an important complication of major abdominal surgery. In the absence of complications, CRP increases rapidly from 6 h after surgical injury (Fig. 12.1), reaching a peak concentration at 48 h and falling with a half-time of about 48 h.[33,63] The same pattern is seen following resection of an inflammatory gut lesion even when this has caused a high concentration of CRP pre-operatively. Complications of surgery such as wound infection, subphrenic abscess, tissue necrosis or thromboembolism result in a sustained rise in CRP which may be of diagnostic value in the absence of other evidence.

Other conditions in which measurement of CRP has proved useful in adults include distinguishing viral from bacterial pneumonia,[64] distinguishing pelvic infection from other causes of pelvic pain or masses,[65] and the management of immunosuppressed patients. The serum CRP concentration may also be raised in smokers[66] and after marathon running.[67]

Infection in immunosuppressed patients

Rapid detection of infection is of particular importance in immunosuppressed patients, who frequently pose a difficult diagnostic and therapeutic problem. It was originally shown,[68] by a radical immunodiffusion technique, that the serum CRP concentration increases to above 100 mg/litre in neutropenic leukaemic patients with bacterial infection. Disease activity, cytotoxic drug therapy and the administration of blood products were associated with lower serum concentrations. This observation became of more immediate diagnostic value when rapid assay techniques for CRP – laser nephelometry[69] and enzyme immunoassay[70] – were found to give confirmatory results.

It is common practice in leukaemia units to prescribe a broad-spectrum antibiotic combination to severely neutropenic patients who remain febrile (≥38°C) for 2 h or more. If there is not a rapid clinical response, stored serum can then be assayed for CRP as the concentration does not fall to below 100 mg/litre until appropriate antibiotics have been administered.[71] Thus the main value of the test lies in the detection of occult or unresolved infection and serial monitoring of the response to therapy. A fall in serum CRP concentration can be used as an objective end-point in clinical trials of antibiotic therapy.

These findings have been confirmed by results from several centres.[72–76] If the CRP concentration remains below 30 mg/litre for 48 h after the onset of fever, infection is unlikely to be the cause.[74] Also, when systemic antibiotics are stopped before the serum CRP falls to below 30 mg/litre, fever may recur.[74]

Acute graft-versus-host disease is usually not associated with a rise in serum CRP concentration to above 40 mg/litre (although this is disputed in one small study)[77] so that values above 100 mg/litre in the presence of graft-versus-host disease are indicative of bacterial infection.[78] Also, in 20 patients with chronic graft-versus-host disease, but without infection, the serum CRP concentration was found to be normal.[79]

Viral and fungal infections seem to increase the serum CRP concentration to a lesser extent than bacterial infection[76,78,80] but this depends on the degree of associated tissue damage.

Collagen vascular disorders

Inflammation is a major part of the pathogenesis of most rheumatic diseases. In some conditions, typified by rheumatoid arthritis, a marked acute-phase response is characteristic, while in others, such as systemic lupus erythematosus, only a minor response is seen.[3] The mechanism of

Table 12.3 Acute-phase Protein Responses in Disease

Diseases with absent or minor responses
   Systemic lupus erythematosus, systemic sclerosis, polymyositis
   Osteoarthrosis
   Periarticular disease and spondylosis
   Ulcerative colitis
   Viral infections

Diseases with major responses
   Bacterial infections
   Trauma (burns, surgery, etc.)
   Malignant disease
   Crohn's disease
   Juvenile chronic arthritis
   Polymyalgia rheumatica
   Rheumatoid arthritis
   Seronegative spondarthritis
   Vasculitis

---

these discrepancies is unclear but, in certain connective tissue disorders, there may be a defect in acute-phase responsiveness.[81] Table 12.3 shows diseases in which a minor or major elevation of acute-phase proteins usually occurs.

In early disease, and in connective tissue disorders of acute onset such as polymyalgia rheumatica, there is often a reasonable correlation between clinical signs and symptoms of active disease and the extent of tissue damage. In chronic disease such as long-standing rheumatoid arthritis, however, chronic damage to tissues will cause pathological changes that reverse only very slowly and an alteration in inflammation itself is not reflected by a change in clinical symptoms. In these circumstances, measurement of acute-phase proteins may be of value in giving early warning of an exacerbation or a response to therapy. Also, in mild early polyarthritis, acute-phase proteins may rise before there is clinically detectable synovitis. In polymyalgia rheumatica and, more importantly, in temporal arteritis, massive acute-phase responses may occur at a time when there is minimal clinical or pathological evidence of inflammatory disease.

Measurement of acute-phase proteins provides useful confirmation of the diagnosis in early rheumatoid arthritis, juvenile chronic polyarthritis (Still's disease), ankylosing spondylitis, psoriatic arthropathy, Reiter's syndrome, and arthritis following jejuno-ileal bypass. In these conditions, but particularly in rheumatoid arthritis, the CRP concentration gives an earlier indication of disease activity than clinical indices and is the single most precise objective laboratory measurement of disease activity. Both CRP and ESR may be measured in this context but the CRP correlates more closely with disease activity than the ESR or the concentration of plasma C3D, rheumatoid factor or immune complexes.[82,83] The major advantage of CRP over the ESR is the speed with which it changes in response to effective therapy. A raised ESR in a patient with inflammatory disease and a normal CRP might indicate early remission.

Arthralgia is a common and non-specific symptom which can be caused by a variety of local, systemic and psychogenic factors. Acute-phase protein assays are helpful in confirming organic disease. Back pain is usually non-specific but the presence of an acute-phase response strongly indicates serious organic disease such as ankylosing spondylitis or carcinomatosis. In the case of ankylosing spondylitis, CRP levels may be raised long before significant clinical or radiological signs make the diagnosis obvious.[84]

Polymyalgia rheumatica is a disorder of elderly people characterized by severe morning stiffness and associated with diffuse systemic symptoms such as depression and malaise. Clinical examination is usually normal and there is no diagnostic test. About 30% of patients will develop cranial arteritis with serious risk to eyesight if untreated. Steroids in adequate dosage produce a rapid complete resolution of symptoms and suppress the arteritis. Indices of the acute-phase response, such as ESR and CRP, are almost invariably raised. Studies have established a good correlation between disease activity and the serum concentration of acute-phase proteins and have demonstrated that CRP falls to normal at a rate which reflects clinical improvement.[85] The ESR also falls, but much more slowly, and may still not be normal after 14 days. CRP measurement may thus be useful in differentiating polymyalgia rheumatica from other causes of myalgia such as anxiety, depression, fibrositis, thyroid disease, Parkinson's disease and others.[86] Full clinical remission is invariably associated with a fall to normal of the CRP concentration. The situation is a strong contrast to that of rheumatoid arthritis where, even in clinical remission, patients almost invariably have raised acute-phase proteins. Confusion has surrounded the relationship between the ESR and CRP in both polymyalgia rheumatica and cranial arteritis, Park *et al.*[87] finding a poor correlation ($r = 0.66$) between the two tests, with occasional cases in which only one test was markedly elevated. Mallya *et al.*,[85] however, found that all patients studied with polymyalgia rheumatica had a raised CRP value which reflected disease activity. It is possible that these discrepancies reflect the different time course of the two acute-phase measures in relation to the time of sampling. In practice, either the ESR or CRP can be used to assess the response to steroids in both of these conditions.

Systemic vasculitis is difficult to assess clinically and, although the ESR is usually raised, the result may vary widely from day to day and appears to be less reliable and sensitive than CRP.[88] In Wegener's granulomatosis, Hind *et al.*[89] showed that CRP was invariably raised during active disease and fell rapidly in association with clinical remission induced by immuno-suppression. Similar evidence for the value of CRP as an objective measure of disease activity has been found in polyarteritis nodosa,[89] microscopic polyarteritis[90] and Behçet's syndrome.[91] In systemic lupus erythematosus, dermatomyositis and progressive systemic sclerosis, acute-phase responses are mild or absent even in apparently active disease.[92] In contrast, however, intercurrent infection provides a brisk response.[93] This has led to the use of CRP measurement for distinguishing exacerbations of disease activity from infection.[94]

Thus the value of measuring acute-phase proteins in rheumatic disorders lies in (a) early detection of synovitis, (b) differential diagnosis of arthralgia, myalgia and atypical back pain, (c) detection of vasculitis, (d) monitoring of the response to therapy, and (e) detection of intercurrent infection in some connective tissue diseases.

Inflammatory gut disease

A number of acute-phase proteins have been used to assess the response of inflammatory gut disease to therapy. Early studies suggested that orosomucoid was the most sensitive measure of the acute-phase response in this condition but recent work suggests that a quantitative assay for CRP is better.[95] The value of acute-phase protein measurements lies in distinguishing organic inflammatory gut disease from symptoms due to irritable colon[96] and in assessing disease activity and the response to treatment. The acute-phase response is less marked in ulcerative colitis than would be expected for the extent of inflammation and CRP levels above 50 mg/litre are rarely encountered. A significant proportion of patients with moderately active ulcerative colitis have normal CRP levels which makes it less useful in the diagnosis and monitoring of this condition than of Crohn's disease.[97] This has led to the suggestion that high CRP levels in gastrointestinal disease may indicate a diagnosis of Crohn's disease.[98]

Malignancy

A number of studies have investigated the relationship between a raised concentration of acute-phase proteins and extent of malignant disease. It is clear that patients with a considerable tumour load may lack an acute-phase response, while others with relatively limited disease may demonstrate an increased concentration of acute-phase proteins. However, despite this, several studies have shown that a raised, or increasing, serum concentration of acute-phase proteins is associated with a poor prognosis and, in many cases, with a greater tumour load or the presence of metastases.[99] Multivariant analysis of a number of laboratory parameters, including acute-phase proteins, has been used in the assessment of several tumours.[100] There is little evidence that such approaches provide clinically useful information. In Hodgkin's disease, however, the ESR can be of prognostic value.[101,102]

The elderly

In asymptomatic individuals, the plasma fibrinogen concentration rises with age[103] and there is also an increase in serum globulin and decrease in albumin.[104,105] These changes are a contributory factor to the higher upper limit with increasing age of the reference (normal) range for the Westergren ESR.[106,107] An upper limit of 35–40 mm/1 h was proposed in elderly healthy individuals[106] and values up to 40 mm/1 h were found without apparent cause in hospital patients aged more than 65 years.[108] Elderly out-patients when studied serially for 1 year or more[109] showed Westergren ESR values ranging from 3 to 69 mm/1 h despite continued good health.

More recently, it was suggested that the reference range could be expressed by dividing the age in years by 2 (for women, the age in years plus 10 is divided by 2).[110] Although this applied only to the range 20–65 years, the formula can probably also be used in the range 60–89 years.[111] A much lower upper limit for the Westergren ESR of 20 mm/1 h[112] or 19–22 mm/1 h[111] has also been proposed for individuals above 60 years.

These conflicting recommendations reflect difficulties in defining health in the elderly; differences between community, retirement home and hospital populations; the presence of occult disease in the elderly; low-grade urinary tract infections and arthropathies; and benign changes in plasma proteins with age. Use of the ESR as a screening test after 65 years clearly has substantial limitations owing to overlap of values in health and disease.

Plasma viscosity is less affected than the ESR by alterations in plasma proteins with age. A slightly higher upper limit in the elderly was found in two small earlier studies[113,114] but, in a recent study of 271 healthy individuals,[115] there was no significant difference in plasma viscosity between the age groups <30, 30–50 and >50 years. Further study of elderly patients is required.

In the elderly, CRP is the acute-phase protein of choice for monitoring acute changes in the inflammatory response to infection.[116] When elderly patients were admitted to an acute geriatric unit, measurement of CRP on days 1 and 5 was a better marker of active disease than the Westergren ESR, which showed a mean of 55 mm/1 h on admission in those with active disease and of 41 mm/1 h in those without active disease.[117] Further comparison of CRP with plasma viscosity and the ESR are indicated in elderly populations, both in hospital and in the community. A reference range for CRP in the elderly is also required.

Vascular disease

Myocardial infarction

As in other disorders associated with tissue necrosis, patients with myocardial infarction show an acute-phase response which includes increases in CRP,[118] plasma fibrinogen,[119] ESR[120] and leucocyte count.[119] In a serial study of five acute-phase proteins (CRP, orosomucoid, α_1-antitrypsin, haptoglobin, and α_2-macroglobulin), CRP was found to be the most sensitive to the tissue damage of myocardial infarction.[80] An increase in serum CRP concentration has been reported, 1–2 h[121] and 4 h[80] after the onset of chest pain, although time of onset of pain may not coincide with that of the initial tissue injury. The peak serum concentration of CRP has been found on the third[80] or fourth[122] post-infarct day.

A rise in CRP appears to be a sensitive marker of myocardial necrosis, being found in 49 of 50 patients with acute infarction,[123] in 100 patients with significant changes in the Q wave on electrocardiography,[124] and in 33 patients who were studied serially.[122] After reaching its peak, the serum CRP concentration returns to normal over 7–10 days and thus may be of diagnostic value once serum creatine kinase MB isoenzyme has returned to normal, which is usually within 3 days.

The acute-phase rise in plasma fibrinogen concentration after myocardial infarction can cause an increase in whole-blood viscosity,[125] which may have rheological implications[126] as the raised fibrinogen appears to correlate with infarct size and be predictive of a poor prognosis.[127] Although hyper-fibrinogenaemia increases the ESR after myocardial infarction, haemoconcentration-induced increases in haematocrit tend to reduce the ESR which is therefore a less satisfactory test and does not reflect clinical severity.[119]

Atherosclerosis

Patients in the steady state of atherosclerotic vascular disease, without clinical symptoms of a recent thrombotic episode, may also have an increase in the blood concentration of various acute-phase reactants and other proteins. These include plasma fibrinogen,[128] which causes secondary increases in erythrocyte sedimentation, plasma viscosity and whole-blood viscosity; a leucocytosis;[129] and an increase in antithrombin III and Factor VIII.[129,130]

Hyperfibrinogenaemia occurs in atherosclerosis to an extent greater than that of advancing age.[128] Plasma fibrinogen concentration correlates with the extent of coronary atherosclerosis,[131] is a risk factor for stroke,[132] and is a prognostic factor in atherosclerotic patients with intermittent claudication.[133] Plasma fibrinogen concentration is also a risk factor for cardiovascular disease in clinically healthy adults.[134,135] The pathogenesis of hyper-fibrinogenaemia in vascular disease is important in view of the possible therapeutic value of inducing a reduction in plasma concentration. Stimulation of monocytes/macrophages, located either within the intima of the vessel wall[136,137] or elsewhere, to release cytokines may be one causative factor.[138] It is still uncertain whether the evidence that a raised plasma fibrinogen concentration in asymptomatic adults is a risk factor for cardiovascular disease[134,135] reflects a genetic predisposition[139] or is merely a persistent acute-phase protein response to occult vessel wall damage, the latter being the primary risk factor. This argument can be extended to explain the rise in plasma fibrinogen concentration with age in apparently healthy individuals.[103]

Pregnancy

Normal pregnancy is associated with an increase in several components of the acute-phase response. Plasma fibrinogen increases in parallel with gestational age[140,141] and contributes to a rise in plasma viscosity,[142] whole-blood viscosity and the ESR.[26,143,144] A rise in serum globulin and fall in albumin[145] also contribute to the increase in ESR which is therefore of no diagnostic value in pregnancy.[146] The upper limit of the reference range for plasma viscosity at 25°C (1.72 mPa s) increases to 1.80 mPa s in pregnancy.[46] An increase in leucocyte count with gestational age also occurs in normal pregnancy.[147] α_1-Antitrypsin and ceruloplasmin show significant increases in pregnancy and α_2-pregnancy-associated glycoprotein shows an increase with gestational age.

Mechanisms causing the acute-phase response in pregnancy are incompletely understood although factors contributing to the change in concentration of plasma proteins include loss of albumin and the effects of oestrogen, progesterone and chorionic gonadotrophin.[146] Experimental evidence in mice suggests that an acute-phase response may be a part of normal embryonic implantation. It is absent or diminished in syngeneic pregnancy which has a concomitant high abortion rate.[148] The response may reflect the activity of immunological recognition systems which are necessary for normal pregnancy.

Sickle-cell anaemia

Patients with homozygous sickle-cell anaemia (SS) suffer intermittent episodes of vaso-occlusion resulting in tissue ischaemia and a painful crisis. The pathogenesis of vaso-occlusion is poorly understood and a number of investigators have therefore studied haematological, rheological and haemostatic changes in the early stages of crisis. In addition to an acute-phase increase in plasma fibrinogen concentration,[149] causing increases in plasma viscosity[150] and whole-blood viscosity,[149] there is an acute-phase increase in leucocyte count[151,152] and usually mild fever. We have not found serial measurements of CRP to be of value in differentiating between SS patients in crisis with and without infection (unpublished). Other changes such as a decrease in the number of irreversibly sickled cells[153] and an improvement in erythrocyte deformability after day 2 of crisis[154] probably reflect selective trapping and removal of poorly deformable dense sickle cells in ischaemic areas[155] and are secondary events unrelated to the acute-phase response itself.

PATHOLOGICAL CONSEQUENCES OF THE ACUTE-PHASE RESPONSE

An acute-phase response, particularly when sustained for a long period, may have pathological consequences.

Secondary amyloidosis

Secondary amyloidosis results from the deposition in tissues of a cleavage fragment of SAA protein.[156] It usually follows chronic inflammatory disease (such as juvenile rheumatoid arthritis, suppurative lesions, tuberculosis or leprosy) in which there is a sustained acute-phase response over many years. It is clear, however, that only a relatively small proportion of such patients eventually develop amyloid. Studies of genetically determined AA amyloidosis, particularly in familial Mediterranean fever, suggest that certain allotypes of the protein may be more likely, on proteolysis, to polymerize to form amyloid fibrils. While measurement of SAA protein has no direct role in diagnosis, the risk of amyloid is greatly reduced if acute-phase protein levels are suppressed by adequate treatment.[157] This is particularly true in juvenile chronic polyarthritis where the risk of ultimately developing amyloid is of the order of 30%. CRP measurement is satisfactory for monitoring responses, measurement of SAA protein showing no advantage.[158]

Thrombotic tendency

As discussed at the beginning of this chapter, the acute phase of an illness may be associated with an increase in blood concentration of proteins that are not classical acute-phase proteins. Interleukin-1 can induce several changes in vascular endothelial cells including increased adhesion of leucocytes,[159] enhanced release of von Willebrand factor,[9] and surface expression of procoagulant activity.[160] These changes on the endothelial surface may predispose to thrombosis at sites of inflammation.

A systemic prothrombotic tendency may also result from the acute-phase hyperfibrinogenaemia, which has rheological consequences at low shear rates by inducing erythrocyte aggregation. Thus the ill patient with an acute-phase response who is relatively immobilized is at increased risk of venous thrombosis. The fibrinolytic suppression following surgery, myocardial infarction and other acute events is associated with an acute-phase increase in the plasma concentration of an inhibitor of tissue plasminogen activator.[161–163] This inhibitor increases in the plasma faster than CRP[163] and contributes to the prothrombotic tendency during the acute phase of illness.

Cryofibrinogenaemia

The presence in serum of cryoprecipitable fibrinogen tends to be associated with inflammatory disorders. Although this phenomenon is poorly understood, there is some evidence to suggest that, in the acute-phase response, newly synthesized fibrinogen is more cryo-unstable (Whicher *et al.* 1988; unpublished). It may, under appropriate circumstances, precipitate in peripheral capillaries and impair blood flow.[164]

CONCLUSION

The acute-phase response to tissue injury is complex in both aetiology and expression. The protein component of the response is of particular value for the detection and monitoring of inflammation. When short-term (<24 h) changes in inflammation are likely, then serial measurement of the serum CRP concentration is the test of choice; a solitary measurement is of limited value. An inflammatory response of longer duration is associated with changes in multiple acute-phase, and other, proteins and it is then preferable to use a test, such as the ESR or plasma viscosity, that is sensitive to the combined effect of several plasma proteins. Alternatively, when acute-on-chronic inflammation is present, serial measurement of serum CRP may again be of value.

A wide variety of pathologies (including infection, ischaemia, trauma, immune damage and malignancy) can initiate an inflammatory response, thus explaining the frequent use of laboratory tests, in both paediatric and adult medicine, for monitoring changes in acute-phase proteins. Because of the ubiquitous nature of inflammation, it is important that these tests be applied selectively, and usually serially, in appropriate clinical conditions and the results interpreted against the relevant clinical background

REFERENCES

1. Dinarello, C.A. Interleukin-1. *Rev. Infect. Dis.* **6**: 51–95, 1984.
2. Gauldie, J., Richards, C., Harnish, D. & Baumann, H. Interferon β_2 is identical to monocyte HSF and regulates the full acute phase protein response in liver cells. In *Progress in Leucocyte Biology* (eds M.C. Powanda, J.J. Oppenheim, M.J. Kluger & C.A. Dinarello), Vol. 8, pp. 15–20. Alan R. Liss, New York, 1988.
3. Whicher, J.T. & Dieppe, P.A. Acute phase proteins. *Clin. Immunol. Allergy* **5**: 425–46, 1985.
4. Whicher, J.T. Functions of acute phase proteins in the inflammatory response. In *Marker Proteins in Inflammation* (eds P. Arnaud, J. Bienvenu & P. Laurent), Vol. 2, pp. 84–98. Walter de Gruyter, Berlin, 1984.
5. Baumann, H., Glibetic, M.D., Onorato, V.A. & Jahreis, G.P. Influence of hepatocyte-stimulating factor on the expression of major acute phase plasma protein genes. In *Protides of the Biological Fluids* (ed. H. Peeters), pp. 231–4. Pergamon Press, Oxford, 1986.
6. Kushner, I. & Feldmann, G. Control of the acute phase response. Demonstration of C-reactive protein synthesis and secretion by hepatocytes during acute inflammation in the rabbit. *J. Exp. Med.* **148**: 466–77, 1978.
7. Kuta, A.E. & Baum, L.C. C-reactive protein is produced by a small number of normal human peripheral blood lymphocytes. *J. Exp. Med* **164**: 321–6, 1986.
8. Ramadori, G., Sipe, J.D. & Colten, H.R. Expression and regulation of the murine serum amyloid A (SAA) gene in extrahepatic sites. *J. Immunol.* **135**: 3645–7, 1985.
9. Schorer, A.E., Moldow, C.F. & Rick, M.E. Interleukin 1 or endotoxin increases the release of von Willebrand factor from human endothelial cells. *Br. J. Haematol.* **67**: 193–7, 1987.
10. Alving, B.M., Bell, W.R. & Evatt, B.L. Fibrinogen synthesis in rabbits: effects of altered levels of circulating fibrinogen. *Am. J. Physiol.* **232**: H478–84, 1977.
11. Mendenhall, H.W. Serum protein concentrations in pregnancy. I. Concentrations in maternal serum. *Am. J. Obstet. Gynec.* **106**: 388–99, 1970.
12. Aronsen, K.-F., Ekelund, G., Kindmark, C.-O. & Laurell, C.-B. Sequential changes of plasma proteins after surgical trauma. *Scand. J. Clin. Lab. Invest.* **29**: Suppl. 124, 127–36, 1972.
13. Laurell, C.-B. Acute phase proteins – a group of protective proteins. *Recent Adv. Clin. Biochem.* **3**: 103–24, 1985.
14. Claus, D.R., Osmand, A.P. & Gewurz, H. Radioimmunoassay of human C-reactive protein and levels in normal sera. *J. Lab. Clin. Med.* **87**: 120–8, 1976.
15. Siboo, R. & Kulisek, E. A fluorescent immunoassay for the quantification of C-reactive protein. *J. Immunol. Methods* **23**: 59–67, 1978.
16. Salonen, E.-M. A rapid and sensitive solid-phase enzyme immunoassay for C-reactive protein. *J. Immunol. Methods* **48**: 45–50, 1982.
17. WHO Expert Committee on Biological Standardization. Human C-reactive protein. World Health Organization Technical Report Series **760**: 21–2, 1987.
18. Hindocha, P., Campbell, C.A., Gould, J.D.M., Wojciechowski, A. & Wood, C.B.S. Sequential study of C reactive protein in neonatal septicaemia using a

latex agglutination test. *J. Clin. Pathol.* **37**: 1014–17, 1984.
19. Chambers, R.E. & Whicher, J.T. Quantitative radial immunodiffusion assay for serum amyloid A protein. *J. Immunol. Methods* **59**: 94–103, 1983.
20. Brandwein, S.R., Medsger, T.A., Skinner, M., Sipe, J.D., Rodnan, G.P. & Cohen, A.S. Serum amyloid A protein concentration in progressive systemic sclerosis (scleroderma). *Ann. Rheum. Dis.* **43**: 586–9, 1984.
21. Sveger, T. & Ekelund, H. Variations of protease inhibitors in foetuses, newborn infants and in some neonatal disorders. *Acta Paediatr. Scand.* **64**: 763–9, 1975.
22. Van Lente, F., Marchand, A. & Galen, R.S. Evaluation of a nephelometric assay for haptoglobin and its clinical usefulness. *Clin. Chem.* **25**: 2007–10, 1979.
23. Carell, R.W. & Owen, M.C. α_1-Antitrypsin; structure, variation in disease. *Essays Med. Biochem.* **4**: 83–119, 1979.
24. Milford Ward, A., White, P.A.E. & Wild, G. Reference ranges for serum α_1 antitrypsin. *Arch. Dis. Childh.* **60**: 261–2, 1985.
25. Reimer, C.B., Smith, S.J., Hannon, W.H., Ritchie, R.F., van Es, L., Becker, W., Markowitz, H., Gauldie, J. & Anderson, S.G. Progress towards international reference standards for human serum proteins. *J. Biol. Stand.* **6**: 133–58, 1978.
26. Fåhraeus, R. The suspension-stability of the blood. *Acta Med. Scand.* **55**: 1–228, 1921.
27. International Committee for Standardization in Haematology. Recommendation for measurement of erythrocyte sedimentation rate of human blood. *Am. J. Clin. Pathol.* **68**: 505–7, 1977.
28. Westergren, A. Studies of the suspension stability of the blood in pulmonary tuberculosis. *Acta Med. Scand.* **54**: 247–82, 1921.
29. British Standards Institution. Westergren tubes and support for the measurement of erythrocyte sedimentation rate. BS 2554: 1987.
30. Stuart, J. The acute-phase reaction and haematological stress syndrome in vascular disease. *Int. J. Microcirc. Clin. Exp.* **3**: 115–29, 1984.
31. Hutchinson, R.M. & Eastham, R.D. A comparison of the erythrocyte sedimentation rate and plasma viscosity in detecting changes in plasma proteins. *J. Clin. Pathol.* **30**: 345–9, 1977.
32. Kenny, M.W., Worthington, D.J., Stuart, J., Davies, A.J., Farr, M., Davey, P.G. & Chughtai, M.A. Efficiency of haematological screening tests for detecting disease. *Clin. Lab. Haematol.* **3**: 299–305, 1981.
33. Colley, C.M., Fleck, A., Goode, A.W., Muller, B.R. & Myers, M.A. Early time course of the acute phase protein response in man. *J. Clin. Pathol.* **36**: 203–7, 1983.
34. Mallya, R.K., Berry, H., Mace, B.E.W., De Beer, F.C. & Pepys, M.B. Diurnal variation of erythrocyte sedimentation rate related to feeding. *Lancet* **1**: 389–90, 1982.
35. Lewis, S.M. Erythrocyte sedimentation rate and plasma viscosity. *Assoc. Clin. Pathologists Broadsheet* **94**, 1980.
36. International Committee for Standardization in Haematology (Expert Panel on Blood Rheology). Guidelines for measurement of blood viscosity and erythrocyte deformability. *Clin. Hemorheol.* **6**: 439–53, 1986.
37. International Committee for Standardization in Haematology (Expert Panel on Blood Rheology). Guidelines on selection of laboratory tests for monitoring the acute phase response. *J. Clin. Pathol.* **41**: 1203–12, 1988.
38. Stoltz, J.F., Paulus, F. & Donner, M. Experimental approaches to erythrocyte aggregation. *Clin. Hemorheol.* **7**: 109–18, 1987.
39. Bull, B.S. & Brailsford, J.D. The zeta sedimentation ratio. *Blood* **40**: 550–9, 1972.
40. Raich, P.C. & Temperly, N. Comparison of the Wintrobe erythrocyte sedimentation rate with the zeta sedimentation ratio. *Am. J. Clin. Pathol.* **65**: 690–3, 1976.
41. Bucher, W.C., Gall, E.P. & Becker, P.T. The zeta sedimentation ratio (ZSR) as

the routine monitor of disease activity in a general hospital. *Am. J. Clin. Pathol.* **72**: 65–7, 1979.

42. Morris, M.W., Pinals, R.S. & Nelson, D.A. The zeta sedimentation ratio (ZSR) and activity of disease in rheumatoid arthritis. *Am. J. Clin. Pathol.* **68**: 760–2, 1977.
43. Friederichs, E., Germs, J., Lakomek, M. & Winkler, H. Increased erythrocyte aggregation in infectious diseases: influence of "acute phase proteins". *Clin. Hemorheol.* **4**: 237–44, 1984.
44. Cooke, B.M. & Stuart, J. Automated measurement of plasma viscosity by capillary viscometer. *J. Clin. Pathol.* **41**: 1213–16, 1988.
45. Stuart, J. & Lewis, S.M. Monitoring the acute phase response. Alternative tests to measuring erythrocyte sedimentation rate. *Br. Med. J.* **297**: 1143–4, 1988.
46. Harkness, J. The viscosity of human blood plasma; its measurement in health and disease. *Biroheology* **8**: 171–93, 1971.
47. Whicher, J.T., Chambers, R.E., Higginson, J., Nashef, L. & Higgins, P.G. Acute phase response of serum amyloid A protein and C reactive protein to the common cold and influenza. *J. Clin. Pathol.* **38**: 312–16, 1985.
48. Hanson, L.A., Jodal, U., Sabel, K.-G. & Wadsworth, C. The diagnostic value of C-reactive protein. *Pediatr. Infect. Dis.* **2**: 87–90, 1983.
49. Peltola, H., Vahvanen, V. & Aalto, K. Fever, C-reactive protein and erythrocyte sedimentation rate in monitoring recovery from septic arthritis. A preliminary study. *J. Pediatr. Orthop.* **4**: 170–4, 1984.
50. Sabel, K.-G. & Hanson, L.A. The clinical usefulness of C-reactive protein (CRP) determinations in bacterial meningitis and septicemia in infancy. *Acta Paediatr. Scand.* **63**: 381–8, 1974.
51. Sabel, K.-G. & Wadsworth, Ch. C-reactive protein (CRP) in early diagnosis of neonatal septicemia. *Acta Paediatr. Scand.* **68**: 825–31, 1979.
52. Shine, B., Gould, J., Campbell, C., Hindocha, P., Wilmot, R.P. & Wood, C.B.S. Serum C-reactive protein in normal and infected neonates. *Clin. Chim. Acta* **148**: 97–103, 1985.
53. Adhikari, M., Coovadia, H.M., Coovadia, Y.M., Smit, S.Y. & Moosa, A. Predictive value of C-reactive protein in neonatal septicaemia. *Ann. Trop. Pediatr.* **6**: 37–40, 1986.
54. Stuart, J. & Whicher, J.T. Tests for detecting and monitoring the acute phase response. *Arch. Dis. Childh.* **63**: 115–17, 1988.
55. Hawrylyshyn, P., Bernstein, P., Milligan, J.E., Soldin, S., Pollard, A. & Papsin, F.R. Premature rupture of membranes: the role of C-reactive protein in the prediction of chorioamnionitis. *Am. J. Obstet. Gynecol.* **147**: 240–6, 1983.
56. Ainbender, E., Cabatu, E.E., Guzman, D.M. & Sweet, A.Y. Serum C-reactive protein and problems of newborn infants. *J. Pediatr.* **101**: 438–40, 1982.
57. Dyck, R.F., Bingham, W., Tan, L. & Rogers, S.L. Serum levels of C-reactive protein in neonatal respiratory distress syndrome. *Clin. Pediatr.* **23**: 381–3, 1984.
58. Mathers, N.J. & Pohlandt, F. Diagnostic audit of C-reactive protein in neonatal infection. *Eur. J. Pediatr.* **146**: 147–51, 1987.
59. Putto, A., Ruuskanen, O., Meurman, O., Ekblad, H., Korvenranta, H., Mertsola, J., Peltola, H., Sarkinnen, H., Viljanen, M.K. & Halonen, P. C-reactive protein in the evaluation of febrile illness. *Arch. Dis. Childh.* **61**: 24–9, 1986.
60. Peltola, H.O. C-reactive protein for rapid monitoring of infections of the central nervous system. *Lancet* **1**: 980–3, 1982.
61. Corrall, C.J., Pepple, J.M., Moxon, E.R. & Hughes, W.T. C-reactive protein in spinal fluid of children with meningitis. *J. Pediatr.* **99**: 365–9, 1981.
62. Benjamin, D.R., Opheim, K.E. & Brewer, L. Is C-reactive protein useful in the management of children with suspected bacterial meningitis? *Am. J. Clin. Pathol.* **81**: 779–82, 1984.

63. Fischer, C.L., Gill, C., Forrester, M.G. & Nakamura, R. Quantitation of "acute-phase proteins" postoperatively. Value in detection and monitoring of complications. *Am. J. Clin. Pathol.* **66**: 840–6, 1976.
64. McCarthy, P.L., Frank, A.L., Ablow, R.C., Masters, S.J. & Dolan, T.F. Value of the C-reactive protein test in the differentiation of bacterial and viral pneumonia. *J. Pediatr.* **92**: 454–6, 1978.
65. Hajj, S.N., Angerman, N.S., Evans, M.I., Moravec, W.D. & Schmacher, G.F. C-reactive protein in the differential diagnosis of gynecologic pathology. *J. Reprod. Med.* **23**: 284–7, 1979.
66. Das, I. Raised C-reactive protein levels in serum from smokers. *Clin. Chim. Acta* **153**: 9–13, 1985.
67. Strachan, A.F., Noakes, T.D., Kotzenberg, G., Nel, A.E. & De Beer, F.C. C-reactive protein concentrations during long distance running. *Br. Med. J.* **289**: 1249–54, 1984.
68. Mackie, P.H., Crockson, R.A. & Stuart, J. C-reactive protein for rapid diagnosis of infection in leukaemia. *J. Clin. Pathol.* **32**: 1253–6, 1979.
69. Rose, P.E., Johnson, S.A., Meakin, M., Mackie, P.H. & Stuart, J. Serial study of C-reactive protein during infection in leukaemia. *J. Clin. Pathol.* **34**: 263–6, 1981.
70. Harris, R.I., Stone, P.C.W., Hudson, A.G. & Stuart, J. C reactive protein rapid assay techniques for monitoring resolution of infection in immunosuppressed patients. *J. Clin. Pathol.* **37**: 821–5, 1984.
71. Schofield, K.P., Voulgari, F., Gozzard, D.I., Leyland, M.J., Beeching, N.J. & Stuart, J. C-reactive protein concentration as a guide to antibiotic therapy in acute leukaemia. *J. Clin. Pathol.* **35**: 866–9, 1982.
72. Williams, M., McCallum, J. & Dick, H.M. The detection of infection in leukaemia by serial measurement of C-reactive protein. *J. Infect.* **4**: 139–47, 1982.
73. Peltola, H., Saarinen, U.M. & Siimes, M.A. C-reactive protein in rapid diagnosis and follow-up of bacterial septicemia in children with leukemia. *Pediatr. Infect. Dis.* **2**: 370–3, 1983.
74. Starke, I.D., De Beer, F.C., Donnelly, J.P., Catovsky, D., Goldman, J.M., Galton, D.A.G. & Pepys, M.B. Serum C-reactive protein levels in the management of infection in acute leukaemia. *Eur. J. Cancer Clin. Oncol.* **20**: 319–25, 1984.
75. Gozzard, D.I., French, E.A., Blecher, T.E. & Powell, R.J. C-reactive protein levels in neutropenic patients with pyrexia. *Clin. Lab. Haematol.* **7**: 307–16, 1985.
76. Grønn, M., Slørdahl, S.H., Skrede, S. & Lie, S.O. C-reactive protein as an indicator of infection in the immunosuppressed child. *Eur. J. Pediatr.* **145**: 18–21, 1986.
77. Rowe, I.F., Worsley, A.M., Donnelly, P., Catovsky, D., Goldman, J.M., Galton, D.A.G., Pepys, M.B. Measurement of serum C reactive protein concentration after bone marrow transplantation for leukaemia. *J. Clin. Pathol.* **37**: 263–6, 1984.
78. Walker, S.A., Rogers, T.R., Riches, P.G., White, S. & Hobbs, J.R. Value of serum C-reactive protein measurement in the management of bone marrow transplant recipients. Part I: early transplant period. *J. Clin. Pathol.* **37**: 1018–21, 1984.
79. Walker, S.A., Riches, P.G., Rogers, T.R., White, S. & Hobbs, J.R. Value of serum C-reactive protein measurement in the management of bone marrow transplant recipients. Part II: late post-transplant period. *J. Clin. Pathol.* **37**: 1022–6, 1984.
80. Voulgari, F., Cummins, P., Gardecki, T.I.M., Beeching, N.J., Stone, P.C.W. & Stuart, J. Serum levels of acute phase and cardiac proteins after myocardial infarction, surgery, and infection. *Br. Heart J.* **48**: 352–6, 1982.
81. Whicher, J.T. & Westacott, C. Are there defects in the production of interleukin 1 in disease. In *Marker Proteins in Inflammation* (eds J. Bienvenu, J.A. Grimaud & P. Laurent) Vol. 3, pp. 27–35. Walter de Gruyter, Berlin, 1986.

82. Mallya, R.K., De Beer, F.C., Berry, H., Hamilton, E.D.B., Mace, B.E.W. & Pepys, M.B. Correlation of clinical parameters of disease activity in rheumatoid arthritis with serum concentration of C-reactive protein and erythrocyte sedimentation rate. *J. Rheumatol.* **9**: 224–8, 1982.

83. Mallya, R.K., Vergani, D., Tee, D.E.H., Bevis, L., De Beer, F.C., Berry, H., Hamilton, E.D.B., Mace, B.E.W. & Pepys, M.B. Correlation in rheumatoid arthritis of concentrations of plasma C3d, serum rheumatoid factor, immune complexes and C-reactive protein with each other and with clinical features of disease activity. *Clin. Exp. Immunol.* **48**: 747–53, 1982.

84. Cowling, P., Ebringer, R., Cawdell, D., Ishii, M. & Ebringer, A. C-reactive protein, ESR, and klebsiella in ankylosing spondylitis. *Ann. Rheum. Dis.* **39**: 45–9, 1980.

85. Mallya, R.K., Hind, C.R.K., Berry, H. & Pepys, M.B. Serum C-reactive protein in polymyalgia rheumatica. A prospective serial study. *Arth. Rheum.* **28**: 383–7, 1985.

86. Mowat, A.G. & Hazleman, B.L. Polymyalgia rheumatica – a clinical study with particular reference to arterial disease. *J. Rheumatol.* **1**: 190–202, 1974.

87. Park, J.R., Jones, J.G. & Hazleman, B.L. Relationship of the erythrocyte sedimentation rate to acute phase proteins in polymyalgia rheumatica and giant cell arteritis. *Ann. Rheum. Dis.* **40**: 493–5, 1981.

88. Parish, W.E. Studies on vasculitis. VII. C-reactive protein as a substance perpetuating chronic vasculitis. Occurrence in lesions and concentrations in sera. *Clin. Allergy* **6**: 543–50, 1976.

89. Hind, C.R.K., Winearls, C.G. & Pepys, M.B. Correlation of disease activity in systemic vasculitis with serum C-reactive protein measurement. A prospective study of thirty-eight patients. *Eur. J. Clin. Invest.* **15**: 89–94, 1985.

90. Hind, C.R.K., Savage, C.O., Winearls, C.G. & Pepys, M.B. Objective monitoring of disease activity in polyarteritis by measurement of C reactive protein concentration. *Br. Med. J.* **288**: 1027–30, 1984.

91. Lehner, T. & Adinolfi, M. Acute phase proteins, C9, factor B, and lysozyme in recurrent oral ulceration and Behçet's syndrome. *J. Clin. Pathol.* **33**: 269–75, 1980.

92. Pepys, M.B. Serum C-reactive protein, serum amyloid P-component and serum amyloid A protein in autoimmune disease. *Clin. Immunol. Allergy* **1**: 77–101, 1981.

93. Honig, S., Gorevic, P. & Weissmann. G. C-reactive protein in systemic lupus erythematosus. *Arth. Rheum.* **20**: 1065–70, 1977.

94. Becker, G.J., Waldburger, M., Hughes, G.R.V. & Pepys, M.B. Value of C-reactive protein measurement in the investigation of fever in systemic lupus erythematosus. *Ann. Rheum. Dis.* **39**: 50–2, 1980.

95. Chambers, R.E., Stross, P., Barry, R.E. & Whicher, J.T. Serum amyloid A protein compared with C-reactive protein, alpha 1-antichymotrypsin and alpha 1-acid glycoprotein as a monitor of inflammatory bowel disease. *Eur. J. Clin. Invest.* **17**: 460–7, 1987.

96. Shine, B., Berghouse, L., Lennard Jones, J.E. & Landon, J. C-reactive protein as an aid in the differentiation of functional and inflammatory bowel disorders. *Clin. Chim. Acta.* **148**: 105–9, 1985.

97. Campbell, C.A., Walker-Smith, J.A., Hindocha, P. & Adinolfi, M. Acute phase proteins in chronic inflammatory bowel disease in childhood. *J. Pediatr. Gastroenterol. Nutr.* **1**: 193–200, 1982.

98. Fagan, E.A., Dyck, R.F., Maton, P.N., Hodgson, H.J.F., Chadwick, V.S., Petrie, A. & Pepys, M.B. Serum levels of C-reactive protein in Crohn's disease and ulcerative colitis. *Eur. J. Clin. Invest.* **12**: 351–9, 1982.

99. Weinstein, P.S., Skinner, M., Sipe, J.D., Lokich, J.J., Zamcheck, N. & Cohen, A.S. Acute-phase proteins or tumour markers: the role of SAA, SAP, CRP and

CEA as indicators of metastasis in a broad spectrum of neoplastic diseases. *Scand. J. Immunol.* **19**: 193–8, 1984.

100. Cooper, E.H. & Stone, J. Acute phase reactant proteins in cancer. *Adv. Cancer Res.* **30**: 1–44, 1979.

101. Vaughan Hudson, B., MacLennan, K.A., Bennett, M.H., Easterling, M.J., Vaughan Hudson, G. & Jelliffe, A.M. Systemic disturbance in Hodgkin's disease and its relation to histopathology and prognosis (BNLI report no. 30). *Clin. Radiol.* **38**: 257–61, 1987.

102. Friedman, S., Henry-Amar, M., Cosset J.-M., Carde, P., Hayat, M., Dupouy, N. & Tubiana, M. Evolution of erythrocyte sedimentation rate as predictor of early relapse in posttherapy early-stage Hodgkin's disease. *J. Clin. Oncol.* **6**: 597–602, 1988.

103. Meade, T.W., Chakrabarti, R., Haines, A.P., North, W.R.S. & Stirling, Y. Characteristics affecting fibrinolytic activity and plasma fibrinogen concentrations. *Br. Med. J.* **1**: 153–6, 1979.

104. Roberts, L.B. The normal ranges, with statistical analysis for seventeen blood constituents. *Clin. Chim. Acta* **16**: 69–78, 1967.

105. Keating, F.R., Jones, J.D., Elveback, L.R. & Randall, R.V. The relation of age and sex to distribution of values in healthy adults of serum calcium, inorganic phosphorus, magnesium, alkaline phosphatase, total proteins, albumin, and blood urea. *J. Lab. Clin. Med.* **73**: 825–34, 1969.

106. Wilhelm, W.F. & Tillisch, J.H. Relation of sedimentation rate to age. *Med. Clin. North Am.* **35**: 1209–11, 1951.

107. Böttiger, L.E. & Svedberg, C.A. Normal erythrocyte sedimentation rate and age. *Br. Med. J.* **2**: 85–7, 1967.

108. Boyd, R.V. & Hoffbrand, B.I. Erythrocyte sedimentation rate in elderly hospital in-patients. *Br Med. J.* **1**: 901–2, 1966.

109. Sharland, D.E. Erythrocyte sedimentation rate: the normal range in the elderly. *J. Am. Geriatr. Soc.* **28**: 346–8, 1980.

110. Miller, A., Green, M. & Robinson, D. Simple rule for calculating normal erythrocyte sedimentation rate. *Br. Med. J.* **286**: 266, 1983.

111. Griffiths, R.A., Good, W.R., Watson, N.P., O'Donnell, H.F., Fell, P.J. & Shakespeare, J.M. Normal erythrocyte sedimentation rate in the elderly. *Br. Med. J.* **289**: 724–5, 1984.

112. Crawford, J., Eye-Boland, M.K. & Cohen, H.J. Clinical utility of erythrocyte sedimentation rate and plasma protein analysis in the elderly. *Am. J. Med.* **82**: 239–45, 1987.

113. Somer, T. The viscosity of blood, plasma and serum in dys- and paraproteinemias. *Acta Med. Scand.* **180**. Suppl. 156, 1–97, 1966.

114. Roe, P.F. & Harkness, J. Plasma viscosity in the elderly. *Geront. Clin.* **17**: 168–72, 1975.

115. Jung, F., Roggenkamp, H.G., Ringelstein, E.B., Leipnitz, G., Schneider, R., Kiesewetter, H. & Zeller, H. Effect of sex, age, body weight, and smoking on plasma viscosity. *Klin. Wochenschr.* **64**: 1076–81, 1986.

116. Kenny, R.A., Hodkinson, H.M., Cox, M.L., Caspi, D. & Pepys, M.B. Acute phase protein responses to infection in elderly patients. *Age Ageing* **13**: 89–94, 1984.

117. Kenny, R.A., Saunders, A.P., Coll, A., Harrington, M.G., Caspi, D., Hodkinson, H.M., & Pepys, M.B. A comparison of the erythrocyte sedimentation rate and serum C-reactive protein concentration in elderly patients. *Age Ageing* **14**: 15–20, 1985.

118. Löfström, G. Comparison between the reactions of acute phase serum with pneumococcus C-polysaccharide and with pneumococcus type 27. *Br. J. Exp. Pathol.* **25**: 21–6, 1944.

119. Losner, S., Volk, B.W. & Wilensky, N.D. Fibrinogen concentration in acute

myocardial infarction. *Arch. Intern. Med.* **93**: 231–45, 1954.

120. Rabinowitz, M.A., Shookhoff, C. & Douglas, A.J. The red cell sedimentation time in coronary occlusion. *Am. Heart J.* **7**: 52–65, 1931.

121. Kushner, I., Broder, M.L. & Karp, D. Control of the acute phase response. Serum C-reactive protein kinetics after acute myocardial infarction. *J. Clin. Invest.* **61**: 235–42, 1978.

122. De Beer, F.C., Hind, C.R.K., Fox, K.M., Allan, R.M., Maseri, A. & Pepys, M.B. Measurement of serum C-reactive protein concentration in myocardial ischaemia and infarction. *Br. Heart J.* **47**: 239–43, 1982.

123. Levinger, E.L., Levy, H. & Elster, S.K. Study of C-reactive protein in the sera of patients with acute myocardial infarction. *Ann. Intern. Med.* **46**: 68–78, 1957.

124. Kozonis, M.C. & Gurevin, I. The value of the C-reactive protein determination in coronary artery disease. *Ann. Intern. Med.* **46**: 79–85, 1957.

125. Ditzel, J., Bang, H.O. & Thorsen, N. Myocardial infarction and whole-blood viscosity. *Acta Med. Scand.* **183**: 577–9, 1968.

126. Biro, G.P., Beresford-Kroeger, D. & Hendry, P. Early deleterious hemorheologic changes following acute experimental coronary occlusion and salutary antihyperviscosity effect of hemodilution with stroma-free hemoglobin. *Am. Heart J.* **103**: 870–8, 1982.

127. Haines, A.P., Howarth, D., North, W.R.S., Goldenberg, E., Stirling, Y., Meade, T.W., Raftery, E.B. & Millar-Craig, M.W. Haemostatic variables and the outcome of myocardial infarction. *Thromb. Haemost.* **50**: 800–3, 1983.

128. Pilgeram, L.O. Relation of plasma fibrinogen concentration changes to human arteriosclerosis. *J. Appl. Physiol.* **16**: 660–4, 1961.

129. Stuart, J., George, A.J., Davies, A.J., Aukland, A., Hurlow, R.A. Haematological stress syndrome in atherosclerosis. *J. Clin. Pathol.* **34**: 464–7, 1981.

130. Van Oost, B.A., Veldhuyzen, B.F.E., van Houwelingen, H.C., Timmermans, A.P.M., & Sixma J.J. Tests for platelet changes, acute phase reactants and serum lipids in diabetes mellitus and peripheral vascular disease. *Thomb. Haemost.* **48**: 289–93, 1982.

131. Lowe, G.D.O., Drummond, M.M., Lorimer, A.R., Hutton, I., Forbes, C.D., Prentice, C.R.M. & Barbenel, J.C. Relationship between extent of coronary artery disease and blood viscosity. *Br. Med. J.* **280**: 673–4, 1980.

132. Wilhelmsen, L., Svärdsudd, K., Korsan-Bengtsen, K., Larsson, B., Welin, L. & Tibblin, G. Fibrinogen as a risk factor for stroke and myocardial infarction. *N. Engl. J. Med.* **311**: 501–5, 1984.

133. Dormandy, J.A., Hoare, E., Colley, J., Arrowsmith, D.E. & Dormandy, T.L. Clinical haemodynamic, rheological, and biochemical findings in 126 patients with intermittent claudication. *Br. Med. J.* **4**: 576–81, 1973.

134. Meade, T.W., North, W.R.S., Chakrabarti, R., Stirling, Y., Haines, A.P., Thompson, S.G. & Brozović, M. Haemostatic function and cardiovascular death: early results of a prospective study. *Lancet* **1**: 1050–4, 1980.

135. Meade, T.W., Mellows, S., Brozovic, M., Miller, G.J., Chakrabarti, R.R., North, W.R.S., Haines, A.P., Stirling, Y., Imeson, J.D. & Thompson, S.G. Haemostatic function and ischaemic heart disease: principal results of the Northwick Park Heart Study. *Lancet* **2**: 533–7, 1986.

136. Gerrity, R.G. The role of the monocyte in atherogenesis. I. Transition of blood-borne monocytes into foam cells in fatty lesions. *Am. J. Pathol.* **103**: 181–90, 1981.

137. Gerrity, R.G., Naito, H.K., Richardson, M. & Schwartz, C.J. Dietary induced atherogenesis in swine. Morphology of the intima in prelesion stages. *Am. J. Pathol.* **95**: 775–86, 1979.

138. Stuart, J. Rheological importance of acute-phase reactants. *Nouv. Rev. Fr. Hematol.* **28**: 33–6, 1986.

139. Humphries, S.E., Cook, M., Dubowitz, M., Stirling, Y. & Meade, T.W. Role of

genetic variation at the fibrinogen locus in determination of plasma fibrinogen concentrations. *Lancet* **1**: 1452–5, 1987.

140. Gram, H.C. On the causes of the variations in the sedimentation of the corpuscles and the formation of the crusta phlogistica ("size", buffy coat") on the blood. *Arch. Intern. Med.* **28**: 312–30, 1921.

141. Plass, E.D. & Matthew, C.W. Plasma protein fractions in normal pregnancy, labor, and puerperium. *Am. J. Obstet. Gynec.* **12**: 347–58, 1926.

142. Inglis, T.C.N., Stuart, J., George, A.J. & Davies, A.J. Haemostatic and rheological changes in normal pregnancy and pre-eclampsia. *Br. J. Haematol.* **50**: 461–5, 1982.

143. Bland, P.B., Goldstein, L. & First, A. The sedimentation test in pregnancy and in the puerperium. A study of five hundred forty patients. *Surg. Gynec. Obstet.* **50**: 429–34, 1930.

144. Malmnäs, C. The erythrocyte sedimentation rate during pregnancy and the puerperium. *Acta Med. Scand.* **161**: 323–39, 1958.

145. Hoch, H. & Marrack, J.R. The composition of the blood of women during pregnancy and after delivery. *J. Obstet. Gynaec. Br. Emp.* **55**: 1–16, 1948.

146. Hamilton, G.M. The erythrocyte sedimentation rate in pregnancy. *J. Obstet. Gynaec. Br. Emp.* **60**: 409–15, 1953.

147. Stuart, J., Kenny, M.W. & Inglis, T.C.M. Erythrocyte filterability in normal pregnancy and pre-eclampsia. *Br. J. Haematol.* **53**: 353–5, 1983.

148. Waites, G.T., Bell, A.M. & Bell, S.C. Acute phase serum proteins in syngeneic and allogeneic mouse pregnancy. *Clin. Exp. Immunol.* **53**: 225–32, 1983.

149. Richardson, S.G.N., Matthews, K.B., Stuart, J., Geddes, A.M. & Wilcox, R.M. Serial changes in coagulation and viscosity during sickle-cell crisis. *Br. J. Haematol.* **41**: 95–103, 1979.

150. Kenny, M.W., Meakin, M., Worthington, D.J. & Stuart, J. Erythrocyte deformability in sickle-cell crisis. *Br. J. Haematol.* **49**: 103–9, 1981.

151. Diggs, L.W. Sickle cell crises. *Am. J. Clin. Pathol.* **44**: 1–19, 1965.

152. Stuart, J. Sickle-cell disease and vascular occlusion – rheological aspects. *Clin. Hemorheol.* **4**: 193–207, 1984.

153. Rieber, E.E., Veliz, G. & Pollack, S. Red cells in sickle cell crisis: observations on the pathophysiology of crisis. *Blood* **49**: 967–79, 1977.

154. Lucas, G.S., Caldwell, N.M. & Stuart, J. Fluctuating deformability of oxygenated sickle erythrocytes in the asymptomatic state and in painful crisis. *Br. J. Haematol.* **59**: 363–8, 1985.

155. Kaul, D.K., Fabry, M.E. & Nagel, R.L. Vaso-occlusion by sickle cells: evidence for selective trapping of dense red cells. *Blood* **68**: 1162–6, 1986.

156. Cohen, A.S., Shirahama, T., Sipe, J.D. & Skinner, M. Amyloid proteins, precursors, mediator, and enhancer. *Lab. Invest.* **48**: 1–4, 1983.

157. De Beer, F.C., Mallya, R.K., Fagan, E.A., Lanham, J.G., Hughes, G.R.V. & Pepys, M.B. Serum amyloid-A protein concentration in inflammatory diseases and its relationship to the incidence of reactive systemic amyloidosis. *Lancet* **2**: 231–4, 1982.

158. Falck, H.M., Maury, C.P.J., Teppo, A.-M. & Wegelius, O. Correlation of persistently high serum amyloid A protein and C-reactive protein concentrations with rapid progression of secondary amyloidosis. *Br. Med. J.* **286**: 1391–3, 1983.

159. Schleimer, R.P. & Rutledge, B.K. Cultured human vascular endothelial cells acquire adhesiveness for neutrophils after stimulation with interleukin 1, endotoxin, and tumor-promoting phorbol diesters. *J. Immunol.* **136**: 649–54, 1986.

160. Bevilacqua, M.P., Pober, J.S., Majeau, G.R., Cotran, R.S. & Gimbrone, M.A. Interleukin 1 (IL-1) induces biosynthesis and cell surface expression of

procoagulant activity in human vascular endothelial cells. *J. Exp. Med.* **160**: 618–23, 1984.

161. Juhan-Vague, I., Aillaud, M.F., De Cock, F., Philip-Joet, C., Arnaud, C., Serradimigni, A. & Collen, D. The fast-acting inhibitor of tissue-type plasminogen activator is an acute phase reactant protein. In *Progress in Fibrinolysis*, Vol. VII (eds J.F. Davidson, M.B. Donati & S. Coccheri), pp. 146–9. Churchill Livingstone, Edinburgh, 1985.

162. Kluft, C., Verheijen, J.H., Jie, A.F.H., Rijken, D.C., Preston, F.E., Sue-Ling, H.M., Jespersen, J. & Aasen, A.O. The postoperative fibrinolytic shutdown: a rapidly reverting acute phase pattern for the fast-acting inhibitor of tissue-type plasminogen activator after trauma. *Scand. J. Clin. Lab. Invest.* **45**: 605–10, 1985.

163. Gram, J., Kluft, C. & Jespersen, J. Depression of tissue plasminogen activator (t-PA) activity and rise of t-PA inhibition and acute phase reactants in blood of patients with acute myocardial infarction (AMI). *Thromb. Haemost.* **58**: 817–21, 1987.

164. Jager, B.V. Cryofibrinogenemia. *N. Engl. J. Med.* **266**: 579–83, 1962.

13

Lymphadenopathy

I.W. Delamore
Consultant Physician, Department of Haematology, Manchester Royal Infirmary, Manchester, UK

D.I. Gozzard
Consultant Haematologist, Ysbyty Glan Clwyd, Bodelwyddan, UK

INTRODUCTION

Lymphadenopathy is a common physical sign in clinical medicine. The diagnostic problem facing the physician is that an enlarged lymph node arises as an end-point of several pathological processes, e.g. inflammation, neoplasia, and this may be a reaction to distant stimuli or direct invasion. The infecting agents or neoplastic cells reach the nodes either through the lymphatic system or via the blood. Localized lymphadenopathy arises following lymphatic spread from the adjacent area of lymph drainage, whereas blood-borne or systemic disease produces generalized lymphadenopathy. Lymph nodes may also become involved due to infiltration by foreign particulate material, by disturbances of metabolism, especially of lipids, and by primary haematological conditions.

Affected lymph nodes are usually amenable to palpation, biopsy and various imaging procedures. Clinical examination may reveal important information regarding the character of enlarged superficial lymph nodes together with the degree and extent of involvement of these nodes. This can produce important evidence as to the site of origin and, in many cases, to the nature of the causative agent. A knowledge of the drainage areas of the various regional lymph nodes of the body is essential for both clinical diagnosis and for planning future therapy.

Lymph nodes contain both immunological and phagocytic cells and are situated at key sites throughout the body to react to any 'insult' whether it is infective, inflammatory, or neoplastic. This accounts for the ubiquitous role of the lymphatic tissues and the finding of lymphadenopathy in a wide variety of disease processes. The spleen, being the largest lymphoid organ in the body, is often affected by these same stimuli to enlarge sufficiently to be demonstrable as clinical splenomegaly. This is reviewed in Chapter 14.

SITES OF LYMPH NODES

The areas of the body in which collections of lymph nodes are to be found are arbitrarily divided into 13 separate 'regions' of which eight are bilateral and five are 'midline'. The former collection include (1) the cervical, supraclavicular, occipital and pre-auricular nodes, (2) infraclavicular, (3) axillary and pectoral, (4) epitrochlear and brachial, (5) hilar, (6) iliac, (7) inguinal and femoral, and (8) popliteal. The single nodal groups include the spleen and the para-aortic, mesenteric and mediastinal lymph nodes and Waldeyer's ring.

FUNCTION AND COMPOSITION OF LYMPH NODES

The lymphoreticular system (LRS) refers to that portion of the mobile and fixed cellular elements which is concerned with body defence involving macrophage activity and immunological mechanisms. However, this excludes the granulocytic cells of various types. The responses of the LRS to any stimulus invariably include increased cellular proliferative activity.

The function of the LRS is to provide an efficient apparatus to defend the body against pathogenic microorganisms and against the growth of cells that have acquired neoplastic characteristics. In order to accomplish this defensive role the system must be flexible, rapidly mobilizable and able to respond appropriately in several different ways. Potentially pathogenic bacteria, fungi and viruses are contained and eliminated by different mechanisms, the former usually eliciting a pyogenic response with cell death due to the release of granulocytic lysosomal toxins. However, there is little or no long-lasting immunity or other input from the lymphoid system. On the other hand, the cooperation of the lymphoid and monocyte–macrophage system is necessary to deal with tuberculous lesions which may lead to the proliferation of charateristic granulomata. The effect of immunity is noted in the difference of degree of response to primary or secondary exposure. Some bacteria and fungi remain viable intracellularly and the LRS serves to deter their multiplication. In general, the manifestations of the encounter between the LRS and the pathogen or incompatible tissue or material depend upon the nature of the cellular response elicited by the pathogen, the degree and site of localization of the pathogenic experience, previously developed immunity, and the functional capability of the various components of the LRS.

In the light of good evidence, particularly from the study of various congenital deficiencies of immune function, it is generally accepted that the lymphoid system comprises two main components. Firstly, lymphocytes that bear surface immunoglobulin and are the precursors to antibody-producing plasma cells. These are the B-lymphocytes, following the nomenclature of the cell-type found in the bursa of Fabricius in birds. Secondly, thymus-derived or T-lymphocytes. These are particularly involved in antigenic memory, delayed hypersensitivity reactions, graft rejection and graft-versus-host disease. Both types of lymphocytes have a recognized maturation scheme and are found not only in the blood, but in the marrow, spleen, regional lymph nodes and thoracic duct. They are situated in certain well-defined regions of the lymph node with the B-lymphocytes found in the paracortical area, medullary cords, and forming the follicles. The T-lymphocytes form the deep cortical and peri-follicular areas. It is now recognized that circulating lymphocytes tend to recirculate to the tissues from which they originated, e.g. gut-associated lymphoid tissue.

AGE CHANGES IN LYMPHOID TISSUE

The general distribution of lymph nodes and amount of lymphoid tissue bear a definite relation to age. The rate of growth of lymphoid tissue is greatest in infancy and continues at a high level throughout childhood. It reaches its peak about puberty and declines thereafter. Measurements of amounts of lymphoid tissue present show that at 2 years of age the child has 50% of the lymphoid tissue of a 20-year-old person; at 4 years, 80%; at 8 years 120%; at 12 years 190%; at 16 years, 120%. The maximal development of lymphoid tissue occurs during the time when acute infections of the respiratory and alimentary tracts are most common, and during the period of greatest increase in weight and height. This suggests that it is part of the natural defence mechanism particularly as a child starts or changes schools with exposure to a different environment of potential pathogens. During infancy and childhood, moreover, lymphoid tissue responds characteristically to infection by prompt and excessive swelling and hyperplasia. Advancing age is associated with less dramatic changes.

Children have more numerous and larger lymph nodes than adults. There is marked hypertrophy during childhood, and involution during adult life. However, there is no real atrophy as a rule since at any age local or generalized infections may induce marked hypertrophy. Involutional changes in the lymph nodes consist in reduction in the size of the nodes and of the germinal centres, accompanied by infiltration with fat. Scarring may occur, particularly in inguinal glands, making them unsuitable for histological analysis.

The fact that certain groups of lymph nodes disappear in adult life and that certain areas of lymphoid tissue, although they do not disappear, undergo involution, is of practical significance since it serves to explain the relative incidence of certain pathological conditions with reference to age. Perhaps the most significant diseases from this point of view are: adenoiditis, tonsillitis, retropharyngeal abscess, appendicitis and mesenteric adenitis.

REACTIONS TO INFECTIONS

Lymph nodes have evolved as sites of interaction, where noxious stimuli, whether cellular or products of metabolism, meet the fixed cellular constituents of the lymphoreticular system. Both the lymph and blood-stream drain through the lymph nodes bringing noxious stimuli to the optimal site for antigenic stimulation. Afferent lymphatic channels enter the lymph node and empty into the marginal or peripheral sinus. The richer reticulin network of the node pulp, in which the lymphocyte aggregations occur, commences at the inner surface of the marginal sinus. The lymph filters through this region, passing through fine sinusoids. On reaching the medulla of the node the lymph is collected by larger sinuses and channelled towards the efferent lymphatic vessel which leaves the hilum.

When antigenic material is engulfed by the sinus macrophages some antigen appears on the cell surface. These antigen-bearing dendritic cells tend to aggregate and they cooperate in lymphocyte transformation producing larger cells with vesicular nuclei, distinct nucleoli and pyrinino-philic cytoplasm. Mitotic figures frequently occur. Germinal, or follicular, centres appear as paler areas in the middle of rather ill-defined collections of small lymphocytes of the cortex, the primary follicles.

From observations of the mixture of lymphoid cells, certain generaliza-tions have been made. Some of the cells have extremely irregular nuclei, often with deep notches in their outline, some of these notched nuclei only being slightly larger than small lymphocytes, but others being considerably larger. These are designated 'cleaved cells', in contradistinction to which are the 'non-cleaved' lymphoid cells of the follicular centres, with large oval to round open nuclei. Most of the lymphoid cells found in the follicular centres have been shown to be B-lymphocytes. Virgin B-cells leave the bone marrow to circulate in the bloodstream, which they leave by adhering to, and then squeezing between, the specialized tall, endothelial cells of post-capillary venules, situated in the interfollicular areas of lymphoid tissues. They then migrate to the cortical areas and pass into the follicular centres to undergo a phase of antigen-driven proliferative activity.

The majority of these processed B-lympocytes drain away in the efferent lymph to enter the bloodstream and then migrate across specialized endothelial sites to pass through other thymus-independent areas of lymphoid tissue. Recently it has been shown that lymphocytes tend to recirculate to specific sites of lymphoid tissue, i.e. lymphocytes originating in the gut-associated lymphoid tissue will tend to return to that tissue.

NEOPLASTIC REACTIONS

Contrary to the sequential changes in lymph node population during reaction to infection, the neoplastic cell population is relatively monotonous. Neoplastic cells result from the uncontrolled proliferation of a malignant clone and are closely related to one another, whereas reactive states represent complex cooperative activity between differing cell types, and thus result in a more mixed appearance. Hodgkin's disease is the exception to this rule in that the cellular reaction to the malignant cells is often florid, and anything but monotonous.

Neoplastic cells ignore tissue boundaries, and often spread beyond the capsule of the node into surrounding tissues.

LYMPHADENOPATHY

Carcinomatous invasion

Carcinoma has a special tendency to spread by the lymphatic system, as evidenced by the preponderance of metastases to the regional lymph nodes. Spread of cancer by the lymphatic route may occur as a result of permeation or cancer cell emboli. In the first of these, the cancer cells, after reaching the lymphatic capillaries, invade their lumina and then spread along the lymph vessels. Embolization is the predominant method of spread. The emboli are filtered from the lymph by the lymph nodes. At first they become arrested in the subcapsular sinus, but eventually may completely replace the node. The metastatic lesion generally has the same morphological characteristics as the primary cancer although the growth may be more florid, with massive neoplastic lymphadenopathy occurring from a relatively small primary neoplasm. Metastatically involved nodes are subject to secondary changes, such as necrosis and fibrosis. Carcinoma in the lymphatic channels also may reach the venous system by lymphaticovenous shunts.

It must be emphasized that the clinical examination of lymph nodes is not sufficient to determine the presence or absence of lymph node metastases. Enlarged lymph nodes are not necessarily involved metastatically; lymph nodes may show reactive hyperplasia before they are invaded by cancer emboli. Such reactive hyperplasia is due to phagocytosis of cellular debris, resulting from necrosis of the primary growth. This is the so-called 'foreign body reaction'. The affected lymph node presents the picture of granulomatous lymphadenitis on microscopy. Enlargement of lymph nodes due to reactive hyperplasia without cancer emboli may indicate an improved prognosis. The primary site may also serve as an entrance site for infection leading to infectious lymphadenopathy. It occurs particularly in lymph nodes some distance from the primary focus. On the other hand, lymph nodes in the immediate vicinity of the primary lesion may show no reactive hyperplasia, and therefore may not be enlarged, and yet may contain neoplastic emboli.

Occasionally atypical lymph nodes may be reached by metastases through lymphatic vessels that drain an organ that has become involved secondarily with carcinoma through the haematogenous route.

Infectious adenopathy

Acute inflammation causes lymph nodes to become enlarged, tender and soft. There may be overlying erythema with oedema and induration of surrounding tissues. This is true for many viral or bacterial causes. However, there are some identifiable syndromes in which the physician can reasonably suggest the aetiological agent from clinical examination and simple laboratory tests.

Acute pharyngitis is usually viral in origin, but may be due to a group A β-haemolytic streptococcus, or occasionally to a pneumococcus or coagulase-positive staphylococcus. Differentiating viral from bacterial pharyngitis on the basis of physical examination alone is difficult. Fever, cervical lymphadenopathy and leucocytosis may be present in both viral and streptococcal infection, although may be more marked in the latter.

Acute tonsillitis is usually due to a streptococcal or, less commonly, a viral infection. In this condition the tonsils are oedematous and hyperaemic. There may be a purulent exudate from the crypts and sometimes membranous formation with the presence of a white, thin, non-confluent membrane confined to the tonsil that peels away without bleeding. The differential diagnosis includes diptheria, Vincent's angina (trench mouth) and infectious mononucleosis. Typical faucial diptheria is always associated with some cervical lymphadenopathy and periadenitis. In the most severe forms gross cervical periadenitis may produce the typical 'bull-neck' appearance. The diptheritic pharyngeal membrane is characteristically adherent and produces bleeding on separation. Vincent's angina is due to infection by a fusiform bacillus and a spirochaete. It is characterized by superficial, painful ulcers with erythematous borders. The glands on the affected side become enlarged and tender and the breath is characteristically offensive.

The triad of infectious mononucleosis, toxoplasmosis and cytomegalovirus are considered together because of the similarity in the clinical syndromes each may produce. Infectious mononucleosis is characterized by symptoms of fever, malaise and headache. Pharyngitis, lymphadenopathy which may be localized or generalized, and splenomegaly are common features. Lymphadenopathy, often detected by patients themselves, is rarely a presenting symptom of infectious mononucleosis but most patients are aware of this abnormality at some time during the illness. Although the nodes are never spontaneously nor exquisitely painful their moderate tenderness may call early attention to their enlargement. Sometimes they are accidentally discovered or are detected during self-examination following the development of systemic symptoms. In about 3% of all cases of infectious mononucleosis the gross cervical lymphadenopathy imparts a 'bull neck' appearance. Enlargement of lymph nodes usually begins 2–3 days after the onset of the first symptoms, by the end of the first week, palpable lymphadenopathy is present in 70–80% of all patients. Sometimes the enlargement persists for several weeks and rarely months or years after the cessation of the acute illness. Palatal petechiae and periorbital swelling with oedema of the eyelids are common early features. The disease occurs chiefly in children and young adults, particularly in those living in institutions such as hospitals and residential colleges. The haematological features include a normal or slightly raised white cell count but with neutropenia associated with the presence of large lymphoid cells, 'atypical lymphocytes', which possess large amounts of basophilic, 'foamy' cytoplasm. The Paul–Bunnell reaction usually becomes positive by the end of the first week, but may not be present until the second or third week in some cases. This reaction depends upon the presence of a heterophile antibody active against sheep red cells.

Toxoplasmosis is an endemic infection in temperate climates. Sexual multiplication occurs in the intestine of cats with oocysts being shed in the stools. The more common form of acquired toxoplasmosis resembles infectious mononucleosis and is characterized by cervical and axillary lymphadenopathy, malaise, muscle pain and irregular low fever. Mild anaemia, hypotension, leucopenia, lymphocytosis and slightly altered liver function may be present. More commonly, it presents as asymptomatic cervical lymphadenopathy. The diagnosis is usually suspected when a 'mononucleosis' is associated with a persistently negative Paul–Bunnell test. Recent acquisition of a family kitten should cause consideration of the diagnosis, which can be confirmed by serological tests. Cytomegalovirus (CMV) is another Paul–Bunnell-negative 'mononucleosis'. Clinical features are shared with infectious mononucleosis, although CMV infrequently causes pharyngitis or lymphadenopathy, differential points of diagnostic importance. The diagnosis can be confirmed by isolation of the virus from body fluids, although since CMV can be excreted several years after infection the results should be interpreted in the light of other evidence. Rising titres of antibodies to CMV may occur during the illness.

In chronic infections, the enlarged lymph nodes are often not accompanied by oedema and tenderness and the nodes are more or less firm, depending on the degree of fibrosis. Tuberculous lymphadenitis has decreased in incidence with the control of bovine tuberculosis (TB); in the past most tuberculous lymphadenitis occurred as scrofula, cervical lymphadenitis due to primary infection in the oropharyngeal lymphatic tissue. Currently, TB of the lymph nodes represents lymphohaematogenous spread from a primary pulmonary focus. The diagnosis is made by an excisional biopsy. The process may be localized or disseminated. Nowadays, the infecting organism is as likely to be an atypical mycobacterium, rather than *Mycobacterium bovis* or *M. tuberculosis*. Syphilis has as a common feature of the second stage of the disease, rubbery, discrete, non-tender enlargement of lymph nodes, particularly those of the posterior triangle of the neck. Leprosy (Hansen's disease) may involve regional lymph nodes and if superficial may rupture to the surface producing chronic ulcers with sinuses discharging bacilli. An acute necrotizing lymphadenitis may be seen in some patients with lepromatous leprosy and erythema nodosum leprosum.

In lymphogranuloma venereum (LV) and cat-scratch fever, both conditions due to chlamydial infection, regional lymph nodes may enlarge. LV is sexually transmitted and, after an incubation period of 3–12 or more days, a small, transient, non-indurated, vesicular lesion is formed that ulcerates quickly, heals and may pass unnoticed. Usually the first symptom is unilateral tender enlargement of the inguinal lymph nodes, which progresses to form a large, tender, fluctuant mass that adheres to the deep tissues and inflames the overlying skin. Multiple sinuses may develop and discharge purulent or blood-stained material. Healing eventually occurs with scar formation, but sinuses can persist or recur. Clinical diagnosis can be confirmed by a complement fixation test to demonstrate a rising antibody titre. Cat-scratch fever produces regional lymphadenopathy within 2 weeks, usually unilaterally and in relation to the scratch site. The nodes are initially firm and tender, but later become fluctuant and may drain with fistula formation. The skin lesion and lymphadenopathy subside completely within 2–5 months. Diagnosis is by history of cat contact, negative studies for other causes of regional lymphadenopathy and characteristic histopathology.

Other causes of lymphadenopathy include brucellosis in which slight or moderate enlargement of lymph nodes may occur several weeks into the illness. *Yersinia enterolitica* may cause acute disease of the ileo-caecal region, often simulating acute appendicitis. At operation the mesenteric lymph nodes are enlarged and may be biopsied. Diagnosis is by serological means. Fungal infections rarely cause lymphadenopathy.

Infiltrative invasion

This type of involvement of the lymphatic system occurs predominantly in the respiratory system and is associated with the inhaling of dust particles (coal, silica, etc.). Such dust particles are removed from the pulmonary alveoli by macrophages. The dust-laden macrophages then migrate into the interalveolar septa and enter the interlobar and perivascular lymphatics. In time the lymphatics of the lung become filled with the dust-laden macrophages with the development of an obstructive lymphangitis. Many of the macrophages eventually migrate to the bronchial lymph nodes. Upon degeneration of the macrophages, the freed dust particles are now taken up by the reticulo-endothelial cells of the nodes.

Infiltrative adenopathy is seen particularly in anthracosis, silicosis and chalicosis. The histological picture of the affected nodes is of a granulomatous lymphadenitis.

Metabolic disturbances

Certain pathological states are associated with disturbances in metabolism of lipids, the reticulo-endothelial cells of the lymph nodes (and other organs) become engorged with various types of lipids. Such lipid-storing reticulo-endothelial cells are very characteristic. They are large and their cytoplasm is filled with globules of lipid, giving the cell a vacuolated appearance. Hence, these cells are called 'foam cells'. The lipids chiefly involved are cerebroside, phosphatide and cholesterol.

The clinical anatomical features of the various types of lipidoses are dominated by the specific lipid involved, by the disturbed fat metabolism, and by the effects of the xanthomatous accumulations in the tissues of the body.

In the primary lipidoses, the anatomic and functional changes related to the lipid storage are so constant and specific that they are recognized as disease entities. There are two major well-defined primary lipidoses: (1) Gaucher's disease, and (2) Niemann–Pick's disease. Both are congenital and familial, being transmitted as an autosomal recessive gene.

In Gaucher's disease, the essential lipid disturbance is the accumulation of cerebroside in reticulo-endothelial cells. Both adult and infantile forms are recognized, the diagnosis in the former usually being recognized in late childhood or early in adult life. The common manifestations are splenomegaly, which is progressive; hepatomegaly; bone pain, due to infiltration of the bone marrow with Gaucher cells, which may expand the bones, particularly the lower end of the femora giving the 'Erlenmeyer' flask deformity; pathological fractures; pigmentation of the skin and pingueculae. Accumulation of foam cells in the lymph nodes causes generalized, but often trivial, enlargement of both superficial and deep nodes. The serum acid phosphatase is raised, and pancytopenia may occur due to hypersplenism. The diagnosis is established by bone marrow examination and the finding of large Gaucher cells, 20–50 µm in diameter with pale cytoplasm showing a wavy pattern of fine fibrils (see also Chapter 14).

In Niemann–Pick's disease there is accumulation of large amounts of phospholipid, especially sphingomyelin. The foam cells are large and yellow. There is slight enlargement of the superficial nodes and may be considerable enlargement of the intra-abdominal nodes, particularly the hepatic, pancreatic, splenic and mesenteric nodes. The onset is in the first year of life with weight loss, vomiting, abdominal distension, hepatosplenomegaly and with neurological lesions leading to weakness, spasticity, blindness and deafness. The diagnosis is established by bone marrow examination and the finding of foam cells containing hyaline droplets (see also Chapter 14).

Histiocytosis X is a group of related disorders characterized by proliferation of histiocytes and affecting primarily children. Whilst eosinophilic granuloma does not cause lymphadenopathy, both Hand–Schuller–Christian disease and Letterer–Siwe disease may cause significant lymph node enlargement. Letterer–Siwe disease occurs before the age of 3 years and is usually fatal. It is the acute form of the Histiocytosis X syndrome and affects skin, bone, liver and spleen as well as causing generalized prominent lymphadenopathy. Hand–Schuller–Christian disease is often detected in early childhood but can appear even in late middle age. The extent of lymph node involvement depends on the severity of the disease, but isolated lymph node enlargement may be the presenting feature.

Primary haemopoietic disorder

Primary disease may involve any of the cellular divisions of the haemopoietic system. Lymph nodes may become involved both by primary tumours of lymphoid tissue (lymphomas) and by constitutional diseases (leukaemias).

The primary tumours of lymph nodes are all malignant. Such tumours may arise from the lymphoid or the reticulo-endothelial elements of the nodes or their derivatives and the tumour may arise from these cells at any stage of their development. Such tumours can be broadly divided into Hodgkin's disease, non-Hodgkin's lymphoma, and true histiocytic neoplasms. Usually the type of neoplasm is identical in all involved nodes (concordant tumour) but occasionally different grades of tumour are found within the same lymph node or involving separate nodes – discordant tumours.

The patient with Hodgkin's disease (HD) most commonly seeks medical attention after becoming aware of an unusual lump or mass in the neck. The superficial cervical lymph nodes are the apparent site of disease origin in 60–80% of patients and the left side is involved somewhat more often than the right. Initial axillary nodal involvement occurs in 6–20% of patients, the mediastinal nodes in 6–11%, and inguinal nodes in 6–12%.[1-7] Enlarged lymph nodes are typically neither painful nor tender and they may have reached a considerable size before becoming noticeable. Enlarged groin nodes are relatively uncommon at presentation and enlarged epitrochlear nodes distinctly unusual, both being more frequently seen with the non-Hodgkin's lymphomas. Involvement of nasopharyngeal or tonsillar lymphoid tissue is rarely encountered in HD. Infraclavicular nodal involvement is associated with an adverse prognosis.[8] The nodes are at first discrete, moveable, smooth, rubbery in consistency and measure up to 3 cm in diameter. Later in the disease they become firm, larger nodular masses that seldom suppurate. Symptoms may arise due to the effect of pressure on vital structures by the enlarging glands, especially from enlarged mediastinal nodes causing tracheobronchial or oesophageal compression (cough, dyspnoea, dysphagia, pain, pleural effusions) or obstruction of the superior vena cava (congestion of the face and neck, headache, papilloedema). There are well-documented instances of waxing and waning in the size of lymph node masses and not infrequently the patient will report diminution in size of lymphadenopathy following treatment with antibiotics. Some patients are febrile at the time of presentation, a feature usually taken to indicate more advanced disease. The fever may be smouldering and low-grade in character. The cyclical Pel–Ebstein bouts of fever, each lasting 1–2 weeks and separated by afebrile periods of similar duration, are rare and now only seen in exceptional patients with far advanced untreated disease. Night sweats characterize advanced HD; these may drench the patient and cause him to wake at night in order to change his night clothes. Weight loss may occur and is thought also to indicate advanced disease. Pruritis when present is usually generalized in character and may be severe enough to cause the patient to scratch extensively. Occasionally patients will report that the consumption of alcohol leads almost immediately to pain in one or more of their enlarged lymph nodes. Alcohol-induced pain is rare in patients with HD, and occurs also in some patients with bony deposits of carcinoma or in patients with eosinopilic granuloma, limiting its diagnostic value. Other symptoms that may lead to a diagnosis of HD include anorexia, generalized weakness and fatigue, back pain, bone pain or jaundice.

Needle aspiration of an enlarged node can yield material that points to or occasionally clinches the diagnosis of HD but excision biopsy of an enlarged node or other appropriate tissue is mandatory in any patient where HD is suspected. A lymph node imprint may produce an early diagnosis.

The peripheral blood picture in patients with untreated HD is frequently normal. Alternatively patients with early disease may show a mild thrombocytosis. A neutrophil leucocytosis also occurs. Both monocyte and eosinophil numbers may be raised, on rare occasions the latter very considerably. In more advanced disease, lymphocyte numbers may be decreased and the degree of lymphopenia may correlate with the stage of the disease. Anaemia may rarely be due to direct bone marrow involvement by Hodgkins tissue or result from haemolysis. In the former case, the blood film may show leucoerythroblastic changes. The erythrocyte sedimentation rate (ESR) is usually but not invariably raised in patients with untreated HD. When raised, it should return to normal after successful specific treatment. Occasionally patients are seen who throughout their course have a normal ESR.

Once the diagnosis of HD has been reached there should be a thorough search for widespread disease. This is because the prognosis using radiotherapy for localized disease is excellent, with chemotherapy being reserved for those cases with disseminated disease (stages 3/4) or with 'B' symptoms (weight loss >10% body weight in the previous 6 months, night sweats or fevers). However, the staging laparotomy has now been shown to be unnecessary.[9]

A patient with non-Hodgkin's lymphoma (NHL) may present with localized or generalized peripheral lymphadenopathy indistinguishable on clinical grounds from HD, but major constitutional symptoms such as fever, night sweats or weight loss occur less commonly in NHL than in HD. The abnormal nodes usually appear first in the cervical, supraclavicular, axillary or inguinal regions, but in about one-quarter of all patients the enlargement of retroperitoneal or mesenteric lymph nodes produces abdominal symptoms, which may require laparotomy for diagnosis. Furthermore, patients with NHL commonly present with features of disease occurring outside the lymphatic system, a further point of distinction from HD. Intrathoracic disease may be manifested by hilar or mediastinal adenopathy, superior vena caval obstruction or pulmonary parenchymal involvement. Unilateral or bilateral pleural effusions are not uncommon at the time of presentation. Involvement of Waldeyer's ring is a relatively common presenting feature. Enlarged nodes in the presacral region may cause symptoms of bowel or urinary tract obstruction, and those in the ileofemoral regions may lead to oedema or thrombophlebitis in the lower extremities.

In chronic lymphocytic leukaemia (CLL) there occurs a progressive accumulation of lymphocytes which are mostly of a normal mature appearance but which are immunologically incompetent. There is a generalized symmetrical lymphadenopathy, a moderate degree of splenomegaly and a variable lymphocytosis in the bone marrow and peripheral blood together with a progressive immunological deficiency which is responsible for a great vulnerability to infections, both bacterial and viral, which plague the later stages of the disease.

The disease is rare below the age of 20 years, becoming gradually more common towards the age of 40–50 years and then the incidence increases steeply until it becomes the commonest type of leukaemia in old age. Between 60 and 75% of cases occur in males and its familial incidence is greater than for any other type of cancer.

In most patients a superficial lymphadenopathy is the most striking clinical feature; this is usually generalized, but the neck nodes are particularly noticeable. The degree of enlargement is very variable with early cases producing a diffuse shotty nodal enlargement only, whereas in advanced cases it may be very great and individual nodes may measure up to 5.0 cm diameter. Characteristically the nodes are firm, discrete and painless, except in areas where there has been previous inflammation, for instance in the tonsillar nodes or in the groins. They are not matted and are neither attached to superficial nor deep structures. The enlargement is by no means limited to superficial nodes, however, for enlargement of mediastinal and abdominal nodes may be found on radiological or clinical examination; very occasionally mediastinal nodes may cause compression of neighbouring structures, and abdominal nodes may cause diverse symptoms. Collections of fluid in the pleural and peritoneal cavities may occur but then usually late in the course of the disease. The diffuse lymph node enlargement in the mesentery may cause steatorrhoea due to lymphatic obstruction. As in cases of malignant lymphoma, tonsillar enlargement may be a presenting symptom, and the finding of tonsillar enlargement with repeated attacks of local infection in an elderly patient should raise the possibility of CLL.

The characterstic feature is the raised lymphocyte count. In early cases values of about 5×10^9 per litre are quite common, the average count is about 100×10^9 per litre but counts of $100–200 \times 10^9$ per litre occur in about one-third and higher counts are rare. In this condition the lymphocytes are very readily damaged in the preparation of smears, and so-called 'smear' cells are very frequently seen.

Patients with acute leukaemia often have enlargement of the superficial lymph nodes, being more common in the lymphoblastic type (80%) than the myeloblastic (10–60%). Children with acute myeloid leukaemia are more likely to exhibit lymphadenopathy than adults. Monocytic leukaemia may be associated with mild enlargement of the cervical lymph nodes.

Angioimmunoblastic lymphadenopathy (AILD) is an uncommon lympho-proliferative disorder. The frequency with which patients have been taking drugs before the onset of AILD and the development of different types of rash suggest that the patient may be allergic to an undefined antigen but the disease may truly be at the interface between a benign reactive condition and a neoplasm, since progression to lymphoma occurs in a minority of cases. Histologically an involved node has three main characteristics: (1) the node is enlarged and the normal structure is effaced, and there is a pleomorphic cellular infiltrate comprising immunoblasts and plasma cells, polymorph neutrophils and histiocytes; (2) there is considerable proliferation of arborizing small blood vessels, characterized as post-capillary venules, with PAS-positive thickened walls; and (3) there is a deposit of amorphous interstitial material possibly derived from cellular debris associated with rapid cell turnover in the node. The absence of Sternberg–Reed cells and the presence of the 'immunoreactive cell' proliferation distinguish the histo-logical picture from that of Hodgkin's disease. Lymphocyte populations and their respective functions have been studied and, although no firm conclusions have yet been reached a suggested production of a B-cell stimulatory factor by T-cells could explain the B-cell hyper-reactivity and autoimmune phenomenon. Suppression of mitogen-induced proliferation and IgG production could explain the predisposition to infection noted in these patients.[10]

Clinically the patients present with an acute or subacute illness characterized by fever, sweating, weight loss, generalized lymphadenopathy and hepatosplenomegaly. A history of drug ingestion is frequent and about one-third have non-specific rashes. The majority of patients have a polyclonal hypergammaglobulinaemia involving especially IgM, a feature in marked contradistinction to the usually normal or depressed immuno-globulin levels in straightforward malignant lymphomas. A cryoglobulin is occasionally present. About half the patients have haemolysis with a positive direct antiglobulin test. The clinical course of the AILD after diagnosis is very variable. About two-thirds of patients have a progressive disease and die eventually from malignant transformation or infectious complications. In the remainder the disease may spontaneously regress or respond to chemotherapy. No special features are recognized that will predict whether a patient will or will not respond and the management of AILD will be guided largely by the clinical response until valid monitors of disease are available.[11]

In 1939 Scott & Robb-Smith[60] introduced the term 'histiocytic medullary reticulosis' to describe a condition characterized by fever, wasting, general-ized lymphadenopathy, hepatosplenomegaly and often jaundice. There was widespread infiltration of tissues by cells resembling 'histiocytes' which were capable of phagocytosing erythrocytes. A characteristic mode of lymph node infiltration suggested the term 'medullary'. In 1966 Rappaport[61] and colleagues introduced the term 'malignant histiocytosis' to describe a disorder involving 'systemic progressive invasion of morphologically atypical histiocytes and their precursors'. He considered the condition synonymous with histiocytic medullary reticulosis.

As in the lymphomas, the aetiology of the condition is unknown. Histopathologically a biopsied lymph node shows replacement of normal architecture to a varying degree by an infiltrate of pleomorphic mononuclear cells that may vary in appearance from that of a typical 'blast cell' with rounded nucleus, dispersed nuclear chromatin and meagre cytoplasm to a large cell with abundant non-pyroninophilic cytoplasm containing phago-cytosed nuclear debris and occasionally ingested erythrocytes. Rarely ingested erythroblasts, polymorphs or platelets are visible in the cytoplasm. The same cell may be present in the bone marrow and at times in the peripheral blood. Cytochemically these cells show positive reactions for naphthol-AS acetate esterase, lysozyme and acid phosphatase, and thereby show features of a true histiocyte.[12]

Clinically the disease is dominated by systemic features. The patient has fever, anorexia, weight loss and sweats when first seen. Examination reveals generalized lymphadenopathy and hepatosplenomegaly. The patient may be anaemic, neutropenic and thrombocytopenic. The serum lysozyme is often raised and the serum cholesterol low. Marrow aspirates show variable infiltration with scattered histiocytes of varying maturity or histiocytic cells gathered into foci. It is the sustained fever and generalized nature of the disease at diagnosis that allows it to be differentiated from the histiocytic ('true' histiocytic) type of malignant lymphoma.

Peripheral lymph nodes may be involved late in the course of mycosis fungoides, and this usually indicates clinical acceleration of the disease, occasionally associated with the leukaemic phase, Sezary syndrome. Enlarged peripheral lymph nodes are also found in Waldenstrom's macroglobulinaemia. The disease should be considered when this finding is associated with hepatosplenomegaly and retinal abnormalities.

Some special conditions

Although the virus responsible for the acquired immunodeficiency syndrome (AIDS) has been identified – human immunodeficiency virus 1 (HIV-1) – patients are characterized as having AIDS on the basis of the opportunistic infections and neoplasia they develop. This definition of AIDS is both stringent and restrictive and fails to include a wide range of clinical conditions and abnormalities that appear to be associated with AIDS but that do not fulfil the diagnostic criteria. These associated conditions are now termed AIDS-related complex (ARC). The clinical features of ARC include prolonged generalized often-painful unexplained lymphadenopathy, fever, oral candida, herpes zoster, unexplained weight loss, night sweats and constitutional symptoms such as malaise, fatigue and myalgia.[13,14] Laboratory abnormalities in ARC are similar to those in AIDS, particularly an absolute lymphopenia, leucopenia, thrombocytopenia and cellular immuno-logic abnormalities. ARC occurs in the same risk groups as AIDS, specifically homosexually active men, haemophiliacs, Haitian immigrants, intravenous drug abusers, female sexual partners of AIDS patients, children of high-risk parents, prostitutes and prisoners. A sub-set of ARC patients have persistent generalized lymphadenopathy, which describes patients with lymphadenopathy (nodes >1 cm) of at least 3 months' duration involving 2 or more extra-inguinal sites confirmed on physical examination (in the absence of any illness or drugs known to cause lymphadenopathy) and the presence of reactive hyperplasia in a lymph node, if a biopsy is done. Primary care physicians are likely to see more patients with the acute non-specific viral syndrome occurring 2–4 weeks after infection with HIV-1. There may be generalized lymphadenopathy associated with fever, malaise, rash and arthralgias followed in 1–3 months by seroconversion.

The histological appearances of the lymph nodes in patients with ARC have recently received much attention. The initial lymphadenopathy in the prodromal stage is associated with intense follicular hyperplasia. Clinical deterioration with 'B' symptoms such as fever, weight loss, night sweats and diarrhoea is associated with development histologically of follicular involution and a reduction in the lymphadenopathy. Some workers have referred to this as lymph node 'burn-out'. Cachexia and weight loss are the cardinal symptoms and signs of the progression of ARC to AIDS.

Clinical management of lymphadenopathy in high-risk individuals is still a controversial matter. Lymph nodes in these patients may wax and wane in size and a thorough evaluation for intercurrent illness associated with lymphadenopathy, such as viral (cytomegalovirus and Epstein–Barr virus) mononucleosis, toxoplasmosis, etc., should be performed. Which lymph nodes should be biopsied, how many should be biopsied, and how frequently should biopsies be repeated are unanswered questions. Patients with AIDS are at risk from Kaposi's sarcoma and non-Hodgkin's lymphomas. Every investigator who has cared for a large number of such patients can attest to the infrequent occurrence of Kaposi's sarcoma or lymphoma serendipitously discovered by lymph-node biopsy in an otherwise asymptomatic individual.

The hydantoin group of drugs, especially diphenylhydantoin used in the prevention of epilepsy, occasionally produce in patients an apparently allergic reaction. The cervical nodes are commonly enlarged, other groups less so, and other features include fever, rash, conjunctivitis, eosinophilia, and often splenomegaly.[15] Lymph node biopsy may be carried out and shows an enlarged node usually with follicular hyperplasia and an inflammatory cell infiltrate comprising immunoblasts, plasma cells, polymorph neutrophils and particularly eosinophils. There may be atypical or binucleate histiocytes but classical Sternberg–Reed cells are lacking. There is a high mitotic rate and the histological picture closely resembles angio-immunoblastic lymphadenopathy. When treatment with hydantoin drugs is discontinued, the lymphadenopathy and other features subside after some weeks. The condition is regarded as benign and sometimes designated pseudolymphoma. Reactions may occur with other drugs, among them para-aminosalicylic acid, phenylbutazone and carbamazepine. Similar appearances may occur in serum sickness, the allergic reaction appearing 7–12 days after administration of a foreign serum or certain drugs, e.g. penicillins. There may be fever, arthralgias, skin rash and lymphadenopathy.

The association of the hydantoins with lymphadenopathy is complicated by the fact that patients have been described in whom the apparent pseudolymphoma fails to regress after stopping the drug but rather progresses in a malignant fashion and terminates in the death of the patient.[16] In other cases the pseudolymphoma has regressed but then recrudesces without further exposure to hydantoins.[17] The histological picture in these cases of apparently of true lymphoma has been both that of HD and NHL.[18] Whether or not the hydantoin drug has directly caused the lymphoma remains uncertain but the association is seen more often than would be expected by chance.

Patients with marked splenomegaly, occasionally lymph node enlargement, eosinophilic leucocytosis, and progressive cardiac disease have been described. Diagnostic features of leukaemia were not present, and death resulted from cardiac failure.[19]

Miscellaneous conditions

Autoimmune disorders may be associated with lymphadenopathy of a minor degree, but in some children massive lymphadenopathy may occur, and the extent of this often parallels the severity of the haemolytic process.[20] In some cases the histological appearances may mimic that of malignant lymphoma.

Generalized lymph node enlargement is common in rheumatoid arthritis and systemic lupus erythematosus. The constitutional symptoms of the collagen–vascular disorders, together with lymph node and/or splenic enlargement, and various cytopenias, such as occurs in Felty's syndrome, can make distinction from malignant lymphoma difficult in some cases. The histological picture of the lymph nodes in rheumatoid arthritis may closely mimic that seen in follicular lymphomas.

Generalized lymphatic hyperplasia may accompany certain endocrine disorders, particularly hyperthyroidism. In this disorder the lymph node enlargement and symptoms of hypermetabolism can be confused with lymphoma. Lymphadenopathy occasionally occurs in hypoadrenalism and hypopituitarism.

Patients with rashes often develop enlarged superficial lymph nodes corresponding to the areas of drainage of affected skin. When the rash is widespread, as in exfoliative dermatitis, the lymphadenopathy is generalized. The lymphadenopathy which occurs is independent of any skin infection, and eczema and psoriasis are the commonest associated diseases. On biopsy these nodes are of normal architecture but show widening of the cortex due to proliferation of macrophages, some containing intracytoplasmic fat (foam cells) and some melanin. There are increased numbers of eosinophils, plasma cells and immunoblasts.[21] The lymph node enlargement regresses with improvement of the dermatitis.[22] Some patients may subsequently be found to have malignant lymphoma.[23]

Sarcoidosis, a disease of undetermined causation characterized by the presence in all affected tissues of epithelioid cell tubercles without granulation, may produce superficial lymph node enlargement in about 70% of American patients, but only about half that number in European cases. This is due to the different pattern of the disease in the North American negro. The cervical (70%), the axillary (40%) and the epitrochlear (20%)

groups are most commonly affected. Individual nodes seldom exceed 3–4 cm in diameter; there is no tenderness, fluctuation, nor periadenitis and they share the tendency to spontaneous remission. The commonest presentation of sarcoidosis is bilateral hilar lymphadenopathy found on routine chest radiography.

Massive lymph node enlargement, predominantly in the cervical region but often generalized, has been described in infants, children and young adults with a unique entity, sinus histiocytosis of the lymph nodes.[24] Splenomegaly is absent but fever and leucocytosis may occur. The disorder is benign but node enlargement may persist for months or years.

The sea-blue histiocyte syndrome may present infrequently with enlarged lymph nodes. Other well-defined clinicopathological entities are angio-follicular lymph node hyperplasia (Castlemann's disease) and sinus histiocytosis with massive lymphadenopathy (Rosai–Dorfman disease).

The principal causes of lymphadenopathy are summarized in Table 13.1.

LABORATORY INVESTIGATION OF LYMPHADENOPATHY

The main question in the clinician's mind when confronted by lymphadeno-pathy is 'reactive or malignant?' Laboratory tests can, in a number of situations, reassure the doctor and patient that an alarming lymph node enlargement is benign in nature, usually infective. The converse, of course, is that negative investigations do not necessarily reassure. Several patho-logical specialties often provide laboratory input for any particular patient, and the following descriptions of laboratory tests are not designed to define what is necessary, but only to indicate what tests might be available for use, clinical information selecting those tests deemed useful.

Haematological

The blood count parameters are the most commonly requested tests but provide little specific information. Both reactive conditions, such as infections or inflammatory disorders, and neoplasia may cause cytopenias. For instance, in Hodgkin's disease anaemia may be due to bone marrow involvement by tumour, hypersplenism, autoimmune haemolytic anaemia, ineffective erythropoiesis or expansion of the plasma volume. The mean corpuscular volume, if raised, could point to folate deficiency arising due to anorexia and malnourishment, bone marrow involvement, or equally well a reticulocytosis, as occurs in immune haemolytic anaemias.

More information may be gleaned from the peripheral blood film. Here, the morphological changes that accompany viral infections, leukaemias or lymphomas may be demonstrated. The typical Downey lymphocytes of infectious mononucleosis are present within a leucocytosis of $10–20 \times 10^9$ per litre, and very exceptionally counts as high as 60×10^9 per litre occur. There is almost invariably a neutropenia from the onset unless there has been some complication such as bacterial infection or splenic rupture. Confirmation of the diagnosis is by the Paul–Bunnell test or the 'Monospot' test. These serological tests are often negative in the first week but become

Table 13.1 Causes of Lymphadenopathy

Malignant
  Haematological
  Acute leukaemia
  CLL
  CGL (rarely)
  Lymphoma
  Angioimmunoblastic lymphadenopathy
  Reactive hyperplasia
  Angiofollicular hyperplasia

Carcinoma
  Non-haematological
  Lung
  Stomach
  Head and neck
  Breast
  Kidney

Infections
  (A) Bacterial
    Streptococcal
    Staphylococcal
    Salmonella
    Tuberculosis
    Brucellosis
    Syphilis
  (B) Non-bacterial
    Cytomeglovirus
    Toxoplasmosis
    Infectious mononucleosis
    Human immunodeficiency virus (HIV)
    Rubella
    Histoplasmosis
    Coccidiomycosis
    Malaria

Connective tissue disorders
  Rheumatoid arthritis
  Dermatomyositis
  SLE

Drug-induced
  Serum sickness
  Hydantoin therapy

Sarcoidosis

Lipid storage
  Nieman–Pick disease
  Gaucher's disease

---

positive after this time and remain so for several months. Young children under the age of 5 years may not develop a positive test, but other tests for specific IgM antibody against the Epstein–Barr virus point to the correct diagnosis. A differential diagnosis of 'Monospot-negative glandular fever cells' include toxoplasmosis and cytomegalovirus for which complement fixation tests are available.

The erythrocyte sedimentation rate (ESR) is a non-specific indicator of disease activity. It has little use for diagnostic purposes, although the ESR would be expected to fall with resolution of the disease process. It is commonly used in the treatment of Hodgkin's disease and the lymphomas to demonstrate satisfactory response to therapy and, in those patients in remission, an early indicator of possible relapse.

Bone marrow aspiration may produce diagnostic material. Visceral leishmaniasis (Kala-azar) is likely to be clinically diagnosed by the history of travel to an area endemic for the protozoa of the genus *Leishmania*, together with a febrile, prostrate patient with progressive hepatosplenomegaly. However, occasionally the disease produces prominent generalized lymph node enlargement, particularly in certain areas, such as the Sudan. The diagnosis depends upon identification of the parasite which can usually be easily found in material withdrawn from bone marrow, spleen or liver, or in the peripheral blood. Although infectious mononucleosis produces florid blood changes, bone marrow examination is unrewarding. An aspirate in Hodgkin's disease is usually normal although an eosinophilia may be noted. The trephine biopsy produces useful information only rarely in HD and recent advice has been to withdraw bone marrow examination as a staging procedure on the grounds that it does not significantly affect survival. However, the bone marrow is often involved in non-Hodgkin's lymphoma, 40% by morphological criteria in follicular lymphoma[25,26] although more by immunological methods.[27,28]

Biochemical

Patients with Hodgkin's disease may have hypercalcaemia and elevated serum alkaline phosphatase levels indicative of bone and liver disease respectively.[29–32] Hypoalbuminaemia and increased α_2-, β- and γ-globulins occur in patients with active Hodgkin's disease and other lymphomas.[33] A low plasma zinc and elevated serum copper levels have been reported.[34] Serum acid phosphatase levels have been reported in some patients with malignant histiocytosis.[35] An elevation of this serum enzyme is a consistent feature of Gaucher's disease.[36] Serum lactic dehydrogenase levels are now recognized as one of the more important prognostic factors in high-grade NHL since high levels indicate a rapid rate of tumour cell proliferation and death and are also associated with involvement of the bone marrow, liver, gastrointestinal tract, pleura/lung and central nervous system.[37,38] Abnormal liver function tests are a major poor prognostic factor in patients with follicular lymphoma.[26]

Immunological

Monoclonal immunoglobulin components are found frequently in patients with lymphomas of all types and in patients with chronic lymphocytic leukaemia.[39] Polyclonal hypergammaglobulinaemia occurs in angio-immunoblastic lymphadenopathy and the acquired immunodeficiency syndrome. Immune paresis is common in CLL, either early in the course of the disease or later, as marrow, spleen and liver infiltration develop.[40] Immunological surface phenotyping of circulating lymphoid cells have revealed malignant B-lymphocytes in some patients with apparently localized high-grade NHL.[28] The relevance of the presence of these cells in terms of relapse-free survival remains to be determined.

There is generally a decrease in the number of OKT4/Leu3 ('helper/inducer') T-lymphocytes in the peripheral blood with a variable decrease in the OKT8/Leu4 ('suppressor/cytotoxic') T-lymphocytes in patients in the later stages of infection with the HIV-1.[16] However, a number of viral disorders will also produce a similar inversion of ratio and this is far from specific for AIDS. Patients with ARC also have a T-cell sub-set imbalance but tend to have ratios greater than 0.5.

Serological

A serological test for syphilis should be performed. If a non-treponemal test is used (VDRL, rapid plasma reagin test) a false-positive result may occur. Confirmation of syphilis should be by a treponemal test (fluorescent treponemal antibody absorption test, treponemal passive haemagglutination test, *T. pallidum* immobilization test). Toxoplasmosis can be detected by either the complement fixation test or by the toxoplasma dye test.

It has recently been recognized that a number of patients in whom lymph node biopsy produces the report of reactive hyperplasia may have rheumatoid arthritis.[41] Lymphadenopathy has been recognized as an early or presenting feature of this disorder.[42] A test for rheumatoid factor may be helpful.

Imaging techniques

All patients with lymphadenopathy should have a chest X-ray. This simple investigation may reveal primary tumour, tuberculosis or bilateral hilar lymphadenopathy typical of sarcoidosis. Mediastinal lymphadenopathy will be demonstrated in 40–50% of patients with Hodgkin's disease at presentation. This typically appears on the chest film as enlarged paratracheal nodes, in some cases associated with hilar lymphadenopathy. Involvement of the lung is present in less than 10% of patients at diagnosis, the most usual form being direct extension out from enlarged hilar nodes. However, miliary mottling, opacities, cavitating lesions or pleural plaques may occur.[43]

Imaging techniques are used extensively in the staging of lymphomas and the following approach has proved useful:[44,45]

1. Sites that are frequently involved with lymphoma should be screened routinely if the imaging test is sufficiently accurate. The choice of technique also depends on local expertise, patient acceptability and the clinician's preference. For example, retroperitoneal lymph nodes which are involved frequently in both HD AND NHL are evaluated readily by computed tomography (CT) or lymphography, either of which may, therefore, be used routinely.
2. Sites involved infrequently (e.g. gastrointestinal tract) are not screened routinely but specific investigations are performed in cases where signs or symptoms suggest involvement.
3. Although some sites are frequently involved (e.g. liver and spleen), available tests such as ultrasound, CT and radionuclides are insensitive and non-specific. In these sites the rigour with which involvement is sought will depend on the degree to which involvement will influence management.

CT has certain advantages over lymphography; it is non-invasive and becoming more widely available; it is safe whereas both mortality and morbidity have been associated with lymphography;[46] mesenteric nodes can be visualized with CT.

Ultrasound, like CT, has the ability to show lymph node enlargement in the region of the coeliac axis, at the splenic hilum;, in the mesentery and at the porta hepatis.[47,48] However, bowel gas may cause obstruction to full imaging of the retroperitoneum and there may be degradation of image resolution by retroperitoneal fat. The role of ultrasound has largely been superseded by CT.

Radionuclides are not routinely used for staging of lymphoma, but can be of value in certain circumstances. Bone scanning with Tc-labelled methylene diphosphonate is more sensitive but less specific than X-rays, and gallium citrate does not specifically identify neoplastic tissue but is taken up also by inflamed tissues and certain normal organs.[49] Nuclear magnetic resonance imaging is still under evaluation for lymphoma staging, and is not widely available.

Histological investigations

When lymph node material is obtained the local circumstances will decide how to investigate the tissue further. The tissue is usually fixed in formalin, but recent developments, particularly with immunological techniques, have dictated that a portion of the node should be sent to the laboratory in a dry container for frozen sections to be made. Some may be placed in glutaraldehyde to fix for resin-embedded sections to be made or for material for electron microscopy.

The field of histological investigation by monoclonal antibodies is too large to enter here, but the diagnosis of lymphoma has been helped by these techniques, the use of which is discussed by Mason & Gatter.[50]

Surgical biopsy

Lymph node biopsies should be performed early rather than late. Certainly an enlarged node should be biopsied within 4 weeks of presentation. Inguinal nodes are the least satisfactory for histological examination; chronic hyperplasia of these nodes is not uncommon, and the classic histological features of malignant disease are often obscured by secondary infection and scarring.

If a lymph node biopsy is to be performed a practical point is to consider whether the probable diagnosis is likely to require a bone marrow aspirate or trephine as these could be arranged during the same anaesthetic.

A lymph node imprint can be easily made at operation by sectioning the node and dabbing its cut surface onto a clean glass slide. Diagnostic information may become available later the same day, whereas histological processing takes 24 h or more.

An alternative to surgical biopsy is needle aspiration of a lymph node. Material may be obtained for cytological analysis.

CLINICAL APPROACH TO THE PATIENT WITH LYMPHADENOPATHY

The age of the patient is of major importance due to the greater reactivity of lymphoid tissue to stimuli in the young. Lymphadenopathy detected beyond the fourth decade usually represents tumour[51] and there is evidence that the probability of malignancy in enlarged peripheral lymph nodes increases steadily with age from late adolescence through to adulthood.[52] Lymphadenopathy in a young child usually represents a bacterial or viral infection, or a developmental anomaly.[53]

The clinical approach to lymphadenopathy should encompass these points:

(a) The areas drained by the involved lymph nodes should be searched for possible primary source of infection or malignant disease.
(b) Other lymph node areas should be examined; if other enlarged nodes are found, then the condition must be part of some generalized lymphadenopathy.
(c) The liver and spleen must be carefully palpated.
(d) The size, tenderness, consistency and mobility of the glands should be noted.

In many instances the cause of the lymphadenopathy will have become obvious. The primary care physician may elucidate the diagnosis further by recourse to certain laboratory investigations:

1. Blood film examination may clinch the diagnosis of infectious mononucleosis or leukaemia. The laboratory will often instigate serological investigations for infectious mononucleosis.
2. Chest X-ray may show evidence of enlarged mediastinal nodes or may reveal a primary occult tumour of the lung, which is the source of disseminated deposits, or may demonstrate the bilateral hilar lymphadenopathy.

3. Serological investigations for syphilis can be undertaken.

Following these investigations the patient should be referred for further investigation. If the lymphadenopathy is tender and an infectious origin is suspected a course of antibiotics may be given, although this should not unduly delay referral. Hodgkin's disease may appear to respond initially to antibiotics, with recurrence a few weeks later.

On referral the physician must decide the urgency of investigation, particularly with respect to surgical biopsy. The necessity for considering the investigations in each particular case was exemplified by the paper of Slap *et al.*[54] They investigated the records and histopathology slides of 123 9–25 year old patients who underwent biopsies of enlarged peripheral lymph nodes. They reviewed the pathological diagnosis and 22 clinical findings. Seventy-two (58%) of patients had biopsy results that did not lead to treatment and 51 (42%) had results that did lead to treatment. By the use of step-wise discriminant analysis, a predictive model was developed that assigned 95% of the cases to the correct biopsy group based on lymph node size; history of recent ear, nose and throat symptoms; and chest X-ray. When this model was tested prospectively on new patients it correctly classified 32 (97%) of 33 patients. The authors point out that this model could be used to check the decision to withhold or proceed to biopsy but should not replace clinical judgement. Of the three variables that made up the function the chest X-ray was found to have the greatest impact on the discriminant score. The strong association between an abnormal chest X-ray and granulomatous or malignant peripheral lymphadenopathy is well-supported in both the paediatric and adult medical literature.[53,55–58] Knight *et al.*[58] found that 78% of children with abnormal chest X-rays had cancer or granulomata on peripheral node biopsy, compared with 18% of children with no X-ray abnormality. Zuelzer & Kaplan[53] noted that enlarged mediastinal nodes in children rarely were caused by common bacterial or viral infections. Salzstein[56] found that 79% of adults with abnormal chest X-rays and non-diagnostic lymph node biopsies subsequently were found to have malignant or granulomatous disease.

More recently Kelly & Malcolm[41] have reviewed 72 patients in whom a diagnosis of reactive hyperplasia had been made at lymph node biopsy. Interestingly, at the end of a mean period of 4.5 years (range 2–10), 18 patients (25%) still had lymphadenopathy for which no cause was apparent. Spontaneous remission had occurred in seven patients. The other 54 patients had developed conditions very likely related to their lymph node hyperplasia. Of these, 41 patients had previous evidence of disease but the relationship had been sufficiently uncertain to justify biopsy. Thirteen subsequently developed new symptoms within 6 months of the biopsy, allowing a firm diagnosis to be made. No patient developed an associated condition later than 6 months after biopsy. The diagnostic categories of the related conditions were rheumatic (22%), neoplastic (21%) infective (14%) and a group of other disorders (18%) such as cystic mastopathy, dermatitis and thrombophlebitis. Lymphoma accounted for only three cases in this study.

The series of Rocchi *et al.*[59] selected 140 patients out of 348 cases referred for evaluation of lymphadenopathy seen over a 2-year period. These represented the non-neoplastic cases (40%) followed over 3 years. A high proportion of Epstein–Barr virus (EBV) infection (27 cases, 19%) and toxoplasma infection (20 cases, 14%) was found, and tuberculous lympha-denopathy was diagnosed in 14 cases (10%). However, for 65 patients (46%) no aetiological diagnosis could be established. Spontaneous regression of the lymphadenopathy occurred within 2–4 weeks and a 6 month follow-up confirmed that the disease was non-neoplastic. Lymph node biopsies were carried out in 30 of these 65 patients and showed either a reactive hyperplasia or normal histological appearance. The effect of age was noted; the ability to make a diagnosis in those aged above 30 years (29/37=78%) was greater than in those younger individuals (44/103=45%) ($P<0.005$). Serological investigations enabled early diagnosis of EBV and toxoplasma infection obviating the necessity for lymph node biopsy. However, the laboratory investigations based upon serological examination of lymph node biopsies failed to identify the cause of lymphadenopathy in approximately one-half of cases. But lymph node material was not cultured for bacteria, mycoplasma or viruses, nor were tests for fungal infections performed in these patients. Therefore, one cannot exclude the fact that laboratory studies in greater depth, including clinical immunological tests, would have enhanced the possibility of identifying other causes in this study.

There is no one feature or combination of features that will single out all patients requiring urgent biopsy without subjecting some patients to unnecessary biopsy. However, certain points should alert the physician:

(a) Most commonly the rate of growth of the gland, the texture to palpation and the site or sites of involvement may indicate the aetiology.

(b) Association with weight loss, night sweats, fevers or pruritus strongly suggests malignant haematological disease. However, tuberculosis should be considered, whilst AIDS will be an increasingly frequent diagnosis.

(c) The older the patient the more likely the association with malignant disease. This reflects the reduced capacity of aged lymphoid tissue for inflammatory response. Childhood lymphadenopathy is frequently inflammatory in aetiology.

(d) A drug history may reveal hydantoin therapy, recent vaccination or methyl DOPA/penicillin therapy (AILD).

(e) Foreign travel may indicate an exotic pathology.

(f) Recent upper respiratory tract infections may be associated with cervical lymphadenopathy. However, this should rapidly regress in a few days, although those due to infectious mononucleosis may persist. A serological test for IM should be performed.

(g) An abnormal chest X-ray often indicates a granulomatous or malignant pathology.

(h) Examination of the blood film may be diagnostic.

(i) Lymph node aspiration may lead to an early diagnosis.

(j) The emergence of AIDS has caused the medical practitioner to examine the possibility of this disease in all patients with lymphadenopathy. An enquiry into the sexual practices of the patient may not be reasonable at the first visit, but unexplained lymphadenopathy in a young, sexually-active patient should prompt discrete enquiries into the possibility of ARC/AIDS prior to invasive biopsy procedures. At the time of writing HIV-testing requires the patient's fully-informed consent.

REFERENCES

1. Rosenberg, S.A. & Kaplan, H.S. Evidence for an orderly progression in the spread of Hodgkin's disease. *Cancer Res.* **26**: 1225–31, 1966.
2. Han, T. & Stutzman, L. Mode of spread in patients with localised malignant lymphoma. *Arch. Intern. Med.* **120**: 1–7, 1967.
3. Banfi, A., Bonnadonna, G., Carnevarli, G., Oldini, C. & Salvini, E. Preferential sites of involvement and spread in malignant lymphomas. *Eur. J. Cancer* **4**: 319–24, 1968.
4. Landberg, T. Clinical course of Hodgkin's disease treated with radiotherapy. *Acta Radiol. (Ther.) (Stockholm)* **8**: 487–504, 1969.
5. Smithers, D.W. Spread of Hodgkin's disease. *Lancet* **i**: 1262–7, 1970.
6. Ultmann, J.E. & Moran, E.M. Clinical course and complication in Hodgkins disease. *Arch. Intern. Med.* **131**: 311–53 (341 refs), 1973.
7. Ultmann, J.E., Cunningham, J.K. & Gellhorn, A. The clinical picture of Hodgkin's disease. *Cancer Res.* **26**: 1047–62, 1966.
8. Peckham, M.J., Guay, J.P., Hamlin, I.M.E. & Lukes, R.J. Survival in localised nodal and extranodal non-Hodgkin's lymphomata. *Br. J. Cancer* **31**, Suppl. 2: 413–24, 1975.
9. Worthy, T.S. Evaluation of diagnostic laparotomy and splenectomy in Hodgkin's disease. *Clin. Radiol.* **32**: 523–6, 1981.
10. Honda, M., Smith, H.R. & Steinberg, A.D. Studies on the pathogenesis of Angioimmunoblastic Lymphadenopathy. *J. Clin. Invest.* **76**: 332–40, 1985.
11. Coupland, R.W., Pontifex, A.H. & Salinas, F.A. Angioimmunoblastic lymphadenopathy with dysproteinaemia: Circulating immune complexes and the review of 18 cases. *Cancer* **55**: 1902–6, 1985.
12. Huhn, D. & Meister, P. Malignant histiocytosis: morphologic and cytochemical findings. *Cancer* **42**: 1341–9, 1978.
13. Centers for Disease Control. Diffuse, undifferentiated non-Hodgkins lymphoma among homosexual males – United States. *Morbidity Mortality Weekly Rep.* **31**: 277–9, 1982.
14. Gottlieb, M.S., Groopman, J.E., Weinstein, W.M., Fahey, J.L. & Detels, R. The acquired immunodeficiency syndrome. *Ann. Intern. Med.* **99**: 208–20, 1983.
15. Siegal, S. & Berkowitz, J. Diphenyldantoin (Dilantin) hypersensitivity with infectious mononucleosis-like syndrome and jaundice. *J. Allergy* **32**: 447–51, 1961.
16. Eyster, E.E., Goedbert, J.J., Poon, M.-C. & Preble, O.T. Acid-labile alpha interferon. A possible marker for the acquired immunodeficiency syndrome in haemophilia. *N. Engl. J. Med.* **309**: 583, 1983.
17. Gams, R.A., Neal, J.A. & Conrad, F.G. Hydantoin-induced pseudolymphoma. *Ann. Intern. Med.* **69**: 557–68, 1968.
18. Hyman, G.A. & Sommers, S.C. Development of Hodgkin's disease and lymphoma during anticonvulsant therapy. *Blood* **28**: 416–27, 1966.
19. Sheperd, A.J.N., Walsh, C.H., Archer, R.K. & Wetherly-Mein, G. Eosinophilia, splenomegaly and cardiac disease. *Br. J. Haematol.* **20**: 233–9, 1971.
20. Zuelzer, W.W., Mastrangelo, R., Stulberg, C.S., Polik, M.O., Page, R.H. & Thompson, R.I. Autoimmune hemolytic anaemia: Natural history and viral-immunologic interactions in childhood. *Am. J. Med.* **49**: 80–93, 1970.
21. Dorfman, R.F. & Warnke, R. Lymphadenopathy simulating the malignant lymphomas. *Human Pathol.* **5**: 519–50 (81 refs), 1974.
22. Nairn, R.C. & Anderson, T.E. Erythrodermia with lipomelanotic reticulum-cell hyperplasia of lymph nodes (dermatopathic lymphadenitis). *Br. Med. J.* **i**: 820–4, 1955.
23. Block, J.B., Edgcomb, J., Eisen, A. & Van Scott, E.J. Mycosis fungoides: Natural history and aspects of its relationship to other malignant lymphomas. *Am. J. Med.* **34**: 228–35, 1963.

24. Rosai, J. & Dorfman, R.F. Sinus histiocytosis with massive lymphadenopathy. A newly recognised benign clinicopathological entity. *Arch. Pathol.* **87**: 63–70, 1969.
25. Chabner, B.A., Johnson, R.E., Young, R.C., Canellos, G.P., Hubbard, S.P., Johnson, S.K. & DeVita, V.T. Sequential surgical and non-surgical staging on non-Hodgkin's lymphoma. *Ann. Intern. Med.* **85**: 149–56, 1976.
26. Gallagher, C.J., Gregory, W.M., Jones, A.E., Stansfeld, A.G., Richards, M.A., Dhaliwal, H.S., Malpas, J.S. & Lister, T.A. Follicular lymphoma. Prognostic factors for response and survival. *J. Clin. Oncol.* **4**: 1470–80, 1986.
27. Ault, K.A. Detection of small numbers of monoclonal B lymphocytes in the blood of patients with lymphoma. *N. Engl. J. Med.* **300**: 1401–5, 1979.
28. Smith, B.R., Weinberg, D.S., Robert, N.J., Towle, M., Luther, E., Pinkus, G.S. & Ault, K.A. Circulating monoclonal B lymphocytes in non-Hodgkins lymphoma. *N. Engl. J. Med.* **311**: 1476–81, 1984.
29. Kabakow, B., Mine, M.F. & King, F.H. Hypercalcaemia in Hodgkin's disease. *N. Engl. J. Med.* **256**: 59–62, 1957.
30. Aisenberg, A.C., Kaplan, M.M., Rieder, S.V. & Goldman, J.M. Serum alkaline phosphatase at the onset of Hodgkin's disease. *Cancer* **26**: 318–26, 1970.
31. Belliveau, R.E., Weirnik, P.H. & Abt, A.B. Liver enzymes and pathology in Hodgkin's disease. *Cancer* **34**: 300–5, 1974.
32. Johnson, R.E., Thomas, L.B., Johnson, S.K. & Johnston, G.S. Correlation between abnormal baseline liver tests and long-term clinical course in Hodgkins disease. *Cancer* **33**: 1123–6, 1974.
33. Arends, T., Coonrad, E.V. & Rundles, W. Serum proteins in Hodgkin's disease and malignant lymphoma. *Am. J. Med.* **16**: 833–41, 1954.
34. Hrgovic, M., Tessmer, C.F., Minckler, T.M., Mosier, B. & Taylor, G.H. Serum copper levels in lymphoma and leukaemia: Special reference to Hodgkin's disease. *Cancer* **21**: 743–55, 1968.
35. White, D.R., Bannayan, G.A., George, J.N. & Sears, D.A. Histiocytic medullary reticulosis with parallel increases in serum acid phosphatase and disease activity. *Cancer* **37**: 1403–11, 1976.
36. Tuchman, L.R., Suna, H. & Carr, J.J. Elevation of serum acid phosphatase in Gaucher's disease. *J. Mt Sinai Hosp.* **23**: 227–9, 1956.
37. Blatt, J., Reaman, G. & Poplack, D.G. Biochemical markers in lymphoid malignancy. *N. Engl. J. Med.* **303**: 918–22, 1980.
38. Koziner, B., Little, C., Passe, S., Thaler, H.T., Sklaroff, R., Strauss, D.J., Lee, B.J. & Clarkson, B.D. Treatment of advanced histiocytic lymphoma: an analysis of prognostic variables. *Cancer* **49**: 1571–9, 1982.
39. Talerman, A. & Haije, W.G. The frequency of M-components in sera of patients with solid malignant neoplasms. *Br. J. Cancer* **27**: 276–82, 1973.
40. Rundles, R.W., Coonrad, E.V. & Arends, T. Serum proteins in leukaemia. *Am. J. Med.* **16**: 842–53, 1954.
41. Kelly, C.A. & Malcolm, A.J. The significance of hyperplastic lymphadenopathy. *Br. J. Hosp. Med.* **37**: 159–60, 1987.
42. Robertson, M.D.J., Dudley Hart, F., White, W.F., Nuki, G. & Boardman, B.L. Rheumatoid lymphadenopathy. *Ann. Rheum. Dis.* **27**: 253–60, 1968.
43. Peckham, M.J. The radiotherapy of Hodgkin's disease. *Br. J. Hosp. Med.* **9**: 457–68, 1973.
44. Castellino, R.L. & Marglin, S.I. Imaging of abdominal and pelvic lymph nodes: lymphography or CT? *Invest. Radiol.* **17**: 433–43, 1982.
45. Bonadonna, G. & Santoro, A. Clinical evolution and treatment of Hodgkin's disease. In *Neoplastic Diseases of the Blood* (eds P.H. Wiernik, G. Canellos, R.A. Kyle & C.A. Schiffer), p. 789. Churchill Livingstone, Edinburgh, 1985.
46. Craig, J.O.M.C. Lymphangiography. In *Textbook of Radiology* (ed. D. Sutton), p. 674. Churchill Livingstone, Edinburgh, 1975.
47. Sutcliffe, S.B.J., Timothy, A.R. & Lister, T.A. Staging in Hodgkin's disease. *Clin.*

Haèmatol. **8**(3): 593–609, 1979.
48. Carroll, B.A. Ultrasound of lymphoma. *Semin. Ultrasound* **III**(2): 144–22, 1982.
49. Turner, D.A., Fordham, E.W., Ali, A. & Slayton, R.E. Gallium-67 imaging in the management of Hodgkin's disease and other malignant lymphomas. *Semin. Nucl. Med.* **VIII**(3): 205–18, 1978.
50. Mason, C.Y. & Gatter, K.C. The role of immunocytochemistry in diagnostic pathology. *J. Clin. Pathol.* **40**: 1042–54, 1987.
51. Lee, J.G. & Helmus, C. Cervical lymph node biopsy. *Mich. Med.* **69**: 581–3, 1970.
52. Lee, Y., Terry, R. & Lukes, R.J. Lymph node biopsy for diagnosis: a statistical study. *J. Surg. Oncol.* **14**: 53–60, 1980.
53. Zuelzer, W.W. & Kaplan, J. The child with lymphadenopathy. *Semin. Haematol.* **12**: 323–34, 1975.
54. Slap, G.B., Brooks, J.S.J. & Schwartz, J.S. When to perform biopsies of enlarged peripheral nodes in young patients. *J. Am. Med. Assoc.* **252**: 1321–6, 1984.
55. Greenfield, S. & Jordan, C. The clinical investigation of lymphadenopathy in primary care practice. *J. Am. Med. Assoc.* **240**: 1388–93, 1978.
56. Salzstein, S.L. The fate of patients with non-diagnostic lymph node biopsies. *Surgery* **58**: 659–62, 1965.
57. Sinclair, S., Beckman, E. & Ellman, L. Biopsy of enlarged superficial lymph nodes. *J. Am. Med. Assoc.* **228**: 602–3, 1974.
58. Knight, P.J., Mulne, A.F. & Vassy, L.E. When is lymph node biopsy indicated in children with enlarged peripheral nodes? *Pediatrics* **69**: 391–6, 1982.
59. Rocchi, G., Volpi, A., Ragona, G., Papa, G., Tripaldi, F. & Mandelli, F. Acute enlargement of lymph nodes: diagnostic dilemma and the role of laboratory investigations. A study on 140 patients. *Haematologica* **70**: 414–18, 1985.
60. Scott, R.B. & Robb-Smith, A.H.T. Histiocytic medullary reticulosis. *Lancet* **ii**: 194–8, 1939.
61. Kindon, H.B., Baron, J.M., Byrne, G.E. & Rappaport, H. Malignant histiocytosis. *Ann. Intern. Med.* **72**: 705–9, 1970.

14

Splenomegaly

J.A. Liu Yin
Consultant Haematologist, Manchester Royal Infirmary, Manchester, UK

The association between enlargement of the spleen and disease had been recognized since Hippocratic times, particularly in Mediterranean countries where malaria was endemic. The spleen has for centuries fascinated and puzzled physicians and philosophers alike. Galen called it 'an organ of mystery' and attributed to it an essential role in the regulation of the psyche. It was only in the seventeenth and eighteenth centuries, with the advent of the microscope, that the structure of the spleen was described in some detail. Its physiological functions soon became recognized. An association with the lymphatic system and the role of the Malpighian follicles in the production of white blood cells were subsequently described. Indeed the important function of the spleen as an organ for filtering and destroying red blood cells was recognized more than a century ago. It thus became apparent that splenic enlargement frequently occurred in disorders of the haemopoietic system and that surgical removal of the spleen could in some cases result in cure. However, it is only recently that there has been a greater understanding of the functions of the spleen in health and disease and this has led to a rational approach to the investigation and management of splenic disorders.

STRUCTURE OF THE SPLEEN

The weight of the spleen varies with age. It is at its maximum at about 200–300 g soon after puberty and decreases to about 100–150 g after the age of 65 years. Based on findings from a large number of autopsies, the average weight of the adult spleen was found to be about 135 g.[1] Thus the weight of an apparently normal spleen can vary from 100 to 250 g. The normal adult spleen has a blood flow of 200–300 ml/min, which represents about 4–5% of the cardiac output. It contains about 140 billion cells, approximately half of which are capable of phagocytosis.[2,3]

The spleen has a complicated structure and is a highly vascular organ which contains specialized vascular channels, lymphatic tissue, lymph channels and cells of the haemopoietic and reticulo-endothelial (RE) systems. It has a thick fibrous capsule from which projects a network of trabeculae which provide a connective tissue scaffolding for the vascular channels within the splenic pulp. The trabeculae carry blood vessels, lymphatic channels and autonomic nerve fibres. The connective tissue of the capsule and trabeculae is made up predominantly of collagen and elastin fibres.

PARENCHYMA

Histologically the spleen can be divided into three parts: the white pulp, the red pulp and the marginal zone lying between the red and white pulp. The white pulp consists of lymphatic tissue organized around the arterial vessels in cylindrical sheaths and adjoining nodular structures which are the lymph follicles of Malpighi, consisting of germinal centres and surrounding mantle layers of small lymphocytes. These nodules consist mainly of B-cells, whereas the lymphocytes in the peri-arterial sheaths are predominantly T-cells. Within the white pulp, the branches from the central arteries take off at right-angles and this facilitates a skimming effect of leucocyte-rich plasma from the outer layer of blood.[4] The red pulp is a spongy compartment which contains two vascular channels, namely the sinuses and cords (Billroth). The sinuses are anastomosing elongated channels 20–40 μm in diameter, which are lined by longitudinally arranged flattened endothelial cells. These are held together by a fenestrated basement membrane which is part of the reticular framework supporting the pulp vessels. The cords, on the other hand, are spaces lined by reticular cells and lie between the sinuses from which they are separated by the basement membrane. They also contain numerous lymphocytes and macrophages.

BLOOD FLOW

The spleen has a unique vascular organization which brings blood from the systemic circulation into very close contact with lymphatic tissue and cells of the RE system. Within the spleen, the splenic artery divides into a series of trabecular and central arteries, giving rise to an arborising pattern of blood supply.[5] Some of the branches from the central arteries terminate in the white pulp while others end in the marginal zone and the red pulp. The arteries in the red pulp are devoid of lymphatic sheaths, muscular or adventitial coats and connect either directly with splenic sinuses or terminate as free endings in the splenic cords. The splenic sinuses drain into collecting and trabecular veins and thence into the splenic vein. The fenestrations of the basement membrane lining the vascular sinuses allow red cells to squeeze through inter-endothelial slits and cross from cords into adjacent sinuses. In addition, blood flow through the inter-endothelial slits is regulated by adventitial reticular cells which lie over the basal surface of the basement membrane.[6] The controversy regarding whether the circulation through the red pulp is 'open' or 'closed' has been largely resolved. The 'open' system refers to the passage of blood from the arterial capillaries through the cordal space before reaching the sinuses whereas in the 'closed' system, the blood flows directly from the capillaries into the sinuses. There is now unequivocal evidence for both open and closed pathways in the human spleen.[6–8] The splenic circulation has thus both a rapid and a slow transit component.

However, in normal subjects, blood kinetic studies have demonstrated that the closed system is physiologically the major pathway of splenic blood flow.[9] Blood flows through the spleen at a rate of 5–10% of the blood volume per minute, which is similar to that in other organs. Under normal conditions less than 2% of red cells entering the spleen traverse the cordal compartment.[9]

FUNCTIONS OF THE NORMAL SPLEEN

The pathophysiological role of the spleen in systemic disease can be readily understood in terms of the diverse and specialized functions of the normal spleen. The main functions ascribed to the normal spleen have included haemopoiesis and its regulation, the destruction of effete blood cells, filtration and phagocytosis of particulate matter, lymphopoiesis and antibody production. Of these the humoral control of haemopoiesis by the spleen has not been clearly demonstrated. In man the storage of red cells is not a function of the normal spleen, which has a red cell pool of 20–60 ml.[10] However, it is a site of storage for platelets, Factor VIII and iron.[11–15] Stored platelets in the spleen comprise some 20–40% of the total circulating platelet pool and these can be readily mobilized in conditions of stress.[12,16] Reticulocytes are also sequestered in the spleen and undergo maturation within the pulp before being released into the circulation.[17,18]

Haematopoiesis

Haematopoiesis, which is present in the foetal spleen from the 12th week, ceases after birth, except for lymphopoiesis. The spleen itself is not a significant site of lymphocyte production although lymphoid proliferation occurs in the germinal centres in response to antigen stimuli. However, the adult spleen retains its capacity for erythropoiesis in conditions of severe haematological stress, for example in thalassaemia major and intermedia and in congenital or acquired chronic haemolytic anaemias. This compensatory extramedullary erythropoiesis should be distinguished from myeloid metaplasia which occurs in myeloproliferative disorders such as idiopathic myelofibrosis and chronic myeloid leukaemia. In the latter conditions, haemopoietic foci become established in the spleen and at other sites outside the bone marrow and presumably are able to proliferate in those sites because of their neoplastic nature.

The normal adult human spleen is not capable of initiating haemopoiesis as it presumably lacks the necessary microenvironment present in the bone marrow. However, experimental studies have demonstrated the presence of pluripotent haemopoietic stem cells (CFU-S) and erythroid progenitor cells (BFU-E) in the spleen as well as in the bone marrow.[19,20] It is thus possible that colony-forming progenitor cells migrate from the bone marrow to the spleen and may represent an important component of the marginal pool of pluripotential stem cells. That the spleen is a site of sequestration of circulating progenitor cells in patients with significant splenomegaly may well explain the clinical observation that such patients develop a disproportionate degree of cytopenia (leucopenia and/or thrombocytopenia) after receiving splenic irradiation.

Filter function and phagocytosis

The spleen performs an essential 'quality control' function through its filtering action of the blood. Its unique vascular structure serves to bring the circulating blood components into very close contact with a high concentration of macrophages and phagocytic reticular cells. It is thus able to modify red cells for recirculation and remove effete or defective cells along with other foreign particulate matter. Unfortunately under certain circumstances these useful physiological functions can become exaggerated and consequently harmful to the host. Three mechanisms or processes have been described:[21] (1) Sequestration is the temporary process whereby cells are held in the splenic pulp before returning to the circulation. (2) Pooling refers to the presence of an increased amount of blood or its components in the spleen; for example a pooling effect has been demonstrated for platelets, whilst pooling of red cells is a common feature of splenomegaly. Unlike sequestered cells, pooled cells are in continuous exchange with the circulation. (3) Phagocytosis is the broad term used to describe the removal of effete or damaged cells or particulate foreign matter by macrophages and reticulum cells or the destruction of viable cells rendered abnormal by processes such as prolonged sequestration and coating by antibody. The term 'culling' has also been used to describe the ability of the spleen to remove defective cells such as sickle cells, spherocytes, parasitized red cells and sensitized platelets.[22-25] In contrast, 'pitting' is the process whereby particulate inclusion bodies are removed from red cells which are then allowed to recirculate. This is the mechanism by which the spleen removes Howell–Jolly bodies, siderotic granules and Heinz bodies from red cells.[13,24,26] 'Pitting' has been well-demonstrated in animal experiments where electron microscopy studies showed that inclusion bodies are removed at the sinus wall when the red cells squeeze through the inter-endothelial slits when passing from the cords to the sinus lumen. These inclusions, whether Heinz bodies or malarial parasites, are trapped in the trailing ends of red cells as they cross the sinus endothelium, become detached and are subsequently ingested by local phagocytes.[26,27]

Splenic blood flow and red cell characteristics are the two important factors which influence the process of phagocytosis. The high haematocrit of the splenic blood leads to a sluggish flow in the red pulp, resulting in a prolonged transit time. Sequestered red cells in the presence of metabolically active macrophages become exposed to an adverse metabolic environment characterized by a low O_2 tension, a low ambient pH and a reduced glucose concentration.[28,29] As a consequence the red cells become depleted of ATP and this results in the membrane becoming unstable and fragmented, leading to the formation of rigid spheres.[30] Red cells which are unduly susceptible to this sequestration effect and consequently become inflexible are those which are already abnormal, fragmented or misshapen. Such abnormal cells include those with an intrinsic metabolic defect (as in certain congenital haemolytic anaemias, e.g. pyruvate kinase deficiency) or with a pre-existing membrane defect such as hereditary spherocytosis or an acquired defect, for example resulting from antibody coating in warm autoimmune haemolytic anaemia. Rigid cells trapped in the cord spaces subsequently undergo phagocytosis.

Immunological function

The spleen is an immunologically competent organ with its lymphoid tissue accounting for a quarter of the total lymphatic mass in the human body. It is a major source of antibody production, in particular of the IgM type, but its loss is compensated by an increased activity of other lymphoid organs. Its structure allows trapping of microorganisms and other particulate antigens by macrophages in the marginal zone and the red pulp, before being delivered to the adjoining immunologically competent lymphocytes. The close integration of cells enables the B-lymphocytes to respond to particulate antigenic challenge by rapid production of neutralizing IgM antibodies.[31,32] Indeed this vital first-line defence against invading encapsulated micro-organisms such as pneumococci and meningococci, is lost in post-splenectomy or hyposplenic patients and may give rise to overwhelming infection. The spleen is also responsible for the generation of the complement component properdin, and the phagocytosis-promoting tetra-peptide, tuftsin, and levels of these factors are reduced in post-splenectomy subjects.[33,34] The spleen may also play a role in the production of auto-antibodies in conditions such as autoimmune thrombocytopenic purpura (ATP) and autoimmune haemolytic anaemia. One study in patients with ATP showed a fall in serum antiplatelet antibody titres following splenectomy.[35] However, as discussed previously, the spleen, irrespective of its size, is a major site of destruction of sensitized platelets and red cells and cure of these conditions can be achieved by splenectomy.

SPLENOMEGALY

General considerations

The normal adult spleen is 8–13 cm long and 4.5–7 cm wide. These figures are based on *in vivo* scan measurements. The spleen has to be enlarged one and a half to twice its normal size before it becomes palpable. In practice, splenic size is assessed by palpation and a palpable spleen usually signifies splenomegaly, although it may be possible to palpate a normal spleen in subjects with a low diaphragm. One study in the USA showed that about 3% of apparently healthy college freshmen had palpable spleens.[36] In the majority of these cases the splenomegaly was attributed to infectious mononucleosis which is endemic in this age group. However in 30% of these students, the spleen remained palpable and a 10 year follow-up in the same students revealed no increased incidence of lymphoreticular malig-nancies.[37] Similarly in about 25% of unselected patients who were found to have a palpable spleen on routine physical examinations, no cause could be found to account for the splenomegaly.[38] Nevertheless, with few exceptions, the presence of splenomegaly implies a pathological process which warrants appropriate and, whenever indicated, exhaustive investigations in an attempt at establishing a diagnosis. In otherwise healthy individuals where a pathological diagnosis cannot be made, careful long-term follow-up is indicated.

When clinically not palpable, for example, in obese subjects, an enlarged spleen can be easily demonstrated by a variety of imaging procedures. These include ultrasonic scan, radionuclide scan, X-ray computerized tomography (CT) and nuclear magnetic resonance imaging. CT examination is particularly useful and effective in the investigation and management of splenomegalic disorders, for example in patients with lymphoma. For further details on splenic imaging techniques the reader is referred to a recent monograph on the spleen.[39]

Causes of splenomegaly

The main causes of splenomegaly are shown in Table 14.1. However, it is worth noting the different pattern of pathological association in patients with splenomegalic disorders in different parts of the world. In Western Europe and the USA, splenomegaly is frequently associated with portal hypertension, haematological malignancies and viral infections, whereas in the tropics it is most commonly due to parasitic infections such as malaria, Kala-azar and schistosomiasis. In the latter cases, the spleen can become very markedly enlarged. Portal hypertension, especially in association with hepatic cirrhosis, is also an important cause of splenomegaly in many tropical countries, parts of India and South East Asia. In other countries, haemoglobinopathies account for a significant proportion of cases. In temperate climates, massive splenomegaly is most commonly due to idiopathic myelofibrosis, chronic myeloid leukaemia, hairy-cell leukaemia and Gaucher's disease. A grossly enlarged spleen can sometimes be seen in patients with chronic lymphatic leukaemia, prolymphocytic leukaemia and non-Hodgkin's lymphoma.

The diverse pathogenetic processes which lead to the development of splenomegaly are summarized in Table 14.2. More than one process may be involved, and in many cases the effects of the splenic enlargement, irrespective of the primary cause, come to dominate the clinical picture. The pathophysiological effects of significant splenomegaly are discussed below.

Red cell pool

In most patients with splenomegaly, the dynamics of splenic blood flow are profoundly altered. Analysis of the uptake curve of the radioactivity over enlarged spleens following an intravenous injection of ^{51}Cr-labelled red cells clearly shows the existence of two distinctive patterns of blood flow. A rapid initial rise of activity over the spleen is followed by a longer second phase of slower accumulation.[40–42] Thus it may take up to 60 min to achieve equilibration of red cells in the spleen with those in the general circulation.

Table 14.1   Causes of Splenomegaly

Infections
  Acute
    Septicaemia, viral hepatitis, infectious mononucleosis, cytomegalovirus infection, typhoid, paratyphoid, brucellosis, typhus, relapsing fever, toxoplasmosis, tularaemia
  Subacute and chronic
    Subacute bacterial endocarditis, tuberculosis, brucellosis, syphilis, malaria[a] leishmaniasis,[a] schistosomiasis,[a] trypanosomiasis, histoplasmosis and other systemic fungal infections, human immunodeficiency virus (HIV) infection

Inflammatory disorders
  Rheumatoid disease, Felty's syndrome, systemic lupus erythematosus, rheumatic fever, serum sickness, sarcoidosis, berylliosis

Congestive splenomegaly
  Intrahepatic portal hypertension
    Portal, post-necrotic and biliary cirrhosis, haemochromatosis, Wilson's disease, congenital fibrosis
  Portal vein obstruction
    Thrombosis, cavernous malformation, obstruction at porta-hepatis
  Splenic vein obstruction
    Thrombosis, angiomatous malformation, obstruction, aneurysm of splenic artery
  Budd–Chiari syndrome
  Cardiac
    Congestive cardiac failure, constrictive pericarditis.

Haematological
  Haemolytic disorders
    Hereditary spherocytosis, hereditary elliptocytosis, autoimmune haemolytic anaemia, thalassaemia, sickle cell disease, haemoglobin-SC disease, sickle-thalassaemia, red cell enzyme defects
  Myeloproliferative disorders
    Idiopathic myelofibrosis,[a] polycythaemia vera, essential thrombocythaemia
  Miscellaneous
    Idiopathic non-tropical splenomegaly,[a] megaloblastic anaemia, iron deficiency anaemia

Malignancy
  Haematological
    Acute leukaemia, chronic myeloid leukaemia,[a] chronic lymphatic leukaemia, hairy cell leukaemia,[a] malignant lymphoma,[a] malignant histiocytosis, systemic mastocytosis, myelodysplastic syndromes, myelomatosis
  Others
    (a) Malignant: angiosarcoma, fibrosarcoma, secondary metastasis from carcinoma and melanoma
    (b) Benign: haemangioma, fibroma, haemartoma

Storage diseases
  Gaucher's disease,[a] Niemann–Pick disease, histiocytosis X, Tangier disease, Hurler's syndrome

Miscellaneous
  Cysts
    Echinococcus, pseudocysts from trauma or post-infarction
    Amyloidosis, osteopetrosis, hereditary haemorrhagic telangiectasia, hyperthyroidism

[a] May be associated with massive splenomegaly.

These findings are in keeping with the concept of two functional pathways in the enlarged spleen, namely the presence of a fast pathway (predominant in the normal spleen) and a second slow pathway in which there is a slow exchange of red cells between the splenic pool and the systemic circulation.[9]

Significant red cell pooling in the spleen occurs in conditions where there is either an abnormality of the splenic structure or of the red cells. Pooling dependent on abnormality of the spleen is seen in myelofibrosis, chronic myeloid leukaemia, lymphoproliferative disorders and portal hypertension. Examples of red cell defects associated with splenic pooling include hereditary spherocytosis, thalassaemia and autoimmune haemolytic anaemia. In these conditions the splenic cords become so grossly distended with red cells that they become indistinguishable from the sinuses, indicating that the cordal compartment is the site of pooling.[29]

The presence of a large splenic pool has important clinical implications. This is seen particularly in myeloproliferative disorders, some lympho-proliferative disorders such as hairy cell leukaemia and prolymphocytic leukaemia, and in the tropical splenomegaly syndrome where the pool may exceed 1–1.5 litres of red cells.[43–45] The splenic red cell pool may thus come to represent a significant fraction (up to half) of the total red cell mass not immediately available for the general circulation and consequently creating a functional anaemia. The latter can be corrected by splenectomy. It is worth noting that in the myeloproliferative disorders, the red cell pool contributes largely to the splenomegaly whereas in lymphomas, tumour infiltration may be the primary cause of the splenic enlargement. In myelofibrosis there is a marked expansion of the sinus compartment while in hairy cell leukaemia the red pulp characteristically contains 'pseudo-sinuses', which are lakes of red cells lined by hairy cells.

The 'whole-body' haematocrit (Hb), measured from separate determina-tions of red cell and plasma volumes, is generally lower than the venous haematocrit (Hv) and in normal subjects the Hb/Hv ratio lies in the range of 0.89–0.924.[46–48] Many patients with splenomegaly have elevated Hb/Hv ratios, which are due to the marked haemoconcentration of red cells in the splenic red cell pool.[49–51]

Table 14.2 Pathogenetic Classification of Splenomegaly

1. Splenic hyperplasia, e.g. haemolytic anaemias, infective and inflammatory disorders
2. Congestive splenomegaly with raised splenic venous pressure
3. Red cell pooling secondary to
   (a) abnormal red cells
   (b) abnormal splenic structure
4. Primary myeloid metaplasia and compensatory extramedullary haemopoiesis
5. Neoplastic proliferation
   Primary and secondary
6. Histiocytic storage disorders
7. Miscellaneous, e.g. amyloidosis, cysts, haemartomas

Portal hypertension

Although splenomegaly commonly results from primary portal hypertension, massive splenomegaly can itself give rise to secondary portal hypertension. In massive splenomegaly, for example, in association with the tropical splenomegaly syndrome, Kala-azar and certain haematological malignancies (Table 14.1), splenic blood flow may exceed 10 times normal, with the enlarged spleen in effect acting as an arteriovenous shunt.[52-53] As a result the intrasplenic pressure is increased, the splanchnic vasculature expanded and the total flow in the portal vein increased several fold. In portal hypertension of the hyperkinetic type, bleeding from oesophageal and gastric varices can occur, despite the absence of obstructive lesions to portal blood flow.

Plasma volume and dilutional anaemia

Splenomegaly is frequently associated with an increase in plasma volume, causing a dilution of the red cell mass and giving rise to an apparent or pseudo-anaemia. This phenomenon was first described by McFadzean *et al.* in patients wth cryptogenic splenomegaly, whose anaemia was significantly improved by splenectomy, provided that there was no significant hepatic disease as well.[54,55] Subsequent studies showed that the expansion of plasma volume causing dilutional anaemia, is a general characteristic of splenomegaly and that it is approximately proportional to the degree of splenic enlargement, irrespective of the cause. It has also been described in patients wth Gaucher's disease, chronic leukaemia, myelofibrosis, hairy cell leukaemia, Felty's syndrome, congestive splenomegaly and tropical splenomegaly.[56-63] The cause for the plasma volume expansion is not entirely clear. One explanation lies in the altered haemodynamics which occur in portal hypertension, regardless of the cause. The rise in portal pressure leads secondarily to an expansion of the splanchnic vasculature which in turn requires an expansion of the blood volume. In conditions where red cell production is reduced or is already at its maximum, any further increase in the red cell mass cannot be met and it is suggested that the plasma volume expands disproportionately to compensate for the red cell deficit in order to maintain the total blood volume. In patients with tropical splenomegaly, high serum globulin levels are usually present and this hypergammaglobulinaemia is believed to be a contributory cause of plasma volume expansion.[60] Dilutional anaemia can be corrected by splenectomy except in cases where there is obstruction to the portal blood flow, for example in hepatic cirrhosis.

Platelet and granulocyte pool

In normal subjects there is pooling of 20–40% of the total circulating platelet mass within the spleen.[11,12,16] The size of the storage platelet pool is roughly proportional to the spleen size and in splenomegalic states, up to 90% of the platelet population may be found in the spleen.[9] The resulting thrombocytopenia causes a compensatory increase in platelet production in the bone marrow but this is often partial, unlike the situation of maximal megakaryopoiesis seen with platelet destruction such as immune thrombocytopenic purpura. This is because the total platelet mass appears to be a more important factor in the control of platelet production than the level of the platelet count. Also, while there is a close correlation between platelet pooling and the size of the spleen, the effect of splenomegaly on platelet survival is variable and usually unremarkable. In congestive splenomegaly the platelet lifespan may be either normal or moderately shortened.[64]

With respect to neutrophils or granulocytes, no significant pool has been demonstrated in the normal spleen. However abnormally large pools, arising from increased margination of granulocytes in splenic blood vessels, can be found in patients with very gross splenomegaly, particularly in association with Felty's syndrome.[65,66] Except in Felty's syndrome, where other immunological mechanisms may be involved, severe neutropenia is rarely seen in splenomegaly.

Hypersplenism

The term 'hypersplenism' was first introduced by Chauffard in 1907 to describe the haemolytic activity of the spleen in hereditary spherocytosis.[64] Although the concept of hypersplenism has caused considerable confusion and controversy over the years, the term itself has been used widely for descriptive purposes. Dameshek[68] had originally described the features of the syndrome which can now be summarized to include the following:

1. splenomegaly;
2. pancytopenia or deficiency of one or more lines in the peripheral blood;
3. normal or increased cellularity of the bone marrow corresponding to the deficiency of the peripheral cell line;
4 increased cell turnover in the affected cell lines resulting in, for example, mild reticulocytosis and an increased population of banded forms in the granulocyte series in the peripheral blood. This, however, is not invariable; and
5. correction of the cell deficits by splenectomy. Thus confirmation of this disorder can only be made on a retrospective basis.

Hypersplenism has been arbitrarily divided into two types: primary and secondary. Primary hypersplenism includes a number of conditions characterized by peripheral cytopenias for which no other recognizable disease is present, at least at the time of diagnosis. Secondary hypersplenism occurs in association with an enlarged spleen as part of a disease process for which a cause is known. The degree of hypersplenism appears to correlate with the size of the enlarged spleen, irrespective of the underlying cause. The main disorders associated with hypersplenism are shown in Table 14.3. It is now customary not to include conditions such as hereditary spherocytosis and idiopathic thrombocytopenic purpura as examples of hypersplenism, as in these disorders the pathogenesis is well-established and the spleen is only performing its normal function. However, in hereditary spherocytosis, secondary hypersplenism can occur if the

Table 14.3 Main Disorders Associated with Hypersplenism

Primary hypersplenism
  Examples include primary splenic neutropenia, non-tropical idiopathic
  splenomegaly, simple splenic hyperplasia

Secondary hypersplenism
  Acute infections with splenomegaly
  Chronic infections: malaria, Kala-azar, tuberculosis, brucellosis
  Inflammatory conditions: Felty's syndrome, systemic lupus erythematosus
  Congestive splenomegaly
  Leukaemias and lymphomas
  Myeloproliferative disorders, e.g. idiopathic myelofibrosis
  Storage disorders: Gaucher's disease, Hurler's syndrome
  Chronic haemolytic disorders, e.g. hereditary spherocytosis, thalassaemia,
  some sickling disorders

spleen becomes markedly enlarged. Thus the term primary hypersplenism may become obsolete in future as the pathogenesis of the cytopenias currently described under this term becomes more clearly defined.

The mechanisms responsible for the features of hypersplenism have been the subject of controversy in the past. Two differing views were expressed to explain the concept of hypersplenism as that of excessive splenic activity. One school of thought, led by Doan,[69] postulated that destruction of blood cells within the spleen was the principal cause of the peripheral cytopenias. Dameshek[68] on the other hand held the opposing view that peripheral blood cell deficits resulted from inhibition of bone marrow activity, this being mediated through humoral factors produced by the spleen. As discussed previously, there is no firm evidence to support the hypothesis that the spleen in any way regulates the production, maturation or release of bone marrow haemopoietic cells. Certainly in hypersplenism, present evidence militates against the existence of a putative regulator involved in the control of haemopoiesis.[42]

It is now well-established that cell destruction within the spleen is responsible for the observed peripheral cytopenias. This has been best demonstrated in conditions where the abnormality, either intrinsic or acquired, lies in the red cell itself (see phagocytosis section). Thus the spleen is seen acting essentially as a filtering organ, facilitating the retention of the abnormal cell which is subsequently destroyed in the splenic pulp. In the majority of splenomegalic disorders, while there is moderate shortening of the red cell survival, haemolysis does not occur to any significant degree as to cause anaemia. The half-life of ^{51}Cr-labelled red cells in such cases is between 18 and 24 days, compared to a normal range of 26–34 days.[42] When anaemia is present, it is usually due to a failure of the compensatory proliferative response of the bone marrow, which is attributed to the underlying disorder. However, in conditions associated with significant splenomegaly, anaemia can be further aggravated by the presence of both a sizeable splenic red cell pool and by the dilutional effect of an expanded plasma compartment. Similarly, thrombocytopenia results from the effect of excessive platelet pooling in the enlarged spleen while platelet survival is not significantly affected. It is thus clear that splenomegaly per se does not cause any significant increase in blood cell destruction, but when peripheral cytopenias are present, there are usually additional defects either of the circulating cells or the compensatory bone marrow response. In addition any deficiencies can be further aggravated by the effect of a large splenic pool. Finally, although there is no convincing evidence that the spleen can elaborate humoral factors which modulate bone marrow activity, it is now recognized that the spleen is able to produce auto-antibodies which, by sensitizing blood cells, can cause their premature destruction not only in the spleen, but also in other parts of the reticulo-endothelial system. However, in the majority of patients with hypersplenism, the presence of reactive auto-antibodies against platelets and red cells cannot be demonstrated.[70]

Specific causes of splenomegaly

Congestive splenomegaly

Congestive splenomegaly results from raised splenic venous pressure which can arise in a wide variety of conditions. The main causes of congestive splenomegaly are shown in Table 14.1. Splenomegaly is frequently associated with portal hypertension, and at autopsy it has been found in approximately 70% of cases of portal cirrhosis.[71] The largest spleen tends to occur in association with the most advanced cases of hepatic cirrhosis. As discussed previously, haemodilution and splenic pooling are largely responsible for the pancytopenia observed in cases of congestive spleno-megaly. Moreover, in the presence of hepatic cirrhosis, anaemia may be accentuated by additional factors such as haemorrhage from varices, impaired erythropoiesis, folate deficiency and haemolysis in the spleen.

Non-tropical idiopathic splenomegaly

This term was first used by Dacie et al.[70] to describe a series of 10 patients who presented with gross splenomegaly and haematological features of hypersplenism but had not been exposed to malaria or other parasitic infections. Clinical findings include anaemia, severe leucopenia and neutro-penia, and moderate thrombocytopenia. The liver was commonly palpable but hepatic cirrhosis or portal hypertension was absent. Evidence of auto-antibody production, including a positive red cell antiglobulin test, may be present. In some patients, malignant lymphoma was present in the spleen at the time of presentation (diagnosis only made retrospectively), while in others the main morphological feature in the spleen was non-malignant lymphoreticular hyperplasia, possibly representing either an exaggerated immunological reaction or an autoimmune process. Splenectomy appeared to be beneficial, with sustained and significant clinical and haematological improvement in 'most' instances, although neutropenia failed to resolve in four out of nine splenectomized patients. In four cases, lymphoma had subsequently developed at periods ranging from 8 months to 6 years after splenectomy, and on reviewing the original splenic histology, with hindsight it was possible to detect cytological changes consistent with a lymphomatous process in three of them.[72] Nowadays with the application of cell marker studies in spleen sections, it may be easier to distinguish between neoplastic and non-neoplastic lymphoreticular proliferation. None-theless it is important to ensure that any patients with the diagnostic label of non-tropical idiopathic splenomegaly be followed up on a long-term basis.

Tropical splenomegaly syndrome

Tropical splenomegaly syndrome (TSS) is found in areas where malaria is endemic and seen commonly in Central, West and East Africa and in parts of New Guinea, where the incidence is particularly high. It is a chronic disorder characterized by usually massive splenomegaly and its diagnosis requires the exclusion of other known causes of splenic enlargement, in particular parasitic infections endemic in the tropics. In the early course of the disease, patients are prone to recurrent febrile episodes resulting from infections with malarial parasites and typically they remain afebrile with the established syndrome. In these patients, parasitaemia is rare. TSS is usually seen in young adults although it may be present in childhood. The spleen may attain a weight in excess of 6–8 kg, extending to the iliac crest and filling the abdominal cavity and through its sheer size cause mechanical symptoms. The liver is also enlarged, with the left lobe being disproportion-ately prominent.[73] TSS remains an important cause of considerable morbidity and mortality in tropical countries.

Mild pancytopenia is frequent, with anaemia being invariably present; the latter resulting mainly from increased splenic red cell pooling and a greatly expanded plasma volume. Mean haemoglobin values of 10.4 g/dl in men and 8.7 g/dl in women, with frequent, periodic, individual fluctuations, have been reported in TSS.[74] Moreover, the dilutional anaemia of TSS may be exacerbated by concurrent nutritional deficiencies and blood loss from hookworm infestation. In addition red cell lifespan is shortened with excess red cell destruction occurring entirely in the enlarged spleen. The mild leucopenia and thrombocytopenia frequently observed in patients with TSS result from pooling of granulocytes and platelets in the massively enlarged spleen.[75] The peripheral cytopenias are usually corrected by splenectomy.[60]

In TSS, the liver and spleen are the two organs which show marked pathological changes. Histological examination of the liver reveals pro-nounced lymphocytic infiltration of the sinusoids and Kupffer cell hyper-plasia, with phagocytosis.[76,77] There may also be infiltration of the portal tracts with lymphoid and plasma cells. In the spleen, the cords and sinuses are greatly dilated with prominent hyperplasia of reticulo-endothelial cells, some of which may show haemophagocytosis. Extensive packing of red cells in the red pulp leads to a significant proportion, in some cases up to 40%, of the total red cell mass being pooled in the spleen.

Patients with TSS have very high levels of serum IgM and may also have other abnormal serological reactions including positive rheumatoid factors, non-organ specific auto-antibodies and high concentrations of cold agglut-inins and cryoglobulins.[78,79] In these patients, the plasma volume expansion is partly due to the presence of the very high levels of IgM and IgG.

Epidemiological evidence suggests that TSS is causally related to chronic malarial infestation. This is further supported by the presence of raised titres of malarial antibody, the beneficial effect of prolonged antimalarial therapy with regression of splenomegaly and relapse with discontinuation of treatment.[80,81] However, only a small fraction of the profuse IgM antibody response seen in TSS is due to malaria. It is likely that TSS results from an abnormal immunological response to malarial antigens leading to intense lymphoreticular proliferation particularly in the spleen. A defect in suppressor T-cell activity has been proposed, although genetic factors are also important. Prolonged treatment with antimalarial drugs is warranted in patients with TSS. Although splenectomy is followed by clinical and haematological improvement, it is worth remembering that such patients are at risk of fulminant malaria after removal of the spleen.[81,82]

Infiltrative splenomegaly: storage diseases

The 'storage diseases' comprise a heterogeneous group of disorders affecting the monocyte–macrophage components of the reticulo-endothelial system and characterized by the development of hepatosplenomegaly and secondary cytopenias. Most of these disorders are hereditary and represent inborn errors of metabolism in which the reticulo-endothelial cells become markedly overloaded with diverse metabolites, especially lipids and mucopolysaccharides. The central defect in the majority of these storage disorders is a deficiency of a lysosomal enzyme involved in the catabolic degradation of the accumulated substance. The lipidoses provide examples of storage disorders in which different ceramide compounds accumulate in the reticulo-endothelial cells, resulting in the wide range of clinical manifestations seen in these conditions. Gaucher's and Niemann–Pick diseases will be described here as two such examples. Clinical features of other storage disorders are well described in standard textbooks of medicine and paediatrics.

Gaucher's disease.   Gaucher's disease is a familial lipidosis due to a deficiency of β-glucocerebrosidase activity, resulting in an excessive accumulation of glucosyl ceramide in tissues and red cells.[83,84] It is inherited as an autosomal recessive disorder and broadly has three main clinical presentations. In the infantile form, severe neurological involvement predominates whilst in the adult type, the nervous system is spared and the presenting features include splenomegaly and pancytopenia. In the juvenile variant, the nervous system may be involved, with hepatosplenomegaly being the dominant feature. There is a particularly high incidence of the adult form in Ashkenazi Jews.

The striking pathological finding is the Gaucher's cell which accumulates in the bone marrow, liver and spleen. It is a large cell, measuring 20–80 μm in diameter and has a small eccentric nucleus and a characteristic fibrillar cytoplasm[85] (see Chapter 1). In the adult type, the spleen can become massively enlarged as a result of extensive infiltration with nests of engorged Gaucher's cells. Haematological abnormalities arise from a combination of impaired haemopoiesis due to marrow infiltration by

Gaucher's cells and secondary hypersplenism. These include anaemia, leucopenia and thromboctyopenia. Thrombocytopenia is common and may give rise to bleeding problems. This can usually be improved by splenectomy, which in addition may correct any coexisting anaemia or haemolysis. Splenectomy also provides symptomatic relief of pain and abdominal discomfort in cases of massive organomegaly. Unfortunately it may be followed by accelerated extension of Gaucher's lesions in bones and the liver.

Niemann–Pick disease.   Of the other lipidoses, Niemann–Pick disease deserves brief mention. This autosomal recessive disorder results from deficiency of sphingomyelinase and affects mostly infants who present with mental retardation and hepatosplenomegaly. The characteristic cell which is present in the bone marrow is 20–90 μm in size and the cytoplasm is uniformly laden with lipid (sphingomyelin) droplets giving it a 'foamy' appearance. Vacuolation of lymphocytes and monocytes is also a feature.[86] With progressive disease, splenomegaly can give rise to significant hypersplenism, usually correctable by splenectomy.

Laboratory and clinical approach to the investigation of splenomegaly

Splenomegaly is often a presenting or dominant feature of systemic disease. In some cases the diagnosis is obvious, while in others it can only be established after extensive investigations. There is indeed much to be gained in adopting a logical and systematic approach to the investigation of splenomegaly. One such approach makes use of algorithms designed to provide a rational and cost-effective diagnostic scheme.[87]

To start with, the importance of taking a full history and carrying out a thorough and careful physical examination cannot be overemphasized. Some important features in the history should include racial origin of the patient, country of abode, foreign travel and family history. It is worth remembering that mild splenomegaly may not be detectable on even the most careful physical examination, with the patient both in the supine and in the lateral decubitus position. In such cases, a diagnostic scan is necessary. An ultrasound scan is a simple and non-invasive procedure to detect splenic enlargement whilst a radioisotopic scan gives additional information on the splenic reticulo-endothelial function. For example, decreased radioisotope uptake in an enlarged spleen may suggest infarction or tumour infiltration. As mentioned previously, CT scanning, however, is the most sensitive method available for detecting small intrasplenic lesions and is particularly useful in detecting small splenic lacerations and should thus be used when splenic trauma is suspected.[88]

A scheme for investigating patients with splenomegaly is briefly outlined here and shown in Figs. 14.1 and 14.2 in the form of flow charts; it is not meant to be a comprehensive approach for diagnosing the more esoteric causes of splenomegaly. From a diagnostic point of view, it is possible to divide splenomegalic disorders into two broad groups, namely those in association with an acute or subacute illness and those with a chronic illness

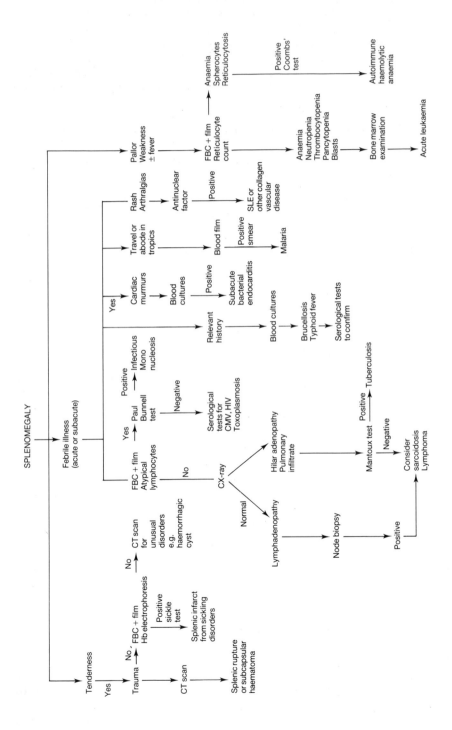

Fig. 14.1. Flowchart for investigating splenomegaly with acute or subacute illness.

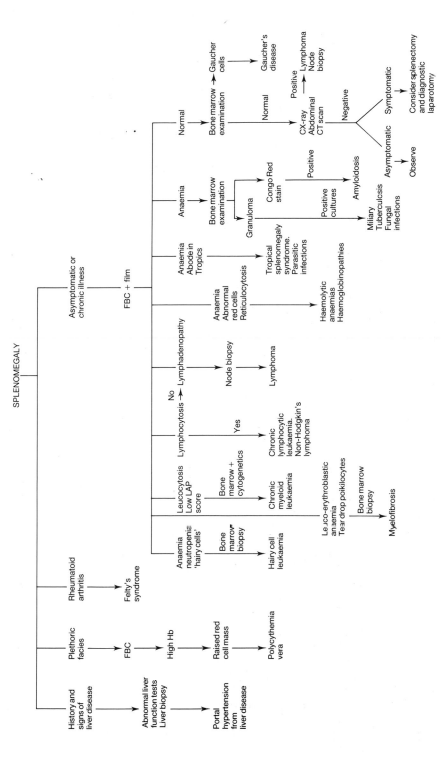

Fig. 14.2. Flowchart for investigating splenomegaly with chronic illness or with symptoms.

or no accompanying symptomatology.[84] In previously healthy patients with a history of trauma and acute left hypochondrial pain, an enlarged tender spleen suggests a subcapsular haematoma or even rupture. However, pathological or spontaneous rupture of the spleen is a well-recognized complication of acute infections, notably infectious mononucleosis, typhoid fever and malaria, but can also occur in acute and chronic leukaemias.[89] In patients presenting with an acute or subacute febrile illness and spleno-megaly, the possibility of infection has to be considered.

Other features from the history and examination will obviously help to narrow down the diagnostic possibilities and the type of infection. For example, a recent history of travel in the tropics would alert the clinician to the possibility of malaria. In these cases, simple examination of the blood film may reveal the diagnosis. On the other hand, if the history is uninformative, specific attention must be paid to physical signs, in particular, the presence of anaemia, jaundice, cardiac murmurs, lymph-adenopathy, hepatomegaly, skin rash and joint pain or swelling. Initial diagnostic tests would include a full blood count, blood film examination, ESR, liver function tests, Monospot or Paul–Bunnell test (useful screening test in young people and those suspected of having infectious mono-nucleosis), blood cultures and a chest X-ray. A blood count may indicate the diagnosis of acute or chronic leukaemia which can be confirmed by examination of the bone marrow. Furthermore, the blood film may show morphological changes which give a direct clue as to the cause of the splenomegaly (see Chapter 1). Serological tests should follow if brucella, salmonella, toxoplasma, fungal or viral infections (e.g. cytomegalovirus or human immunodeficiency virus) is suspected. In addition, appropriate cultures of body fluids and stools may yield useful information. In the presence of a rash and joint involvement, systemic lupus erythematosus and other collagen vascular disorders should be considered. Finally, in patients with lymphadenopathy in whom a lymphoma is suspected, a lymph node biopsy is indicated.

In the diagnostic assessment of splenomegaly in patients who are either asymptomatic or who have a chronic illness, the main disorders which need to be considered include: liver disease with portal hypertension, lympho-proliferative and myeloproliferative disorders, myelodysplastic syndromes (especially in the elderly), storage disorders, congenital haemolytic anaemias, amyloidosis and splenic cysts. In the tropics, however, parasitic infestations such as malaria, Kala-azar and schistosomiasis remain the predominant causes of splenomegaly, although hepatic cirrhosis and haematological malignancies should be included in the differential diag-nosis. Liver disease as the cause of portal hypertension and congestive splenomegaly may be obvious from the physical examination. Abnormal liver function tests support the diagnosis which can be confirmed by a liver biopsy. Examination of the peripheral blood and a bone marrow aspirate with trephine biopsy, coupled with a lymph node biopsy where indicated, will reveal the great majority of lymphoproliferative and myeloproliferative disorders. The application of cell marker studies has, in addition, greatly facilitated the diagnosis of lymphoid neoplasms.

Lipid storage disorders, for example, Gaucher's disease, can be diagnosed by the presence of typical storage cells in the bone marrow. Felty's syndrome would be obvious in a patient with rheumatoid arthritis and neutropenia. Anaemia with abnormalities of the red cell and reticulocytosis would point towards a chronic haemolytic process. Additional tests such as haemoglobin electrophoresis, sickling test, osmotic fragility, acidified serum lysis test and red cell enzyme assays may be required to diagnose the type of haemolytic anaemia involved.

The patient who presents with splenomegaly as an isolated abnormal finding poses a more difficult management problem. Routine investigations may give no clue as to the underlying disorder. One possibility is the presence of occult liver disease with a well-compensated portal hypertension. A liver biopsy with appropriate investigations for portal hypertension including upper gastrointestinal tract endoscopy or barium studies may therefore be necessary. Investigations for an underlying lymphoma should include a chest X-ray, CT scan of the abdomen and spleen, and bone marrow examination (aspirate and trephine biopsy). However, despite extensive investigations, the cause of splenomegaly remains undiagnosed in a number of cases. A high proportion of these patients will turn out to have isolated intrasplenic lymphoma, congestive splenomegaly or other pathology which can only be diagnosed by a diagnostic laparotomy and splenectomy. The decision to proceed to surgical exploration and splenectomy will depend on the patient's clinical condition. If the patient is well and asymptomatic and has no other signs of disease, a sensible approach would be to keep the patient under regular and careful observation. Such a pragmatic approach can be justified on the grounds that splenectomy is unlikely to alter the management of the patient. Moreover, splenectomy carries both short- and long-term risks which have to be balanced against the potential benefits of splenectomy to the patient. On the other hand, in the ill patient with signs of disease, splenectomy as a diagnostic procedure is justified.[90] Furthermore, the removal of a very large spleen may correct any secondary hypersplenism and provide symptomatic relief from the mechanical discomfort of a huge intra-abdominal organ.

REFERENCES

1. Krumbhaar, E.B. & Lippincott, S.W. The postmortem weight of the "normal" human spleen at different ages. f90Am. J. Med. Sci. **197**: 344–58, 1939.
2. Koyama, K. Haemodynamics of the spleen in Banti's Syndrome. *Tohoku J. Exp. Med.* **93**: 199–217, 1967.
3. Jandl, J.H., Files, N.M., Barnett, S.B. & MacDonald, R.A. Proliferative response of the spleen and liver to haemolysis. *J. Exp. Med.* **122**: 299–325, 1965.
4. Weiss, L. The structure of fine splenic arterial vessels in relation to hemoconcentration and red cell destruction. *Am. J. Anat.* **111**: 131–79, 1962.
5. Lewis, O.J. The blood vessels of the adult mammalian spleen. *J. Anat.* **91**: 245–50, 1957.
6. Weiss, L. The red pulp of the spleen: structural basis of blood flow. *Clin. Haematol.* **12**: 375–93, 1983.
7. Chen, L.T. & Weiss, L. Electron microscopy of the red pulp of the human spleen. *Am. J. Anat.* **134**: 425–57, 1972.
8. Barnhart, M.I., Baechler, C.A. & Lusher, J.M. Arteriovenous shunts in the human spleen. *Am. J. Hematol.* **1**: 105–14, 1976.

9. Jandl, J.H. The spleen and hypersplenism. In *Blood, Textbook of Hematology*, pp. 407–32. Little, Brown & Co., Boston/Toronto, 1987.

10. Hegde, U.M., Williams, E.D., Lewis, S.M. *et al.* Measurement of splenic red cell volume and visualisation of the spleen with ^{99m}Tc. *J. Nucl. Med.* **14**: 769–71, 1973.

11. Aster, R.H. & Jandl, J.H. Platelet sequestration in man. I Methods. *J. Clin. Invest.* **43**: 843–55, 1964.

12. Penny, R., Rozenberg, M.C. & Firkin, B.G. The splenic platelet pool. *Blood* **27**: 1–16, 1966.

13. Crosby, W.H. Siderocytes and the spleen. *Blood* **12**: 165–70, 1957.

14. Libre, E.P., Cowan, P.H., Watkins, S.P. Jr & Shulman, N.R. Relationships between spleen, platelets and Factor VIII levels. *Blood* **31**: 358–68, 1968.

15. Norman, J.C., Lambilliotte, J.P., Kojima, Y. & Sise, H.S. Anti-hemopoetic factor release by perfused liver and spleen. Relationship to hemophilia: *Science* **158**: 1060–61, 1967.

16. Aster, R.H. Pooling of platelets in the spleen: role in the pathogenesis of "hypersplenic" thrombocytopenia. *J. Clin. Invest.* **45**: 645–57, 1966.

17. Berendes, M. The proportion of reticulocytes in the erythrocytes of the spleen as compared with those of circulating blood with special reference to hemolytic states. *Blood* **14**: 558–63, 1959.

18. Song, S.H. & Groom, A.C. Immature and abnormal erythrocytes present in the normal healthy spleen. *Scand. J. Haematol.* **8**: 487–93, 1971.

19. Schofield, R. The pluripotent stem cell. *Clin. Haematol.* **8**: 221–37, 1979.

20. Murphy, M.J. (ed.) In *In Vitro Aspects of Erythropoiesis*, pp. 75–80. Springer, New York, 1978.

21. Lewis, S.M. The spleen – Mysteries solved and unsolved. *Clin. Haematol.* **12**: 363–73, 1983.

22. Crosby, W.H. Normal functions of the spleen relative to red blood cells: a review. *Blood* **14**: 399–408, 1959.

23. Schnitzer, B., Sodeman, T.M., Mead, M.L. & Contacos, P.G. An ultrastructural study of the red pulp of the spleen in malaria. *Blood* **41**: 207–18, 1973.

24. Rifkind, R.A. Heinz body anaemia and ultrastructural study II. Red cell sequestration and destruction. *Blood* **41**: 433–48, 1965.

25. Tavassoli, M. & McMillan, R. Structure of spleen in idiopathic thrombocytopenic purpura. *Am. J. Clin. Pathol.* **64**: 180–91, 1975.

26. Koyama, S., Aoki, S. & Deguchi, K. Electron microscopic observations of the splenic red pulp with special reference to the pitting function. *Mie Med. J.* **14**: 143–88, 1964.

27. Schnitzer, B., Sodeman, T., Mead M.L. & Contacos, P.G. Pitting function of the spleen in malaria: Ultrastructural observations. *Science* **177**: 175–7, 1972.

28. Jandl, J.H. & Aster, R.H. Increased splenic pooling and the pathogenesis of hypersplenism. *Am. J. Med. Sci.* **253**: 383–97, 1967.

29. Murphy, J.R. The influence of pH and temperature on some physical properties of normal erythrocytes and erythrocytes from patients with hereditary spherocytosis. *J. Lab. Clin. Med.* **69**: 758–75, 1967.

30. Weed, R.I., LaCelle, P.L. & Merrill, E.W. Metabolic dependence of red cell deformability. *J. Clin. Invest.* **48**: 795–809, 1969.

31. Rowley, D.A. The formation of circulating antibody in the splenectomised human being following intravenous injection of heterologous erythrocytes. *J. Immunol.* **65**: 515–21, 1950.

32. Brown, E.J., Hosea, S.W. & Frank, M.M. The role of the spleen in experimental pneumococcal bacteremia. *J. Clin. Immunol.* **67**: 975–82, 1981.

33. Carlisle, H.N. & Saslaw, S. Properdin levels in splenectomised persons. *Proc. Soc. Exp. Biol.* **102**: 150–5, 1959.

34. Spirer, Z. VI, Zakuth, V., Dramant, S. *et al.* Decreased tuftsin concentrations in patients who have undergone splenectomy. *Br. Med. J.* **2**: 1574–6, 1977.

35. Karpatkin, S., Strick, N. & Siskind, G.W. Detection of splenic antiplatelet antibody synthesis in idiopathic autoimmune thrombocytopenic purpura (ATP). *Br. J. Haematol.* **23**: 167–76, 1972.
36. McIntyre, O.R. & Ebaugh, F.G. Jr. Palpable spleens in College freshmen. *Ann. Intern. Med.* **66**: 301–6, 1967.
37. Ebaugh, F.G. Jr & McIntyre, O.R. Palpable spleens: ten-year follow-up. *Ann. Intern. Med.* **90**: 130–1, 1979.
38. Schloesser, L.L. The diagnostic significance of splenomegaly. *Am. J. Med. Sci.* **245**: 84–90, 1963.
39. Myers, M.J. Spleen imaging. *Clin. Haematol.* **12**: 395–420, 1983.
40. Harris, I.M., McAlister, J. & Prankerd, T.A.J. Splenomegaly and the circulating red cell. *Br. J. Haem.* **4**: 97–102, 1958.
41. Motulsky, A.G., Casserd, F., Giblett, E.R., *et al.* Anaemia and the spleen. *N. Engl. J. Med.* **259**: 1164–9, 1215–19, 1958.
42. Bowdler, A.J. Splenomegaly and hypersplenism. *Clin. Haematol.* **12**: 467–88, 1983.
43. Richmond, J., Donaldson, G.W., Williams, R. *et al.* Haematological effects of the idiopathic splenomegaly seen in Uganda. *Br. J. Haematol.* **13**: 348–63, 1967.
44. Bagshawe, A. A comparative study of hypersplenism in reactive and congestive splenomegaly. *Br. J. Haematol.* **19**: 729–37, 1970.
45. Pryor, D.S. The mechanism of anaemia in tropical splenomegaly. *Q. J. Med.* **34**: 337–56, 1967.
46. Bowdler, A.J. The spleen in disorders of the blood. In *Blood and its Disorders* (eds R.M. Hardisty & D.J. Weatherall), pp. 751–97. Blackwell Scientific Publications, Oxford, 1982.
47. Chaplin, H. Jr, Mollison, P.L. & Vetter, H. The body/venous hematocrit ratio: its constancy over a wide hematocrit range. *J. Clin. Invest.* **32**: 1309–16, 1953.
48. Hicks, D.A., Hoppe, A., Turnbull, A.L. & Verel, D. The estimation and prediction of normal blood volume. *Clin. Sci.* **15**: 557–65, 1956.
49. Bowdler, A.J. Regional variations in the proportion of red cells in the blood of man. *Br. J. Haematol.* **16**: 557–71, 1969.
50. Fudenberg, H.H., Baldini, M., Mahoney, J.P. & Dameshek, W. The body haematocrit/venous haematocrit ratio and the "splenic reservoir". *Blood* **17**: 71–82, 1961.
51. Loria, A., Sanchez-Medal, L., Kauffer, N. & Quintaner, E. Relationship between body haematocrit and venous haematocrit in normal, splenomegalic and anaemic states. *J. Lab. Clin. Med.* **60**: 396–408, 1962.
52. Williams, R., Parsonson, A., Somers, K., Hamilton, P.J.S. Portal hypertension in idiopathic splenomegaly. *Lancet* **1**: 329–33, 1966.
53. Garnett, E.S., Markby, D., Goddard, B.A. & Weber, C.E. The spleen as an arteriovenous shunt. *Lancet* **1**: 386–8, 1969.
54. McFadzean, A.J.S., Todd, D. & Tsang, K.C. Observations on the anemia of cryptogenic splenomegaly. II. Expansion of the plasma volume. *Blood* **13**: 524–32, 1958.
55. McFadzean, A.J.S. & Todd, D. The blood volume in post-necrotic cirrhosis of the liver with splenomegaly. *Clin. Sci.* **32**: 339–50, 1967.
56. Bowdler, A.J. Dilutional anaemia corrected by splenectomy in Gaucher's disease. *Ann. Intern. Med.* **58**: 664–9, 1963.
57. Weinstein, V.F. Haemodilution anaemia associated with simple splenic hyperplasia. *Lancet* **ii**: 218–23, 1964.
58. Bowdler, A.J. Dilutional anaemia associated with enlargement of the spleen. *Proc. R. Soc. Med.* **58**: 664–9, 1967.
59. Bowdler, A.J. Blood volume changes in patients with splenomegaly. *Transfusion* **10**: 171–81, 1970.
60. Pryor, D.S. Splenectomy in tropical splenomegaly. *Br. Med. J.* **ii**: 825–8, 1967.
61. Blendis, L.M., Ramboer, C. & Williams, R. Studies on the haemodilution

anaemia of splenomegaly. *Eur. J. Clin. Invest.* **1**: 54–64, 1970.

62. Hess, C.E., Ayers, C.R., Wetzel, R.A. *et al.* Dilutional anaemia of splenomegaly: an indication for splenectomy. *Ann. Surg.* **173**: 693–9, 1971.

63. Castro-Malaspina, H., Najean, Y. & Flandrin, G. Erythrokinetic studies in hairy cell leukaemia. *Br. J. Haematol.* **42**: 189–97, 1979.

64. Burger, T. & Schmelczer, M. Comparative study of platelet kinetics with [75]Semethionine and ^{51}Cr in ITP and congestive splenomegaly. *Folia Hematol. (Leipz.)* **100**: 278–89, 1973.

65. Fieschi, A. & Sacchetti, C. Clinical assessment of granulopoiesis. *Acta Haematol. (Basel)* **31**: 150–62, 1964.

66. Scott, J.L., McMillan, R., Davidson, J.G. & Marino, J.V. Leukocyte labelling with [51]chromium. II. Leukocyte kinetics in chronic myelocytic leukaemia. *Blood* **38**: 162–73, 1971.

67. Chauffard, M.A. Pathogene de l'ictere congenital de l'adulte. *Semaine Medicale, Paris* **27**: 25, 1907.

68. Dameshek, W. Hypersplenism. *Bull. N.Y. Acad. Med.* **31**: 113–36, 1955.

69. Doan, C.A. Hypersplenism. *Bull. N.Y. Acad. Med.* **25**: 625–50, 1949.

70. Dacie, J.V., Brain, M.C., Harrison, C.V. *et al.* 'Non-tropical idiopathic splenomegaly' (primary hypersplenism): a review of ten cases and their relationship to malignant lymphomas. *Br. J. Haematol.* **17**: 317–33, 1969.

71. Armas-Cruz, R., Yazigi, R., Lopez, O. *et al.* Portal cirrhosis: an analysis of 208 cases with correlations of clinical, laboratory and autopsy findings. *Gastroenterology* **17**: 327–43, 1951.

72. Dacie, J.V., Galton, D.A.G., Gordon-Smith, E.C. & Harrison, C.V. Non-tropical 'idiopathic splenomegaly': a follow-up study of ten patients described in 1969. *Br. J. Haematol.* **38**: 185–93, 1978.

73. Pitney, W.R. The tropical splenomegaly syndrome. *Trans. R. Soc. Trop. Med. Hyg.* **62**: 717–28, 1968.

74. Pryor, D.S. Tropical splenomegaly in New Guinea. *Q. J. Med.* **36**: 321–36, 1967.

75. Marsden, P.D., Hutt, M.S.R., Wilks, N.E. *et al.* An investigation of tropical splenomegaly at Mulago Hospital, Kampala, Uganda. *Br. Med. J.* **i**: 89–92, 1965.

76. Pitney, W.R., Pryor, D.S. & Tait, S.M. Morphological observations on livers and spleens of patients with tropical splenomegaly in New Guinea. *J. Pathol. Bacteriol.* **95**: 417–22, 1968.

77. Leather, H.M. Portal hypertension and gross splenomegaly in Uganda. *Br. Med. J.* **i**: 15–18, 1961.

78. Wells, J.V. Serum immunoglobulin levels in tropical splenomegaly syndrome in New Guinea. *Clin. Exp. Immunol.* **3**: 943–51, 1968.

79. Fakunle, Y.M. Tropical splenomegaly Part 1. Tropical Africa. *Clin. Haematol.* **10**: 963–75, 1981.

80. Gebbie, D.A.M., Hamilton, P.J.S., Hutt, M.S.R. *et al.* Malarial antibodies in idiopathic splenomegaly in Uganda. *Lancet* **ii**: 392–3, 1964.

81. Watson-Williams, E.J. & Allen, N.C. Idiopathic tropical splenomegaly syndrome in Ibadan. *Br. Med. J.* **iv**: 793–6, 1968.

82. Watson-Williams, E.J., Allan, N.C. & Fleming, A.F. 'Big spleen' disease. *Br. Med. J.* **iv**: 416–17, 1967.

83. Patrick, A.D. A deficiency of glucocerebrosidase in Gaucher's disease. *Biochem. J.* **97**: 17c–18c, 1965.

84. Brady, R.O., Kanfer, J.N., Bradley, R.M. & Shapiro, D. Demonstration of a deficiency of glucocerebroside-clearing enzyme in Gaucher's disease. *J. Clin. Invest.* **45**: 1112–15, 1966.

85. Pennelli, N., Scaravilli, F. & Zacchello, F. The morphogenesis of Gaucher cells investigated by electron microscopy. *Blood* **34**: 331–47, 1969.

86. Crocker, A.C. & Farber, S. Niemann–Pick disease: a review of eighteen patients. *Medicine* **37**: 1–95, 1958.

87. Eichner, E.R. & Whitfield, C.L. Splenomegaly: an algorithmic approach to diagnosis. *J. Am. Med. Asscoc.* **246**: 2858–61, 1981.
88. Mall, J.C. & Kaiser, J.A. CT diagnosis of splenic laceration. *Am. J. Roent.* **134**: 265–9, 1980.
89. Liu Yin, J.A. Spontaneous splenic rupture in acute monocytic leukaemia. *Eur. J. Haematol.* **40**: 279, 1988.
90. Hermann, R.E., DeHaven, K.E. & Hawk, W.A. Splenectomy for the diagnosis of splenomegaly. *Ann. Surg.* **168**: 896–900, 1968.

15

Cytogenetic abnormalities

J.D.M. Richards
Consultant Haematologist and Physician, University College Hospital, London, UK

S.J. Russell
Clinical Research Fellow, Chester Beatty Research Institute, London, UK

H. Walker
Senior Cytogeneticist, University College Hospital, London, UK

This chapter describes the two categories of cytogenetic disease – congenital and acquired – which are relevant to haematological and other malignancies. It is nearly 30 years since the first syndrome with an associated cytogenetic abnormality, trisomy 21 or Down's syndrome was described.[1] It had been recognized that children with Down's syndrome showed an increased frequency of acute leukaemia and it is now well-established that cytogenetic abnormalities both congenital and acquired are associated with haematological malignancies.

The Philadelphia chromosome (Ph[1]) first described in 1960[2] was recognized in 1973 as a balanced translocation,[3] by means of banding techniques described in 1971.[4] It was the only cytogenetic abnormality identified with a haematological malignancy, until new and improved techniques[5,6] led to the discovery of other chromosome abnormalities with specific associations. These include 5q−, inversion (inv)16, monosomy 7 and translocation (t), t(15;17). Many others with less specificity have been described such as t(8;21), trisomy 8, t(8;14) and i(17q).

The latest aids in the field of cytogenetics and molecular genetics are radioactive or fluorescent probes which are used to detect sub-microscopic rearrangements of genes known as oncogenes which play a major role in the leukaemogenic process.

CONGENITAL CYTOGENETIC ABNORMALITIES

Congenital and inherited cytogenetic abnormalities include Down's syndrome, trisomy 18, Turner's and Klinefelter's syndromes and diseases of DNA repair mechanisms such as Fanconi's anaemia and Bloom's syndrome which exhibit distinct cytogenetic abnormalities in the form of chromosome damage.

Down's syndrome

Down's syndrome (DS) was the first congenital chromosome abnormality to be described (in 1959), but long before the cytogenetic abnormality trisomy 21 was discovered the increased risk of leukaemia in patients with DS was apparent, but unexplained.[7] Children and adolescents with DS appear to have a 10- to 30-fold increased incidence of leukaemia, but proportionally, DS is seen with equal frequency among patients with acute lymphoblastic leukaemia (ALL) and acute non-lymphoblastic leukaemia (ANLL).[9]

A hypothesis for the underlying mechanism for the development of leukaemia in patients with DS has been proposed. In AML M2 type (French–American–British classification) about 18% of individuals have a t(8;21) wth the breakpoint localized to q22 on chromosome 21. Trisomy 21 is a commonly observed chromosome abnormality in leukaemia, particularly in children.

Leukaemia is thought to be caused by an alteration in the activity of oncogenes and an oncogene *ets*-2 has been mapped to the region of q22 involved in the t(8;21) translocation. Trisomy 21 or its involvement in the t(8;21) translocation may lead to the alteration of the *ets*-2 oncogene activity or, in the case of trisomy 21, to its amplification and thus lead to leukaemia.[9]

Retinoblastoma

Retinoblastoma is the classic inherited tumour, but it also occurs sporadically. It occurs at a frequency of 1:80,000 and is the cause of 1% of cancer deaths in children and 5% of blindness. Forty per cent of cases are hereditary and tend to appear earlier and are often bilateral. The remaining cases are sporadic and unilateral.

Children with retinoblastoma in association with congenital malformations and mental retardation almost always have a specific abnormality of chromosome 13, a deletion at 13q14. They appear to be hemizygous for a gene relating to retinoblastoma formation so that a subsequent spontaneous mutation or chromosome abnormality at the same place on the homologous chromosome, or even loss of this homologous chromosome starts the tumour.

The gene for esterase D is closely linked to the retinoblastoma gene and is included in this step-wise decrease in dosage of the latter.[10]

Abnormalities involving chromosomes other than 13 have been reported, and in a recent review of some 82 cases of retinoblastoma, recurrent abnormalities of chromosomes in addition to those of 13 (21% of cases) included copies of chromosome 1q material (44%), isochromosome 6p (45%), monosomy 16 (18%), marker 1p$^+$ (13%) and homogeneously staining regions and double minutes (9%).[11]

Cured retinoblastoma patients do run an increased risk of developing secondary tumours, especially osteogenic sarcomas. Cases of ALL have been reported.[12]

Diseases of DNA repair

There is a group of systemic diseases loosely grouped together, as they are associated with increased sensitivity to one or more of the DNA-damaging agents which include ionizing radiation, UV light and chemical mutagens. This sensitivity can be manifested cytogenetically as chromosome damage in cultured lymphocytes or fibroblasts or as molecular lesions measured as excision repair using chemical or enzymatic means.

These diseases include ataxia telangiectasia, Bloom's syndrome, Cockayne syndrome, Fanconi's anaemia and xeroderma pigmentosum. Individually these diseases occur very infrequently varying from 1:40,000 for ataxia telangiectasia to 1:250,000 for xeroderma pigmentosum. They are autosomally recessively inherited, but together form an interesting group, some of which frequently progress to some form of malignancy.

Table 15.1 indicates the common features of these diseases including cytogenetic abnormalities and cellular sensitivity to various damaging agents.

Ataxia telangiectasia

Ataxia telangiectasia (AT) is a multi-system disorder characterized by cerebellar ataxia, oculocutaneous telangiectasia, paranasal and pulmonary infections, high incidence of neoplasia and variable immunodeficiency. It is associated with disordered cell growth and shows chromosome sensitivity to chemical and physical agents and ionizing radiation. The thymus in these patients has an embryonic appearance and is associated with disorders of T-cell-mediated immunity.

Most patients with AT have an immunodeficiency that includes the inability to produce antigen-specific, self-restricted cytotoxic T-lymphocytes to viral pathogens. This lack of immune cytotoxic killer production may contribute to the incidence of increased infections and neoplasia seen in these patients. Progression to Hodgkin's disease, non-Hodgkin's lymphoma, acute or chronic lymphocytic leukaemia is common. In fact several workers have described a chromosome abnormality in AT involving the terminal band of chromosome 14q, the site of the t(8;14) seen in lymphomas.

Chromosome damage in the form of fragments, chromatid breaks and gaps, and dicentrics is increased in patients with AT, but may not be seen in all patients.[13] However, chromosomal rearrangements or translocations occur more often, i.e.frequency about 40 times higher than in normal cells, with chromosomes 7 and 14 frequently involved.[14] As previously mentioned, cells from patients with AT are hypersensitive to induction of chromosome aberrations by ionizing radiation and show 3- to 15-fold increase in chromosome deletions, gaps, breaks and exchanges compared with normal controls. The proportion of clonally abnormal cells in patients with AT may vary during the course of the disease and in patients who develop T-cell lymphocytic leukaemia the appearance of the abnormalities may well precede the leukaemia.

Table 15.1 Cytogenetic Features of Diseases of DNA Repair and Their Sensitivities

| | Intrinsic chromosome damage | SCE raised | Cells sensitive to UV light | Cells sensitive to X-ray | Malignancies | |
					Solid	Haematological
Ataxia telangiectasia	+	−	−	+	Infrequent	Common
Bloom's syndrome	+	+	−	+	Infrequent	Common
Cockayne syndrome	−	−	+	−	N/A	N/A
Fanconi's anaemia	+	−	+	−	Infrequent	Common
Xeroderma pigmentosum	−	−	+	−	Common	Infrequent

SCE = Sister chromatid exchange

Bloom's syndrome

Patients with Bloom's syndrome (BS) characteristically present with dwarfism of low birth weight type and adults rarely reach a height of 5 feet. There is severe immune deficiency leading to respiratory and gastro-intestinal infections. The face is thin with a relatively large nose and a sun-sensitive erythema. Clinodactyly and vitiligo or 'spotty' hyperpigmentation may occur.[15] As with other diseases of DNA repair there is an increased risk of cancer, predominantly acute leukaemia, with approximately one-quarter of reported cases developing a malignancy.

Cytogenetically the disease is characterized by spontaneously occurring chromosome damage with homologous chromatid exchange. Both sister chromatid exchange and mitotic crossing over may lead to formation of tri- or quadriradial chromosomes. There is a tendency for somatic cells to fuse spontaneously, a phenomenon usually seen only when one cell is malignant. Evidence for this is the presence of prematurely condensed chromosomes (PCC).[16] The most characteristic cytogenetic features in BS are the increased rate of sister chromatid exchange (SCE) (the exchange of chromatin between sister chromatids) and the high incidence of mitotic chiasmata, crossing of chromatids, both occurring during mitosis.[17] SCE is demonstrated by growing phytohaemagglutinin (PHA)-stimulated lympho-cytes in the presence of 5-bromodeoxyuridine (BrdU), a thymidine substitute, for two entire replication cycles. The BrdU-substituted DNA fluoresces less intensely than the non-substituted DNA, when stained with a fluorochrome dye such as 33258 Hoechst and appears pale when subsequently stained with Giemsa. The points of exchange can be clearly seen as a harlequin pattern.[18]

If BS cells are hybridized with normal cells the high level of SCE can be corrected. However, if BS cells are merely cocultivated with normal cells, different effects have been shown. Some workers have found SCE rates in the BS cells to be corrected but others have found that the SCE rate in the normal cells increases.[19]

The non-random mitotic chiasmata seen in the Q dark regions on chromosomes may be important in leading the homozygosity of some cancer-causing genes[20] or to rearrangements or amplification of these genes. It has been suggested that there is some association between oncogenes, consistent cancer chromosome breakpoints and chiasma-rich regions as seen in BS, and these factors may be related to the very high frequency of cancers seen in BS patients.[21]

Cockayne syndrome

Cockayne syndrome (CS) is characterized clinically by cachetic dwarfism, progressive mental and physical retardation, unsteady gait and tremor, intracranial calcification, perceptive deafness, retinitis pigmentosa and a loss of facial adipose tissue giving a premature ageing appearance.

Cultivated fibroblasts from patients with CS are sensitive to UV light but not to ionizing radiation, sharing this latter feature with xeroderma pigmentosum (XP) cells. CS cells have the ability to excise UV light-induced pyrimidine dimers with the same efficiency as normal cells.[22]

Unlike the other diseases of DNA repair with their associated chromosome damage CS is not associated with spontaneous chromosome damage or an increased rate of carcinogenesis.[23]

Fanconi's anaemia

Fanconi's anaemia (FA) is characterized by a diversity of clinical manifestations with a progressive failure of the bone marrow in combination with one or more congenital malformations which include failure to thrive, hypoplastic thumbs, absent pinnae, renal abnormalities and cafe-au-lait pigmentation.[24] The bone marrow failure involves all series and patients who do not die from marrow failure have an increased risk of developing leukaemia or solid tumours.[25]

Cytogenetically the diagnosis of FA is made because of the intrinsic chromosome damage seen in cultured lymphocytes. In the absence of any of the classic clinical features of FA but where there is an aplastic anaemia, a cytogenetic stress test using a bifunctional alkylating agent, mitomycin C (MMC), can be used in the differential diagnosis of FA. With this test patients with FA show chromosome damage up to 50 times the spontaneous breakage rate. The increase in exchange figures is up to 200 times higher than seen spontaneously. Patients with acquired aplastic anaemia show a response to the MMC stress test comparable with control subjects.[26]

Antenatal diagnosis of FA is possible as the intrinsic chromosome damage is apparent before the disease is manifest.[27]

Unlike other diseases of DNA repair, the bone marrow failure of FA can be treated. The patients usually will respond to treatment with androgens and corticosteroids early in their disease. Bone marrow transplantation (BMT) offers the chance of a cure for the bone marrow aplasia.[28]

A careful study of sibling donors is done to exclude the possibility of transplanting with a non-manifest affected homozygote. Detection of the obligate heterozygote condition is more problematical than was imagined.[29]

Xeroderma pigmentosum

Xeroderma pigmentosum (XP) is clinically manifested by abnormal skin pigmentation which develops in response to exposure to sunlight. Malignant tumours, especially basal cell and squamous cell carcinomas, subsequently develop. Less frequently XP patients have neurological abnormalities and mental retardation.[30] The most striking feature of these patients and what indeed may be the underlying cause of the malignant clinical manifestations is the inability of XP cells *in vivo* and *in vitro* to repair DNA damaged by UV light.[31]

Chromosome damage has not been described as occurring with high frequency in XP, and SCE in XP has been shown to be normal.[15] Most work on XP has been done on cultivated fibroblast lines derived from patients and their families. There is a class of XP patients who clinically manifest the disease, but whose cells do not show the repair defects. However, these variant XP patients when tested with a host-cell reactivation technique showed defects in the repair of DNA damaged by irradiation when compared with normal cells.[32]

Repair replication of DNA occurs at a reduced rate or not at all in XP cells after UV irradiation. XP cells are defective in the endonuclease-mediated chain breakage which constitutes the initial step in dimer excision after UV irradiation and subsequent repair of the affected DNA strand.[33] Double strand breaks induced by ionizing radiation in XP fibroblasts do not differ in production or repair when compared with normal cells.

Clearly these five syndromes are not the only diseases to fall into the broad category of diseases of DNA repair. There are other conditions which demonstrate one or more of the characteristics seen in the diseases described. Unlike the syndromes discussed they do not necessarily have a higher incidence of neoplasia than the general population. These diseases include incontinentia pigmenti,[34] scleroderma,[35] porokeratosis of Mibelli,[36] glutathione reductase deficiency,[37] Kostmann's agranulocytosis,[38] and basal cell naevus (Gorlin's) syndrome.[39]

FRAGILE SITES AND ONCOGENES IN HAEMATOLOGICAL MALIGNANCIES

The study of fragile sites and oncogenes has intensified during the last 4 years since the localization of the c-*abl* oncogene to the breakpoint on chromosome 9 involved in the t(9;22) seen in CGL.[69] Fragile sites and oncogenes seem to be linked with the neoplastic process and an introduction to them precedes the section on the acquired cytogenetic abnormalities in haematological disease.

Fragile sites were discovered in 1965,[40] but active interest in them began in the late 1970s when the fragile X was recognized in association with, or possibly the cause of, one form of X-linked mental retardation in both males and females.[41] Fragile sites can be divided into two major groups: heritable and common.[42] The heritable fragile sites are classified according to the culture conditions under which they are expressed and fall into three groups: folate-sensitive sites, Distamycin A-inducible fragile sites and 5-bromodeoxyuridine-requiring fragile sites. Common fragile sites are usually only seen in a small percentage of metaphases but are weakly induced by the same conditions that induce the folate-sensitive sites and are more strongly induced by aphidicolin.[43]

Cytologically the appearance of fragile sites is variable but there are several essential properties of heritable fragile sites.[44,45]

1. the fragile site is a non-staining gap of varying width, usually involving both chromatids;
2. the fragile site is always at the same point in an individual or kindred;
3. the fragile site is inherited in a Mendelian co-dominant fashion; and
4. the fragile site is evidenced by acentric fragments, deleted chromosomes, figures, etc.

The fragile X chromosome is of particular interest clinically as alone among fragile sites it appears to disturb development. Males with fragile X are usually mentally retarded and a sizeable proportion of females with fragile X are also affected. The fragile X is second only to trisomy 21 (DS) as the most common abnormality among the mentally retarded. However, the majority of fragile sites have not been associated with disease, though fragile sites have been implicated in the pathogenesis of human neoplasia.

A relationship between the fragile sites and breakpoints that occur in the non-random abnormalities associated with leukaemia and lymphoma has been found by several workers[46-48] and a statistically significant association between 21 fragile sites and 50 cancer-specific breakpoints was accepted by the Seventh Human Gene Mapping Workshop 1983.[49] Of 11 fragile sites which occur in chromosome bands that are involved in non-random abnormalities in human neoplasias, ten are recognized heritable fragile sites and one is a common fragile site (see Table 15.2 and Fig. 15.1).

Certain fragile sites at cancer breakpoints appear to involve oncogenes and transforming sequences.[50] In addition, other genes have been mapped to chromosomal regions which are breakpoints in cancer cells and are also the location of fragile sites. These genes include the α- and β-interferons and the metallothionein family of genes.[51,52]

There are many unanswered questions in the field of fragile sites and cancer. The function and identity of genes located at the fragile sites are unknown. Some fragile sites are inherited and may be related to a genetic predisposition to the development of malignancies.

Table 15.2   Leukaemia, Lymphoma and Other Tumour Breakpoints Coinciding with Fragile Sites

Fragile site	Rearrangement	Neoplasia
3p14[a]	[del(3)(p14p23)]	Solid tumours
6p23	t(6;9)(p23;q34)	ANLL
7p11	t(1;7)(p11;p11)	ANLL, MPD, MDS
8q22	t(8;21)(q22;q22)	AML-M2
9p21	t(9;11)(p21p22;q23)	AMoL
	del(9p)	ALL
10q25	t(10;14)(q24-25;q11)	ALL, NHL (T-cell origin)
11q13	t(10;11)(p14;q13-14)	AMoL
	t(11;14)(q13;q32)	ALL, NHL, CLL
11q23	t with 2,4,6,9,10,14,17,19	NHL, ALL, ANLL, AMoL, AMML
12q13	del(12q) t(12q)	Salivary gland tumours
	dup(12)(q13;q22)	NHL
16q22	inv(16)(p13;q22)	AMML
	del(16)q22	AMML
	t(16;16)(q13;q22)	AMML
17p12	iso,dic(17p)	CML, ANLL

[a] Common fragile site.

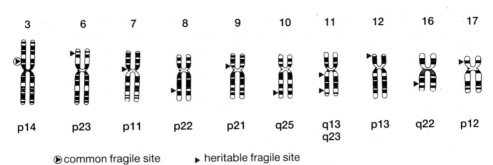

Fig. 15.1. Diagram showing 11 fragile sites coinciding with breakpoints in human tumours.

Oncogenes and tumour suppressor genes

The processes of cell proliferation and differentiation are subject to complex networks of control processes which vary according to cell type and involve both positive and negative regulatory proteins. Genetic alterations may change the level of expression or specific activity of the proteins involved in such networks, sometimes resulting in increased tendency to proliferate with loss of ability to differentiate. Accumulation of genetic alterations of this nature may transform the cell to a malignant phenotype with serious consequences for the organism.

Oncogenes

Oncogenes are dominantly or co-dominantly acting genes with cellular transforming activity (for comprehensive reviews see Refs 53–55). They are often derived from normal cellular counterparts (proto-oncogenes) through a variety of genetic alterations which result either in altered control of gene expression or altered activity of the protein for which the gene codes. The mechanisms whereby oncogenes may be derived from proto-oncogenes include retroviral transduction, insertional mutagenesis, chromosomal translocation, gene amplification and point mutation.

Retroviral insertional mutagenesis.   When retroviral RNA enters a cell it is copied into DNA which integrates at a random site into a host-cell chromosome, and subsequently directs synthesis of its own RNA. If integration happens to occur close to or within a normally regulated cellular proto-oncogene, the viral DNA can direct uncontrolled transcription of the oncogene, resulting in cell transformation. This process is termed insertional mutagenesis and occurs, for example, in murine mammary tumour virus (MMTV)-induced breast cancer in mice through activation of the proto-oncogenes *int*-1 and *int*-2.[56]

Retroviral transduction.   Recombination between retroviral and cellular genomes may result in implantation of a cellular proto-oncogene (which may be mutated in the process) into the viral genome. Such a virus can direct synthesis of the transforming oncogene product. Many of the currently known proto-oncogenes were discovered as a result of the study of these 'acutely transforming retroviruses'. When the viral oncogenes had been identified, it was possible to construct DNA probes with which to scan the cellular genome for homologous proto-oncogenes. Examples include c-*ras*, c-*abl*, c-*myc*, c-*sis* and c-*myb*.

Chromosomal translocation.   The study of retroviral transduction and insertional mutagenesis facilitated the discovery of many of the currently known proto-oncogenes, but although these processes contribute to tumorigenesis in laboratory animals there is very little evidence to date to suggest that they are important in humans. However, this situation may change as a result of the recent discovery of possible retroviral particles in the monocytes of patients with breast cancer.[57]

Chromosomal translocations, on the other hand, are common in a variety of human malignancies and careful molecular analysis of the chromosomal breakpoints has revealed the frequent involvement of proto-oncogenes whose level of expression or specific activity is increased as a result of translocation to a new genetic environment. Several specific examples such as c-*myc* translocation in Burkitt's lymphoma and c-*abl* translocation in chronic granulocytic leukaemia are discussed in the following sections. In addition, new proto-oncogenes have been discovered as a result of the study of translocation breakpoints, such as *bcl*-2 in non-Hodgkin's lymphoma.[58]

Gene amplification.   Cytogenetic studies of human malignancies sometimes reveal double-minute chromosomes or homogenously staining regions which disrupt the normal banding patterns of chromosomes. These abnormalities are due to amplification of specific domains within chromosomes, often containing proto-oncogenes. Such proto-oncogene amplification often affects genes with homology to c-*myc* (N-*myc*, L-*myc*) and is thought to be important in progression, rather than initiation, of the neoplastic phenotype.

Point mutations.   Transfection of DNA from malignant cells into cell lines such as NIH 3T3 may result in transformation to neoplastic growth. Such gene transfer experiments have resulted in the discovery of oncogenes which have arisen by mutation of normal cellular genes. The most commonly identified oncogene in these assays is a mutant c-*ras* containing point mutations which result in amino acid substitutions at positions 12, 13 or 61 in the protein product.[59] It should be pointed out that NIH 3T3 cells are abnormal, immortalized mouse fibroblasts which are teetering on the brink of neoplastic transformation. The transfected oncogene merely provides the final step required for truly neoplastic growth.

How do oncogenes transform cells?   As was mentioned earlier, proto-oncogenes code for proteins which are important in the complex process of growth control. The expression of these genes is switched on and off at appropriate moments during the lifetime of the cell in response to diverse signals which are transduced via cell membrane, cytoplasmic or nuclear receptors. The finer details of these growth signal transduction pathways have not yet been worked out, but are sufficiently understood to allow some insight into the mechanism of oncogene action.

Oncogenes may be divided into four broad categories based on their mechanisms or site of action within the cell:

1. Nuclear proteins, e.g. c-*myc*, c-*fos*, c-*myb*,
2. Protein kinases
   a. Tyrosine, e.g. c-*erb*B, c-*fms*, c-*abl*, c-*src*
   b. Serine-threonine, e.g. c-*mos*, c-*raf*
3. GTP-binding proteins, e.g. c-Ha-*ras*, c-Ki-*ras*
4. Growth factors, e.g. c-*sis*

Nuclear proteins.   The mechanism of action of these nuclear proteins is very poorly understood, but they are believed to bind to DNA, possibly regulating the transcription of other sets of genes. Their importance in cellular proliferation is suggested by higher levels of expression in dividing cells and activation of transcription following exposure of cells to appropriate growth factors. However, high levels of *myc* are also seen in mature macrophages.

The best example of a cell cycle-dependent gene is *myb*, with maximal expression during G1.[60] It seems likely that continued non-suppressible (constitutive) expression of these genes is responsible for their cell-transforming activity. Activation of c-*myc* in Burkitt's lymphoma is a good example which is discussed in the section on lymphomas.

Protein kinases.   The activity of a vast number of cellular enzymes may be regulated by phosphorylation and dephosphorylation. It is therefore not surprising that protein kinases represent an important component of cellular signal transduction pathways.

(a) Tyrosine kinases. The first tyrosine protein kinase to be identified was the 60 kDa protein encoded by the *src* oncogene of Rous sarcoma virus.[61] Since then, several other oncogene proteins have been shown to possess tyrosine kinase activity. In general, the normal cellular homologues of these enzymes have lower activity, which suggests that increased oncogene-directed phosphorylation of some critical protein contributes to cell transformation. However, although several proteins are known to be phosphorylated on tyrosine, the critical target protein(s) has not yet been identified.

Two of the oncogenes in this class bear a close resemblance to cellular growth factor receptors, *erb*B with epidermal growth factor (EGF) receptor[62] and *fms* with the macrophage colony stimulating factor (M-CSF) receptor. The *erb*B oncogene represents a truncated EGF receptor which has lost its ligand-binding domain but retains the intracytoplasmic domain which is necessary for tyrosine kinase activity.

(b) Serine-threonine kinases. Serine/threonine protein kinases are activated as part of two important transmembrane signalling pathways, both of which involve G-proteins. Membrane G-proteins may activate either adenylate cyclase or phospholipase C. Adenylate cyclase catalyses generation of cyclic-AMP (cAMP) which is an activator of protein kinase A.

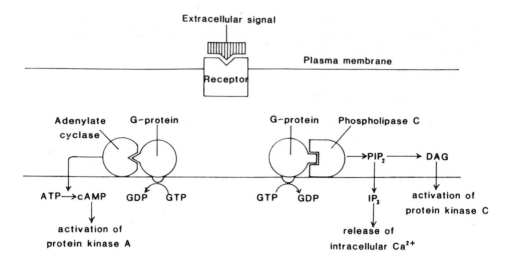

Fig. 15.2. Diagram illustrating the central role played by membrane G-proteins in the transduction of extracellular signals to the cell interior (see text for details). PIP₂, phosphatidylinositol-6-phosphate; IP₃, inositol triphosphate; DAG, diacylglycerol; cAMP, cyclic-AMP.

Phospholipase C cleaves membrane phosphatidylinositol biphosphate (PIP_2) into inositol triphosphate (IP_3) and diacylglycerol (DAG). IP_3 stimulates release of calcium from intracellular stores, while DAG activates protein kinase C (see Fig. 15.2).

Many cellular signals are transduced via these two pathways. It is therefore not surprising that oncogenes with serine/threonine kinase activity have been identified.

GTP (guanosine triphosphate)-binding proteins.   The cell membrane GTP-binding or G-proteins consist of α, β and γ subunits. The α subunit has GTP-binding and GTPase activity and in the resting state binds to the β/γ subunit. Upon stimulation of the appropriate cellular receptor, the α subunit binds GTP, dissociates from the β/γ subunit and activates either adenylate cyclase or phospholipase C. The intrinsic GTPase activity of the α subunit ensures hydrolysis of bound GTP to GDP with consequent loss of catalytic activity and reassociation with the β/γ subunit.

Mutant *ras* oncogenes possess GTP-binding and GTPase activity and are associated with the cytoplasmic side of the plasma membrane. The amino acid substitutions at positions 12, 13 and 61 which confer oncogenic activity on the *ras* proteins are known to result in decreased GTPase activity and hence persistent activation following GTP binding. In contrast to the G-proteins mentioned earlier, the signal transmitted by the activated *ras* protein has not been clearly identified although recent evidence suggests activation of phospholipase C.[63]

Growth factors.   As the amino acid sequence of platelet-derived growth factor (PDGF) was being fed into a computer database, it became clear that the oncogene *sis* had extensive homology with the PDGF B chain.[64] Also, the oncogene *int*-2 resembles fibroblast growth factor.

Tumour suppressor genes

There is an increasing body of evidence for the existence of genes which are capable of suppressing the malignant phenotypes.[65] These genes presumably code for proteins whose function is to regulate cell proliferation and/or to stimulate differentiation. Loss or inactivation of both copies of these genes appears to contribute to the multi-step process of carcinogenesis. Evidence for tumour suppressor genes and their involvement in carcinogenesis comes from the study of tumours for which a predisposition is inherited, somatic cell hybridization, 'normal' revertants of transformed cell lines, and induction of differentiation of tumour cell lines.

Hereditary tumours

Retinoblastoma (discussed in detail earlier) is the prototype for the model of carcinogenesis resulting from loss of both alleles of a tumour suppressor gene located on chromosome 13q14. The gene from this locus has recently been cloned and lack of expression has been demonstrated in both retinoblastoma and osteosarcoma. Cytogenetic evidence exists for similar homozygous or hemizygous recessive mutations affecting tumour suppressor genes in several other tumours such as small cell lung carcinoma, Wilms' tumour and hepatoblastoma.

Somatic cell hybridization

When malignant cells are fused with normal fibroblasts the resulting hybrids are non-tumorigenic provided they retain certain specific chromosomes donated by the fibroblast. Loss of these chromosomes is associated with re-emergence of the malignant phenotype.[66] The inference is that there are tumour suppressor genes on these critical chromosomes which are inactivated in the original tumour. The 'critical' chromosome may vary between different tumours.

Revertants

It is possible *in vitro* to isolate normal revertants of transformed cell lines and to study the mechanisms of reversion. Inactivation of the transforming oncogene may be responsible for reversion, but more interesting revertants continue to express the transforming protein and are resistant to retransformation by the same oncogene. This suggests that the malignant phenotype has been suppressed either by a suppressor protein or by mutational inactivation of an important protein in the transformation pathway. A recent study of revertants of v-*fos* transformed rat fibroblasts gave support to the latter possibility.[66]

Differentiation of tumour cell lines

Strong differentiation signals may result in terminal differentiation of tumour cell lines derived from promyelocytic leukaemia, erythroleukaemia and a variety of other tumours. This suggests that genes which cause cell differentiation can suppress the response to a strong proliferative stimulus.

Conclusion

In summary, cancer may be viewed as a breakdown in the normal regulation of cell growth and differentiation due to the accumulation of genetic changes. Mutation or overexpression of genes which stimulate cell division (proto-oncogenes) and deletion or inactivation of genes which inhibit cell division and stimulate differentiation (tumour suppressor genes) are the building blocks of cell transformation. Understanding of these genetic changes is advancing at a very rapid pace.

ACQUIRED CYTOGENETIC ABNORMALITIES IN HAEMATOLOGICAL MALIGNANCIES

Since the Philadelphia chromosome was originally described in chronic granulocytic leukaemia (CGL),[2] it has become clear that the majority of haematological malignancies may be associated with acquired clonal cytogenetic abnormalities. Many specific cytogenetic–clinicopathological associations have been discovered, contributing greatly to the classification of leukaemias and lymphomas and providing important prognostic information which frequently influences treatment strategy.

More detailed studies of the chromosomal breakpoints and rearrangements at the genetic and molecular level are providing exciting new insights into the mechanisms of malignant transformation of cells.

Space precludes a detailed consideration of all the clonal cytogenetic abnormalities identified to date in haematological malignancies but an attempt has been made to give the reader an overview of the more common examples, with more detailed discussion of abnormalities which illustrate important principles or advances in our understanding of the mechanisms producing leukaemia and lymphoma.

Chronic granulocytic leukaemia

Chronic granulocytic leukaemia (CGL) is a disease characterized by malignant proliferation of a pluripotent bone marrow stem cell. Initially the disease runs a chronic course but eventual acceleration and/or blastic transformation results in rapid clinical deterioration and death. Allogeneic bone marrow transplantation during the chronic phase currently gives the best chance of a cure.

In 1960 Nowell and Hungerford described a shortened chromosome 22, designated the Philadelphia (Ph[1]) chromosome in CGL.[2] This cytogenetic abnormality has subsequently been identified as a balanced reciprocal translocation between chromosomes 9 and 22 (t(9;22)(q34;q11))[68] and is seen in 90% of cases of CGL.[3] The translocation results in the movement of two known cellular oncogenes into a new genetic environment. The c-*sis* oncogene which codes for one of the two chains constituting platelet-derived growth factor moves with the long arm of chromosome 22 to chromosome 9, while the c-*abl* oncogene (cellular homologue of the v-*abl* oncogene product of Abelson murine leukaemia virus) moves from the long arm of chromosome 9 to chromosome 22. Studies of variant translocations have indicated that the consistent rearrangement is translocation of genetic material from chromosome 9 to chromosome 22,[69] and c-*sis* transcription has not been demonstrated in the malignant cells of patients with CGL.[70] It has therefore been concluded that c-*sis* is not important in the pathogenesis of CGL, although this view has been contested.[71]

The breakpoint on chromosome 22 occurs at a variable site within a 5.8 kilobase segment of DNA termed the breakpoint cluster region or *bcr*.[72] The 5' end of the c-*abl* oncogene from chromosome 9 fuses with the *bcr*, resulting in production of a hybrid *bcr/abl* mRNA coding for a 210 kDa protein (p210[*bcr/abl*]) with higher tyrosine-specific protein kinase activity than the normal 145 kDa c-*abl* gene product.[73,74] This protein is thought to be critical in the pathogenesis of CGL and can transform cells of the haemopoietic lineage *in vitro*.[75] The *bcr/abl* rearrangement has been demonstrated in Ph[1]-negative CGL, further supporting the importance of p210[*bcr/abl*]. However, it has recently been argued that the initial pathogenetic event in CGL is not the Ph[1] translocation, but an increase in the activity of platelet DNA polymerase (PDP), an enzyme with reverse transcriptase activity which could cause the Ph[1] translocation.[71]

From the clinical point of view the Ph[1] translocation remains an important disease marker, both for confirming the diagnosis and for assessing the response to various forms of treatment. The significance of the presence of some cytogenetically normal clones in some cases of Ph[1]-positive CGL remains undecided. If such clones represent normal haemopoietic precursors which are not involved in the leukaemic process, then cure using high-dose chemotherapy might be possible. If, on the other hand, such cytogenetically normal clones represent pre-Ph[1]-positive leukaemic cells, then modification of cell behaviour or allogeneic bone marrow transplantation would appear to be more logical approaches to treatment.

Blastic transformation of CGL

Progression of CGL from chronic phase to blast crisis is usually associated with the acquisition of new cytogenetic abnormalities in addition to the Ph[1] chromosome. This chromosome clonal evolution is non-random, with three major changes (+8, +Ph[1], i(17q)) occurring either alone or in combination in 70% of cases.[76] The i(17q) abnormality is associated with myeloid differentiation of blasts and a marked basophilia but +8 and +Ph[1] are not strongly associated with any one type of blast crisis. Combinations of the above abnormalities or complex changes are associated with a worse prognosis, while loss of the Y chromosome seems to protect the cell against further clonal evolution. Between 10 and 20% of cases of CGL have abnormalities additional to the Ph[1] at the time of diagnosis and in general these patients have more aggressive disease.

Thirty per cent of patients with CGL eventually develop a lymphoid blast transformation[77] and the Ph[1] chromosome has been detected in 17–25% of adult patients with acute lymphoblastic leukaemia (ALL).[78,79] Molecular studies of Ph[1] positive ALL have revealed cases with and without the *bcr* rearrangement. The p210$^{bcr/abl}$ gene product is expressed in *bcr*-positive ALL, which is thought to represent a lymphoid blast crisis following a clinically silent phase of CGL. Conversely, *bcr*-negative ALL is characterized by a distinct p190^{c-abl} tyrosine kinase and is thought to represent ALL arising *de novo* in a more restricted precursor, since the Ph[1] translocation disappears during remission.

Research into the molecular biology of Ph[1]-positive leukaemias is moving at a rapid pace and it is hoped that it will not be long before the advent of new and effective treatment based on improved understanding of these diseases.

Myelodysplastic syndromes

The myelodysplastic syndromes (MDS) are a group of diseases characterized by disordered myelopoiesis with consequent marrow failure. There is a high incidence of progression to AML after a variable period of time. The most widely accepted classification of the MDS is the FAB classification[80] which is based on the morphological findings on peripheral blood smears and bone marrow aspirates. Five categories are recognized, all of which may be associated with dyserythropoiesis, dysgranulopoiesis or dysmegakaryo-poiesis. They are differentiated on the basis of the percentage of blasts in the bone marrow and blood, presence of ring sideroblasts and peripheral blood monocytosis (see Table 15.3).

As can be seen from Table 15.3, the most consistent cytogenetic findings in the MDS are 5q−, monosomy 7 and trisomy 8. The presence of a cytogenetic abnormality appears to place the patient in a less favourable prognostic category with increased risk of progression to acute leukaemia.[83] 5q− is easily the most common cytogenetic finding in all MDS groups except for CMML and secondary MDS. Monosomy 5, monosomy 7 and structural changes of 12p are associated with secondary MDS and hence with a particularly poor prognosis. Little is known of the mechanisms whereby cytogenetic changes in MDS contribute to disease pathogenesis but the 5q-abnormality has been most studied in this regard and will therefore be discussed in some detail.

Table 15.3 Myelodysplastic Syndromes: FAB Classification and Cytogenetic Associations

Category	Blood	Bone marrow	% with abnormal cytogenetics	Major cytogenetic abnormalities
RA – refractory anaemia	<1% blasts	< 5% blasts <15% ring sideroblasts	32[81]	5q–, +8, –7
RAS – refractory anaemia with ring sideroblasts	<1% blasts	< 5% blasts ≥15% ring sideroblasts	21[81]	5q–, +8, –7, 20q–, 11q–
RAEB – refractory anaemia with excess of blasts	<5% blasts	5–20% blasts	45[81]	5q–, +8, –7, –5
RAEB-T – refractory anaemia with excess of blasts in transformation	≥5% blasts	20–30% blasts	60[81]	
CMML – chronic myelomonocytic leukaemia	<5% blasts >1 × 10^9 monocytes	<20% blasts excess monocyte precursors	30[82]	–7, +8, 12p–

5q−

This cytogenetic abnormality is encountered in a variety of acquired haematological disorders including the MDS and both primary and secondary leukaemias. When 5q− is the sole abnormality, the patient is likely to have a stable refractory anaemia (the 5q− syndrome), while cytogenetic abnormalities additional to 5q− are more frequently found in refractory anaemia with excess of blasts (RAEB) and AML.[84]

The 5q− syndrome has been described as 'the association of an interstitial deletion of the long arm of chromosome 5 and refractory anaemia'[85] and is usually characterized by macrocytic anaemia, normal or high platelet count and hypolobulated megakaryocytes in the bone marrow smear (Fig. 15.3).

All chromosomal bands between 5q11 and 5q35 have at some time been implicated as 5q− breakpoints but altered staining of the breakage regions (prosomization) may result in inaccurate interpretation. Precise characterization of the chromosomal morphology in 15 patients with RA and 5q− revealed interstitial deletions in all patients with breakpoints consistently at sub-bands 5q13.3 proximally and 5q33.1 distally.[86]

The important result of the deletion could be either loss of a gene with anti-oncogenic activity or activation of a quiescent oncogene, although there is currently little hard evidence to support either theory. The c-*fms* oncogene, which codes for a transmembrane glycoprotein with tyrosine-specific protein kinase activity,[87] has been mapped to 5q31–33[88] and is thus deleted in 5q−. The c-*fms* gene product shows extensive homology with the

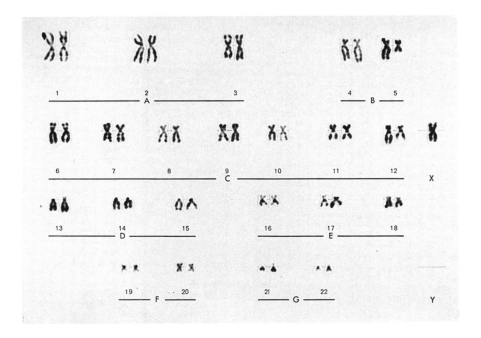

Fig. 15.3.   45,X,-X,del(5)(q13-q35) Karyotype from a patient with 5q− syndrome, also one X chromosome is missing.

receptor for granulocyte–macrophage colony stimulating factor, but it is not known how its deletion may disturb cell differentiation and proliferation.

Acute myeloid leukaemia

Acute myeloid leukaemia (AML) is a disease characterized by arrested maturation and continued proliferation of primitive bone marrow precursor cells of the myeloid lineage. The clinical features are largely secondary to the associated bone marrow failure. AML may arise suddenly in a previously fit, healthy adult (*de novo* AML) or more insidiously following a previous haematological malignancy or myelodysplastic syndrome or following chemoradiotherapy for another malignancy (secondary AML).

The disease may be classified according to morphology and cytochemical staining into seven major groups which reflect the predominant cell lineage involved and the stage at which maturation is arrested (FAB classification,[89,90] see Table 15.4). Occasionally, the disease may be unclassifiable according to this system.

Cytogenetic studies in AML have revealed some striking cytogenetic–clinicopathological associations which are emerging as important prognostic indicators, on which treatment modifications may be based. Predictably, such studies are also providing important insights into the mechanisms of leukaemogenesis.

Cytogenetic abnormalities were first related to prognosis in 1973[91] and the association has been studied by many workers since then. The most comprehensive study to date included 305 (of 660) AML cases collected at the Fourth International Workshop on Chromosomes in Leukaemia.[92] Approximately 60% of AML patients have a clonal cytogenetic abnormality, although a figure closer to 100% has been claimed by Yunis[93] with the use of methotrexate cell synchronization to give higher resolution of chromosome banding patterns. The abnormalities may broadly be divided into two groups. The first category includes those cases with fairly gross chromosomal damage, loss or gain of part or all of a chromosome or chromosomes (e.g. -7, $7q-$, -5, $5q-$, $+8$), and complex combinations of abnormalities. These findings are associated with an older age group, secondary and

Table 15.4 FAB Categories of AML

M1 Acute myeloblastic
M2 Acute myeloblastic with differentiation
M3 Promyelocytic
   M3v Microgranular variant
M4 Myelomonocytic
   M4Eo With abnormal eosinophils
M5 Monocytic
   M5a Poorly differentiated
   M5b Well-differentiated
M6 Erythroleukaemia
M7 Megakaryoblastic

Table 15.5   Prognostic Significance of Some Cytogenetic Abnormalities in AML

Low grade	inv(16), t(16;16), del(16)
Intermediate grade	t(15;17), t(8;21), t(9;11), t(6;9), +8, normal chromosomes
High grade	−7, del 7q, complex abnormalities

treatment-related AML. Tri-lineage dysplasia is frequently seen on the bone marrow smear, indicating involvement of a more primitive precursor cell and the prognosis is poor, particularly for complex abnormalities (Table 15.5).

The second broad category includes the specific recurring chromosomal rearrangements – translocations and inversions [e.g. inv(16), t(15;17), t(8;21)], which are associated with abrupt onset *de novo* AML often in patients under 60 years of age. This type of AML is associated with relatively high remission rates and intermediate or long survivals. Certain of these recurring rearrangements have been very closely associated with a specific clinico-pathologic picture. Most notable in this respect are t(15;17) and inv(16).

t(15;17)

t(15;17) was first described in M3 AML (acute promyelocytic leukaemia) in 1977[94] and since then the association has become firmly established not only in M3 AML,[95] but also in acute promyelocytic transformation of both CGL[96] and AMML.[97]

t(15;17) has never been reported in any other sub-type of leukaemia. M3 AML is a clearly identifiable sub-type in which marrow replacement by hyper- or less frequently hypogranular promyelocytes is associated with disseminated intravascular coagulation. It therefore seems that this chromosomal rearrangement leads to a specific block to maturation beyond the promyelocyte stage. The gene encoding granulocyte colony stimulating factor (G-CSF)[98] and the c-*erb*A oncogene[99] have been mapped proximal to the breakpoint on chromosome 17. It is possible that the translocation could deregulate the expression of either of these genes (Fig. 15.4).

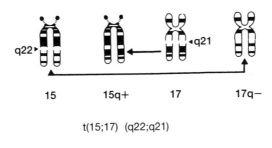

q22▸

◂q21

15   15q+   17   17q−

t(15;17) (q22;q21)

breakpoints ▸

Fig. 15.4.   Translocation between chromosomes 15 and 17.

inv(16) (Fig. 15.5)

Acute myelomonocytic leukaemia (AMML) with abnormal eosinophils (designated M4Eo by the French–American–British Co-operative Group[90]) accounts for approximately 9% of AML cases[100,101] and is invariably associated with structural abnormalities of chromosome 16 involving band q22 [(inv(16)(p13;q22)[102], t(16;16)(p13;q22),[103] del(16)(q22)[104]]. The most distinctive morphological feature of this disease is the presence of large, strongly basophilic granules in the abnormal bone marrow eosinophil myelocytes, which are present in increased numbers.[105]

AMML (M4Eo) is the best prognostic category of AML identified to date with high first and second remission rates and a median survival of greater than 2 years in those patients achieving remissions. The usual presentation is *de novo* acute leukaemia with no preceding myelodysplastic syndrome. A high incidence of CNS relapse has been observed, manifesting as leptomeningeal disease and intracerebral granulocytic sarcomas, and 'prophylactic' CNS therapy has therefore been recommended.[106]

The breakpoint on the long arm of chromosome 16 (q22) splits the metallothionein gene cluster[52] and corresponds to a recently identified chromosomal fragile site which occurs in one in 100 of the population studied and is inherited in Mendelian co-dominant fashion.[107] This fragile site has been demonstrated in the peripheral blood lymphocytes of most

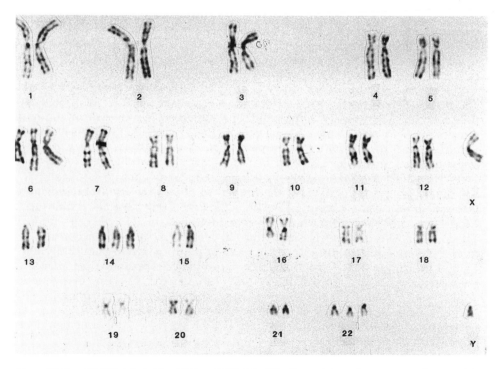

Fig. 15.5. 49,XY,+6,+14,+22,inv(16)(p13q22) Karyotype from a patient with AMML (M4Eo) with inverted chromosome 16 and additional chromosomes 6, 14 and 22.

patients with this type of AML who have been tested in remission and in their families. It has therefore been suggested that the fragile site serves as a heritable factor predisposing to chromosomal rearrangement and the development of AMML (M4Eo).

How can one explain the involvement of the metallothionein genes in leukaemogenesis? The metallothioneins are ubiquitous low molecular weight proteins which bind heavy metal ions.[108] They are probably involved in the control of cell differentiation and proliferation, scavenging of free radicals and protection against heavy metal toxicity. They can potentially modulate the activity of many metallo-enzymes.

A recently proposed mechanism for leukaemogenesis[109] suggests that phosphorylation of DNA topoisomerase by tyrosine protein kinases inhibits binding of the enzyme to DNA, thus preventing the strand breakage and ligation processes which are required for cell differentiation. It is possible that in AMML (M4Eo) disruption of the metallothionein genes results in reduced topoisomerase activity by altering the availability of heavy metal ions. Alternatively, the transcriptional control elements of the metallo-thionein gene may activate an unidentified oncogene on the short arm of chromosome 16.

Acute lymphoblastic leukaemia

Acute lymphoblastic leukaemia (ALL) is a disease characterized by malignant proliferation of a primitive lymphoid stem cell, presumably due to loss of its ability to differentiate or respond to normal growth-regulatory signals. The disease is heterogeneous and may be classified morphologically as L1, L2 or L3,[110] or with immunological markers as B, T or 'non-B non-T' (B-cell precursor).[111]

Cytogenetic studies in ALL are hampered by poor quality of metaphase preparations with highly contracted chromosomes of 'fuzzy' ill-defined morphology. Nevertheless, clonal cytogenetic abnormalities have been identified in approximately two-thirds of ALL cases and have emerged as an important prognostic indicator.[112]

At The Third International Workshop on Chromosomes in Leukaemia[113] 330 newly diagnosed patients were studied to determine the frequency and type of chromosome abnormalities in ALL and their clinical significance. Clonal chromosomal abnormalities were identified in 218 patients (66%). The patients were then classified into 10 karyotypic groups according to modal chromosome number (normal, <46-hypodipoloid, 46-pseudodiploid, 47–50-hyperdiploid A, >50-hyperdiploid B) and presence of specific recurring structural abnormalities (see Table 15.6). Certain cytogenetic abnormalities were strongly correlated with specific morphology or immunophenotype and at the most recent follow-up of this group of patients in 1985,[112] it was clear that high- and low-risk categories could be identified cytogenetically.

The best prognostic category appears to be hyperdiploidy B, while the recurring structural abnormalities carry a uniformly dismal prognosis, and the remaining categories (hypodiploid, normal, pseudodiploid and hyper-diploid A) carry an intermediate prognosis.

Table 15.6 ALL Prognosis by Karyotype From the Third International Workshop on Chromosomes in Leukaemia

Cytogenetic group	Percentage of patients (n=330)	Median survival (months)
Normal	34	31
Hyperdiploidy B	9	57
Hyperdiploidy A	8	18
Pseudodiploid	12	22
Hypodiploid	5	12
t(9;22)	12	12
t(4;11)	5	7
t(8;14)	5	5
14q+	4.5	9
6q−	4	29

The prognostic value of cytogenetic studies appears to be greater in children than in adults who, as a group tend to do worse. Several cytogenetic–clinicopathological associations have emerged. For example t(8;14)(q24;q32) is associated with B-cell ALL of L3 morphology and carries a very bad prognosis. Molecular studies of this translocation have led to a detailed understanding of the genetic rearrangements which give rise to B-cell malignancies (see discussion of Burkitt's lymphoma). Philadelphia positive ALL is another extensively studied category which is discussed more fully in the section on CGL.

t(4;11) Acute leukaemia (Figs. 15.6 and 15.7)

Acute leukaemia with the t(4;11)(q21;q23) is a fascinating disease with features of both B-cell (rearranged immunoglobulin heavy chain genes[114]) and monocytic lineage (monocytic cell-surface antigen expression and limited ability to differentiate along monocytic pathway).[115]

It presents with a very high white blood cell count and carries a very bad prognosis with conventional treatment, but better results may be achieved in the future by a combination of ALL- and AML-type treatment.

In summary, analysis of the leukaemic cell karyotype in ALL at presentation provides important prognostic information and may be diagnostically helpful. Identification of high-risk cytogenetic abnormalities allows selection of patients for more aggressive treatment programmes.

Lymphomas

Lymph node biopsy is the best cellular material for study of lymphoma cytogenetics. It should be transported in culture medium and minced with a sharp scalpel to release cells which may then be treated as bone marrow, setting up direct and short-term cultures.

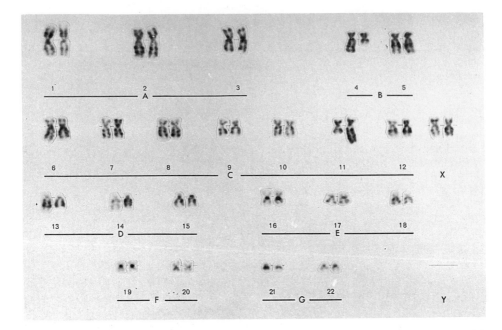

Fig. 15.6   46,XX,t(4;11)(q21;q23) Karyotype from a patient with ALL with translocation between chromosomes 4 and 11.

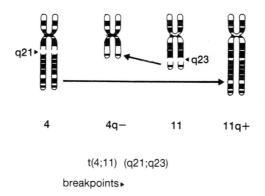

4   4q−   11   11q+

t(4;11) (q21;q23)

breakpoints▸

Fig. 15.7. Translocation between chromosomes 4 and 11.

Hodgkin's disease

Hodgkin's disease is the most common type of malignant lymphoma but although random numerical and structural chromosome anomalies are common, no characteristic cytogenetic changes have yet been described.[116]

Non-Hodgkin's lymphoma

Non-Hodgkin's lymphomas (NHL) represent a large group of diseases for which several classifications are available. For most cytogenetic discussions an international working formulation[117] is used with further sub-division according to cell lineage (B or T) (see Table 15.7).

In contrast to Hodgkin's lymphomas, clonal cytogenetic abnormalities are frequently identified in NHL and some major patterns are emerging.[118,119] Trisomy 12 is seen in small lymphocytic and small cleaved cell lymphomas (also the most frequently observed abnormality in CLL), and 6q− in diffuse large cell lymphomas.[120]

The most important group of abnormalities are reciprocal translocations involving the immunoglobulin heavy- (14q32) and light-chain kappa (2p11) and lambda (22q11) gene regions and the T-cell receptor alpha (14q11) and beta (7q34) chain gene regions. For example, t(14;18)(q32;q21) is strongly associated with follicular lymphomas,[121] t(11;14)(q13;q32) with small lymphocytic lymphoma and its leukaemic counterpart CLL,[120] t(8;14) (q24;q32), t(2;8)(p11;q24), and t(8;22)(q34;q11) with small non-cleaved cell lymphomas[122] and inv(14)(q11;q32), t(7;9)(q34;q32) with T-cell lymphomas,[123] and T-cell prolymphocytic leukaemia.[124] In addition non-

Table 15.7 International Working Formulation of NHL

Low grade
  Small lymphocytic
  Follicular, predominantly small cleaved
  Follicular, mixed small cleaved and large cells

Intermediate grade
  Follicular predominantly large cell
  Diffuse small cleaved cell
  Diffuse mixed small and large cell
  Diffuse large cell

High grade
  Large cell – immunoblastic
  Lymphoblastic
    Convoluted
    Non-convoluted
  Small non-cleaved cell
    Burkitt's
    Non-Burkitt's

Miscellaneous, including mycosis fungoides, composite lymphomas

recurring translocations involving these same gene regions are frequently observed.

Immunoglobulin gene rearrangement

The following brief discussion of IgH gene rearrangement (reviewed by Tonegawa[125]) will help to illustrate the mechanisms of such translocations, and the way in which they lead to cell transformation.

Variable gene region (Fig. 15.8).   The IgH gene region lies on the long arm of chromosome 14 and consists of variable and constant regions which code respectively for the variable and constant regions of the immunoglobulin heavy chain. In the earliest B-cell, the variable region consists of multiple V_H, D and J_H gene segments. During B-cell development, a single D segment recombines first with a J_H segment and then with a V_H segment to produce a $V_H DJ_H$ gene which codes for a unique antigen recognition site. The recombinase enzyme which engineers this gene rearrangement recognizes specific heptamer–nonamer signal sequences which are present on the 3' and 5' ends of the D segment, at the 3' end of the V_H segment and at the 5' end of the J_H segment. The recognition sequences consist of a seven-base palindrome abutting on the relevant gene segment, a space of 11 or 23 nucleotides (one or two turns of the DNA helix) and then an AT-rich nine-base sequence. D segments are flanked by recognition sequences with 11-base spacers while V_H and J_H segments have recognition sequences with 23-base spacers. The recombinase enzyme joins a segment with an 11-base spacer to one with a 23-base spacer recognition sequence, thus avoiding V_H to J_H or D to D recombination. There are hundreds of V_H segments, about 20 D segments and 4 J_H segments, thus allowing an enormous number of possible $V_H DJ_H$ recombinations. Antibody diversity is further contributed to by two processes at the site of gene segment recombination. Firstly random loss of nucleotides occurs at the site of recombination and secondly addition of nucleotides (N-regions) at the site of recombination is catalysed by a template-independent DNA polymerase (terminal deoxynucleotide transferase).

Constant gene region.   Returning to the constant region of the IgH gene, it consists of eight segments, each of which codes for a different class of antibody. At the time of B-cell activation, the cell may switch, for instance, from production of IgM to IgA, IgG or IgE. This change is brought about by another recombination event named switch recombination, in which C regions between the VDJ unit and the C region to be used are deleted. The isotype switching enzyme for this rearrangement recognizes switch, or S regions which lie 5' to each C region.

Recombinase mistakes and lymphomagenesis.   How do these processes relate to the transformation into lymphomas?

    Analysis of follicular lymphomas characterized by t(14;18) has revealed heptamer–nonamer recognition sequences in relation to the breakpoint on chromosome 18, while the breakpoint on chromosome 14 is at the 5' end of a

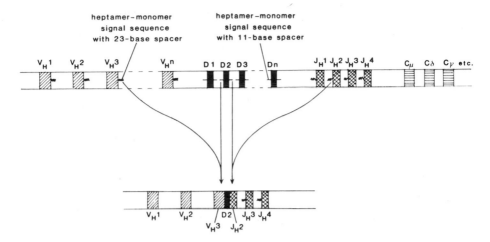

Fig. 15.8. Variable immunoglobulin heavy-chain region rearrangement. Recombinase enzyme recognizes heptamer–monomer signal sequences and catalyses D to J_H recombination, followed by V_H to DJ_H recombination. Random nucleotide loss and terminal deoxynucleotide transferase catalysed nucleotide addition generate a further diversity at sites of recombination.

J_H segment, i.e. at the recombinase recognition site.[126] N regions were also demonstrated.

Similar data are available for t(11;14) in CLL and t(8;14) in Burkitt's lymphoma (BL), strongly implicating recombinase mistakes in the genesis of these translocations.

The three commonly observed translocations in BL [t(8;14), t(2;8), t(8;22)] each result in movement of the c-*myc* proto-oncogene from the long arm of chromosome 8 into an immunoglobulin gene region. Subsequent deregulation of c-*myc* expression is thought to be the major reason for cell transformation. Indeed, it has been demonstrated *in vitro* that lymphoblastoid cell lines transfected with c-*myc* attached to an SV40 promoter subsequently become tumorigenic in nude mice.[127]

Comparison of chromosome breakpoints in endemic African BL and sporadic BL reveals important differences[120] which suggest that endemic BL arises as a result of recombinase mistakes at an early stage of B-lymphocyte development, while sporadic BL results from isotype-switching enzyme mistakes at a later stage of B-cell development.

BL is common in regions of Africa where malaria is endemic and childhood EBV infection is rife. It is therefore hypothesized that EBV-induced polyclonal B-cell activation proceeds unchecked in a patient whose T-suppressor cell response is dampened by malarial infection. The increased pool of proliferating B-cells with active recombinases increases the chance of recombinase mistakes, and hence the risk of one of the critical translocations which may cause BL.

The story is not so clear for the other gene rearrangements seen in NHL. For instance the genes on chromosomes 11 (*bcl*-1) and 18 (*bcl*-2) which are translocated to the IgH region in t(11;14) and t(14;18) have been cloned.

However, they are not related to any known oncogenes and it is not known whether they have cell transforming activity.

Solid tumour cytogenetics

The study of solid tumour cytogenetics has been hampered by technical difficulties caused by low mitotic index of tumour cells, infected tissue specimens especially from gastrointestinal tract, lung and cervix, poor chromosome morphology and difficulty identifying the 'critical' rearrangement amongst a large number of gross karyotypic changes. However, according to a recent comprehensive review,[129] such problems are rapidly being overcome and some interesting patterns are emerging.

Benign tumours

Despite their low mitotic rate, certain benign tumours have been linked to specific recurring cytogenetic abnormalities. For example, loss of a chromosome 22 has been seen in over 50% of meningiomas,[130] but it is too early to say whether the presence of a cytogenetic abnormality is linked to malignant progression.

Adenocarcinomas

Recurring cytogenetic abnormalities have been identified in carcinomas of bladder, prostate, lung, colon, kidney, endometrium and ovary. For example, carcinoma of bladder is associated with five specific recurring abnormalities [i(5p), +7, −9, 9q+, 11p−][131] but the aetiological and prognostic significance of these findings is still unclear.

Sarcomas

Some clear cytogenetic–pathologic associations have been identified in this group of tumours. For example, t(12;16) in myxoid liposarcoma[132] and t(X;18) in synovial sarcoma.[133] Cytogenetic studies may thus occasionally provide a helpful lead when attempting to determine the tissue of origin of a metastasis.

Germ cell and embryonal tumours

The specific deletions associated with retinoblastoma [del(13)(q14)] and Wilms' tumour [del(11)(p13)] have been mentioned earlier in relation to the possibility that loss of 'anti-oncogenes' may be important in their pathogenesis.

   Interestingly, testicular germ cell tumours consistently show i(12p) despite their varied phenotype (chorioncarcinoma, seminoma, embryonal cell cancer)[129] which suggests that i(12p) causes malignant transformation of the germ cell while other factors influence the pathway of differentiation taken by the tumour.

Specific rearrangements have also been identified in Ewing's sarcoma and peripheral epithelioma [t(11;22)][134] and in neuroblastoma [del(1p)].

Conclusion

Cytogenetic studies in haematological malignancies and solid tumours provide useful diagnostic and prognostic information in the individual case and aid disease classification. The study of specific chromosomal rearrangements at the molecular level is helping to elucidate the mechanisms whereby cells are transformed to a malignant phenotype. It is hoped that improved understanding will lead to the development of new effective treatments.

REFERENCES

1. Lejeune, J., Turpin, R. & Gautier, M. Le Mongolisme, premier example d'aberration autosomique humaine. *Ann. Genet. (Paris)* **1**: 41–9, 1959.
2. Nowell, P.C. & Hungerford, D.A. A minute chromosome in human granulocytic leukaemia. *Science* **132**: 1497–517, 1960.
3. Rowley, J.D. A new consistent chromosomal abnormality in chronic myelogenous leukaemia identified by quinacrine fluorescence and Giemsa banding. *Nature* **243**: 289–93, 1973.
4. Caspersson, T., Lomokka, G. & Zech, L. The 24 fluorescence patterns of the human metaphase chromosomes. Distinguishing characters and variability. *Hereditas* **67**: 89–102, 1971.
5. Yunis, J.J. High resolution of human chromosomes. *Science* **191**: 1268–70, 1976.
6. Weber, L.M. & Garson, O.M. Fluorodeoxyuridine synchronisation of bone marrow cultures. *Cancer Genet. Cytogenet.* **8**: 123–32, 1983.
7. Krivit, W. & Good, R.A. Simultaneous occurrence of mongolism and leukemia, a report of a nationwide survey. *Am. J. Dis. Childh.* **94**: 289–93, 1957.
8. Robinson, L.L., Nesbit, M.E. Jr, Sather, H.N. *et al.* Down syndrome and acute leukemia in children: a 10-year retrospective survey from Childrens Cancer Study Group. *J. Paediatr.* **105**(2): 235–42, 1984.
9. Patterson, D. The causes of Down syndrome. *Sci. Am.* **257**(2): 42–8, 1987.
10. Littlefield, J.W. Genes, chromosomes and cancer. *J. Paediatr.* **104**(4): 489–94, 1984.
11. Potluri, V.R., Helson, L., Ellsworth, R.M., Reid, T. & Gilbert, F. Chromosomal abnormalities in human retinoblastoma. A review. *Cancer* **58**(3): 663–71, 1986.
12. Hoefnagel, D., McIntyre, O.R., Storrs, R.C., Sullivan, P.B. & Maurer, L.H. Retinoblastoma followed by acute lymphoblastic leukemia. *Lancet* **1**: 725, 1973.
13. Waldmann, T.A., Misiti, J., Nelson, D.L. & Kraemer, K.H. Ataxia telangiectasia: a multisystem hereditary disease with immunodeficiency, impaired organ maturation, X-ray hypersensitivity, and a high incidence of neoplasia. (Clinical conference): *Ann. Intern. Med.* **99**(3): 367–79, 1983.
14. Taylor, A.M.R., Oxford, J.M. & Metcalfe, J.A. Spontaneous cytogenetic abnormalities in lymphocytes from thirteen patients with ataxia telangiectasia. *Int. J. Cancer* **27**: 311–19, 1981.
15. German, J. Bloom's syndrome. II. The prototype of human genetic disorders predisposing to chromosome instability and cancer. In *Chromosomes and Cancer*

(ed. J. German), pp. 616–36. Wiley, New York, 1974.

16. Otto, P.G. & Therman, E. Spontaneous cell fusion and PCC formation in Bloom's syndrome. *Chromosoma* **85**: 143–8, 1982.

17. Chaganti, R.S.K., Schonberg, S. & German, J. A manifold increase in sister chromatid exchanges in Bloom's syndrome lymphocytes. *Proc. Natl. Acad. Sci. U.S.A.* **71**: 4508–12, 1974.

18. Latt, S.A. Microfluorometric detection of deoxyribonucleic acid replication in human metaphase chromosomes. *Proc. Natl. Acad. Sci. U.S.A.* **70**: 3395–9, 1973.

19. Shiraishi, Y., Matsui, S. & Sandberg, A.A. Normalization by cell fusion of sister chromatid exchange in Bloom's syndrome lymphocytes. *Science* **212**: 820–2, 1981.

20. Kuhn, E.M. Localisation by Q-banding of mitotic chiasmata in cases of Bloom's syndrome. *Chromosoma* **57**: 1–11, 1976.

21. Kuhn, E.M., Therman, E. & Denniston, C. Mitotic chiasmata, gene density, and oncogenes. *Hum. Genet.* **70**(1): 1–5, 1985.

22. Hoar, D.I. & Waghorne, C. DNA repair in Cockayne syndrome. *Am. J. Hum. Genet.* **30**: 590–601, 1978.

23. Fujimoto, W., Greene, M. & Seegmiller, J. Cockayne's syndrome: report of a case with hyperlipoproteinemia, hyperinsulinemia, renal disease and normal growth hormone. *J. Paediatr.* **75**: 881–4, 1969.

24. Swift, M.R. Fanconi's anaemia in the genetics of neoplasia. *Nature* **230**: 370–3, 1971.

25. Bloomfield, C.D. & Brunning, R.D. Acute leukemia as a terminal event in non-leukemic hematopoietic disorders. *Semin. Oncol.* **3**(3): 297–317, 1976.

26. Cervanka, J., Arthur, D. & Yasis, C. Mitomycin C test for diagnostic differentiation of idiopathic aplastic anemia and Fanconi anemia. *Paediatrics* **67**: 119–27, 1981.

27. Shipley, J., Rodeck, C.H., Garrett, C., Galbraith, J. & Gianelli, F. Mitomycin C induced chromosome damage in fetal blood cultures and prenatal diagnosis of Fanconi's anaemia. *Prenatal Diagnosis* **4**: 217–21, 1984.

28. Gluckman, E., Devergie, A., Schaison, G. *et al.* Bone marrow transplantation in Fanconi anaemia. *Br. J. Haematol.* **45**: 557–64, 1980.

29. Cohen, M.M., Simpson, S.J., Honig, G.R., Maurer, H.S., Nicklas, J.W. & Martin, A.O. The identification of Fanconi anaemia genotypes by clastogenic stress. *Am. J. Hum. Genet.* **34**: 794–810, 1982.

30. Robbins, J.H., Kraemer, K.H., Lutzner, M.A., Festoff, B.W. & Koon, H.G. Xeroderma pigmentosum. An inherited disease with sun sensitivity, multiple cutaneous neoplasms and abnormal DNA repair. *Ann. Intern. Med.* **80**: 221–48, 1974.

31. Andrews, A.D., Barrett, S.F. & Robbins, J.H., Xeroderma pigmentosum neurological abnormalities correlate with colony-forming ability after ultra violet light radiation. *Proc. Natl. Acad. Sci. U.S.A.* **75**: 1984–8, 1978.

32. Fornace, A.J. Jr, Kohn, K.W. & Kann, H.E. Jr. DNA single-strand breaks during repair of UV damage in human fibroblasts and abnormalities of repair in xeroderma pigmentosum. *Proc. Natl. Acad. Sci. U.S.A.* **73**: 39–43, 1976.

33. Huang, C.C., Banerjee, A. & Hon. Y. Choromsomal instability in cell lines derived from patients with xeroderma pigmentosum. *Proc. Soc. Exp. Biol. Med.* **148**: 1244–8, 1975.

34. Hecht, F. & McCaw, B.K. Chromosome instability syndromes. In *Genetics of Human Cancer* (eds J.J. Mulvihill, R.W. Miller & J.F. Fraumeni Jr), pp. 105–24. Raven Press, New York, 1977.

35. Emerit, I. Chromosomal breakage in systemic sclerosis and related disorders. *Dermatologica* **153**: 145–56, 1976.

36. Taylor, A.M.R., Harnden, D.G. & Fairburn, E.A. Chromosomal instability associated with susceptibility to malignant disease in patients with porokera-

tosis of Mibelli. *J. Natl. Cancer Inst.* **51**: 371–8, 1976.

37. Hampel, K.E., Lohr, G.W., Blume, K.G. & Rudiger, H.W. Spontane und chloramphenicolinduzierte Chromosomemutationen und biochemische Befunde bei zwei Fallen mit glutathion-reduktasemangel (NAD(P)H glutathione oxido-reductase E.C.I. 642) *Humangenet.* **7**: 305–13, 1969.
38. Matsamiotis, N., Kiossoglou, K.A., Karpouzas, J. & Anastasea-Vlachou, K. Chromosomes in Kostmann's disease. *Lancet* **2**: 104, 1966.
39. Happle, R. & Hoehn, H. Cytogenetic studies on cultured fibroblast like cells derived from basal cell carcinoma tissue. *Clin. Genet.* **4**: 17–34, 1973.
40. Dekaban, A. Persisting clone of cells with an abnormal chromosome in a woman previously irradiated. *J. Nucl. Med.* **6**: 740–6, 1965.
41. Sutherland, G.R. The fragile X chromosome. *Int. Rev. Cytol.* **81**: 107–43, 1983.
42. Sutherland, G.R. & Hecht, F. *Fragile Sites on Human Chromosomes.* Oxford University Press, New York, 1985.
43. Glover, T.W., Berger, C., Coyle, J. & Echo, B. DNA polymerase A inhibition by aphidicolin induces gaps and breaks at common fragile sites in human chromosomes. *Hum. Genet.* **67**: 136–42, 1984.
44. Sutherland, G.R. Heritable fragile sites on human chromosomes. 1. Factors affecting expression in lymphocyte culture. *Am. J. Hum. Genet.* **31**: 125–35, 1979.
45. Sutherland, G.R. Heritable fragile sites on human chromosomes. 2. Distribution, phenotypic effects, and cytogenetics. *Am. J. Hum. Genet.* **31**: 136–48, 1979.
46. Yunis, J.J. The chromosomal basis of neoplasia. *Science* **221**: 227–36, 1983.
47. Le Beau, M.M. & Rowley, J.D. Heritable fragile sites in cancer. *Nature* **308**: 607–8, 1984.
48. Yunis, J.J. Fragile sites and predisposition to leukemia and lymphoma. *Cancer Genet. Cytogenet.* **12**: 85–8, 1984.
49. Human Gene Mapping 7 (1983). International Workshop on Human Gene Mapping, Los Angeles. *Cytogenet. Cell Genet.* **37**: 1–616, 1984.
50. Arthur, D.C. & Bloomfield, C.D. Possible association of fragile site 16q22 with development of acute leukemia. *Blood* **62**: 165, 1983 (Abstr.).
51. Trent, J.M., Olson, S. & Lawn, R.M. Chromosomal location of human leukocyte, fibroblast and immune interferon genes by means of *in situ* hybridization. *Proc. Natl. Acad. Sci. U.S.A.* **79**: 7809–13, 1982.
52. Le Beau, M.M., Diaz, M.O., Karin, M. & Rowley, J.D. Metallothionein gene cluster is split by chromosome 16 rearrangements in myelomonocytic leukaemia. *Nature* **313**: 709–11, 1985.
53. Marshall, C. Human oncogenes. In *RNA Tumour Viruses* (eds R. Weiss, N. Teich, H. Varmus & J. Coffin), Vol. 2, pp. 487–558. Cold Spring Harbor Laboratory, Cold Spring Harbor, New York, 1985.
54. Bishop, J.M. The molecular genetics of cancer. *Science* **235**: 305–11, 1987.
55. Mushinski, J.F. Davidson, W.F. & Morse, H.C. Activation of cellular oncogenes in human and mouse leukemia-lymphomas: Spontaneous and induced oncogene expression in murine B lymphocytic neoplasms. *Cancer Invest.* **5**: 345–68, 1987.
56. Teich, N., Wyke, J. & Kaplan, P. Pathogenesis of retrovirus induced disease. In *RNA Tumour Viruses* (eds R. Weiss, N. Teich, H. Varmus & J. Coffin), Vol. 2, pp. 187–248. Cold Spring Harbor Laboratory, Cold Spring Harbor, New York, 1985.
57. Al-Sumidaie, A.M., Leinster, S.J., Hart, C.A., Green, C.D. & McCarthy, K. Particles with properties of retroviruses in monocytes from patients with breast cancer. *Lancet* **i**: 5–8, 1988.
58. Tsujimoto, Y., Cossman, J., Jaffe, E. *et al.* Involvement of the bcl-2 gene in human follicular lymphoma. *Science* **228**: 1440–3, 1985.
59. Tabin, C.J. & Weinberg, R.A. Analysis of viral and somatic activation of the cHa-ras gene. *J. Virol.* **52**: 260–5, 1985.
60. Thompson, C.B., Challoner, P.B., Neiman, P.E. *et al.* Expression of the c-myb

proto-oncogene during cellular proliferation. *Nature* **319**: 374–80, 1986.
61. Bishop, J.M. & Varmus, H. Functions and origins of retroviral transforming genes. In *RNA Tumour Viruses* (eds R. Weiss, N. Teich, H. Varmus & J. Coffin), Vol. 2, pp. 249–356. Cold Spring Harbor Laboratory, Cold Spring Harbor, New York, 1985.
62. Downward, J., Yarden, Y., Mayes, E. *et al.* Close similarity of epidermal growth factor receptor and v-erbB oncogene protein sequences. *Nature* **307**: 521–7, 1984.
63. Marshall, C.J. Meeting report; oncogenes and growth control 1987. *Cell* **49**: 723–5, 1987.
64. Doolittle, R.F., Hunkapiller, M.W., Hood, L.E. *et al.* Simian sarcoma virus onc gene, v-sis, is derived from the gene (or genes) encoding a platelet derived growth factor. *Science* **221**: 275–7, 1983.
65. Klein, G. The approaching era of the tumour suppressor genes. *Science* **238**: 1539–45, 1987.
66. Harris, H. The genetic analysis of malignancy. *J. Cell. Sci.* Suppl. **4**: 431–44, 1986.
67. Zarbl, H., Latreille, J. & Jolicoeur, P. Revertants of v-fos-transformed fibroblasts have mutations in cellular genes essential for transformation by other oncogenes. *Cell* **51**: 357–69, 1987.
68. Rowley, J.D. Identification of the constant chromosome regions involved in human haematologic malignant disease. *Science* **216**: 749–51, 1982.
69. Bartram, C.R., de Klein, A., Hagemeijer, A. *et al.* Translocation of c-abl oncogene correlates with the presence of a Philadelphia chromosome in chronic myelogenous leukaemia. *Blood* **58**: 158–63, 1983.
70. Gale, R.P. & Canaani, E. An 8-kilobase abl RNA transcript on chronic myelogenous leukaemia. *Proc. Natl. Acad. Sci. U.S.A.* **81**: 5648–52, 1984.
71. Brodsky, I., Hubbell, H.R., Strayer, D.R. & Gillespie, D.H. Implications of retroviral and oncogene activity in chronic myelogenous leukaemia. *Cancer Genet. Cytogenet.* **26**: 15–23, 1972.
72. Groffen, J., Stephenson, J.R., Heisterkamp, N. *et al.* Philadelphia chromosomal breakpoints are clustered within a limited region, bcr, on chromosome 22. *Cell.* **36**: 93–9, 1984.
73. Shtivelman, E., Lifshitz, B., Gale, R.P. & Canaani, E. Fused transcript of abl and bcr genes in chronic myelogenous leukaemia. *Nature* **315**: 550–4, 1985.
74. Konopa, J.B., Watanabe, S.M. & Witte, O.N. An alteration of the human c-abl protein in K562 leukaemia cells unmasks associated tyrosine kinase activity. *Cell* **37**: 1035–42, 1984.
75. Daley, G.Q., McLaughlin, J., Witte, O.N. & Baltimore, D. The CML-specific P210 bcr-abl protein, unlike v-abl does not transform NIH 3T3 fibroblasts. *Science* **237**: 532–5, 1987.
76. Alimena, G., De Cuia M.R., Divero, D., Gastaldi, R., Nanni, M. The karyotype of blastic crisis. *Cancer Genet. Cytogenet.* **26**: 39–50, 1987.
77. Koefler, H.P. & Golde, D. Chronic myelogenous leukaemia – new concepts. *N. Engl. J. Med.* **304**: 1201–9, 1981.
78. Kurzrock, R., Shtalrid, M., Romero, P. *et al.* A novel c-abl protein product in Philadelphia positive acute lymphoblastic leukaemia. *Nature* **325**: 631–5, 1987.
79. Chan, L.C., Karhi, K.K., Rayter, S.I. *et al.* A novel abl protein expressed in Philadelphia chromosome positive acute lymphoblastic leukaemia. *Nature* **325**: 635–7, 1987.
80. Bennett, J.M., Catovsky, D., Daniel, M.T. *et al.* Proposals for the classification of the myelodysplastic syndromes. *Br. J. Haematol.* **51**: 189–99, 1982.
81. Knapp, R.H., Dewald, G.W. & Pierre, R.V. Cytogenetic studies in 174 consecutive patients with preleukaemic or myelodysplastic syndromes. *Mayo Clin. Proc.* **60**: 507–16, 1985.
82. Groupe Francais de Cytogenetique Hematologique: Cytogenetics of chronic

myelomonocytic leukaemia. *Cancer Genet. Cytogenet.* **21**: 11–30, 1986.

83. Heim, S. & Mitelman, F. Chromosome abnormalities in the myelodysplastic syndromes. *Clin. Haematol.* **15**: 1003–21, 1986.

84. Van den Berghe, H., Vermaelen, K., Mecucci, C., Barbieri, D. & Tricot, G. The 5q− anomaly. *Cancer Genet. Cytogenet.* **17**: 189–225, 1985.

85. Carbonell, F., Heimpel, H., Kubanek, V. & Fliecher, T.M. Growth and cytogenetic characteristics of bone marrow colonies from patients with 5q− syndrome. *Blood* **66**: 463–5, 1985.

86. Mitelman, F., Manolova, Y., Manolov, G. *et al.* High resolution analysis of the 5q− marker in refractory anaemia. *Hereditas* **105**: 49–54, 1986.

87. Nienhuis, A.W., Franklin Bunn, H., Turner, P.H. *et al.* Expression of the human c-fms proto-oncogene in hematopoietic cells and its deletion in the 5q− syndrome. *Cell* **42**: 421–8, 1985.

88. Le Beau, M.M., Westbrook, C.A., Diaz, M.O. *et al.* Evidence for the involvement of GM-CSF and FMS in the deletion (5q) in myeloid disorders. *Science* **231**: 984–7, 1986.

89. Bennett, J.M., Catovsky, D., Daniel, M.T. *et al.* Proposals for the classification of the acute leukaemias. *Br. J. Haematol.* **33**: 451–8, 1976.

90. Bennett, J.M., Catovsky, D., Daniel, M.T. *et al.* Proposed revised criteria for the classification of acute myeloid leukaemia: A report of the French–American–British Co-operative Group. *Ann. Intern. Med.* **103**: 620–5, 1985.

91. Sakurai, M. & Sandberg, A.A. Prognosis of acute myeloblastic leukaemia: chromosomal correlation. *Blood* **41**: 93–104, 1973.

92. Fourth International Workshop on Chromosomes in Leukaemia (1982): Clinical significance of chromosomal abnormalities in acute non-lymphocytic leukaemia. *Cancer Genet. Cytogenet.* **11**: 332–50, 1984.

93. Yunis, J.J., Bloomfield, C.D. & Ensrud, K. All patients with acute non-lymphocytic leukemia may have a chromosomal defect. *N. Engl. J. Med.* **305**: 135–9, 1981.

94. Rowley, J.D., Golomb, H.M. & Dougherty, C. 15/17 translocation, a consistent chromosomal change in acute promyelocytic leukaemia. *Lancet* i: 549, 1977.

95. Fourth International Workshop on Chromosomes in Leukaemia (1982): Chromosomes in acute promyelocytic leukaemia. *Cancer Genet. Cytogenet.* **11**: 288–93, 1984.

96. Misawa, S., Lee, E., Schiffer, C.A., Liu, Z. & Testa, J.R. Association of the translocation (15;17) with malignant proliferation of promyelocytes in acute leukaemia and chronic myelogenous leukaemia at blastic crisis. *Blood* **67**: 270–4, 1986.

97. Moir, D.J., Pearson, J.H. & Buckle, V.J. Acute promyelocytic transformation in a case of acute myelomonocytic leukaemia. *Cancer Genet. Cytogenet.* **12**: 359, 1984.

98. Simmers, R.N., Webber, L.M., Shannon, M.F. *et al.* Localisation of the G-CSF gene on chromosome 17 proximal to the breakpoint in the t(15;17) in acute promyelocytic leukaemia. *Blood* **70**: 330–2, 1987.

99. Mitelman, F, Manolov, G., Manolova, Y. *et al.* High resolution chromosome analysis of constitutional and acquired t(15;17) maps c-erb A to subband 17q11.2 *Cancer Genet. Cytogenet.* **22**: 95–8, 1986.

100. Yunis, J.J. & Brunning, R.D. Prognostic significance of chromosomal abnormalities in acute leukaemias and myelodysplastic syndromes. *Clin. Hematol.* **15**: 789–90, 1986.

101. Larson, R.A., Williams, S.F., Le Beau, M.M., Bitter, M.A., Vardiman, J.W. & Rowley, J.D. Acute myelomonocytic leukaemia with abnormal eosinophils and inv(16) or t(16;16) has a favourable prognosis. *Blood* **68**: 1242–9, 1986.

102. Le Beau, M.M., Larson, R.A., Bitter, M.A., Vardiman, J.W., Golomb, H.M. & Rowley, J.D. Association of an inversion of chromosome 16 with abnormal

marrow eosinophils in acute myelomonocytic leukaemia. A unique cytogenetic-clinicopathologic association. *N. Engl. J. Med.* **309**: 630–6, 1983.

103. Testa, J.R., Hogge, D.E., Misawa, S. & Zaudparsa, N. Chromosome 16 rearrangements in acute myelomonocytic leukaemia with abnormal eosinophils. *N. Engl. J. Med.* **310**: 468–9, 1984.

104. Arthur, D.C. & Bloomfield, C.D. Partial deletion of the long arm of chromosome 16 and bone marrow eosinophilia in acute non-lymphocytic leukaemia: a new association. *Blood* **61**: 994–8, 1983.

105. Bitter, M.A., Le Beau, M.M., Larson, R.A. *et al.* A morphologic and cytochemical study of acute myelomonocytic leukaemia with abnormal marrow eosinophils associated with inv(16)(p13;q22). *Am. J. Clin. Path.* **81**: 733–41, 1984.

106. Holmes, R., Keating, M.J., Cork, A. *et al.* A unique pattern of central nervous system leukaemia in acute myelomonocytic leukaemia associated with inv(16)(p13;q22). *Blood* **65**: 1071–8, 1985.

107. Le Beau, M.M. Chromosomal fragile sites and cancer-specific rearrangements. *Blood* **67**: 849–58, 1986.

108. Karin, M. Metallothioneins: Proteins in search of function. *Cell* **41**: 9–10, 1985.

109. Francis, G.E. Leukaemogenesis: A postulated mechanism involving tyrosine protein kinase and DNA topoisomerase. *Med. Hypotheses* **22**: 223–35, 1987.

110. Bennett, J.M., Catovsky, D., Daniel, M.T. *et al.* The French–American–British (FAB) Co-operative Group. The morphological classification of acute lympho-blastic leukaemia: concordance among observers and clinical correlations. *Br. J. Haematol.* **47**: 553–61, 1981.

111. Foon, K.A., Schraff, R.W. & Gale, R.P. Surface markers in leukaemia and lymphoma cells: recent advances. *Blood* **60**: 1–19, 1982.

112. Bloomfield, C.D., Goldman, A.I., Alimena, G. *et al.* Chromosomal abnormal-ities identify high-risk and low-risk patients with acute lymphoblastic leukaemia. *Blood* **67**: 415–20, 1986.

113. Third International Workshop on Chromosomes in Leukaemia: Chromosomal abnormalities and their clinical significance in acute lymphoblastic leukaemia. *Cancer Res.* **43**: 868–73, 1983.

114. Crist, W.M., Cleary, M.L., Grossi, C.E. *et al.* Acute leukaemias associated with the 4:11 chromosome translocation have rearranged immunoglobulin heavy chain genes. *Blood* **66**: 33–8, 1985.

115. Strong, R.C., Korsmeyer, S.J., Parkin, J.L., Arthur, D.C. & Kersey, J.H. Human acute leukaemia with the t(4;11) chromosomal rearrangement exhibits B lineage and monocytic characteristics. *Blood* **65**: 21–31, 1985.

116. Kristoffersson, U., Heim, S., Mandahl, N. *et al.* Cytogenetic studies in Hodgkin's disease. *Acta Pathol. Microbiol. Immunol. Scand.* **95**: 289–95, 1987.

117. The non-Hodgkin's lymphoma pathologic classification project; National Cancer Institute sponsored study of classification of non-Hodgkin's lymphoma; Summary and description of a working formulation for clinical usage. *Cancer* **49**: 2112–35, 1982.

118. Koduru, P.R.K., Filippa, D.A., Richardson, M.E. *et al.* Cytogenetic and histologic correlations in malignant lymphoma. *Blood* **69**: 97–102, 1987.

119. Levine, E.G., Arthur, D.C., Gajl-Peczalska, K.J. *et al.* Correlations between immunological phenotype and karyotype in malignant lymphoma. *Cancer Res.* **46**: 6482–8, 1986.

120. Yunis, J.J., Oken, M.M., Theoglides, A., Howe, R.B. & Kaplan, M.E. Recurrent chromosomal defects are found in most patients with non-Hodgkin's lymphoma. *Cancer Genet. Cytogenet.* **13**: 17–28, 1984.

121. Speaks, S.L., Sanger, W.G., Linder, J. *et al.* Chromosomal abnormalities in indolent lymphoma. *Cancer Genet. Cytogenet.* **27**: 335–44, 1987.

122. Croce, C.M. Role of chromosome translocations in human neoplasia. *Cell* **49**: 155–6, 1987.

123. Reynolds, T.C., Smith, S.D. & Sklar, J. Analysis of DNA surrounding the breakpoints of chromosomal translocations involving the beta T cell receptor gene in human lymphoblastic neoplasms. *Cell* **50**: 107–17, 1987.
124. Brito-Babapulle, Pomfret, M., Matutes, E. & Catovsky, D. Cytogenetic studies on prolymphocytic leukemia. II. T cell prolymphocytic leukemia. *Blood* **70**: 926–31, 1987.
125. Tonegawa, S. Somatic generation of antibody diversity. *Nature* **302**: 575–81, 1983.
126. Tsujimoto, Y., Gorham, J., Cossman, J., Jaffe, E. & Croce, C.M. The t(14;18) chromosome translocation involved in B cell neoplasms results from mistakes in VDJ joining. *Science* **229**: 1390–3, 1985.
127. Sherr, C.J. Leukaemia and lymphoma 1987; Meeting report. *Cell* **48**: 727–9, 1987.
128. Haluska, F.G., Tsujimoto, Y. & Croce, C.M. Mechanisms of chromosome translocation in B and T cell neoplasia. *Trends Genet.* **3**: 11–15, 1987.
129. Sandberg, A.A. & Turc-Carel, C. The cytogenetics of solid tumours. Relation to diagnosis, classification and pathology. *Cancer* **59**: 387–95, 1987.
130. Zang, D.K. Cytological and cytogenetic studies on human meningioma. *Cancer Genet. Cytogenet.* **6**: 249–74, 1982.
131. Sandberg, A.A. Chromosome changes in bladder cancer. Clinical and other correlations. *Cancer Genet. Cytogenet.* **19**: 163–75, 1986.
132. Turc-Carel, C., Limon, J., Dal Cin, P., Rao, U., Karakousis, C. & Sandberg, A.A. Cytogenetic studies of adipose tissue tumors: II. Recurrent reciprocal translocation t(12;16)(q13;p11) in myxoid liposarcomas. *Cancer Genet. Cytogenet.* **23**: 291–300, 1986.
133. Turc-Carel, C., Dal Cin, P., Limon, J., Li, F. & Sandberg, A.A. Translocation X;18 in synovial sarcoma. *Cancer Genet. Cytogenet.* **23**: 93, 1986.
134. Turc-Carel, C., Philip, I., Berger, M.-P., Philip, T. & Lenoir, G.M. Chromosome study of Ewing's (ES) cell lines: Consistency of a reciprocal translocation t(11;22)(q24;q22). *Cancer Genet. Cytogenet.* **12**: 1–19, 1984.

APPENDIX: GLOSSARY OF TERMS AND ABBREVIATIONS

Chiasmata: the points of exchange of chromatid segments

Deletion (del): loss of portion of chromosome following breakage

Dicentric (dic): abnormal chromosome with two centromeres

Inversion (inv): reversal of chromosome segment following breakage altering the gene sequence

Isochromosome (i): metacentric chromosome formed from duplication of long or short arms due to transverse separation of the chromosome at the centromere

Monosomy: missing chromosome designed by − sign before the chromosome, e.g. monosomy 7, −7

Sister chromatid exchange: reciprocal exchange of blocks of chromatin between sister chromatids

Translocation (t): transfer of chromosome material from one chromosome to another following chromosome breakage

Trisomy: extra chromosome designated by a + sign before chromosome, e.g. trisomy 8, +8

p and q arms: p is the short arm, q is the long arm of a chromosome

Index

Figures in *italic* type; tables in **bold** type.

Secondary hypersplenism 476–7, **477**, 481, 485
Secondary leukaemia 508
Secondary myelofibrosis 16
Secondary polycythaemia 17, 21, **68**, 70, 72, 73, 88, 97
Secondary pulmonary vascular disease 82
Sedormid 356
Seizures 100
Self-bleeding **35**, 36
Senile purpura 226, 229
Sensorimotor peripheral neuropathy 321
Sepsis 133, **175**, 239–42, **240**, **241**
Septic abortion 251
Septic arthritis 311
Septicaemia 137, **137**, 350, **473**
  DIC 198, 238, 239, 249
  HIV 389, 390
Septrin 335, 337, 352
Sequestration, spleen 470
Serine 126, 222
Serine proteases 239, 252
Serine-threonine 501–2
Serology
  AIHA 282–4, *283*
  lymphadenopathy 459
Seronegative spondarthritis **425**
Serotonin 179, 181, 182, 221, 222
  drugs and toxins, effect of 209
  thrombocytopenia 357
  thrombocytosis 192
  uraemia 194
  vasospastic disorders 205, 206
Serum amyloid A protein (SAA) **414**, 415, 416, 417, 422
Serum haptoglobins 282
Serum iron 13, 34, 53, **69**
Serum lactate dehydrogenase 282
Serum protein, 300–1, *300*, 308
  amyloid A protein **414**, 415, 416, 417, **422**
Serum sickness **155**, 164, 172, **457**, **473**
Seventh Human Gene Mapping Workshop 498
Severe combined immunodeficiency (SCID) **167**, 168
Sex hormones 51
Sezary's syndrome **155**, **161**, 164, 311, 453
Sherpas, Tibet 81
Shingles 380
Shock **240**, 243, 244, 249, 388–9
Sialic acid 196, 255
Sick sinus syndrome, amyloidosis 321

Sickle cell disease 9, 47, **52**, **186**, 388, 430, **473**
Sickling test osmotic fragility 485
Sideroblastic anaemia (SA) 39, 41–4, **43**, 55
  alcohol and drugs 24, **25**, 42–3, **58**, 59, **329**, 337–8
  CTD 43, **276**, 279, *285*, 286
  malignancy **2**, **4**, 5
  myelodysplastic syndromes 192, 506, **507**
Siderotic granules 13, 38, 470
SIg 313
Silicosis 448
Sinus histiocytosis 456
Sinuses, spleen 468, 479
Sister chromatid exchange (SCE) 495, 496
Sjögren's syndrome 287
Skin 23
  infection 135, 455
  necrosis 231
  pigmentation 37, 448
  rashes 10
  trauma 229
SLE *see* Systemic lupus erythematosus
Sleep apnoea syndrome 88, 89, 102
'Slim disease' 390
Small cell lung carcinoma 503
Small joint arthralgia 47
Smallpox 388
'Smear' cells 451
Smoking 82
  acute-phase response 424
  anaemia 33
  atherosclerosis 205
  lymphocyte abnormalities 153
  platelet function **188**, **189**
  polycythaemia 70, **71**, 72, 88–9, 93, 102
    arterial hypoxaemia 82, 84, 85
Smooth muscle antibody 383
Smouldering multiple myeloma (SMM) **301**, 308, 309, 314
Smudge cells 162
Snake venom 24, 239, **240**, **241**, 244
Snoring 70
Sodium aurothiomalate 360
Sodium valproate **349**
Solid tumours 259, 518–9
Solitary myeloma 318
Solitary plasmacytoma of bone 318
Somatic cell hybridization 503
Somnolence 88
Sorbitol 134
Specific granules, neutrophils **123**, 124, 125, 126, 127, 131, 132, **132**